Vagal Control of the Heart: Experimental Basis and Clinical Implications

The Bakken Research Center Series
Volume 7

Edited by

Matthew N. Levy, M.D.
Chief, Investigative Medicine
Mt. Sinai Medical Center
Cleveland, Ohio
and
Professor Emeritus of Physiology and Biophysics
and of Biomedical Engineering
Case Western Reserve University
Cleveland, Ohio

and

Peter J. Schwartz, M.D.
Professor of Medicine
University of Pavia
Pavia, Italy
and
Professor of Physiology and Biophysics
University of Oklahoma
Oklahoma City, Oklahoma

FUTURA

Futura Publishing Company, Inc.
Armonk, NY

Other volumes in the Bakken Research Center Series:

Volume I, Part I. The Foundation of Cardiac Pacing: An Illustrated Practical Guide to Basic Pacing, by Richard Sutton, DSc Med, FRCP, FACC and Ivan Bourgeois, MS, MBA

Volume II. Transformed Muscle for Cardiac Assist and Repair, edited by Ray Chu-Jeng Chiu, MD, PhD and Ivan Bourgeois, MS, MBA

Volume III. Cardiomyoplasty, edited by Alain Carpentier, MD, PhD, Juan-Carlos Chachques, MD, and Pierre A. Grandjean, MS

Volume IV. Challenges in Cardiology I, edited by Charles E. Rackley, MD

Volume V. Practical Aspects of Staged Therapy Defibrillators, edited by Lukas J. Kappenberger, MD and Fred W. Lindemans, PhD

Volume VI. Tachycardias: Mechanisms and Management, edited by Mark E. Josephson, MD and Hein J.J. Wellens, MD

Dedication

To our wives, Ruth and Luisella, for their continuous and sympathetic support of our commitment to research.

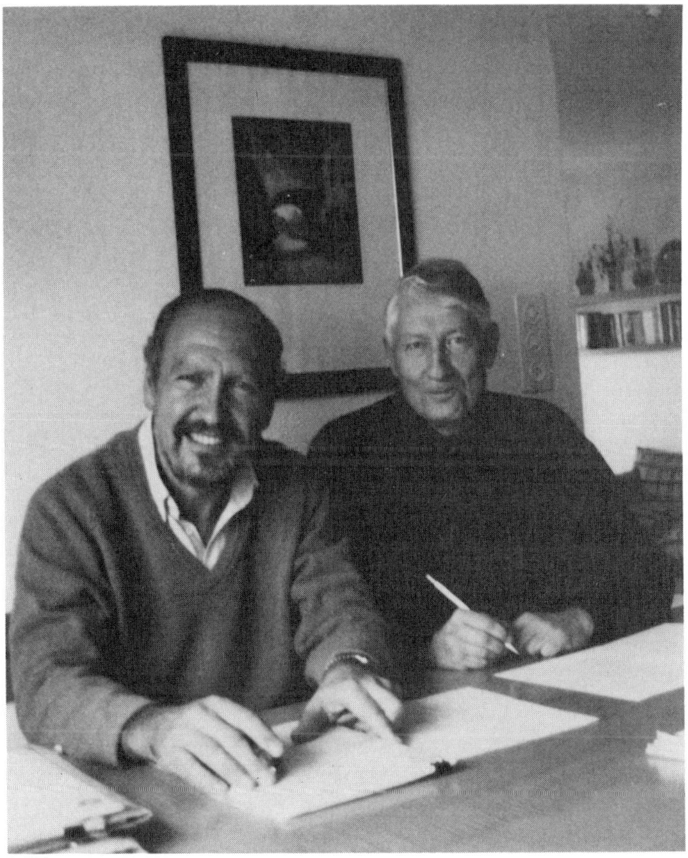

Peter J. Schwartz, M.D. and Matthew N. Levy, M.D.

Library of Congress Cataloging-in-Publication Data

Vagal control of the heart : experimental basis and clinical implications / edited by Matthew N. Levy and Peter J. Schwartz.
p. cm. — (The Bakken Research Center series ; v. 7)
Includes bibliographical references and index.
ISBN 0-87993-561-8
1. Heart—Innervation. 2. Vagus nerve. 3. Arrhythmia—Pathophysiology. I. Levy, Matthew N., 1922– . II. Schwartz, Peter J.. III. Series.
[DNLM: 1. Vagus Nerve—physiology. 2. Heart—innervation. 3. Heart Diseases—physiopathology. W1 BA4794 v.7 1993 / WG 200 V126 1993]
QP113.4.V44 1993
612.1′78—dc20
DNLM/DLC
for Library of Congress 93-23821
CIP

Published by
Futura Publishing Company, Inc.
135 Bedford Road
Armonk, New York 10504-0418

LC#: 93-23821
ISBN #: 0-87993-561-8

Printed in the United States of America.

This book is printed on acid-free paper.

Contributors

Francois M. Abboud, MD, MACP Edith King Pearson Professor of Cardiovascular Research, Professor, Departments of Medicine and Physiology and Biophysics, Director, Cardiovascular Research Center, University of Iowa College of Medicine, Iowa City, Iowa

J. Thomas Bigger, Jr., MD Professor of Medicine and of Pharmacology, Division of Cardiology, Department of Medicine, Columbia University, New York, New York

Vernon S. Bishop, PhD Professor, Department of Pharmacology, The University of Texas Health Science Center at San Antonio, San Antonio, Texas

P.A. Brooks, BSc, PhD Research Fellow, Department of Physiology, Royal Free Hospital School of Medicine, University of London, London, England

Arthur M. Brown, MD, PhD Professor and Chairman, Department of Molecular Physiology and Biophysics, Baylor College of Medicine, Houston, Texas

Douglas Cameron, MD Assistant Professor of Medicine, University of Toronto, Physician, The Toronto Hospital, Toronto Hospital Division, Toronto, Ontario, Canada

Donatella Cerati, MD Research Associate, Centro di Fisiologia Clinica e Ipertensione, Istituto di Clinica Medica Generale e Terapia Medica, University of Milan, Milan, Italy

Margaret J. Chandler, PhD Research Associate, Department of Physiology, College of Medicine, The University of Oklahoma Health Sciences Center, Oklahoma City, Oklahoma

Richard J. Cohen, MD, PhD Professor of Health Sciences and Technology, Director, Harvard-MIT Center for Biomedical Engineering, Massachusetts Institute of Technology, Harvard University, Cambridge, Massachusetts

Gaetano M. De Ferrari Clinical Assistant Professor, Department of Cardiology, Ospedale Maggiore Policlinico, IRCCS, Milan, Italy and Research Associate, Centro di Fisiologia Clinica e Ipertensione, Istituto di Clinica Medica Generale e Terapia Medica, University of Milan, Milan, Italy

Mark E. Dibner-Dunlap, MD Assistant Professor of Medicine, Department of Medicine, Department of Veterans Affairs, Case Western Reserve University, Cleveland, Ohio

Stephen E. DiCarlo, PhD Assistant Professor, Department of Physiology, Northeastern Ohio Universities, College of Medicine, Rootstown, Ohio

Linda W. Dickerson, PhD Instructor, Department of Pharmacology, Georgetown University School of Medicine, Washington, D.C.

Dario DiFrancesco, PhD Professor, Dipartimento di Fisiologia e Biochimica Generali, Università degli Studi di Milano, Milan, Italy

Eric O. Feigl, MD Professor, Department of Physiology and Biophysics, University of Washington Medical School, Seattle, Washington

Joseph L. Fleiss, PhD Professor of Biostatistics, Columbia University, New York, New York

Robert D. Foreman, PhD Professor and Chair, Department of Physiology, The University of Oklahoma Health Sciences Center, Oklahoma City, Oklahoma

Ramesh C. Gupta Department of Medicine and Krannert Institute of Cardiology, Indiana University School of Medicine, Indianapolis, Indiana

P.N. Izzo, BSc, DPhil Department of Physiology, Royal Free Hospital School of Medicine, University of London, London, England

José Jalife, MD Professor and Chairman, Department of Pharmacology, SUNY Health Science Center at Syracuse, Syracuse, New York

Maria Teresa La Rovere, MD Department of Cardiology, Centro Medico Montescano, Fondazione Clinica del Lavoro, IRCCS, Pavia, Italy

Matthew N. Levy, MD Chief, Investigative Medicine, Mt. Sinai Medical Center, Cleveland, Ohio and Professor Emeritus of Physiology and Biophysics and of Biomedical Engineering, Case Western Reserve University, Cleveland, Ohio

Ruth Lindmar, PhD Academic Director, Department of Pharmacology, University of Mainz, Mainz, Germany

Konrad Löffelholz, MD Professor, Department of Pharmacology, University of Mainz, Mainz, Germany

Federico Lombardi, MD Associate Professor of Medicine, Ospedale "L. Sacco," University of Milan, Milan, Italy

Alberto Malliani, MD Professor of Medicine, Ospedale "L. Sacco," University of Milan, Milan, Italy

Paul J. Martin, PhD Associate Chief, Division of Investigative Medicine, Mt. Sinai Medical Center, Cleveland, Ohio

D.I. McCloskey, FRACP FTS FAA Director, Prince of Wales Medical Research Institute, Prince of Wales Hospital, Randwick, Sydney, New South Wales, Australia

Donald C. Michaels, PhD Associate Professor, Department of Pharmacology, SUNY Health Science Center at Syracuse, Syracuse, New York

Andrea Mortara, MD Department of Cardiology, Centro Medico Montescano, Fondazione Clinica del Lavoro, IRCCS, Pavia, Italy

Joachim Neumann, Privatdozent Dr. Med., Abteilung Allgemeine Pharmakologie, Universitäts-Krankenhaus Eppendorf, Hamburg, Federal Republic of Germany

Massimo Pagani, MD, FACC Established Investigator, Ospedale "L. Sacco," University of Milan, Milan, Italy

Achilles J. Pappano, PhD Professor of Pharmacology, The School of Medicine of the University of Connecticut Health Center, Farmington, Connecticut

Erica K. Potter, BSc, PhD Associate Professor, Prince of Wales Medical Research Institute, Prince of Wales Hospital, Randwick, Sydney, New South Wales, Australia

W.C. Randall, PhD Biology Department, Taylor University, Upland, Indiana

William R. Roeske, MD Associate Chief, Section of Cardiology, Professor of Medicine and Pharmacology, Department of Medicine and Pharmacology, University of Arizona Health Science Center, Tucson, Arizona

Michael R. Rosen, MD Gustavus A. Pfeiffer Professor of Pharmacology, Professor of Pediatrics, Department of Pharmacology, College of Physicians and Surgeons of Columbia University, New York, New York

Lino Rossi, MD L.D. Professor, Institute of Pathology, University of Milan, Milan, Italy

J. Philip Saul, MD Associate in Cardiology, Children's Hospital, Boston, Boston, Massachusetts and Assistant Professor of Pediatrics, Harvard Medical School, Boston, Massachusetts

Michael Schimerlik, BS, PhD Professor of Biochemistry, Department of Biochemistry and Biophysics, Oregon State University, Corvallis, Oregon

Peter J. Schwartz, MD Professor of Medicine, University of Pavia, Pavia, Italy, and Professor of Physiology and Biophysics, University of Oklahoma, Oklahoma City, Oklahoma

Michael L. Smith, PhD Assistant Professor of Medicine, Department of Medicine, University Hospitals of Cleveland, Case Western Reserve University, Cleveland, Ohio

Virend K. Somers, MD, DPhil Assistant Professor, Department of Internal Medicine, Division of Cardiovascular Diseases, Cardiovascular Research Center, University of Iowa College of Medicine, Iowa City, Iowa

K.M. Spyer, BSc, PhD, DSc, MD(Hon) Head of Department and Chairman of Division, Department of Physiology, Division of Basic Medical Sciences, Royal Free Hospital School of Medicine, University of London, London, England

Marc D. Thames, MD Chief, Division of Cardiology, University Hospitals of Cleveland, Cleveland, Ohio

Emilio Vanoli, MD Research Assistant, Centro di Fisiologia Clinica e Ipertensione, Istituto di Clinica Medica Generale e Terapia Medica, University of Milan, Milan, Italy and Assistant Professor of Medicine, Section of Cardiology, University of Oklahoma, Oklahoma City, Oklahoma

Richard L. Verrier, PhD Professor of Pharmacology, Department of Pharmacology, Georgetown University School of Medicine, Washington, D.C.

Robert W. Wald, MD Associate Professor of Medicine, University of Toronto, Physician, Mount Sinai Hospital, Toronto, Ontario, Canada

Margaret R. Warner, PhD Assistant Professor of Pharmacology and Medicine, Indiana University School of Medicine, Krannert Institute of Cardiology, Indianapolis, Indiana

August M. Watanabe, MD Professor of Medicine and Pharmacology, Indiana University School of Medicine, Indianapolis, Indiana and Group Vice President, Lilly Research Laboratories, A Division of Eli Lilly and Company, Indianapolis, Indiana

Menashe B. Waxman, MD Professor of Medicine, University of Toronto, Physician, The Toronto Hospital, Toronto Hospital Division, Toronto, Ontario, Canada

R.D. Wurster, PhD Professor, Department of Physiology, Stritch School of Medicine, Loyola University Chicago, Maywood, Illinois

Henry I. Yamamura, PhD Professor, Departments of Pharmacology, Biochemistry and Psychiatry, University of Arizona Health Science Center, Tucson, Arizona

Douglas P. Zipes, MD Professor of Medicine, Indiana University School of Medicine, Krannert Institute of Cardiology, Indianapolis, Indiana

Preface

The publication of this book is prompted mainly by abundant recent investigations that indicate that efferent vagal activity exerts a salutary effect on serious ventricular arrhythmias in both human patients and experimental animals. Only a few decades ago, authorities believed that efferent vagal fibers did not innervate the ventricles in mammalian hearts. For example, in the fifth edition of Wiggers' *Physiology in Health and Disease,* published in 1949, the author asserted that "the evidence seems indisputable that the vagus nerves do not directly affect the ventricles."[1]

A study conducted by one of us about 30 years ago, in collaboration with R.M. Berne and H. DeGeest, revealed that vagal stimulation attenuated the systolic reduction in coronary blood flow in anesthetized dogs.[2] This finding suggested that the vagal activity might have diminished the extravascular compression that is ordinarily exerted by the ventricular contraction; that is, that vagal activity might have exerted a negative inotropic effect on the ventricles. DeGeest and Levy, together with other collaborators, then tested this heretical hypothesis in a group of dogs that we placed on total heart bypass, so that we could rigorously control all the important confounding variables. We did indeed find that the vagus nerves can depress ventricular contractility appreciably.[3] Furthermore, we learned that the magnitude of the negative inotropic effect of the vagal activity depended critically on the prevailing level of sympathetic activity.[4,5] The greater the sympathetic activity, the more pronounced was the inhibitory effect. When sympathetic activity was negligible, however, the vagal influence on ventricular contractility was minimal and often undetectable.[6] More details about the vagal effects on ventricular contractility and of the nature of the sympathetic-vagal interaction are provided in Chs. 11 and 15.

The complexity of this interaction was further highlighted 20 years ago when one of us found that stimulation of cardiac sympathetic afferent fibers inhibited the activity in cardiac vagal efferent fibers.[7] The clinical relevance of the above findings was provided by the demonstration that baroreflex sensitivity, a marker of vagal reflexes, was depressed in a subgroup of conscious dogs that had a healed myocardial infarction and that developed ventricular fibrillation during a transient myocardial ischemia while performing an exercise stress test.[8] In another subgroup of animals in which baroreceptor sensitivity was not depressed, ventricular fibrillation rarely occurred. The subsequent confirmation of this finding in patients with myocardial infarction,[9] combined with the observation that heart rate variability is diminished in patients with a higher mortality rate,[10] has given impetus to the assessment of vagal tone and reflexes as a new tool for risk stratification. At the same time, evidence has been accruing that vagal activation, induced either by exercise training,[11] by direct vagal stimulation,[12] or by muscarinic agonists,[13] has a powerful antifibrillatory effect.

On the basis of this background and of the rapid advances in technics for investigating this important problem, we thought it appropriate and timely to edit a book that would encompass the current basic and clinical knowledge about the vagal control of the heart.

Matthew N. Levy, M.D.
Peter J. Schwartz, M.D.

References

1. Wiggers CJ: Physiology in Health and Disease. 5th ed. Philadelphia, PA, Lea & Febiger, 1949, p. 530.
2. Berne RM, DeGeest H, Levy MN: Influence of the cardiac nerves on coronary resistance. Am J Physiol 208:763–769, 1965.
3. DeGeest H, Levy MN, Zieske H, et al: Depression of ventricular contractility by stimulation of the vagus nerves. Circ Res 17:222–235, 1965.
4. Levy MN, Ng M, Martin P, et al: Sympathetic and parasympathetic interactions upon the left ventricle of the dog. Circ Res 19:5–10, 1966.
5. Levy MN: Sympathetic-parasympathetic interactions in the heart. Circ Res 29:437–445, 1971.
6. Levy MN: Neural control of the heart: Sympathetic-vagal interactions. In J Baan, A Noordergraaf, J Raines (eds): Cardiovascular System Dynamics. Cambridge, MA, MIT Press, 1978, pp. 365–370.
7. Schwartz PJ, Pagani M, Lombardi F, et al: A cardio-cardiac sympatho-vagal reflex in the cat. Circ Res 32:215–220, 1973.
8. Schwartz PJ, Vanoli E, Stramba-Badiale M, et al: Autonomic mechanisms and sudden death: New insights from the analysis of baroreceptor reflexes in conscious dogs with and without myocardial infarction. Circulation 78:969–979, 1988.
9. La Rovere MT, Specchia G, Mortara A, et al: Baroreflex sensitivity, clinical correlates and cardiovascular mortality among patients with a first myocardial infarction. A prospective study. Circulation 78:816–824, 1988.
10. Kleiger RE, Miller JP, Bigger JT Jr, et al: Heart rate variability: A variable predicting mortality following acute myocardial infarction. Am J Cardiol 59:256–262, 1987.
11. Billman GE, Schwartz PJ, Stone HL: The effects of daily exercise on susceptibility to sudden cardiac death. Circulation 69:1182–1189, 1984.
12. Vanoli E, De Ferrari GM, Stramba-Badiale M, et al: Vagal stimulation and prevention of sudden death in conscious dogs with healed myocardial infarction. Circ Res 68:1471–1481, 1991.
13. De Ferrari GM, Salvati P, Grossoni M, et al: Pharmacologic modulation of the autonomic nervous system in the prevention of sudden cardiac death. J Am Coll Cardiol 22:283–290, 1993.

Contents

PART I

Anatomy and Central Integration

CHAPTER 1

Histology of Cardiac Vagal Innervation in Man

L. Rossi

A comprehensive study of cardiac vagal innervation on human autopsy material is exceedingly difficult. Therefore, the histologic substrates of the heart's control by the vagus, whether normal or diseased, are almost always extrapolated from animal experiments, with all the inherent drawbacks. Trying to progress through such a lamentable gap in basic knowledge of the autonomic nervous regulation of the human heart, the present treatment of the subject will consider the morphology of the barochemoreflex arc, encompassing both the components of it (brain stem centers and peripheral receptors) and the nerves and ganglia. The overall importance of barochemoreflexes for the assessment of the vagal control of the heart, at the patient's bedside and in the physiology laboratory[1,2] alike, can explain this pragmatic choice by the neuropathologist.

Materials and Methods

In 80 autopsy cases of ascertained, or plausibly suspected, arrhythmogenic cardiac death (20 of sudden infant death included), and in 15 control cases (of noncardiac death), histologic observations were carried out on the following structures:

1. the brain stem neuronal circuitry that conducts cardioinhibitory impulses into the vagus;
2. the cervical and mediastinal ganglionated and paraganglionated nerve circuitry, with its mechano (chemo?-) receptor terminals (particularly intercarotid in location), and the ill-understood glomera annexed to the extrinsic cardiac plexus; and
3. the vagal (or supposedly so) intrinsic cardiac nerves, from the sinoatrial (SA) plexus to the mechanoreceptor endings in the right atrium, that hitherto were not clearly recognizable histologically.

From *Vagal Control of the Heart: Experimental Basis and Clinical Implications* edited by MN Levy, PJ Schwartz © 1994, Futura Publishing Co. Inc., Armonk, NY.

In all cases that exhibit an impairment in SA impulse formation or in atrioventricular (AV) conduction, the entire conduction system was also controlled. Serial or subserial sections were cut from the excised fragments that had been formalin-fixed, paraffin-embedded, and stained with hematoxylin-eosin (HE), trichromic Heidenhain (azan), Weigert's elastic fibers, Klüver-Barrera, Bielschowsky's, Gros-Schultze (frozen sections), Grimelius, S-100, and neurofilaments (DAKO) (immunohistochemical); one surgical and two animal specimens were added.

Normal Histology

Brain Stem Cardioinhibitory Structures

In man, as in experimental mammals, two main vagus (X) visceromotor nuclei are located beneath the ependyma of the fourth ventricle, close to the obex (Fig. 1): the dorsal nucleus of the vagus (DNV) (Fig. 2) and the

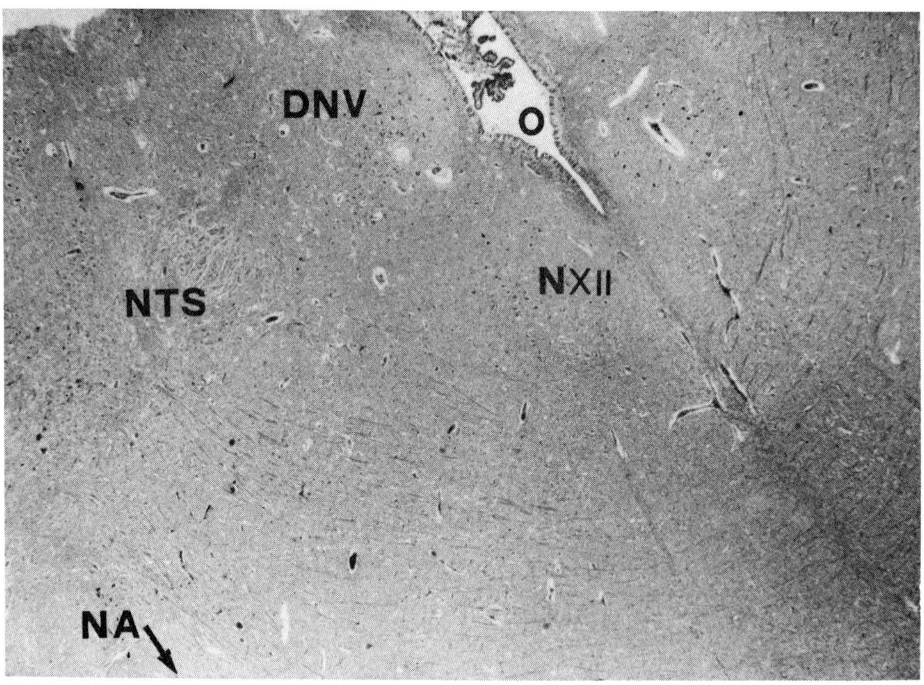

Figure 1. *Brain stem: beneath the obex (0) ependyma, the nucleus hypoglossus (NXII) is the landmark of the "parahypoglossal area," the site of the neuronal circuitry for the barochemoreflex control of the heart. Also shown is the dorsal nucleus of the vagus (DNV), the nucleus tractus solitarii (NTS) and, below them, the nucleus ambiguus (NA). Bielschowsky's, × 20.*

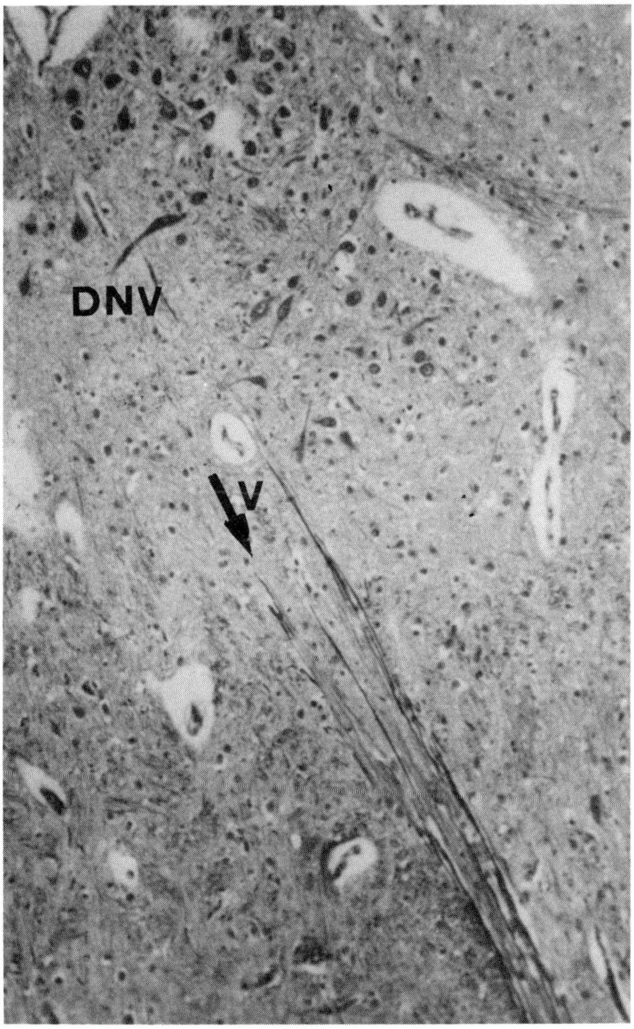

Figure 2. *The dorsal motor nucleus of the vagus (DNV), with the root of its efferent nerve (V, arrow). Bielschowsky's, × 200.*

nucleus ambiguus (NA) (Fig. 3). This latter structure is shared with the glossopharyngeal nerve (IX), and shows close anatomical-functional interrelationships with the ventrolateral respiratory (mainly inspiratory) reticular formation. From the intercarotid and mediastinal barochemoreceptors, viscerosensory fibers of the glossopharyngeal are conveyed (via the tractus solitarius) to the nucleus tractus solitarii (NTS) (Fig. 1).[3–7] The important function of this nucleus in the modulation of baroreflexogenesis discloses intimate anatomical connections with the nearby vagus nuclei (DNV and NA), the adjacent reticular formation, and the upper centers (the locus coeruleus, namely).[3]

Likewise, viscerosensory vagal fibers descend over the spinal trigeminal route to terminate in the nucleus of the spinal tract of the trigeminal nerve, close to the NA.[6]

The nucleus of the hypoglossus (XII) (Fig. 1), with its large-bodied neurons packed at either side of the obex indentation, is a useful landmark epitomized as the "parahypoglossal area,"[3] which is cogent to the central vagal control of heartbeat (Fig. 1).

The cytologic components of the human brain stem nuclei are remarkably different from one another. The neuronal bodies of the NA are as big (Fig. 3) as those of the nucleus hypoglossus, whereas those of the NTS are smaller, and those of the DNV are of medium size (Fig. 2). The latter are similar to the nerve cells of the inferior oliva, whose dorsal accessory nucleus is adjacent to the NA. The vagus root, stemming from the DNV (Fig. 2), is either unmyelinated or poorly myelinated.

The richness in neuronal appendages, the myelinization of axon cylinders,[8] and the thick interweaving of the respiratory reticular formation (poorer in babies) vary with age. Dendritic spines, when present, are longer in babies.[9]

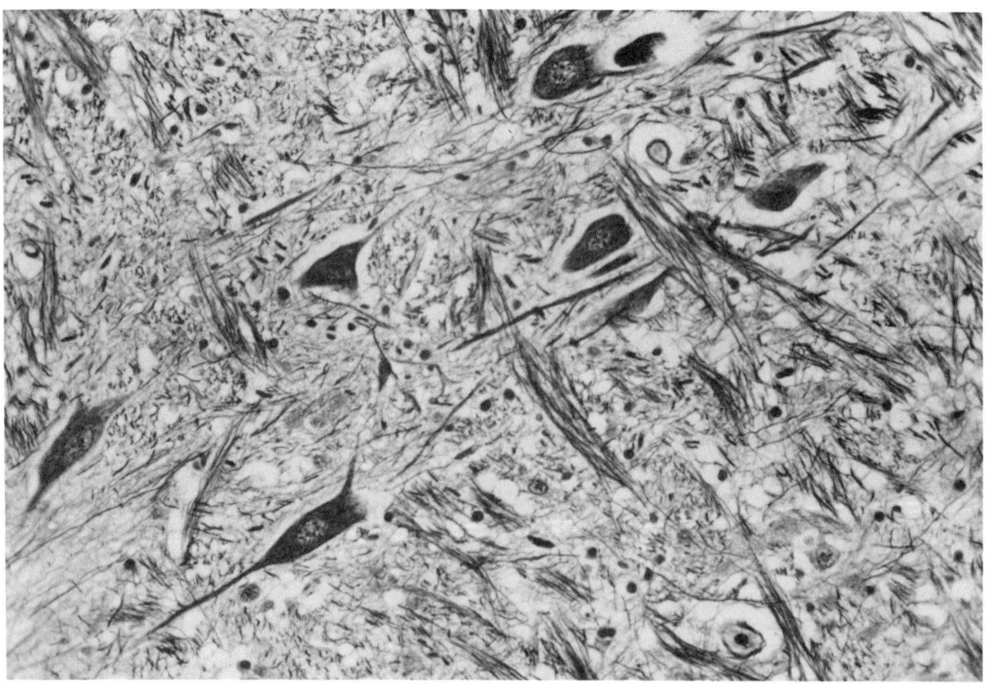

Figure 3. *The big neurons of the NA and the ventrolateral reticular formation (respiratory). Bielschowsky's, × 400.*

Cardiac Vagus

From the superior (jugular) and inferior (nodosum) ganglia downwards, the cervical trunk of the vagus shows a decreasing myelinization of fibers.[10] The vagus' cardiac branches are mostly given off in the thorax, near the origin of the recurrent (inferior) laryngeal nerve. Below this, they are also labelled craniovagal and caudovagal (or cardiopulmonary) nerves, on both sides,[11] or only on the left side.[12] These cardiac nerves, converge into an intricate ganglionated plexus in the mediastinum. This plexus is grossly subdivided into a ventral and a dorsal (cardiopulmonary) plexus,[12] characterized by an elusive main ganglion with the eponymous of Wrisberg's.[13] The plexus consists of a variable interlacing of nerves, equipped with ganglia and nerve cells internal to nerves, distributed throughout the interstitium of the aortic arch, pulmonary artery trunk, and bronchial bifurcation. Its prevailing vagal component anastomoses with sympathetic cardiac branchings in an undetermined fashion. The afferent vagal fibers from the aortic arch constitute a so-called "depressor nerve," better recognizable in animals than in man.[13]

This complex and variable ganglionated aorto-pulmonary plexus in the anterior mediastinum can be regarded as the "extrinsic cardiac plexus," even though a precise anatomical boundary has not been established for it.

One of the most remarkable and least understood features of the cardiac plexus consists of the richness in intraneural and paraneural receptors, with a mixed ganglio-paraganglionic structure.[14,15]

INTERCAROTID CARDIOINHIBITORY RECEPTORS

Carotid Body. The carotid body, or glomus, is well known as the classic chemoreceptor paraganglion. Its peculiar functional cytotype is the chief cell, neural in origin, with the cytoplasm laden with argyrophilic neurotransmitter granules. The chief cells are grouped in clusters, attended by the sustentacular cells (glial-Schwannian in nature), and supplied with a rich carotid-derived vasculature and a mixed glossopharyngeal-vagal innervation. The sympathetic component is minor in man.[10,16] Preterminal nerve fibers, poorly myelinated and with Schwannian sheaths, wrap up the chief-cells clusters, and join them with a substantial synaptic protein.

Carotid Sinus. Contrary to the carotid body, which is a paraganglionic organule, and despite some misunderstanding of terms, the human carotid sinus is not an organ-like differentiated structure, but is composed of loosely interwoven nerve endings throughout the outer media of the initial tract of the internal carotid artery, just above the carotid bifurcation. The slight bulging of the internal carotid artery, the proper "sinus," is attended by a thinning of the elastic and smooth muscle media.[16] This thinning probably enhances the sinus' compliance, and promotes the excitation of the local mechanoreceptor nerve endings (Fig. 4).[10] As such, these features are not strictly specific to the carotid

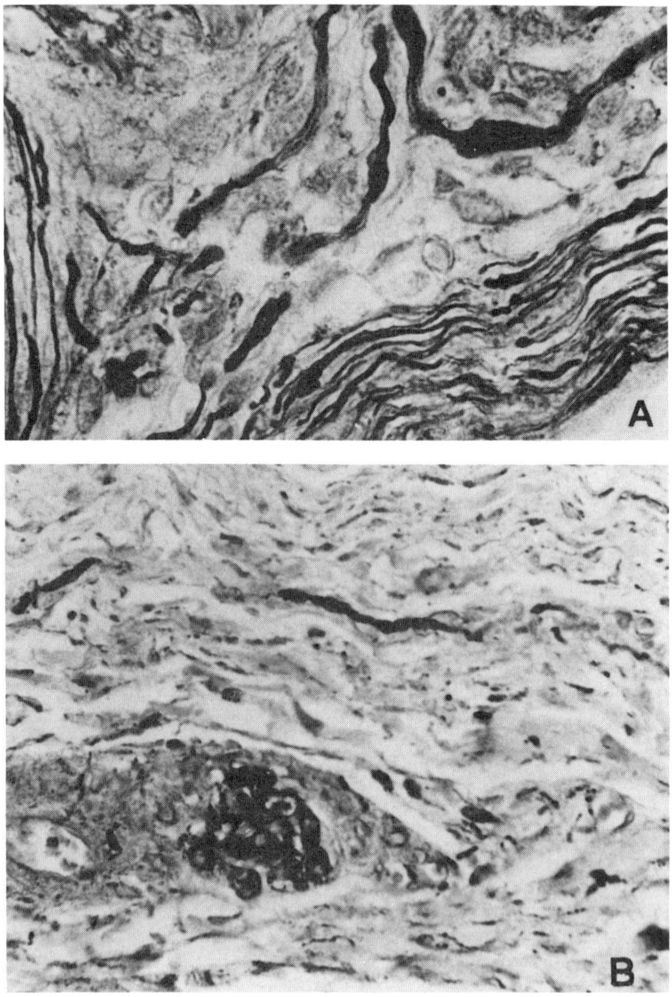

Figure 4. *A: Mechanoreceptor nerve endings (Krause's bulbs) in the carotid sinus, with fibers of the glossopharyngeal nerve and B: A small paraganglion in the inner adventitia of the carotid sinus, close to mechanoreceptor nerve endings of the outer media. Grimelius, × 1000 and × 400.*

sinus, but they are similar to other stretch-sensitive nerve terminals observed in the cardiovascular system. The afferent sinus' fibers in man belong to the glossopharyngeal nerve, with a minor vagal component.[3,10] They present as thick, varicose fibers,[17] attended by Schwann cells (well demonstrated by S.100 immunohistochemistry) either grouped and encapsulated in the so-called "Krause's bulbs" (Fig. 4),[10] or scattered throughout the sinus' media.

Paradoxically, the striking structural difference between the carotid body and the carotid sinus does not correspond to a clear-cut anatomical-functional separation between chemoreception and baroreception, inside or outside the intercarotid area (Fig. 4).[16,17] In some cases, a small paraganglion is embedded in the inner adventitia of the carotid sinus close to, and sharing, the same innervation with Krause's bulbs (Fig. 4). Isolated argyrophilic cells, similar to the chief paraganglionic cytotype, can also be observed nearby.

Moreover, inside the vagus trunk, at the level of the carotid bifurcation, a paraganglion may be present,[15] which adds to the amazing complexity of the intercarotid cardiocirculatory receptor structures. These ill-understood histologic findings seem to be mirrored in the uncertain physiological separation of baroreflexogenesis from chemoreflexogenesis at the level of the glossopharyngeal-vagal neuronal circuitry in the brain stem (Fig. 1).[3,16]

RECEPTOR STRUCTURES OF THE CARDIAC PLEXUS

The current classification of mediastinal glomera pertains to the fourth through the sixth branchial arches, and it defines an aortic body, or paraganglion supracardiale aorticum (sometimes separated into superius and inferius), an aortopulmonary body[10] and, occasionally, a coronary (left) paraganglion.[18] This classification lends credibility to the concept that the aorto-pulmonary paraganglia system consists of a few, easily detectable glomera of the classic carotid-body type.[10] Yet, specialized studies,[14–16] and the present one, have recently shown that this baroreceptor-chemoreceptor system is much more conspicuous, complex, and variable in location and structure than currently held, and that it is closely associated with the heart's innervation.

Actually, a myriad of small glomera is distributed throughout the cardiac plexus. Some glomera present as typical paraganglia that are close to, but anatomically separated from, the walls of mediastinal arteriolae. Many show a mixed ganglionic-paraganglionic composition, with neuronal cells intermingled with chief cells.[15,17] They are located beneath the perineurium or inside the endoneurium of mediastinal nerves,[15] especially in between the ascending aorta and the pulmonary artery trunk, near the first branch of the left coronary artery. This branch runs cranially and is termed intertruncal artery.

Another important morphological-functional topic is that some of these composite paraganglia are arranged as an arch or an entire circle around the tunica media of mediastinal arteriolae (Fig. 5), altogether reminiscent of what is observed in the carotid sinus-glomus complex (Fig. 4).[17] The perivascular layout of such structures may make them sensitive to both modifications in caliber of the vessel, and to chemical variations of the circulating blood. Anew, this arrangement adds to the extant uncertainties about the formal distinction of anatomical substrates for baroreception and, respectively, chemoreception, in the afferent abutment of the baroreflex arc. These arguments may also apply to the mechanoreceptor structures of the thoracic aorta. These terminal nervous structures resemble those of the carotid sinus but, in man, are less conspicuous and more widespread in the outer media and innermost adventitia of the aortic arch. In most cases, their afferent fibers gather in the cardiac plexus, without reuniting into a discernible depressor nerve.[13]

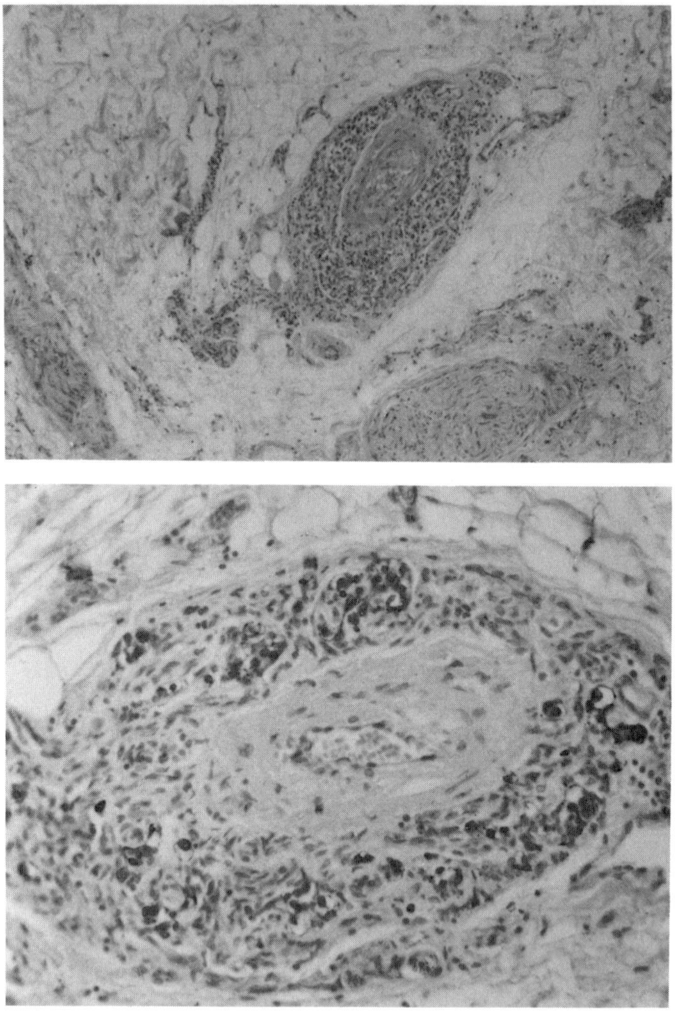

Figure 5. *A mediastinal glomus completely encircling a small artery (baroreception ?). Grimelius, × 20 and × 200.*

The Vagus in the Heart

The vagal innervation intrinsic to the heart is so richly and diffusely intermingled with the sympathetic ramifications that it would be hazardous to draw a clear-cut scheme of the vagus nerve in human cardiac anatomy. Immunohistochemistry alone can, within certain technical limits, make it possible to discern sympathetic from vagal periphery. With regard to the "coarse" subepicardial plexus,[19] one can surmise that the numerous nerves and ganglia in the area of the SA node and intercaval bridge are mainly vagal. In turn, the vagus nerve supply to the ventricles is sparse, with few fibers that travel with the much richer sympathetic innervation. In the AV groove,

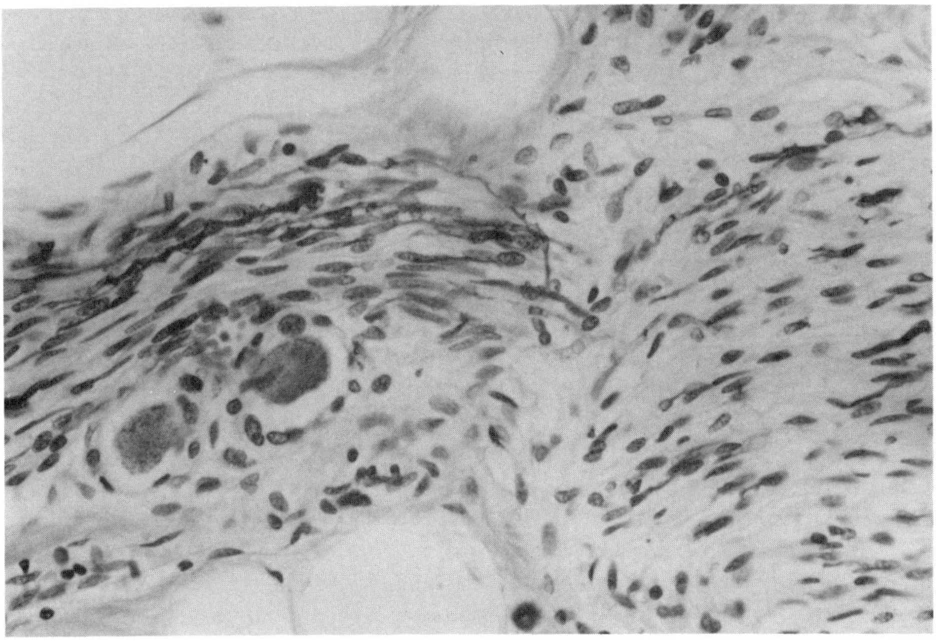

Figure 6. *Myelinated preganglionic fibers (left) and unmyelinated postganglionic fibers (right) in the prevailingly vagal SA plexus. Klüver-Barrera,* × *400.*

however, the vago-sympathetic input is more balanced, with some sympathetic prevalence in the area of the AV node.[20]

Recently, physiological and pharmacological experiments indicated that the vagal fibers beyond the AV groove cross proximally toward the endocardium and send fibers into the myocardium and epicardium only distally (near the apex).[21] This interesting finding still awaits anatomical-histologic demonstration.

Afferent and efferent vagal fibers are indistinguishable in human histology, whereas myelinated preganglionic fibers in the SA plexus may be distinguished from unmyelinated postganglionic fibers (Fig. 6).[6]

VAGAL RECEPTOR ENDINGS IN THE HEART

The presence of afferent vagus terminals in the heart is still an open question in human neurohistology.[11–20] Pathophysiological evidence suggests that vagal receptors prevail in the right atrium and in the inferior wall of the ventricles.[15,21] Some confusion may arise from the functional interpretation of the morphological term "receptor."[22] The solution of such a question is not facilitated by the misuse of the term "neuron,"[23] the long-standing classification of the nerve-cell's body,[24] to denote the peripheral innervation of the heart which, in man, is almost devoid of nerve cells. Moreover, some neuroanatomists maintain that the viscerosensory afferent fibers cannot be labelled vagal or sympathetic, insofar as this basic distinction only applies to efferent autonomic innervation.[6]

To avoid confusion, the term receptor is used here in its physiological sense of a sensory element responsive to special stimuli, without any biochemical-pharmacological implication of a protein binding certain agonists to elicit a response.

Receptors in the human heart seem to develop and differentiate late in fetal life and for several months into the postnatal period.[25] An imbalanced development of vago-sympathetic ventricular receptors may underlie arrhythmias in infants.[25] Recent results from animal experiments are consistent with this hypothesis, and they may help to explain high-risk arrhythmias in infants.[26]

Presynaptic agranular vesicles are well known in vagal cardiac fibers, and they may be associated with granular vesicles along individual sympathetic axons.[6] Attention has recently been centered on those unmyelinated afferent C-fibers at the extreme vagal periphery.[27] They seem to exhibit a mechanoreceptor arrangement and may participate in cardiac baroreflexes.

To increase the probability of visualizing vagal endings, classic frozen-section silver impregnations were used[15] to study the pericaval and intercaval right atrium (SA nodal plexus).[27] Thereby, a reliable histologic demonstration of cardiac mechanoreceptors was obtained that is comparable with, but much less elusive than, the current drawings of them. Convoluted, thin terminal fibrils are seen, sometimes continuous with thicker, varicose, or button-tipped fibers (Fig. 7) scattered throughout the subepicardium, the myocardium, and

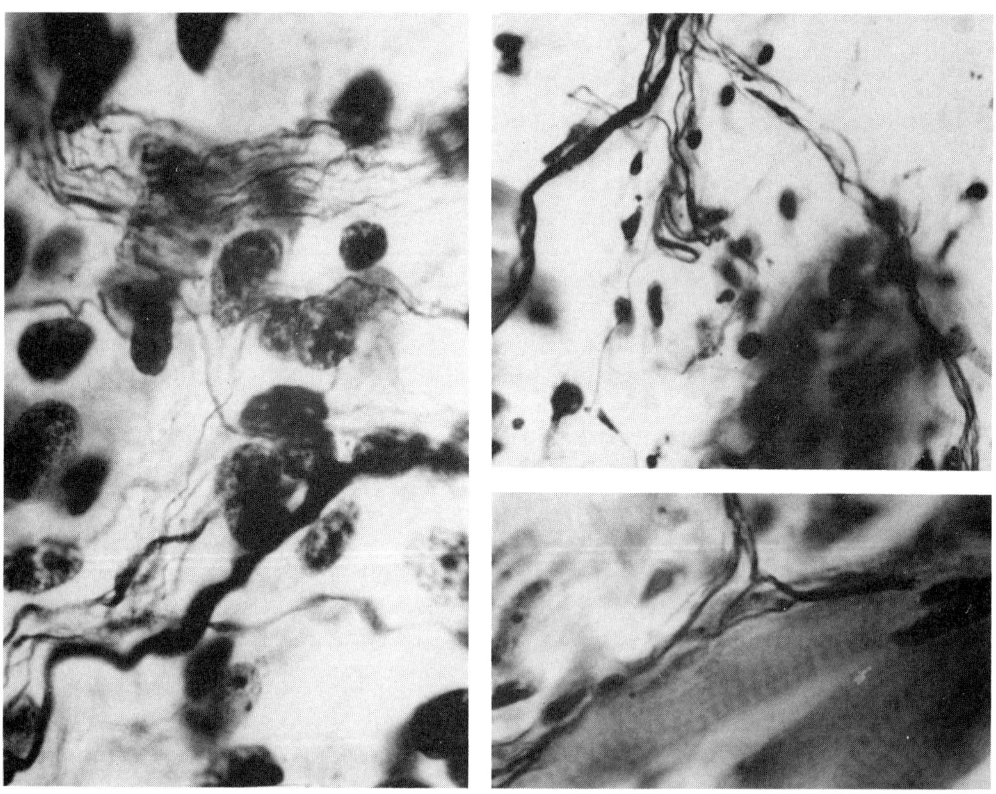

Figure 7. *The finest nerve endings in the intercaval wall of the right atrium, arranged in "brushes" and clusters, probably mechanoreceptor in nature. Gros-Schultze, × 100.*

the subendocardium. These histologic features resemble those sympathetic fibrils observed in ventricles.[10,28]

Histopathology of Cardiac Vagal Innervation

Basic information about cardioneuropathology of the vagus in human disease is inadequate. In the brain stem, the vagal neuronal cell bodies can undergo degeneration (chromatolysis, necrosis) with reactive participation of glial cells (neuronophagia) which, in turn, can proliferate pathologically (gliosis).[24] Edema is very common, but difficult to discriminate from post-mortem artifacts, particularly in human autopsy specimens. Encephalitic round cell infiltration is often superimposed on focal gliosis and neuronophagia (Fig. 8). The neuronal appendages may also grow pathologically; long dentritic spines in infants are regarded as a sign of immaturity.[9]

Autonomic nerve fibers can be disrupted or damaged by degenerative or

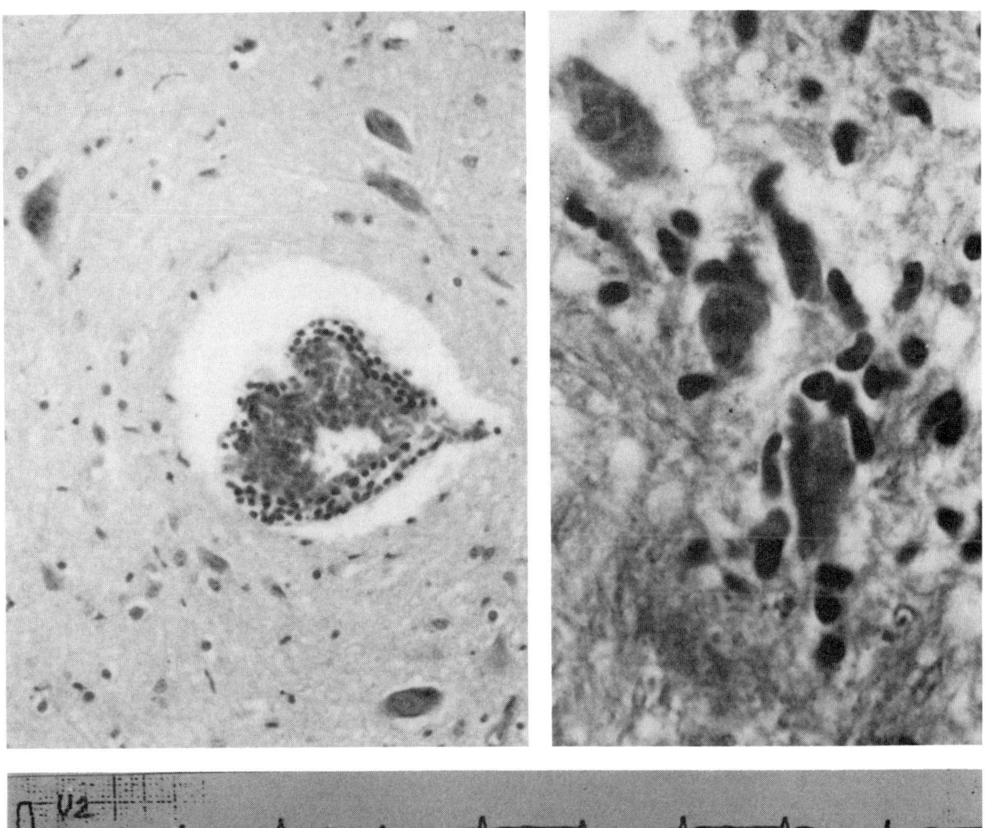

Figure 8. *Brain stem encephalitis: perivascular round cell infiltrate (left) and focal neuronophagia (right) in the DNV and in the NTS, manifesting with intermittent accelerated AV junctional escape (below). Hematoxylin-eosin, × 400 and × 1000.*

inflammatory changes, hemorrhage, amyloid deposits, tumor, and trauma. The classic features of wallerian degeneration (distal to interruption)[29] are not observed in the autonomic nerves of man, probably due to the rich interlacing of nerve networks and to the numerous intercalated and visceral ganglia of peripheral plexuses. Yet, wallerian degeneration of individual fibers can be observed in the experimentally disrupted vagus trunk in animals.

Note that autonomic nerves can withstand the inflammation intrinsic to acute myocardial infarctions. Axonal disruptions may be a consequence of local massive endoneural granulocytic infiltration[15] (enzymic proteolytic action), while tracts of preserved nerves can be found in postinfarction scars.[15,17]

The autonomic peripheral ganglia frequently exhibit ageing or pathological changes, characterized by either degeneration (hydropic swelling) or atrophy of the neuronal body and by nodular proliferation of satellite cells. These cells gather eccentrically in the neuronal space and, when the neuron disappears, they present as compact glomerule-like "Terplan nodules" (Figs. 9, 10).[15,30] Such clusters of satellite cells countersign the "neuronal scar" so precisely that any suspected neuronal depletion of ganglia[31] not based on such evidence is highly questionable.

These pathological features can be appreciated by routine stainings, whereas the demonstration of abnormal growths of appendages close to the neuron (baskets, convolutes)[30] or far from it (thickenings, fragmentation) requires special methods.

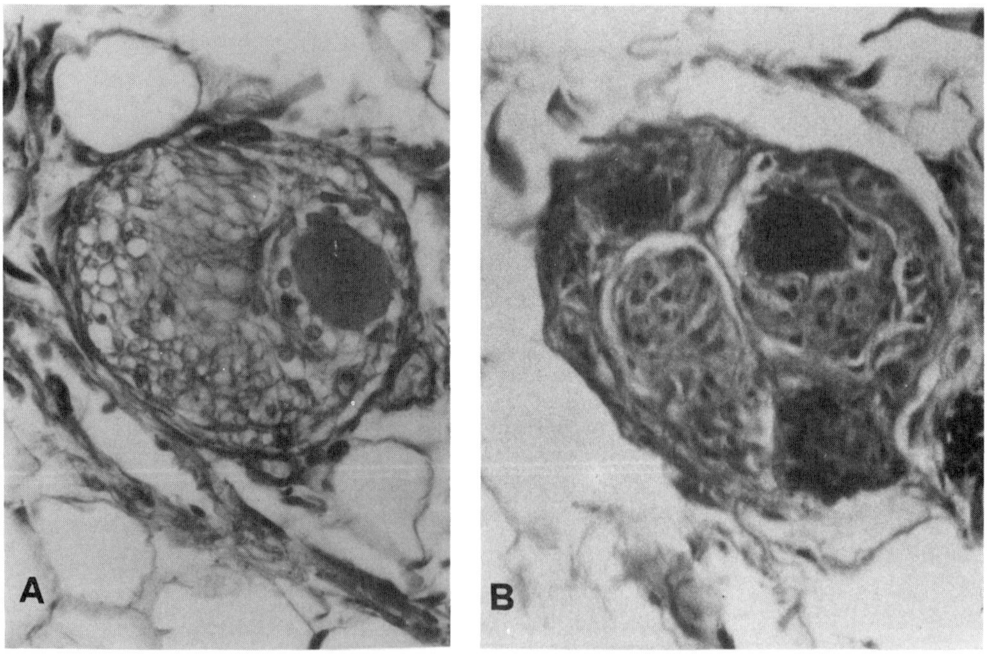

Figure 9. *A: A normal neuron of the AV groove's plexus, in chronic Chagasic cardiopathy and B: Damaged neurons undergoing replacement by Terplan nodules of satellite cells in a SA ganglion in a case of hypertrophic cardiomyopathy. Azan, × 1000.*

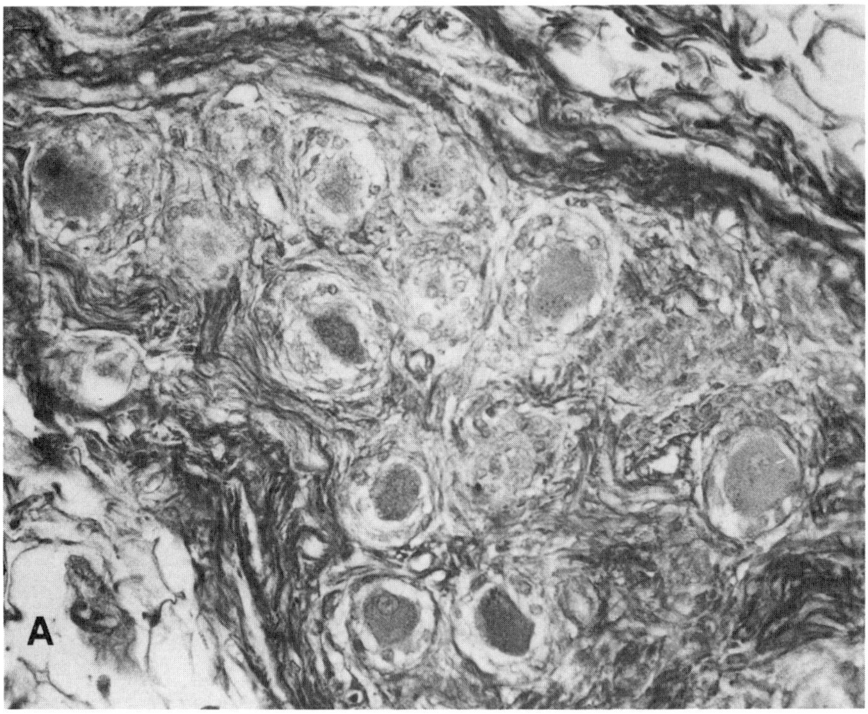

Figure 10. *Diffuse neuronal degeneration with nodular growth of satellite cells (Terplan nodules) in a SA ganglion of a case of human immunodeficiency virus (AIDS).*

The pathology of the extreme periphery of the cardiovascular vagus in man is largely ignored. The only exceptions are those involving the carotid body[16] and some mediastinal paraganglia (chemodectomas)[32] and inflammation[14] or invasion of the neuroreceptors of the carotid sinus or the aortic arch by local tumors.

It is very often impossible to draw any precise anatomical-clinical correlate between the foregoing neuropathological findings and the concomitant dysfunctional manifestations. The evidence of neuronal loss, as well as of axonal interruptions, entails a severe disruptive damage to the innervation, whereas slighter changes may temporarily impair, or even "irritate," the neural efferent and/or afferent activity.[15] These changes result in a vagosympathetic imbalance in the heart. Such an imbalance may underlie the pathophysiological-clinical hazards that are much more grave than the complete cardiac extrinsic denervation resulting from heart transplantation.[33]

Histopathology of Vagal Brain Stem Centers

Four cases were examined in which brain stem lesions (three from viral encephalitis and one from scleroderma vasculitis) seemed to correlate with a disordered vagal control of the heart. In the cases of encephalitis (28- and 36-year-old women and an infant of 2 months), perivascular round cell infiltrates and foci of gliosis and neuronophagia were detected in the DNV, the NTS[34] (Fig. 8) and, in the infant, in the reticular formation close to the NA (Fig. 11). Two patients had exhibited cardiac arrhythmias (sinus arrest with accelerated junctional escape and, respectively, paroxysms of ventricular tachycardia). Both were attended by severe gastroesophageal dyskinesis and profuse salivation, and had succumbed to cardiac arrest. The patient with scleroderma (a 19-year-old man) and the infant also died suddenly from cardiac arrest without previous records of severe arrhythmic manifestations. In all four cases, the conduction system and its innervation revealed no changes.

Pathology of Intercarotid Receptors

Cardioinhibitory or hypotensive manifestations are well known in both carotid sinus syndrome and glossopharyngeal neuralgia.[35] In a case of intractable carotid sinus syndrome, both carotid bodies were surgically ablated. These showed only a moderate increase in periglomerular sustentacular cells; such a change is common in hypoxic states.[36] The clinical symptoms relapsed after a temporary amelioration.

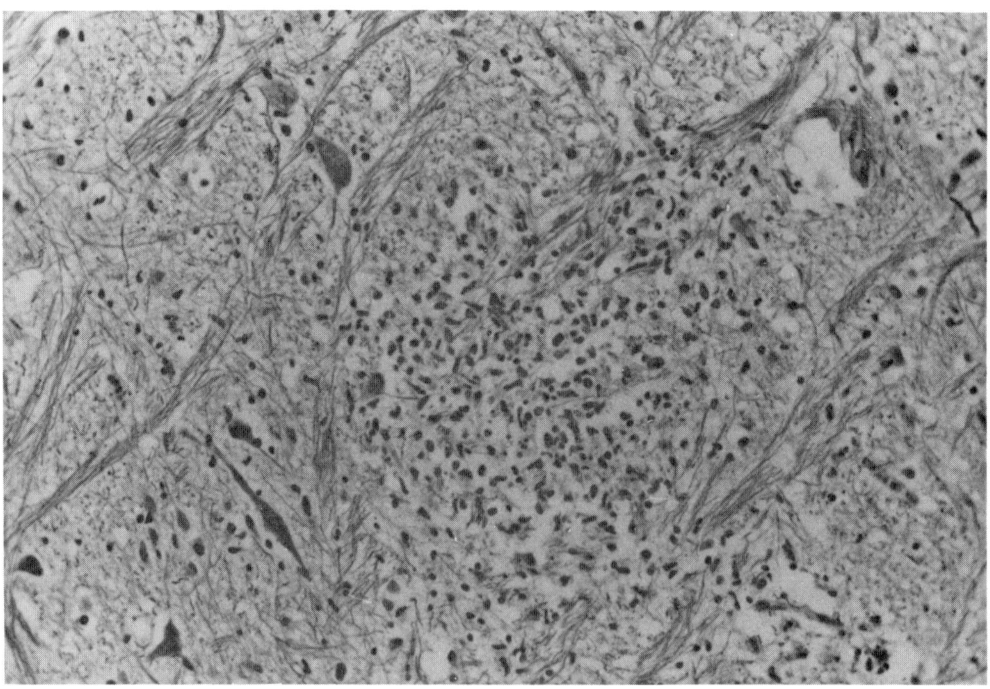

Figure 11. *Brain stem encephalitis, with focal gliosis and round cell infiltration, in the ventrolateral reticular formation adjacent to the NA in a dyspneic infant succumbed to sudden cardiac arrest. Bielschowsky's, × 200.*

Modifications of cardiac rhythm have been accounted for by baroreceptor stations other than those in the carotid area.[37] Some pathological features seem consistent with this concept; for example, arrhythmogenic implications were suspected in three cases with changes of the mediastinal vagus and of the aorto-coronary glomera.[14–16]

Amyloidosis of the cardiac plexus and of the annexed paraganglia, with a panconductional syndrome from amyloidosis in the SA and AV nodal regions, were described in a 62-year-old man. This patient developed severe orthostatic hypotension after he was given nifedipine, which selectively binds with amyloid.[17,38] Another man, 40 years of age, suffered severe dizziness and palpitations whenever he was subjected to strong barochemoreflex stimulation while travelling in airplanes. He succumbed to ventricular fibrillation upon landing.[15,17] Hyperacute ischemia and patchy infarction (from preceding silent heart attacks) were detected, but the epicardial coronary arteries were patent. The intertruncal artery alone was occluded by an organized-calcified thrombus, and the annexed left coronary glomus was almost completely depleted of chief cells, with the extant cells being devoid of neurotransmitter granules. Sclerotic atrophy of the intertruncal coronary glomus was also found in a 61-year-old patient who had severe anginal attacks and infarcts and who had undergone aorto-coronary saphenous graft bypass. Postoperatively, he had experienced temporary systemic hypertension, but the ischemic attacks had become silent. The patient succumbed to another infarct two months after surgery.[15]

The exact mechanism for such lethal cardioneuropathological derangements cannot be established, but a severe impairment of barochemoreflexogenesis, with imbalanced vago-sympathetic input in the heart, may be suspected from the histopathological findings.

Pathology of Atrial Intrinsic Plexuses

In cases of atrial fibrillation or of sick sinus syndrome, degeneration and loss of ganglion cells, variable in degree and extension, were observed in the SA plexus.[34] Changes of this kind, however, are also common in elderly patients who do not present with arrhythmias. Hence, no sound clinical-pathological correlate can be put forward, but only the inference of a disordered cardiac vago-sympathetic balance. This suggestion seems to be strengthened by the finding of severe changes of the SA nerve plexus in two cases (one infected by the human immunodeficiency virus, HIV) (Fig. 10),[17] in which the patients succumbed to torsades de pointes and long QT intervals.

In turn, severe damage to the cardiac vagal ganglia has been held to characterize chronic Chagas' heart disease,[31,39] with ensuing arrhythmias; similar parasympathetic changes of the visceral plexuses would account for the frequent megacolon in Chagasic patients. Nevertheless, it has been pointed out that cardiac vagal lesions are much more frequent and peculiar in cases from Argentina and Venezuela when compared to cases from Brazil.[40,41] Moreover, having realized that the histologic criteria adopted to diagnose neuronal loss in autoptic Chagasic hearts are wide open to criticism, a reexamination of the material is under way.[39] Left ventricular neuritis (close to the pathognomonic apical aneurysm) has been seen,[17] whereas the emphasized neuronal depletion has not yet been confirmed (Fig. 9).[39]

The same applies to the alleged neuronal loss in the right atrial plexus in dilated cardiomyopathy,[31] whereas degeneration of neurons, with nodular proliferation of satellite cells, was observed in cases of hypertrophic cardiomyopathy (Fig. 9). Extensive denervation of the right atrium due to massive infiltration by an epicardial mesothelioma which spared the SA node, entailed only a sinus tachycardia (from probable suppression of the strong local vagus input).[17]

Diabetic cardiac neuropathy, involving the vagus and imbalancing the autonomic input with loss of rhythm modulation[42] (not rarely attended by a prolongation of QT interval),[43] has been recognized in clinics, but not in human histopathology laboratories. Recent observations of the gastric vagus from operated patients showed degeneration and regeneration of myelinated fibers,[44] fairly similar to the findings in spontaneously diabetic rats with heart rate variability.[45] Such neural lesions are mainly attributed to microvascular damage.

Pathology of atrial and ventricular vagal terminals, whether efferent or afferent, in human disease is questionable.[20] However, the hazardous arrhythmogenic implications of postinfarction impairments of baroreflexogenesis has recently been emphasized,[2] and an experimental approach has been devised to prevent it.[46]

The cardiac intrinsic nerve network may survive both the acute infarct damage and the ensuing scarring[15,17] because of the diminished oxygen dependence and different metabolic sources of nerves as compared to the surrounding muscle. Yet the finest nerve endings, namely the receptors (Fig. 7), which lie "naked" in the midst of the necrotic area and in the subsequent dense scarring, may undergo complete obliteration and may not be recognized histologically.

References

1. Schwartz PJ, Billman GE, Stone HL: Autonomic mechanism in ventricular fibrillation induced by myocardial ischemia during exercise in dogs with healed myocardial infarction. Circulation 69:790, 1984.
2. Schwartz PJ, Zaza A, Pala M, et al: Baroreflex sensitivity and its evolution during the first year after myocardial infarction. J Am Coll Cardiol 12:629, 1988.
3. Spyer KM: Neural organization and control of the baroreceptor reflex. Rev Physiol Biochem Pharmacol 88:23, 1981.
4. Manning JW: Intracranial mechanism of regulation. In WC Randall (ed): Neural Regulation of the Heart. New York, Oxford University Press, 1977, p. 189.
5. Zuleger S, Staubesand J: Atlas of the Central Nervous System in Sectional Planes. Baltimore, Urban & Schwarzenberg, 1977, p. 70.
6. Kahle W: Nervous system and sensory organs. In W Kahle, K Leonhardt, W Platzer (eds): Color Atlas and Textbook of Human Anatomy; III. Stuttgart, Georg Thieme, 1986, pp. 138,274.

7. Nieuvenhuis R, Voogd J, van Huijzen C: The Human Central Nervous System: A Synopsis and Atlas. Berlin, Springer, 1988, p. 124.
8. Guntheroth WG: The Sudden Infant Death Syndrome. Mount Kisco, NY, Futura Publishing Company, 1989, p. 50.
9. Quattrocchi JJ, McBride PT, Yates AJ: Brain stem immaturity in sudden infant death syndrome: A quantitative rapid Golgi study of dendritic spines in 95 infants. Brain Res 325:39, 1985.
10. Stohr P Jr: Pathologische anatomie der vegetativen nervensystem, 4. In Wv Möllendorf, W Bargman (eds): Handbuch der mikroskopischen Anatomie des Menschen Nervensystem. Berlin, Springer, 1957, pp. 179,213.
11. Randall WC, Armour AJ: Gross and microscopic anatomy of the cardiac innervation. In WC Randall (ed): Neural Regulation of the Heart. New York, Oxford University Press, 1977, p. 13.
12. Janes RD, Brandys C, Hopkins DA, et al: Anatomy of human extrinsic cardiac nerves and ganglia. Am J Cardiol 57:299, 1986.
13. Mitchell GAG: Cardiovascular Innervation. Edinburgh, E & S Livingstone, 1956, p. 209.
14. Rossi L: Cardioneuropathy and extracardiac neural disease. J Am Coll Cardiol 5:66B, 1985.
15. Rossi L: Neuroanatomopathology of the cardiovascular system. In HE Kulbertus, G Franck (eds): Neurocardiology. Mount Kisco, NY, Futura Publishing Company, 1988, p. 25.
16. Heath D, Smith P: The Pathology of the Carotid Body and Sinus. London, Edward Arnold, 1985, pp. 19,112.
17. Rossi L, Matturri L: Clinicopathological Approach to Cardiac Arrhythmias. Torino, Centro Scient Torinese (distributed by Mount Kisco, NY, Futura Publishing Company), 1990, p. 54.
18. James TN, Isobe JH, Urthaler F: Hemodynamic components of a cardiogenic hypertensive chemoreflex. Circ Res 42:135, 1978.
19. Botar J: The Autonomic Nervous System. Budapest, Akademiai Kiadò, 1966, p. 291.
20. Randall WC, Ardell JL: Nervous control of the heart: Anatomy and pathophysiology. In DP Zipes, J Jalife (eds): Cardiac Electrophysiology: From Cell to Bedside. Philadelphia, Saunders, 1990, p. 291.
21. Zipes DP, Miyazaki T: The autonomic nervous system and the heart: Basis for understanding interactions and effects on arrhythmia development. In DP Zipes, J Jalife (eds): Cardiac Electrophysiology: From Cell to Beside. Philadelphia, Saunders, 1990, p. 312.
22. Karlson P: Historical development of the receptor concept. In G Seifert (ed): Cell Receptors: Morphological Characterization and Pathological Aspects. Berlin, Springer, 1991, p. 3.
23. Sisson JC, Lynch JJ, Johnson J, et al: Scintigraphic detection of regional disruption of adrenergic neurons in the heart. Am Heart J 116:67, 1988.
24. Okazaki H: Fundamentals of Neuropathology. New York, Igaku-Shoin, 1989, p. 10.
25. Wolff GS, Han J, Curran G: Wolff-Parkinson-White syndrome in the neonate. Am J Cardiol 41:559, 1978.
26. Malfatto G, Rosen TS, Steinberg SF, et al: Sympathetic neural modulation of cardiac impulse initiation and repolarization in the newborn rat. Circ Res 66:427, 1990.
27. Linden RJ: Sensory endings in the heart with comment on excitatory reflexes. In B Lown, A Malliani, M Prosdocimi (eds): Neural Mechanisms and Cardiovascular Disease. Berlin, Springer, 1986, p. 11.
28. Rossi L: Structures of the human baroreflex arc in health and disease: An anatomofunctional survey. Eur JCPE 2:53, 1992.
29. Bennington JL: Pathology of Peripheral Nerves. Philadelphia, Saunders, 1978, p. 50.

30. Feyrter F: Über die Pathologie der vegetativen nervösen Peripherie und ihrer ganglionären Regulationsstätten. Wien, Maudrich, 1951, p. 139.
31. Olsen EGJ: Atlas of Cardiovascular Pathology. Lancaster, MTP Press, 1987, p. 81.
32. Glenner GG, Grimley PM: Tumors of the extra-adrenal paraganglion system (including chemoreceptors). In Atlas of Tumor Pathology II/9. Washington DC, Armed Forces Institute of Pathology, 1974, p. 39.
33. Smith ML, Ellenbogen KA, Eckberg DL, et al: Subnormal parasympathetic activity after cardiac transplantation. Am J Cardiol 66:1243, 1990.
34. Rossi L: Histopathologic correlates of atrial arrhythmias. In P Touboul, AL Waldo (eds): Atrial Arrhythmias: Current Concepts and Management. St. Louis, Mosby Year Book, 1990, p. 27.
35. Johnston RT, Redding VJ: Glossopharyngeal neuralgia associated with cardiac syncope: Long term treatment with permanent pacing and carmabazepine. Br Heart J 64:403, 1990.
36. Bencini C, Pulera N: The carotid bodies in bronchial asthma. Histopathology 18:195, 1991.
37. Mancia G, Ferrari A, Gregorini L, et al: Baroreceptor control of heart rate in man. In PJ Schwartz, AM Brown, A Malliani, et al (eds): Neural Mechanisms in Cardiac Arrhythmias. New York, Raven Press, 1978, p. 323.
38. Volpi A, Cavalli A, Maggioni AP, et al: Cardiac amyloidosis involving the conduction system and the aortocoronary neuroreceptors: Clinicopathological correlates. Chest 90:619, 1986.
39. Milei J, Storino RA, Beigelman R, et al: Histopathology of specialized and ordinary myocardium and nerves in chronic Chagas' disease, with a morphometric study of inflammation and fibrosis. Cardiologia 36:107, 1991.
40. Lopes ER, Tafuri WL: Involvement of the autonomic nervous system in Chagas' disease. Rec Soc Brasil Med Tropic 16:206, 1983.
41. Wyrme J, Braunwald E: The cardiomyopathies and myocarditides. In E Braunwald (ed): Heart Disease: A Textbook of Cardiovascular Medicine. Philadelphia, Saunders, 1988, p. 1446.
42. Maser RE, Pfeifer MA, Dorman JS, et al: Diabetic autonomic neuropathy and cardiovascular risk. Pittsburg epidemiology of diabetes complications study III. Arch Intern Med 150:1218, 1990.
43. Ewing DJ, Boland OM, Cho CG, et al: QT interval, diabetic neuropathy and unexpected death. Diabetologia 33(suppl):A33, 1990. Abstract.
44. Britland ST, Young RJ, Sharma AK, et al: Vagus nerve morphology in diabetic gastropathy. Diabetic Med 7:780, 1990.
45. Zhang WX, Chakrabarti S, Greene D, et al: Diabetic autonomic neuropathy in BB rats and effect of ARI treatment on heart rate variability and vagus nerve structure. Diabetes (US) 39:613, 1990.
46. Vanoli E, De Ferrari GM, Stramba-Badiale M, et al: Vagal stimulation and prevention of sudden death in conscious dogs with a healed myocardial infarction. Circ Res 68:1471, 1991.

CHAPTER 2

Peripheral Innervation of the Heart

W.C. Randall, R.D. Wurster

The rich innervation of the sinoatrial (SA) and atrioventricular (AV) nodal regions of the mammalian heart has been emphasized by nearly all anatomical and/or electrophysiological studies during the past century. The effective regulation of these critical control regions is of obvious importance, and is therefore subject to much speculation (both basic and clinical), but to relatively little carefully controlled laboratory experimentation. The key role of the autonomic nervous system in this control system is universally recognized, but very little is known about differential neuronal distributions from either sympathetic or parasympathetic limbs to individual automatic (pacemaker), conductile, or contractile cells. Only sparse information exists relating the organization of neural elements regulating SA versus AV performance. Perhaps it is generally assumed that both control regions are simultaneously and similarly influenced by either, or both, sympathetic and parasympathetic inputs. Simple, series-like connections from either autonomic limb could conceivably feed into the SA, AV, and contractile mechanisms. Since most of the ganglion complexes have been reported to be located around the base of the aorta, venae cavae, and pulmonary artery, these locations have generally been assumed to represent the sites of pre-postganglionic synapses mediating changes in chronotropic, dromotropic, and inotropic responses.

Selective Anatomical Pathways

A concept of anatomical-functional separation of the SA and AV innervations is a recent development in the understanding of autonomic regulation of cardiac performance. The *selective* distribution of vagal preganglionic pathways to the SA node via ganglia situated in the pulmonary vein fat pad (PVFP), in contrast to those located in the fat pad overlying entry of the coronary sinus into the inferior interatrial septum at the junction of the inferior vena cava-inferior left atrium (IVC-ILA) and supplying the AV region of the canine

The research was supported by the National Heart, Lung, and Blood Institute Grant HL-27595 and the James Depauw Fund of Chicago.
From *Vagal Control of the Heart: Experimental Basis and Clinical Implications* edited by MN Levy, PJ Schwartz © 1994, Futura Publishing Co. Inc., Armonk, NY.

heart,[1,2] provides distinctly different insight into autonomic control of cardiac performance. Since relatively few ganglia are found in ventricular tissues, exceptions being recently reported by Butler et al,[3] it is presumed that ventricular activity is largely influenced by vagal ganglia located within the atria and by sympathetic postganglionic distributions from the middle cervical and stellate ganglia.[4] Additional neurons are known to be present (small intensely fluorescent [SIF] cells, interconnecting fibers, peptidergic fibers) but their functions are not yet understood.[5]

The actual anatomical pathways into and through the several "cardiac plexuses" have remained almost totally unknown until the past few years. Indeed, one can hardly picture a discrete pathway through a true plexus. Therefore, it has been necessary to speak in generalities concerning specific distribution of either sympathetic or parasympathetic fibers to target tissues such as SA or AV nodes, coronary blood vessels, or contractile tissues. Combined structure-function studies, however, have revealed the separate anatomical course of sympathetic and vagal pathways of nerves through the pericardium and transepicardially to some of the critically important control regions of the heart (SA, AV, and conductile and contractile tissues). Staged surgical dissection of small segments of tissues around and along the great vessels entering the heart, with accompanying supramaximal stimulation of proximal portions of the sympathetic and/or parasympathetic cardiac innervation between each stage, permitted systematic descriptions of successive deletions of neurally-induced changes in cardiac performance including specific interventions such as selective interruption of right (or left) vagal inputs to the SA (or AV) region evolved. Thus, it became apparent that electrical stimulation of individual cardiac nerves, or stimulation of a cervical vagus before and after highly specific dissections around the common pulmonary artery, revealed very restricted responses in SA discharge frequency (heart rate), AV conduction, or in localized contractile force.[6] In the canine heart, vagal innervation of the SA node was shown to be derived primarily from vagal branches following the superior vena cava, superior pulmonary veins, and distal portions of the right pulmonary artery. These pathways were interrupted surgically without jeopardizing major vagal inputs to the AV regions. Conscious animal models sustaining selective SA parasympathectomy show marked AV block without sinus slowing during baroreceptor stimulation.[7]

Selective parasympathectomy of the AV region is accomplished by destruction of the fat pad overlying the junctional bridge between the IVC-ILA. Supramaximal stimulation of the cervical vagi elicits profound inhibition in sinus discharge rates without change in AV conduction following such surgical procedures. Negative inotropic changes are partially attenuated by excision of either the PVFP, which obliterates vagal slowing in heart rate, or the IVC-ILA fat pad, which removes vagal inhibition of AV conduction and block. Equally important, all of these parasympathetic interventions may be performed without serious interference with sympathetic distributions to either SA or AV regions in the dog. These experiments demonstrated that both sympathetic and parasympathetic nerves are distributed to highly restricted regions of the heart over discrete anatomical pathways, and that the central nervous system

(CNS) thus, at least potentially, has *selective anatomical pathways* for control of automatic (SA) or conductile (AV) mechanisms. Whether and how the CNS actually utilizes such paths under normal physiological conditions remains open.

Injection of horseradish peroxidase (HRP) into either PVFP or IVC-ILA fat pads in dogs elicited retrograde axoplasmic transport of the marker to preganglionic cell bodies in the medulla oblongata, 98% in the nucleus ambiguus (NA), and 2% in the dorsal motor nucleus (DMN) and intermediate zones.[8] Simultaneous injection of two different markers into both PVFP and IVC-ILA pads resulted in comparable distribution of both markers in NA and DMN, but thus far, no dually labelled preganglionic cells have been detected. This result further indicates CNS ability to selectively activate either SA or AV changes either together or independently.

Figure 1 represents a ventral view of the dog's right atrium. The figure shows the relationships between the PVFP that overlies entry of the right pulmonary veins into the atrium and the course of the sinoatrial nodal artery (SANA) branch off the right coronary artery to the sulcus terminalis, where the branch turns rostrally to supply the SA nodal and neighboring regions. The base of the triangular-shaped PVFP nearly covers the pulmonary vein complex, while its apex approximates the SANA in the sulcus terminalis. Large and small ganglia may be found throughout the corpus of the fat pad, but density is greatest along its rostro-medial borders. The ganglia are generally immersed in fatty tissue, closely adjacent to the epicardial surface with modest extensions rostrally along nerves coursing parallel to the sulcus terminalis. If ganglia are surrounded by muscle, they are generally enveloped within a fatty-connective tissue sac.[9,10]

Using a small, bipolar, concentric exploring electrode to stimulate intramural nerves, Bluemel et al[11] mapped the right atrial freewall for vagal postganglionic nerves from the PVFP to SA node with short duration bursts from a small, bipolar-exploring electrode. Results showed that the primary vagal postganglionic pathways to the SA node are subepicardial and parallel to the SANA along the sulcus terminalis. Hexamethonium in PVFP abolished SA inhibition during right or left cervical vagal excitation, but it did not interrupt vagal suppression of AV conduction. SA slowing, however, continued to occur after hexamethonium administration (either in PVFP or systemically) when the exploring electrode was applied directly over intramural fibers between the PVFP and the SA node. A few ganglia were also identified along the course of the sulcus terminalis and the caudal end of the SA node. These experiments were interpreted to indicate that the PVFP is the primary site for vagal synapses mediating reflex regulation of SA function, rather than the conventionally identified concentration of ganglia located on the posterior right atrium. Comparable exploration of epicardial surfaces between the posterior right atrial ganglia (PAFP), together with histologic tracing of neuronal markers injected into the SA node, confirms these conclusions,[12] although a few subepicardial ganglia on the posterior right atrium at the base of the superior vena cava contain some synapses which mediate vagal inputs to the SA node.

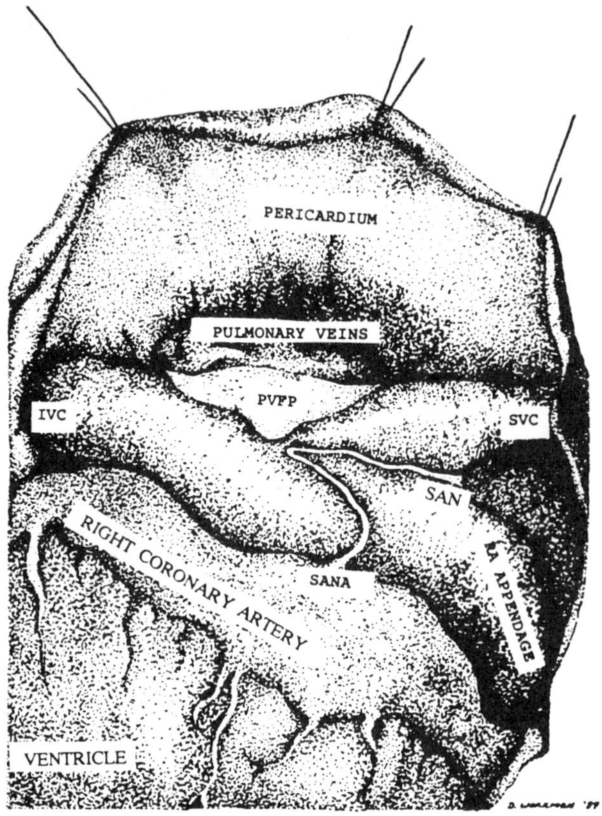

Figure 1. *Location of the pulmonary vein fat pad (PVFP) on the right side of the canine heart, containing the ganglia that innervate the sinoatrial node (SAN). The inferior vena cava (IVC) and superior vena cava (SVC) are caudal and rostral to the PVFP, which is adjacent to the right pulmonary veins. The sinoatrial nodal artery (SANA) loops near the PVFP before turning toward the SAN.*

Cardiac performance is continuously modulated by tonic activity in both sympathetic and parasympathetic limbs. Contrary to earlier doctrine, however, there is not necessarily a "reciprocal balance" between them; opposing influences are not simply algebraically additive but, rather, are governed by complex interactions.[13–15] Thus, a controlled stimulation of the vagus nerves induces a greater inhibition in automaticity and conductivity when prevailing sympathetic input (tone) is high, or conversely, a lesser response is elicited by sympathetic stimulation when concomitant vagal input is elevated.[13] In contrast to the marked cholinergic predominance in modulation of sinus and junctional automaticity and atrial and ventricular contractility, it appears that comparable autonomic interactions are practically absent in the control of AV conduction.[16] Thus, the nature and extent of parasympathetic-sympathetic interactions vary considerably, depending on which cardiac target tissues are studied. AV conduction is especially sensitive to modulation by sympathetic inputs, whereas sinus node automaticity is especially responsive to cholinergic influences.

Physiology of Intracardiac Ganglia

Many reviews of neural control of the heart rarely mention that the vagus nerve does not actually terminate on myocardial cells but rather on nerve cells in intracardiac ganglia. Even when these reviews consider the intracardiac ganglia, they presume that ganglion cells function merely as relay neurons. These assumptions are based upon a lack of electrophysiological understanding of the structure and function of these cells. Due to the difficulty in locating these ganglia and their seeming inaccessibility in mammals, knowledge of the electrophysiological characteristics have been, until recently, largely limited to amphibians. These amphibian studies have indicated that an array of neurophysiological mechanisms are available for integrative functions of these ganglia; these ganglia do not function as simple relays.[17–20]

In the last few years, electrophysiological studies of mammalian intracardiac ganglia have used dissociated, adult cells and neonatal preparations.[21–25] Our laboratory was able to localize adult canine intracardiac ganglia in the PVFP[10] and was able to remove a small piece of the PVFP and dissect away much of the fat until a plexus of ganglia and their intraganglionic nerves could be visualized.[26] It was revealed that these ganglia still have afferent or preganglionic terminals innervating the ganglion cells. Stable resting membrane potentials, action potentials, and synaptic potentials have been recorded (Fig. 2). In addition, ganglion cells whose physiological properties have been characterized[5,26] have been labelled intracellularly. Compared to amphibian cells, these canine intracardiac ganglion cells have a far more complicated morphology with numerous complex dendrites, varicosities, and spines (Fig. 3). The electron micrographs display cells bodies almost entirely covered by satellite or supportive cell processes.[27] Synaptic boutons were restricted to the processes or spines; none were found on the soma proper.

Based upon responses to intracellularly injected, depolarizing currents, these ganglion cells have been classified into three different functional cell types:

1. single discharging cells (S-cells) (Fig. 2A);
2. repetitive responding cells (R-cells) (Fig. 2B); and
3. nonresponding cells (N-cells).[26,28]

The morphological and physiological properties of these cell types were compared. The order of the resting membrane potentials and input capacitances was N- > S- > R-cells. The capacitance characteristics correlated with the size of the cell bodies as measured from identified, HRP-labelled cells. The input resistance of these cells, however, had the reverse relationship. Thus, larger cells (e.g., the N-cells) required a larger current to depolarize; thus they were less excitable than the smaller cells (e.g., the R-cells). Some of these physiological differences may be related to the nature of the afterpotential currents.

What is the physiological significance of these different cell types? The R-cells are capable of maintaining continuous activity and, hence, may play an

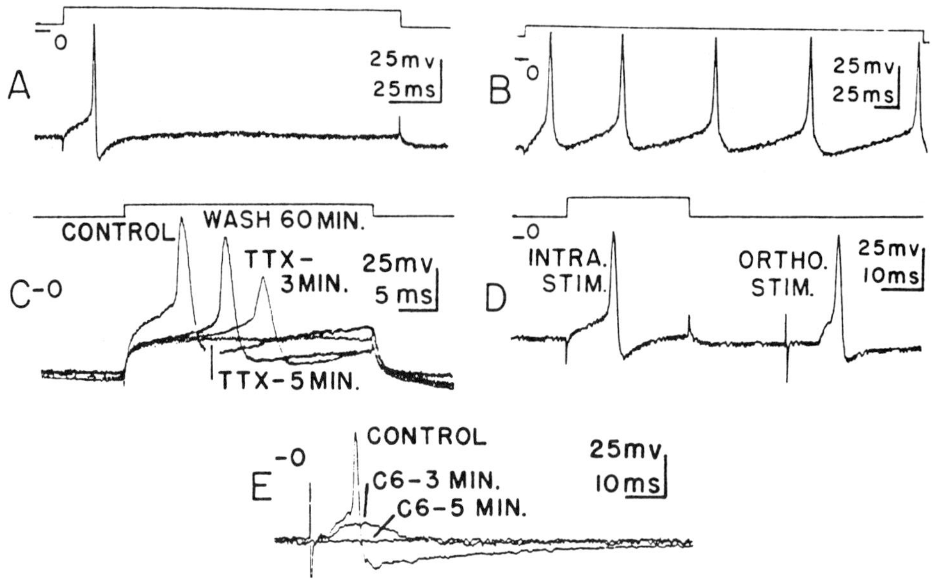

Figure 2. *Intracellular recordings from intracardiac ganglion cell bodies. Lower tracings are membrane potentials. 0 potential line indicated on the ordinate. The upper tracings indicate injection of depolarizing currents (1.25 nA). A: Single discharging cell (S-cell) responded with a single action potential to a maintained depolarization. B: Repetitive responding cell (R-cell) responded with repetitive action potentials. C: The responses before (CONTROL) and 3 and 5 min after the administration of tetrodotoxin (TTX) as well as 60 min following washout of the TTX (WASH 60 MIN). The action potential was reversibly blocked by TTX. D: Responses to orthodromic stimulation (ORTHO. STIM.) as well as to intracellular stimulation (INTRA. STIM.). The amplitude and shape of these action potentials were similar. E: Responses to orthodromic activation before (CONTROL) and 3 and 5 min following hexamethonium administration (C6-1 MIN and C6-3 MIN). Reproduced with permission from Xi X, Thomas JX, Randall WC, et al: Intracellular recordings from canine intracardiac ganglion cells. J Auton Nerv Syst 32:177–182, 1991.*

important role in vagal control of cardiac functions such as heart rate. The S-cells may play an important role in control of phasic cardiac responses. Studies of phasic and tonic sympathetic ganglion cells offer another interesting possibility for the different cell types in the canine intracardiac ganglia.[29,30] The phasic sympathetic ganglion cells were proposed to receive synaptic inputs primarily from the CNS, whereas the tonic units received input from visceral afferent fibers. However, the actual role of these different cell types in intracardiac ganglia awaits further experimental testing. It has been thought that N-cells were nonneuronal cells or damaged neurons. HRP-labelling, however, indicated that these cells were indeed morphologically neurons which apparently were undamaged, for they had stable, high-resting membrane potentials.[5]

When canine ganglion cells were intracellularly labelled with HRP, most of these cells had long axons which either exited the ganglion to innervate the surrounding myocardium directly or entered interganglionic nerves.[5] These

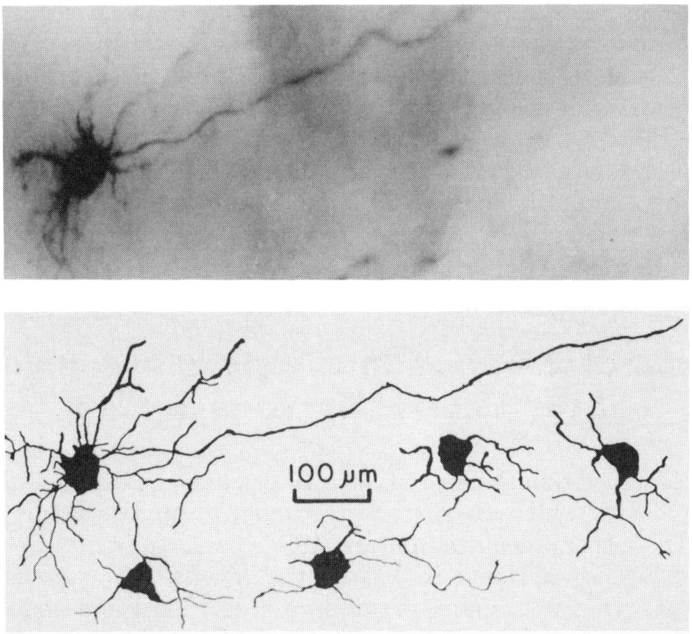

Figure 3. *Five intracardiac ganglion cells that were intracellularly labelled with horseradish peroxidase (HRP) reaction products. Top: Photomicrograph of a labelled cell taken from a 1-mm thick, whole-tissue mount specimen. Portions of the cell pass out of the plane of focus. Bottom: Camera lucida drawings of five labelled intracardiac ganglion cells taken from different preparations. The upper cell is the same cell as in the photomicrograph. Reproduced with permission from Xi X, Thomas JX, Randall WC, et al: Intracellular recordings from canine intracardiac ganglion cells. J Auton Nerv Syst 32:177–182, 1991.*

nerves contained postganglionic fibers that ran through other ganglia to innervate other myocardial regions or possibly to terminate on other ganglion cells (i.e., interganglionic interneurons). Some of the labelled ganglion cells had short axons that did not exit the ganglion. These ganglion cells may have been either inadequately filled with HRP or may have been intraganglionic cells or possibly intraganglionic interneurons. The presence of interneurons would make the intracardiac ganglia more capable of complex integrative functions. If these cells are interneurons, careful electron micrographic evidence will be required to show that these ganglion cells have synaptic boutons on other ganglion cells.

Stimulation of the interganglionic nerves produced antidromic as well as orthodromic action potentials in these ganglion cells (Fig. 2D).[26] Most of these action potentials were sensitive to the fast sodium channel blocker, tetrodotoxin (TTX) (Fig. 2C), and to low Ca^{2+}/high Mg^{2+} solutions (not shown). These responses implicate the role of sodium and calcium channels in the generation of the action potential. Even a single stimulation of these nerves which presumably contain vagal preganglionic axons, produced excitatory postsynaptic potentials (EPSPs) that were usually large enough to reach threshold (Figs. 2D, 2E). These findings are in contrast to extracellular recordings from the same ganglia, where trains of stimuli of preganglionic axons were usually necessary to activate canine intracardiac ganglion cells.[31–34] Previous in vivo studies in several species, however, have shown that single orthodromic preganglionic stimulation is capable of being transmitted through the cardiac ganglion to activate ganglion cells and slow the heart.[35] In addition, the stimulation-evoked excitatory postsynaptic potential and the resultant action potential was blocked by the nicotinic cholinergic antagonist, hexamethonium (C6) (Fig. 2E).

Intracardiac Ganglionic Activity Independent of the Central Nervous System

It was observed that these ganglion cells frequently exhibited spontaneous miniature EPSPs, which often reach threshold to initiate action potentials (Fig. 4).[36] These spontaneous miniature EPSPs occurred in 59% of the R-cells, 50% of the S-cells, and only in 10% of the N-cells. Although most of the spontaneous activity consisted of miniature EPSPs, some cells displayed biphasic or triphasic potential changes. A few cells displayed rhythmic EPSP-like depolarization. This rhythmic activity, however, seemed to correlate with rhythmic contractions of cardiac muscle cells that were sometimes isolated with the ganglion preparation. Almost all of the spontaneous EPSPs were blocked by low Ca^{2+}/high Mg^{2+} solutions (Fig. 4A) and by hexamethonium, but persisted in the presence of action potential blockade with TTX (not shown). These observations suggested that these EPSPs were mediated by vesicular release of acetylcholine acting on nicotinic receptors and did not require

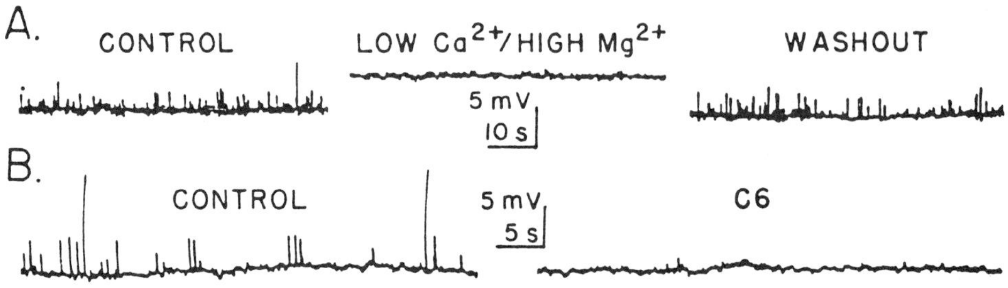

Figure 4. *Effects of synaptic and nicotinic blocking solutions on spontaneous activity. A: Slow oscillograph tracing of spontaneous miniature excitatory postsynaptic potential-(EPSP-)like activity before, during, and following washout of a low Ca^{2+}/high Mg^{2+} synaptic blocking solutions. In addition to a small resting potential depolarization, most of the spontaneous miniature EPSP-like activity was blocked in the presence of the synaptic blocking solution. B: Slow oscillograph recording of spontaneous miniature EPSP-like activity before and during the application of the nicotinic blocking agent hexamethonium (C6) (10^{-4}M). Reproduced with permission from Xi X, Randall WC, Wurster RD: Intracellular recording of spontaneous activity of canine intracardiac ganglion cells. Neurosci Lett 128:129–132, 1991.*

presynaptic action potentials, which might have been produced by injury currents from cut fibers. These studies differed from those of the cultured guinea pig or rat cells that have lost their processes and synapses due to enzymatic and mechanical dissociation.[21–24] Cardiac ganglion cells from neonatal rats sometimes displayed small amplitude miniature EPSPs but not spontaneous action potentials.[25]

Spontaneous action potentials have been recorded extracellularly in the intact anesthetized canine and cat intracardiac ganglia that were decentralized from the CNS.[31–34,37] In the dog, this spontaneous activity was highly correlated with pulmonary and cardiac mechanical changes and was not blocked by hexamethonium.[31] Presuming that this activity was not due to mechanical distortion of the ganglion cells by the recording electrode, this apparently spontaneous activity suggests the involvement of intracardiac reflexes. Accordingly, this spontaneous activity might be, in part, responsible for some of the "vagal tone" reported after vagotomy.[36,38]

Chemical Nature of Synaptic Transmission in Intracardiac Ganglia

Recently, a preliminary report of slow EPSPs and slow inhibitory postsynaptic potentials as well as the fast EPSPs discussed above has been presented.[39] The slow synaptic potentials followed tetanic excitation of the presynaptic fibers that terminate on the intracardiac ganglion cells and persisted for as long as several seconds. The fast EPSP, as well as the orthodromic action potentials, were blocked by the ganglionic blocking drug hexamethonium; this suggests nicotinic ganglionic transmission similar to that in other autonomic ganglia. The slow synaptic potentials involved muscarinic cholinergic mechanisms. These observations contrast with the predominance of noncholinergically-mediated activity recorded extracellularly in canine intracardiac ganglion cells.[31]

Cholinergic and noncholinergic mechanisms may be involved in the control of the intracardiac ganglion cells. The presence of catecholaminergic and peptidergic innervation in the ganglion has been reported.[40,41] Some of the catecholaminergic innervation is associated with postganglionic sympathetic innervation, possibly from SIF cells in the ganglia. The peptidergic innervation, e.g., calcitonin gene-related peptide, may be associated with afferent fibers or with the ganglion cells themselves. Actual synaptic contacts of ganglion cells, however, remains to be validated by electron microscopy.

"Cardiac Brain:" A Hypothesis

The following possible scheme for the organization of the intracardiac ganglia is presented (Fig. 5). The cardiac ganglia contain principal cells (P), which send their axons to pacemaker cells, cardiac conductile cells, and the working myocardium. Some of the ganglion cells may be interneurons (IN),

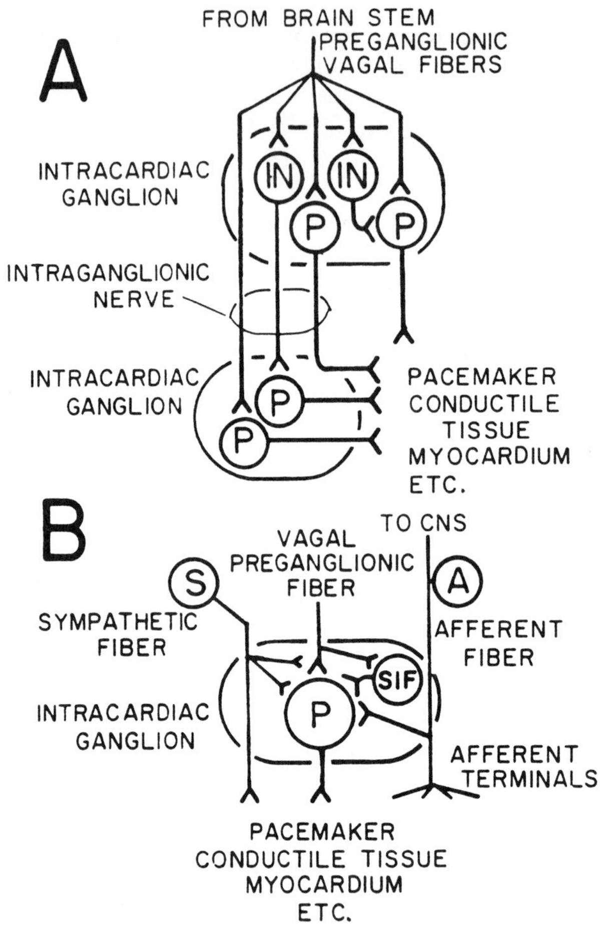

Figure 5. *Model of possible integration within the intracardiac ganglia. A: Vagal preganglionic fibers from the brain stem terminate on principal cells (P) or possibly on interneurons (IN) which may send connections to P cells. Some preganglionic fibers course between ganglia as well as postganglionic fibers and possible axons of IN cells via a intraganglionic nerve. B: In addition to preganglionic and possible IN axons, P cells may receive inputs from small intensively fluorescent (SIF) cells and cardiac afferent (A) fibers. Postganglionic sympathetic fibers (S) may possibly influence P cells via presynaptic or postsynaptic influences.*

which terminate within the ganglia, while others may send their axons to other ganglia in the intracardiac plexus. SIF cell processes may interact with the P cells or the IN. Sympathetic (S) postganglionic axons pass through the intracardiac ganglia, although it is possible that some may terminate on ganglion cells or presynaptically on preganglionic parasympathetic fiber terminals. Cardiac afferent (A) fibers containing various peptides traverse the ganglion also. These afferent fibers may synapse on cells within the intracardiac ganglion, possibly accounting for intracardiac reflexes[31,37,42] similar to those in some sympathetic ganglia.[29,30,43] Thus, within the intracardiac ganglia, there exists a rich potential for complex integration of activity controlling cardiac function. A complex nervous system may exist within the heart—a "cardiac brain" - similar to the enteric nervous system within the gut[44] or the so-called gut or enteric brain. Many of these questions serve as fascinating challenges for future research.

References

1. Ardell JL, Randall WC: Selective vagal innervation of sinoatrial and atrioventricular nodes in the canine heart. Am J Physiol 251:H764, 1986.
2. Randall WC, Ardell JL: Selective parasympathectomy of automatic and conductile tissues of the canine heart. Am J Physiol 248:H61, 1985.
3. Butler CK, Smith FM, Nicholson J, et al: Cardiac effects induced by chemically activated neurons in canine intrathoracic ganglia. Am J Physiol 259:H1108, 1990.
4. Takahashi N, Barber MJ, Zipes DP: Efferent vagal innervation of the canine left ventricle. Am J Physiol 248:H89, 1985.
5. Xi X, Randall WC, Wurster RD: Morphology of intracellularly labeled canine intracardiac ganglion cells. J Comp Neurol 314:396, 1991.
6. Randall WC, Ardell JL: Differential innervation of the heart. In DP Zipes, J Jalife (eds): Cardiac Electrophysiology and Arrhythmias. New York, NY, Grune & Stratton, 1985, p. 137.
7. Randall DC, Randall WC, Brown DR, et al: Heart rate control in awake dog after selective SA-nodal parasympathectomy. Am J Physiol 262:H1128, 1992.
8. Plecha DM, Randall WC, Geis GS, et al: Localization of vagal preganglionic somata controlling the sinoatrial and atrioventricular nodes. Am J Physiol 255:R703, 1988.
9. Randall WC, Ardell JL, Calderwood D, et al: Parasympathetic ganglia innervating the canine atrioventricular nodal region. J Auton Nerv Syst 16:311, 1986.
10. Randall WC, Ardell JL, Wurster RD, et al: Vagal postganglionic innervation of the canine sinoatrial node. J Auton Nerv Syst 20:13, 1987.
11. Bluemel KM, Wurster RD, Randall WC, et al: Parasympathetic postganglionic pathways to the sinoatrial node. Am J Physiol 259:H1504, 1990.
12. Mick J, Wurster RD, Duff M, et al: Epicardial sites for vagal mediation of sinoatrial function. Am J Physiol 262:H1401, 1992.
13. Urthaler F, Neely BH, Hageman GR, et al: Differential sympathetic-parasympathetic interactions in sinus node and AV junction. Am J Physiol 250:H43, 1986.
14. Warner MR, Levy MN: Neuropeptide Y as a putative modulator of the vagal effects on heart rate. Circ Res 64:882, 1989.
15. Warner MR, Levy MN: Inhibition of cardiac vagal effects by neurally released and exogenous neuropeptide Y. Circ Res 65:1536, 1989.
16. Levy MN, Martin PJ: Neural control of the heart. In RM Berne, N Sperelakis (eds): Handbook of Physiology, The Cardiovascular System, The Heart, Vol. 1, Section 2. Bethesda, MD, Am Physiological Society, 1979, p. 581.
17. Clark RB, Tse A, Giles WR: Electrophysiology of parasympathetic neurones isolated from the interatrial septum of bull-frog heart. J Physiol (Lond) 427:89, 1990.
18. Konopka LM, McKeon TW, Parsons RL: Galanin-induced hyperpolarization and decreased membrane excitability of neurones in mudpuppy cardiac ganglia. J Physiol (Lond) 410:107, 1989.
19. Parsons RL, Konopka LM: Analysis of the Galanin-induced decrease in membrane excitability in mudpuppy parasympathetic neurons. Neuroscience 43:647, 1991.
20. Tse A, Clark RB, Giles WR: Muscarinic modulation of calcium current in neurones from the interatrial septum of bull-frog heart. J Physiol (Lond) 427:127, 1990.

21. Allen TGJ, Burnstock G: Intracellular studies of the electrophysiological properties of cultured intracardiac neurones of the guinea pig. J Physiol (Lond) 388:349, 1987.
22. Allen TGJ, Burnstock G: M1 and M2 muscarinic receptors mediate excitation and inhibition of guinea-pig intracardiac neurones in culture. J Physiol (Lond) 422:463, 1990.
23. Fieber LA, Adams DJ: Acetylcholine-evoked currents in cultured neurones dissociated from rat parasympathetic cardiac ganglia. J Physiol (Lond) 434:215, 1991.
24. Fieber LA, Adams DJ: Adenosine triphosphate-evoked currents in cultured neurones dissociated from rat parasympathetic cardiac ganglia. J Physiol (Lond) 434:239, 1991.
25. Seabrook GR, Fieber LA, Adams SJ: Neurotransmission in neonatal rat cardiac ganglion in situ. Am J Physiol 259:H997, 1990.
26. Xi X, Thomas JX, Randall WC, et al: Intracellular recordings from canine intracardiac ganglion cells. J Auton Nerv Syst 32:177, 1991.
27. Mostafa MH, Xi X, Wurster RD, et al: Light and electron microscopic study of neurons in cardiac ganglia of the rat and dog. Soc for Neurosci 16:860, 1990. Abstract.
28. Wurster RD, Xi X, Thomas JX, et al: Electrical properties of mammalian intracardiac ganglion cells. FASEB J 4:A707, 1990.
29. Cassel JF, Clark AL, McLachlan EM: Characteristics of phasic and tonic sympathetic ganglion cells of the guinea-pig. J Physiol (Lond) 372:457, 1986.
30. Meckler RL, McLachlan EM: Axons of peripheral origin preferentially synapse with tonic neurones in the guinea-pig coeliac ganglion. Neurosci Lett 86:189, 1988.
31. Gagliardi M, Randall WC, Bieger D, et al: Activity of in vivo canine cardiac plexus neurons. Am J Physiol 255:789, 1988.
32. Armour JA, Hopkins DA: Activity of in vivo canine ventricular neurons. Am J Physiol 258:H326, 1990.
33. Armour JA, Hopkins DA: Activity of canine in situ left atrial ganglion neurons. Am J Physiol 259:H1207, 1990.
34. Ardell JL, Butler CK, Smith FM, et al: Activity of in vivo atrial and ventricular neurons in chronically decentralized canine hearts. Am J Physiol 260:H713, 1991.
35. Levy MN, Martin PJ, Hano T, et al: Effects of single vagal stimuli on heart rate and atrioventricular conduction. Am J Physiol 218:1256, 1970.
36. Xi X, Randall WC, Wurster RD: Intracellular recording of spontaneous activity of canine intracardiac ganglion cells. Neurosci Lett 128:129, 1991.
37. Nozdrachev AD, Pogorelov AG: Extracellular recordings of neuronal activity of the cat heart ganglia. J Auton Nerv Syst 6:73, 1982.
38. Rigel DF, Lipson D, Katona PG: Excess tachycardia: Heart rate after antimuscarinic agents in conscious dogs. Am J Physiol 15:H168, 1984.
39. Xi X, Randall WC, Wurster RD: Muscarinic synaptic transmission in canine intracardiac ganglia. Soc for Neurosci 17:1322, 1991. Abstract.
40. Wurster RD, Xi X, Weber M, et al: Morphological organization of ganglion cells and small intensely fluorescent (SIF) cells of the canine intracardiac ganglia. Soc for Neurosci Abst 16:860, 1990.
41. Xi X, Duff MJ, Weber M, et al: In vivo effects of calcitonin gene-related peptide (CGRP) on intracardiac vagal ganglia. FASEB J 3:A413, 1989.
42. Priola DV: Intrinsic innervation of the canine heart. Circ Res 47:74, 1980.
43. Szurszewski JH: Physiology of mammalian prevertebral ganglia. Ann Rev Physiol 43:53, 1981.
44. Wood JD: Physiology of the enteric nervous system. In LR Johnson (ed): Physiology of the Gastrointestinal Tract. New York, NY, Raven Press, 1987, p. 67.

CHAPTER 3

Development of Cardiac Vagal Innervation

A.J. Pappano

Regulation of the heartbeat by the vagus nerve and its transmitter, acetylcholine (ACh), has been recently reviewed.[1-6] A better understanding of the anatomical distribution of the vagus nerve in cardiac tissues, of the effects of selective stimulation of this nerve in discrete cardiac regions, and of the various ionic and metabolic mechanisms that govern the response to vagal stimulation have also emerged. This information has allowed a greater reliability in predicting the consequences of vagus nerve action on the heart of adult vertebrates where it is dominated by negative chronotropic, dromotropic, and inotropic effects.

The development of vagal innervation and the establishment of its mechanisms for regulation of the heartbeat in embryonic vertebrates have also been examined. While the advances in these aspects have lagged behind those made through the study of adult hearts, the pace has quickened. Several articles have appeared in which systematic descriptions of the development of vagal innervation and its regulation of cardiac electrophysiological and contractile properties have been documented in the mammalian heart.[7-9]

This chapter discusses two areas, namely, development of vagal innervation and molecular transformations in the muscarinic receptor (mAChR) transduction process that may be associated with innervation. The embryonic chick heart model is the primary focus of discussion here because it has lent itself to experimental manipulations that have proved very useful in answering some of the questions raised in previous reviews of this subject.[10,11] Additionally, salient features of this topic from a rat heart model are presented in a comparative manner.

Vagal Innervation of the Heart

Morphology

The details of ontogenesis of the vagal innervation of the embryonic chick heart have been summarized.[12] By the end of the third incubation day, vagus

This work was supported by USPHS Grant HL-13339.

nerve elements reach the truncus arteriosus.[13] It cannot be excluded, however, that these neuronal elements represent the sensory portion of the vagus nerve which, in the adult, is found in the nodose ganglion.[14] According to Kuratani and Tanaka,[15] vagal innervation of the embryonic chick heart can be traced to branchial (pharyngeal arches) and intestinal (gut) branches of a ganglionic crest of the vagus-glossopharyngeal complex in the lateral aspect of the hindbrain (stage 21, 3.5 days). Vagal innervation of the truncus arteriosus (stage 25, 4.5 to 5 days) was attributed to the superior cardiac nerve from the branchial division. Innervation of the sinus venosus (primary pacemaker area) appeared at stage 24 (4.5 days) and stemmed from an intestinal division of the vagus that also provided nerves to the posterior ventricular wall. This finding is noteworthy because the onsets of vagal neuroeffector transmission to sinus venosus and ventricle occur within one day of each other (see the section entitled Ontogenesis of Vagal Transmission).

Vagal nerve branches were reported in the sinus venosus of the fetal rat heart on the 15th gestational day and ganglion cells were present in the atrium on the 16th day.[16,17] As in the avian heart, the presence of vagal nerve branches provided no information about their activity. The need to identify the function of the vagus nerve elements during ontogenesis has prompted experiments that utilize specific chemical markers for the presence and function of cholinergic nerves.

Chemical Indices

Nerves and ganglia that stained for cholinesterase activity were found along the pulmonary artery on the 9th incubation day; by the 13th incubation day, such nerves were present on the epicardial surface of the embryonic chick heart.[18] Cholinesterase-positive neurons are not necessarily an indication of the presence of cholinergic nerves. A morphological study of neurogenesis, however, reported the presence of cardiac parasympathetic ganglia with a mature appearance by the 11th incubation day.[19] This observation was taken to indicate that the vagal ganglionic synaptic connections were present at this time.

Choline acetyltransferase (ChAT) activity could not be detected in embryonic chick hearts on the 4th or 10th incubation day.[20,21] ChAT activity was present in atria and ventricles, however, on the 11th incubation day; the ventricles displayed about 35% to 50% of the activity seen in the atria. Atrial ChAT activity increased three fold between the 12th and 15th incubation days and then did not change through the day of hatching.[21] The ontogenetic appearance of ChAT, an essential enzyme for ACh synthesis, serves as an important marker of cholinergic nerves. The authors also measured carnitine acetyltransferase activity that can be mistakenly assumed to represent ChAT; this factor was rigorously excluded in their experiments.[20,21]

ChAT activity was first detected on the 19th gestational day in atria and ventricles of the rat heart.[21] At all ages studied (up to 21 days postnatally), ChAT activity was greater in atrial tissue. Stepwise increments in atrial ChAT activity occurred between the 20th gestational day and the day of birth and again between the 7th and 14th postnatal days. No change in atrial ChAT activity was detected between the 14th and 21st postnatal days in the rat.[21] Similar measurements of specific atrial ChAT activity were reported beginning on the day of birth and continuing through 3 months postnatally.[22] On the day of birth, specific ChAT activity accounted for the synthesis of about 150 nmol $ACh.g^{-1}.h^{-1}$. Assuming that homogenate protein accounts for 10% of tissue wet weight, atrial ChAT activity reported for the day of birth by Marvin et al,[21] given as about 15 pmol ACh mg $protein^{-1}$, would equal 90 nmol $ACh.g^{-1}.h^{-1}$. This finding agrees reasonably well with the data of Slavíková and Tuček.[22] Comparison of ChAT activity at later times yields data that are not in accord quantitatively; the values of Marvin et al are about one third those of Slavíková and Tuček. Among the factors contributing to this discrepancy is the estimated ratio of protein to tissue wet weight. In spite of these uncertainties, the qualitative agreement between the studies is heartening.

The presence of a high-affinity choline uptake mechanism has also been used as a marker of cholinergic nerves in the adult avian heart.[23] As shown in Figure 1, high-affinity choline uptake in the embryonic chick atrium was first detected on the 7th incubation day, increased to a plateau by the 10th to 12th incubation days, and then declined to levels that remained relatively constant from the 17th incubation day through four weeks after hatching.[24] The uptake of choline was attributed to cardiac ganglia that originated from neural crest at somite levels 1 to 3. Extirpation of the neural crest reduced choline uptake substantially (up to 60%), but not completely. Residual high-affinity choline uptake was attributed to preganglionic cholinergic nerve terminals arising from the dorsal motor nucleus (DMN) of the vagus.[24] These elegant experiments provide very strong evidence for the presence of cholinergic nerves in the embryonic heart at about the same time that vagal neuroeffector transmission is first detected (see the section entitled Ontogenesis of Vagal Transmission).

Taken altogether, these chemical indices indicated that the cholinergic nerve phenotype rapidly appears at the beginning of the second week of life in ovo. Systematic measurements of ACh content during development of cardiac vagal innervation have not been reported. In hearts from 15-day chick embryos, ACh content was 4.04 ± 0.38 and 3.06 ± 0.25 nmol/mg protein in atria and ventricles, respectively.[25] There is a substantial amount of ACh in ventricles as compared to atria at this age when vagal neuroeffector transmission can be observed in both tissues (see below). ACh content decreased by 31% (atria) and 39% (ventricles) in hearts from embryos whose neural crests (somites 1-3) had been removed at stage 10 (35 hours). In all lesioned animals, conotruncal malformations occurred that were attributed to loss of ectomesenchymal elements. This finding contrasts with the partial denervation of the vagus caused by removal of the neural crest. The production of cardiac malformations by neural crest ablation has been recently reviewed.[26]

Measurements of ACh content in rat atria have been reported in the postnatal period.[27] In this tissue, atrial ACh content (μg/g tissue) was: 0.93 ± 0.15 (3rd to 4th day), 1.10 ± 0.10 (9th to 10th day), 3.31 ± 0.31 (17th to 18th day), 3.82 ± 0.26 (25th day), 5.75 ± 0.34 (53rd day), and 5.69 ± 0.25 (adult).

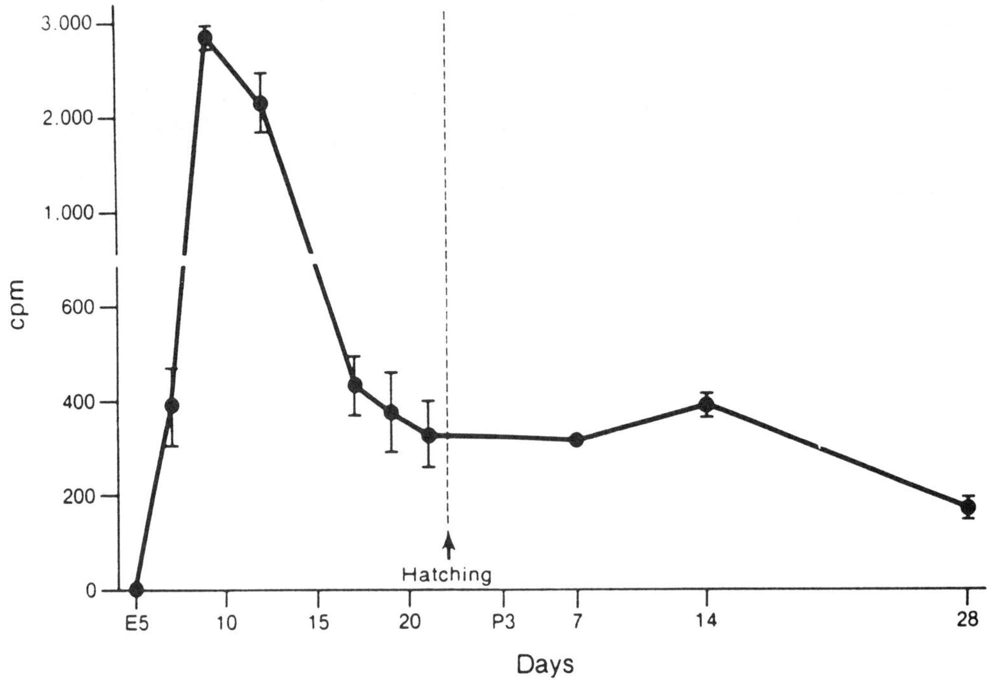

Figure 1. *Activity of high-affinity choline uptake system in developing chick heart. Ordinate: specific activity of neuronal high-affinity uptake (cpm.mg^{-1} tissue relative to incubation medium and Abscissa: age in days (E = embryonic, P = posthatching). Reproduced with permission from Kirby M, Stewart DE: Neural crest origin of cardiac ganglion cells in the chick embryo: Identification and extirpation. Dev Biol 97:433–443, 1983.*

Clearly, there is a strong correlation between the amounts of ACh present in rat atria and the activity of ChAT up to the 25th postnatal day.

Cholinergic Neuroeffector Transmission

Transmission of the signal from postganglionic cholinergic nerves to cardiac tissues requires:

1. synthesis, storage, and release of ACh by the nerve, and
2. postjunctional mAChR connected to cellular effectors by appropriate transducers.

Ontogenesis of Vagal Transmission

Sufficient amounts of ACh are released to inhibit automaticity in the sinoatrial (SA) node and contractions in β-adrenoceptor agonist-stimulated ventricular tissue on the 12th and 13th incubation days, respectively.[28,29] An example of SA node inhibition caused by stimulation of intrinsic cholinergic nerves is shown in Figure 2. Atropine, a mAChR antagonist, prevents the pacemaker inhibition (SA node) and negative inotropic effect (ventricle) caused by field stimulation of intrinsic vagal neurons.

The ontogenetic development of vagal inhibition in the embryonic chick SA node is illustrated in Figure 3. In the presence of physostigmine, which inhibits acetylcholinesterase and thereby prevents ACh hydrolysis, inhibitory transmission could be detected as early as the 10th incubation day.[28] The ACh sensitivity of the SA node increased (ED_{50} decreased from 22 μM to 6 μM) between the 9th and 10th incubation days and did not change (ED_{50} = 4.1 μM) on the 11th incubation day.[30] It was concluded that the onset of vagal transmission to the SA node was delayed until the 12th incubation day by the amount of ACh available for release because postjunctional sensitivity to ACh was the same on the 11th and 12th incubation days. The failure of field stimulation to inhibit the SA node on the 9th incubation day could not be attributed to a lack of impulse conduction because the cervical vagus nerve displayed propagated action potentials at this time.

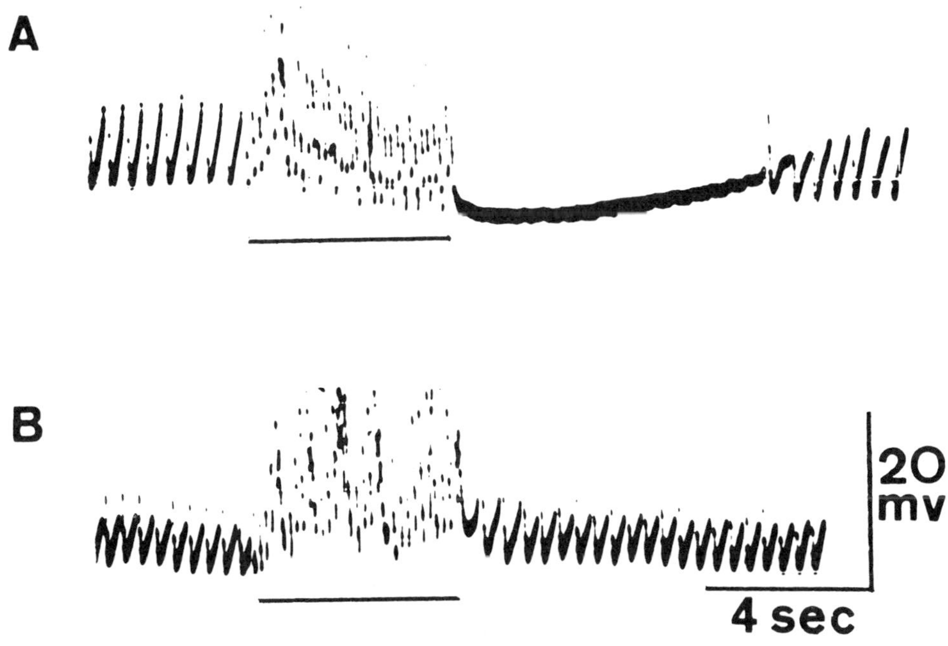

Figure 2. *Suppression of sinoatrial (SA) node pacemaker activity caused by field stimulation in an embryonic chick heart (12th incubation day). A: Lower portion of membrane potential records from one cell shows hyperpolarization and cessation of pacemaker activity caused by 5-s period of field stimulation (30 Hz, 50 V, 0.5 ms) and B: Records from another cell in the same preparation in the presence of atropine (2.8 × 10^{-7}M) that suppressed the inhibition caused by field stimulation. Reproduced with permission from AJ Pappano, K Löffelholz: Ontogenesis of adrenergic and cholinergic neuroeffector transmission in chick embryo heart. J Pharmacol Exp Ther 191:468–478, 1974, © by the American Society for Pharmacology and Experimental Therapeutics.*

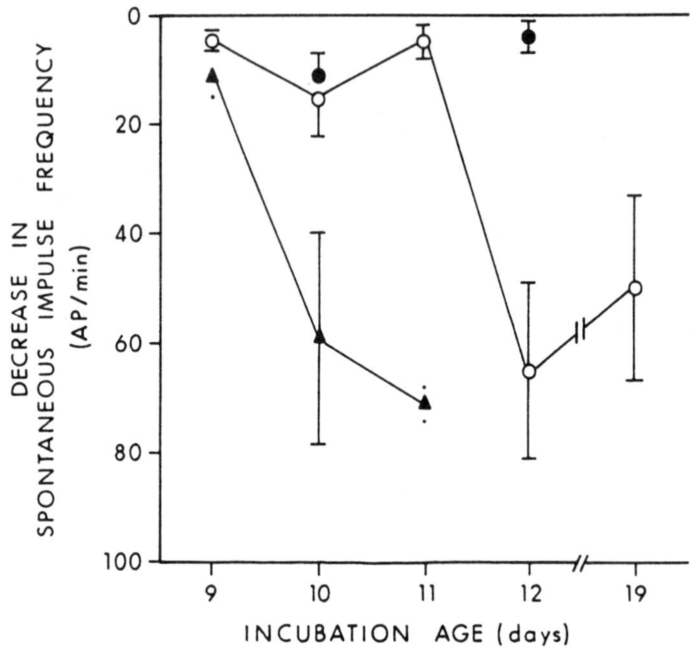

Figure 3. *Onset of cardioinhibitory transmission to the embryonic chick SA node. Ordinate: decrease in spontaneous SA node rate in action potentials (AP)/min and Abscissa: embryonic age in days.* ○, *chronotropic response to field stimulation (30 Hz, 50 V, 0.5 ms) for 5 s in untreated preparations;* ● *in the presence of atropine* (2.8×10^{-7}*M*)*; and* ▲ *in the presence of physostigmine* (3.6×10^{-6}*M*)*. Note: physostigmine allowed detection of pacemaker inhibition caused by intrinsic cardiac nerve stimulation on the 10th incubation day. Reproduced with permission from AJ Pappano, K Löffelholz: Ontogenesis of adrenergic and cholinergic neuroeffector transmission in chick embryo heart. J Pharmacol Exp Ther 191:468–478, 1974, © by the American Society for Pharmacology and Experimental Therapeutics.*

In a series of ablation experiments, removal of neural crest (somites 1 to 3) did not suppress the development of vagal neuroeffector transmission (measured on the 14th and 15th incubation days). This result was attributed to reconstitution of vagal ganglia by neurons arising from the nodose placodes.[31] When the nodose placodes, however, were ablated together with the neural crest, the hearts were parasympathetically aneural and did not display atropine-sensitive responses to field stimulation on the 11th incubation day in contrast to control (sham-operated) embryos. Interestingly, the parasympathetically aneural chick embryos did not survive beyond the 12th incubation day. These experiments underscore the view that vagal transmission to the SA node occurs around the 12th incubation day. Moreover, the data also emphasized that extirpation of neural crest (somites 1 to 3) did not produce parasympathetically aneural hearts because nodose placode cells could reconstitute cardiac ganglia as indicated by reactivity to ChAT antibody[32] and maintenance of near normal ACh concentrations.[25] None of the reports on cholinergic transmission has addressed the problem of ascertaining when the two-neuron efferent vagal system is established.

The ontogenesis of cholinergic neuroeffector transmission has also been studied in the rat heart. In this organ, atropine-sensitive inhibition (30% to 60%) of spontaneous contraction rate occurred on the 21st gestational day (day of birth), but not before this time.[21] A somewhat later onset of vagal transmission to the SA node of the rat heart was reported by Vlk[33] who detected inhibition at the 10th postnatal day. In these experiments, the magnitude of vagally-induced pacemaker inhibition increased up to 24 to 34 days after birth, after which it declined slightly. In spite of the apparent discrepancy between these two reports, it seems reasonable to conclude that the maturation of vagal neuroeffector transmission to the rat SA node occurs between the day of birth and about three weeks postnatally. In contrast to the results in the embryonic chick heart, the sensitivity of the rat SA node was greater at the 12th gestational day ($ED_{50} = 17$ nM) than at the 15th, 18th, and 21st gestational days ($ED_{50} = 100$ nM).[21] Therefore, both the postjunctional ACh sensitivity and transmitter availability limit the onset of cholinergic transmission in the rat heart.

Muscarinic Receptors

In this section, particular attention is given to mAChR properties at the time of cholinergic innervation. The maximum binding (B_{max}) of [^{3}H]-quinuclidinyl benzilate (^{3}H-QNB), a potent mAChR antagonist, to homogenates of embryonic chick atrial membranes averaged approximately 350 pmol/mg protein on the 9th and 12th incubation days.[34] By the 15th incubation day, the B_{max} for ^{3}H-QNB-binding increased by 30% and this was judged to be coincident with the onset of cholinergic neuroeffector transmission. The proportion of mAChR displaying high-agonist affinity for carbachol (CCh) also increased during this three-day interval. Moreover, exposure of hearts to atropine, a mAChR antagonist, prevented the increase in mAChR that occurred between the 12th and 15th incubation days. Summarily, these observations were taken to indicate that the onset of cholinergic neuroeffector transmission was a critical period during which mAChR properties changed. Parenthetically, it is surprising that the number of mAChR did not increase as a result of treatment with atropine because the receptors generally up-regulate when they are treated chronically with antagonist. Perhaps receptor regulation by antagonist treatment does not adhere to this pattern when neuroeffector transmission is first established.

The B_{max} for ^{3}H-QNB-binding to a plasma membrane-enriched fraction from embryonic chick ventricles displayed two increases during development in ovo.[29] The first increase (1.6-fold) occurred between the 11th and 13th incubation days. As shown in Figure 4, vagal transmission to the ventricle was first detected on the 13th incubation day; it was registered as atropine-sensitive inhibition by field stimulation of the positive inotropic effect of β-adrenoceptor agonist. As such, this finding is an expression of the

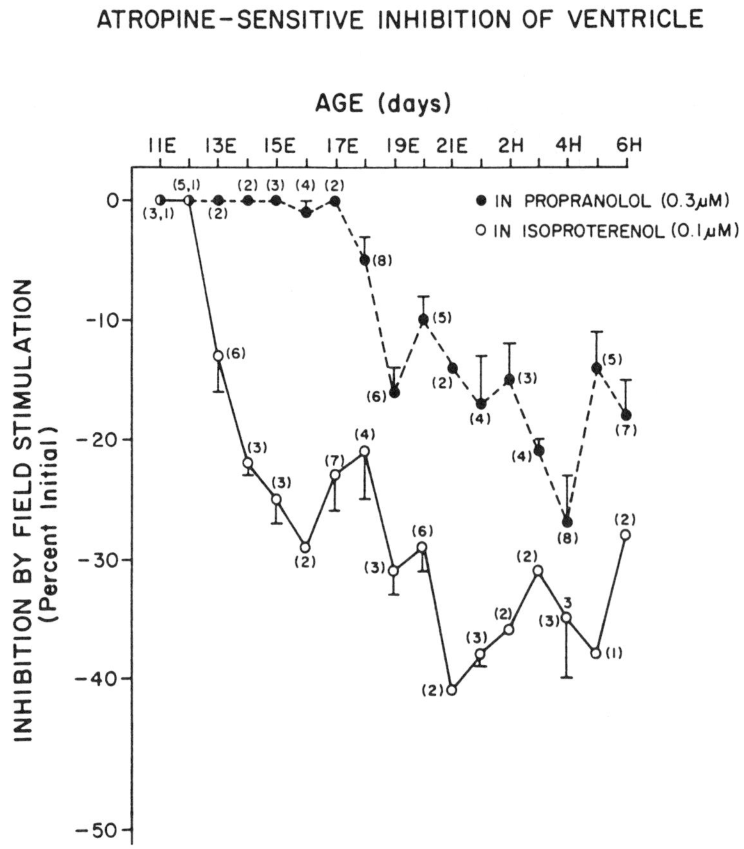

Figure 4. *Vagal inhibition of ventricular contractions in chick ventricle during ontogenesis. Ordinate: percent inhibition of contraction force caused by field stimulation (6 Hz, 50 V, 5 ms) for 5 s in paced (3 Hz) ventricular strips and Abscissa: age in days (E = embryonic; H = hatched). In the presence of isoproterenol (○), field stimulation inhibited ventricular contractions as early as the 13th incubation day. This "accentuated antagonism" of field stimulation was blocked by atropine (3 × 10^{-7}M). In the presence of the β-adrenoceptor antagonist propranolol (●), field stimulation first inhibited contractions on the 18th incubation day. These results indicate that the vagus nerve directly inhibits ventricular contractions in the avian heart. Reprinted by permission of the publisher from Sullivan JK, Sorota S, Zotter C, et al: Is muscarinic receptor number in avian ventricle regulated by vagal innervation. In VJ Ferrans, G Rosenquist, C Weinstein (eds): Cardiac Morphogenesis, New York, NY, Elsevier Science Publishing Co. Copyright 1985 by Elsevier Science Publishing Co., Inc.*

phenomenon of "accentuated antagonism"[35] because there was no effect of field stimulation on contraction force in the absence of β-adrenoceptor agonist. While the increased number of mAChR at this time may be induced on ventricular myocytes by the vagus nerve, one cannot exclude the possibility that the increased mAChR density arises from receptors on vagal nerve terminals.

A second increase in B_{max} of mAChR occurred between the 19th and 21st (day of hatching) incubation days.[29] This observation confirmed those findings made by others[36] and it is suggested that the change arose from an increased density of mAChR per myocyte because cellular hyperplasia has ceased by this time and hypertrophy is evident. It is considered unlikely that the increased B_{max} of mAChR arose from the presence of these receptors on adrenergic nerve terminals because treatment with 6-hydroxydopamine, which removed adrenergic nerve terminals, did not reduce but rather increased B_{max} of mAChR. This observation confirmed those findings made by Renaud et al[37] in the same laboratory. As noted elsewhere,[29] the increased density of mAChR between the 19th and 21st incubation days coincided with the onset of "direct" inhibition of ventricular contractions by the vagus nerve (Fig. 4). At this time, ACh inhibits adenylyl cyclase and Ca^{2+}-dependent action potentials in the presence of β-adrenoceptor antagonist.[38] No more than a coincidental relationship, however, can be inferred for these phenomena.

Development of mAChR in the embryonic rat heart has also been examined in relation to the onset of vagal transmission to atria. The B_{max} of atrial mAChR, as indicated by specific ^{3}H-QNB-binding, increased from approximately 300 pmol/g protein on the 15th gestational day to >600 pmol/g protein on the 19th gestational day.[39] Whereas no change of B_{max} was detected between days 19 and 21, B_{max} declined gradually after birth and, in the adult, was approximately 350 pmol/g protein. The abrupt increase of mAChR between the 15th and 19th gestational days was viewed as related to the onset of innervation reported by others.[21,33] It was also suggested that the onset of vagal transmission to rat atria was effected, at least in part, by the increased density of atrial mAChR.[39]

A tonic inhibition of the heart rate in the rat was reported to occur on the 18th postnatal day.[22] At this age, injection of atropine was associated with a significant (>30.min^{-}1) increase in heart rate. If correct, this would indicate that tonic vagal regulation of the SA node is not evident until 2.5 weeks after vagal neuroeffector transmission. In other words, the final element required to exert tonic vagal regulation of the rat heart is the establishment of central nervous system connections.

Cellular Effectors

The relationship among mAChR, G-proteins, ion channels, and second messengers during ontogenesis has been reviewed.[40] At present, there are no reports concerning the occurrence of changes in any of these muscarinic-regulated processes at the onset of vagal neuroeffector transmission. Suffice it to state that mAChR, G-proteins, ion channels, and second messenger systems are already present and capable of activation *before* the onset of vagal neuroeffector transmission.[40–42]

References

1. Löffelholz K, Pappano AJ: The parasympathetic neuroeffector junction of the heart. Pharmacol Rev 37:1, 1985.

2. Hartzell HC: Regulation of cardiac ion channels by catecholamines, acetylcholine and second messenger systems. Prog Biophys Mol Biol 52:165, 1988.
3. Pappano A: Parasympathetic control of cardiac electrical activity. In DP Zipes, J Jalife (eds): Cardiac Electrophysiology: From Cell to Bedside. Philadelphia, PA, WB Saunders Co, 1990, p. 271.
4. Randall WC, Ardell JL: Nervous control of the heart: Anatomy and pathophysiology. In DP Zipes, J Jalife (eds): Cardiac Electrophysiology: From Cell to Bedside. Philadelphia, PA, WB Saunders Co, 1990, p. 291.
5. Levy M, Warner MR: Autonomic interactions in cardiac control: Role of neuropeptides. In DP Zipes, J Jalife (eds): Cardiac Electrophysiology: From Cell to Bedside. Philadelphia, PA, WB Saunders Co, 1990, p. 305.
6. Sorota S, Pappano AJ: Muscarinic receptor-effector coupling in the heart. In MR Rosen, MJ Janse, AL Wit (eds): Cardiac Electrophysiology: A Textbook. Mount Kisco, NY, Futura Publishing Co, 1990, p. 803.
7. Gootman PM: Neural regulation of cardiovascular function in the perinatal period. In N Gootman, PM Gootman (eds): Perinatal Cardiovascular Function. New York, NY, Marcel Dekker, Inc, 1983, p. 265.
8. Gootman PM: Developmental Neurobiology of the Autonomic Nervous System. Clifton, NJ, Humana Press, 1986.
9. Roskoski R Jr: Cholinergic muscarinic receptor characterization and regulation in tissues innervated by the autonomic nervous system. Rev in Clin Basic Pharmacol 6:1, 1987.
10. Pappano AJ: Ontogenetic development of autonomic neuroeffector transmission and transmitter reactivity in embryonic and fetal hearts. Pharmacol Rev 29:3, 1977.
11. Higgins D: The ontogeny of the response of the avian embryo heart to autonomic neurotransmitters and to neurotransmitter-like drugs. Pharmac Ther 20:53, 1983.
12. Romanoff AL: The Avian Embryo: Structural and Functional Development. New York, NY, The MacMillan Co, 1960.
13. Szepsenwol J, Bron A: L'origine et la nature de l'innervation primitive du coeur chez les embryons d'Oiseaux, (Canard et Poulet). Rev Suisse Zool 43:1, 1936.
14. Walkey GK, Bower AJ: The distal vagal ganglion of the hen (Gallus domesticus). A histological and physiological study. J Anat 132:95, 1981.
15. Kuratani S, Tanaka S: Peripheral development of the avian vagus nerve with special reference to the morphological innervation of heart and lung. Anat Embryol 182:435, 1990.
16. Hall EK: Intrinsic contractility in the embryonic rat heart. Anat Rec 111:381, 1951.
17. Gomez H: The development of the innervation of the heart in the rat embryo. Anat Rec 130:53, 1958.
18. Rickenbacher J, Müller E: The development of cholinergic ganglia in the chick embryo heart. Anat Embryol 155:253, 1979.
19. Kirby ML, Weidman TA, McKenzie JW: An ultrastructural study of the cardiac ganglia in the bulbar plexus of the developing chick heart. Dev Neurosci 3:174, 1980.
20. Roskoski R Jr, McDonald RI, Roskoski LM, et al: Choline acetyltransferase activity in heart: Evidence for neuronal and not myocardial origin. Am J Physiol 233:H642, 1977.
21. Marvin WJ Jr, Hermsmeyer K, McDonald RI, et al: Ontogenesis of cholinergic innervation in the rat heart. Circ Res 46:690, 1980.
22. Slavíková J, Tuček S: Postnatal changes of the tonic influence of the vagus nerve on the heart rate, and of the activity of choline acetyltransferase in the heart atria of rats. Physiol Bohemoslov 31:113, 1982.
23. Lindmar R, Löffelholz K, Weide W, et al: Neuronal uptake of choline following release of acetylcholine in the perfused heart. J Pharmacol Exp Ther 215:710, 1980.
24. Kirby M, Stewart DE: Neural crest origin of cardiac ganglion cells in the chick embryo: Identification and extirpation. Dev Biol 97:433, 1983.
25. Kirby ML, Aronstam RS, Buccafusco JJ: Changes in cholinergic parameters

associated with failure of conotruncal septation in embryonic chick hearts after neural crest ablation. Circ Res 56:392, 1985.

26. Kirby ML: Alteration of cardiogenesis after neural crest ablation. Ann NY Acad Sci 588:289, 1990.
27. Kuntscherová J, Vlk J: Postnatal changes in the amount of acetylcholine in the atrial tissue of the albino rat heart. Physiol Bohemoslov 28:569, 1979.
28. Pappano AJ, Löffelholz K: Ontogenesis of adrenergic and cholinergic neuroeffector transmission in chick embryo heart. J Pharmacol Exp Ther 191:468, 1974.
29. Sullivan JK, Sorota S, Zotter C, et al: Is muscarinic receptor number in avian ventricle regulated by vagal innervation? In VJ Ferrans, G Rosenquist, C Weinstein (eds): Cardiac Morphogenesis. New York, NY, Elsevier Science Publishing Co, Inc, 1985, p. 253.
30. Löffelholz K, Pappano AJ: Increased sensitivity of sinoatrial pacemaker to acetylcholine and to catecholamines at the onset of autonomic neuroeffector transmission in chick embryo heart. J Pharmacol Exp Ther 191:479, 1974.
31. Kirby ML, Creazzo TL, Christiansen JL: Chronotropic responses of chick atria to field stimulation after various neural crest ablations. Circ Res 65:1547, 1989.
32. Kirby ML: Nodose placode contributes autonomic neurons to the heart in the absence of cardiac neural crest. J Neurosci 8:1089, 1988.
33. Vlk J: Postnatal development of postganglionic parasympathetic neurones in the heart of the albino rat. Physiol Bohemoslov 28:561, 1979.
34. Kirby ML, Aronstam RS: Atropine-induced alterations of normal development of muscarinic receptors in the embryonic chick heart. J Mol Cell Cardiol 15:685, 1983.
35. Levy M: Cardiac sympathetic-parasympathetic interactions. Fed Proc 43:2598, 1984.
36. Hosey MM, Fields JZ: Quantitative and qualitative differences in muscarinic cholinergic receptors in embryonic and newborn chick hearts. J Biol Chem 256:6395, 1981.
37. Renaud J-F, Kazazoglou T, Schmid A, et al: Differentiation of receptor sites for [^{3}H] nitrendipine in chick hearts and physiological relation to the slow Ca^{2+} channel and to excitation-contraction coupling. Eur J Biochem 139:673, 1984.
38. Pappano AJ, Biegon RL: Mechanisms for muscarinic inhibition of calcium-dependent action potentials and contractions in developing ventricular muscle: The role of cyclic AMP. In AP Paes de Carvalho, BF Hoffman, M Lieberman (eds): Normal and Abnormal Conduction of the Heartbeat. Mount Kisco, NY, Futura Publishing Co, 1982, p. 327.
39. Nedoma J, Slavíková J, Tuček S: Muscarinic acetylcholine receptors in the heart of rats before and after birth. Pflügers Arch 406:45, 1986.
40. Pappano AJ: Development of postjunctional cardiac autonomic receptors and their regulation of cardiac function during fetal and neonatal life. In N Sperelakis (ed): Physiology and Pathophysiology of the Heart. 2nd ed. Boston, Kluwer Academic Publishers, 1989, p. 381.
41. Barnett J, Shamah SM, Galper JB: The development of physiologic responsiveness to muscarinic stimulation in embryonic chick heart. Ann NY Acad Sci 588:145, 1990.
42. Nathanson NM: Regulation of muscarinic receptor and G-protein expression during cardiac development. Ann NY Acad Sci 588:185, 1990.

CHAPTER 4

Vagal Preganglionic Neurons Supplying the Heart

K.M. Spyer, P.A. Brooks, P.N. Izzo

Heart rate is determined largely by the level of activity of the vagal innervation of the atrial nodal tissue which provides for a beat-by-beat adjustment of rate. This control is dependent on inputs, both excitatory and inhibitory, to the preganglionic cardiac vagal motoneurons (CVMs) that arise from peripheral receptors, among which the arterial baroreceptors are probably the most important.[1] In addition, arterial chemoreceptors, some cardiac receptors, and pulmonary and airway receptors contribute to the reflex regulation of the heart. These inputs are supplemented by central nervous inputs that promote adjustment of heart rate, and hence cardiac output, to support behavioral activities. The effectiveness of these inputs is often modulated by respiratory activity, presumably as a homeostatic mechanism, to maintain a balance between cardiac output and respiratory minute volume. This chapter provides a contemporary review of the localization and morphology of the CVMs within the lower brain stem of the mammal and describes their physiological properties.

CVMs are nearly unique among preganglionic neurons destined to influence the cardiovascular system in that their role can be specified with some certainty; sympathetic preganglionic neurons that innervate the adrenal medulla form the only comparable group. Whether the same neuron acting via postganglionic parasympathetic neurons can also affect inotropic state remains to be resolved. Accordingly, it is somewhat surprising that, at present, considerable uncertainties remain regarding the specific biophysical, pharmacological, and physiological properties of CVMs. Indeed, even their localization within the medulla oblongata was only resolved within the last two decades. Notwithstanding these deficiencies this chapter provides a foundation on which to base a rational hypothesis of the role of the central nervous system (CNS) in cardiovascular control, with CVMs being used as the model.

These studies were supported by Programme Grants from the British Heart Foundation and Medical Research Council. Professor Spyer was in receipt of a Wolfson University Award.
From *Vagal Control of the Heart: Experimental Basis and Clinical Implications* edited by MN Levy, PJ Schwartz © 1994, Futura Publishing Co. Inc., Armonk, NY.

The Localization and Morphology of Cardiac Vagal Motoneurons

CVMs are distributed between two nuclei in the medulla oblongata: the dorsal vagal motonucleus (DVN) and the nucleus ambiguus (NA).[2] This conclusion arose from studies of the neuronal degeneration following vagal nerve section. The evidence suggested that CVMs were located with the DVN[3,4] although earlier evidence had implicated the NA as supplying the innervation of the heart.[5–7] A series of electrophysiological experiments finally demonstrated that, in the cat[8] and other mammalian species, CVMs were primarily distributed within the NA (Fig. 1), although in some species there was a restricted distribution extending dorsomedially from the NA to the DVN.[9] Subsequent detailed anatomical studies using neuronal tracing techniques have confirmed this description and have illustrated the morphology and some of the inputs received by CVMs (see below).

Using the retrograde transport of horseradish peroxidase (HRP), a plethora of studies have reexamined the organization and central representation of CVMs.[2] These investigations have now established both the efferent and afferent vagal innervation of the viscera, and have shown that the DVN is the major source of the vagal efferent fibers supplying the subdiaphragmatic structures,[10] whereas the innervation of thoracic structures (particularly the striated muscles of the soft palate, the pharynx, esophagus, and larynx) arises from the NA. The initial studies with HRP suggested that the vagal innervation of the heart arose from the DVN and nucleus tractus solitarii (NTS),[11] but the majority of recent papers described them to be located in the NA, the DVN, and an area in between these two nuclei.[12–14] The major representation in all species remains the NA, where CVMs appear to be located in the more ventral regions of this dispersed nucleus and not within its compact nuclear component.[15] More recent studies, using the more sensitive retrograde transport of cholera toxin injected directly into the myocardium of the right atrium, have supported this contention (see Fig. 2).[2]

One notable feature of CVMs in all species is the great variation in perikaryal dimension. The largest neurons are found in the principal column of the NA and the smallest neurons are in the ventral region of the NA.[15] Although these differences are so apparent, and may reflect the type of muscle that they innervate, ultrastructural examination of the CVMs reveals no differences in morphology. All CVMs have unindented nuclei cytoplasms rich in organelles (Fig. 2), and are similar morphologically to other motoneurons.[16–18] The synaptic organization of inputs to vagal preganglionic neurons has received attention in studies with both the monkey and cat.[17,18] These studies show that CVMs retrogradely labelled with HRP have marked synaptic inputs, the density of which is directly related to the size of their perikarya. The relationship between function and distribution of input on the soma and dendrites remains to be resolved, as does both the chemistry and origin of synaptic inputs.

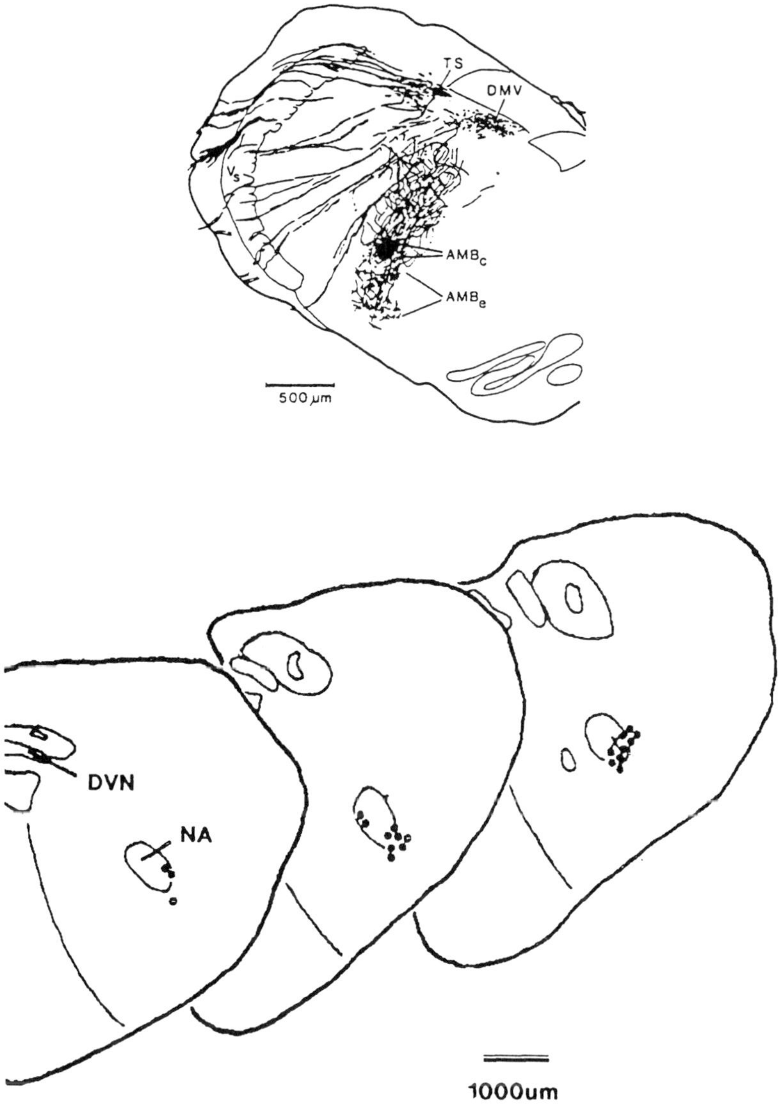

Figure 1. *Upper: Transverse section of rat medulla oblongata, showing retrograde cell body labelling of vagal motor neurons after injection of horseradish peroxidase (HRP) into the cervical vagus nerve. Vagal motor neurons lie in the dorsal vagal nucleus (DMV) as well as within two portions of the nucleus ambiguus (the compact part 0 AMB_e). TS: tractus solitarius; V_s: spinal trigeminal tract. Lower: The position of 21 CVMs (●) are shown on three standard sections of the medulla taken at obex level and 1 and 2 mm rostral to the obex. DVN: dorsal motor nucleus of the vagus; NA: nucleus ambiguus. Reproduced from Bieger D, Hopkins DA: Viscerotopic representation of the upper alimentary tract in the medulla oblongata in the rat; the nucleus ambiguus. J Comp Neurol 262:546, 1987. Copyright © 1987 Wiley-Liss. Reprinted by permission of Wiley-Liss, a division of John Wiley and Sons, Inc.*

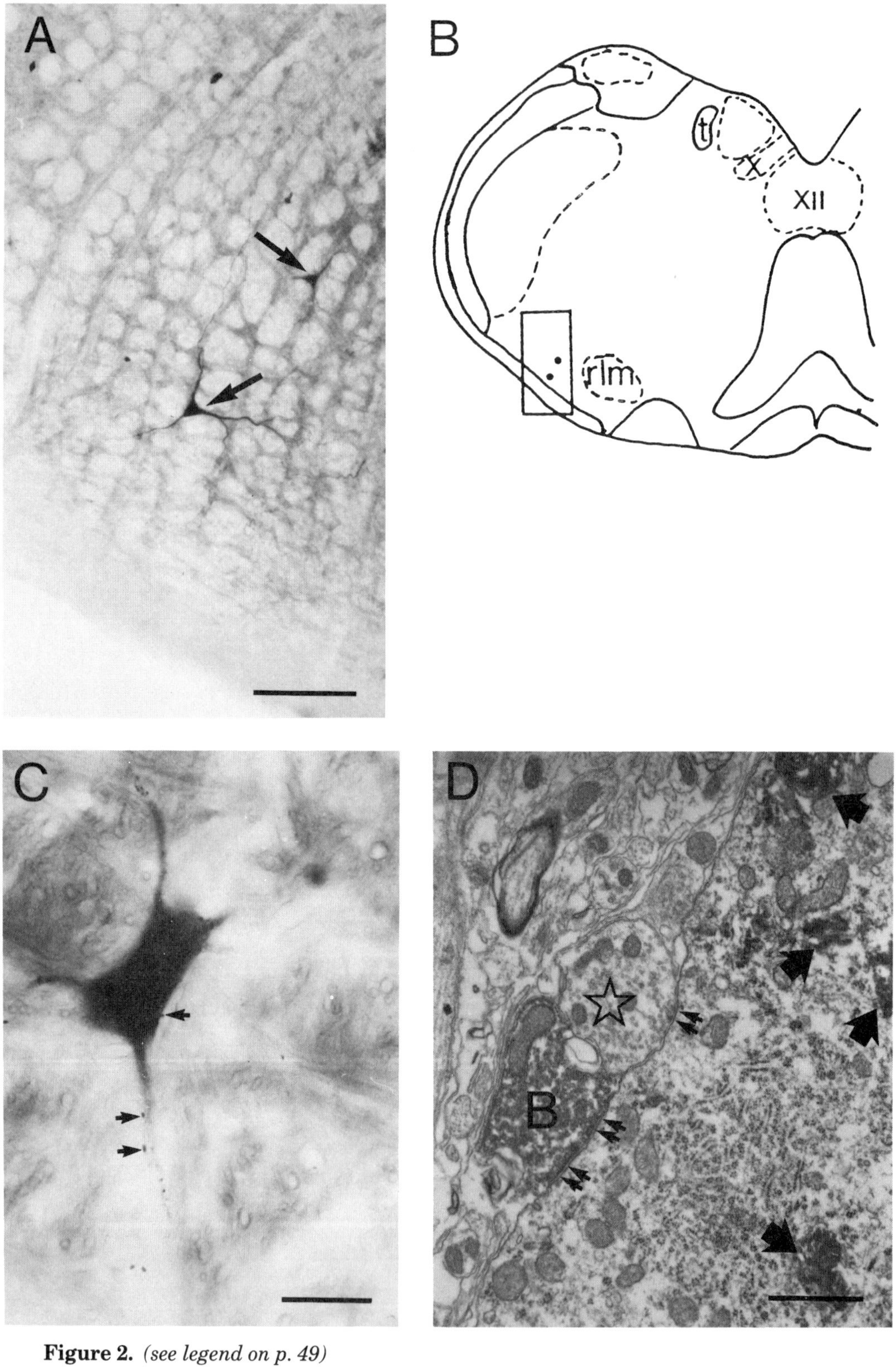

Figure 2. *(see legend on p. 49)*

Afferent Inputs to Cardiac Vagal Motoneurons

As yet, relatively little is known of the specific afferent inputs to CVMs, while considerable data exist from anatomical tracing studies regarding the innervation of both the DVN and NA, in general.[2] These data are only secure with regard to CVMs located in the DVN as a consequence of its relatively homogeneous arrangement. For the NA, considerable uncertainty exists concerning the afferent input to the CVMs located within it because this region receives a heterogeneous mixture of fibers that are widely distributed throughout the ventrolateral medulla. Both the DVN and NA receive input from the NTS, the primary site of termination of afferent inputs that provide the major reflex regulation of the cardiovascular and respiratory systems (see Fig. 2).[2] There are widespread connections from the medullary reticular formation to the two nuclei, and evidence suggests that the medullary raphe nuclei also provide significant inputs to them. The pontine parabrachial nucleus also sends fibers to both the DVN and NA, and the latter also receives a significant input from the neighboring Kölliker-Fuse nucleus. The mesencephalic central gray has descending connections to both DVN and NA, which may be an important relay for subcortical and forebrain inputs to the lower brain stem. There are, however, indications of hypothalamic, amygdaloid, and insular cortical pathways impinging on both vagal nuclei. The details of these connections have been reviewed elsewhere (Fig. 3).[2] In general, it appears that any region of the CNS that exerts an influence on the cardiovascular system has direct, or indirect, connections with these vagal neurons.

While these data are indicative of connections that may be important in the control of CVM activity, it is essential to recall that the evidence does not relate specifically to CVMs. Indications have been obtained, however, (using the anterograde transport of biocytin following ionophoretic application to restricted regions of the NTS), of fibers that innervate previously retrogradely labelled vagal motoneurons in the NA of the cat (Fig. 2).[19] These data establish the existence of monosynaptic connections between the NTS and CVMs and has been further illustrated in studies employing the transynaptic retrograde transport of pseudorabies virus after injections into the myocardium of the rat. CVMs are labelled in the NA after 24 hours following the injection and, subsequently, neurons in the dorsomedial NTS, the raphe obscurus and

Figure 2. *A: Low-power light micrograph showing retrogradely labelled neurons (arrows) in the ventrolateral medulla following the injection of cholera toxin-horseradish peroxidase into the myocardium of the rat. Scale bar = 200 μm. B: Drawing illustrating the position of the neurons shown in A (●). C: High-power light micrograph of a retrogradely labelled vagal preganglionic motoneuron in the ventral NA of the cat. In this material, axons are also present (arrows) that have been labelled following the injection of an anterograde tracer (biocytin) into an area of the NTS electrophysiologically identified as receiving afferents from the carotid sinus nerve. Scale bar = 25 μm. D: Electron micrograph showing a biocytin labelled NTS afferent bouton (B) synapsing (small arrows) to the soma of the retrogradely labelled vagal motoneuron illustrated in C, identified by the granular reaction product in the cytoplasm (large arrows). The soma of this cell is also contacted by an unlabelled bouton (star). Scale bar = 0.5 μm.*

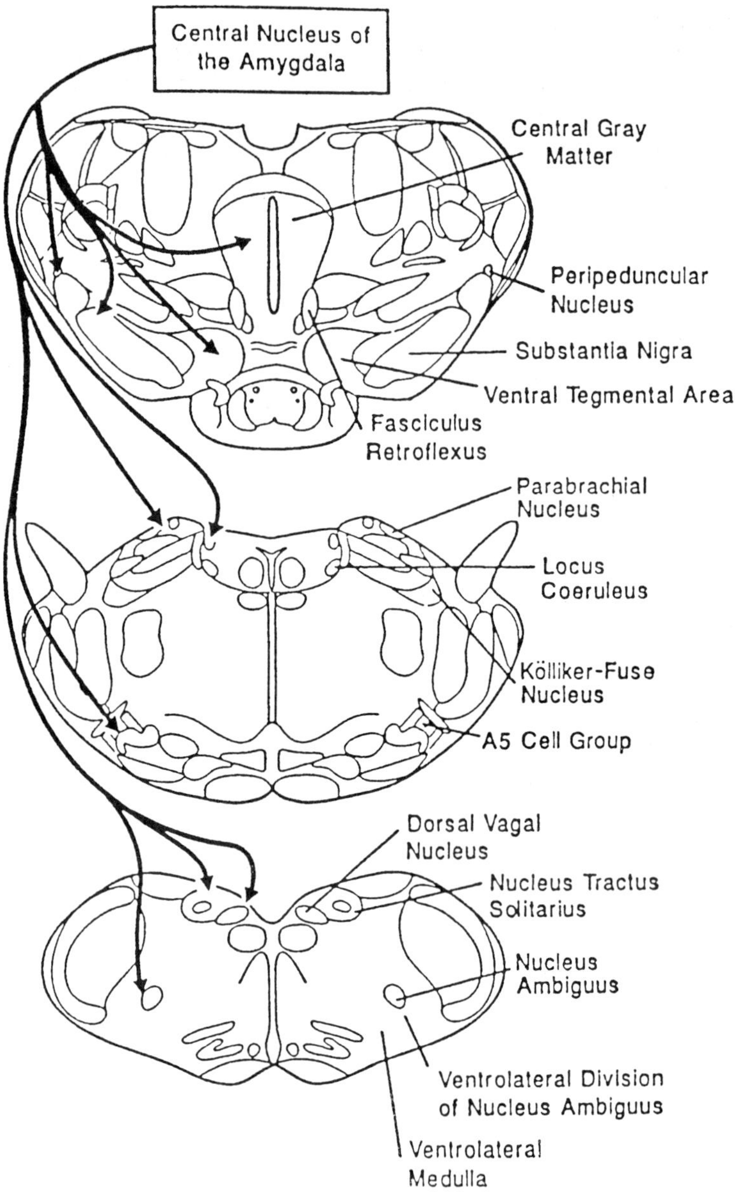

Figure 3. *Series of drawings showing the descending projections from the central nucleus of the amygdala that innervate the brain stem. Reproduced with permission from AD Loewey: Central autonomic pathways. In AD Loewy, KM Spyer (eds): Central Regulation of Autonomic Functions. New York, NY, Oxford University Press, 1990, p. 88.*

magnus are shown to contain the virus. These findings confirm some of the suggestions derived from earlier studies of significant afferent inputs arising from these medullary structures (although transport over sympathetic pathways was not eliminated in this study).[14]

Reflex Inputs to Cardiac Vagal Motoneurons

A considerable body of evidence demonstrates that vagal efferent fibers in the cardiac branches of the vagus[20] or dissected from the cervical vagus[21–30] have pulse-related rhythm of discharge, which indicates that they are powerfully excited by baroreceptor inputs. They are also excited by arterial chemoreceptor, trigeminal, superior laryngeal, and unmyelinated vagal cardiac afferent inputs, but appear unaffected by stimulation of myelinated atrial afferents.[31] Lung inflation inputs silence these efferents and, in addition, the efferents tend to fire in expiration.[20,27–30,32] These observations are supplemented by considerable additional information from investigations on the reflex effects of these various inputs on heart rate. Such effects have been shown to be mediated via the vagus. In particular, Daly and his colleagues,[33,34] in a long series of studies, have shown the facilitatory interactions between these various inputs in evoking vagal bradycardias and the particularly potent effects of ventilatory inputs—central respiratory rhythm and lung inflation inputs—on the efficacy of receptor activation to evoke heart rate responses. If inspiration is arrested by either laryngeal or trigeminal inputs, vagally-mediated responses are potentiated, while lung inflation exerts differential, but largely inhibitory, actions on these inputs. A single inflation of the lungs in the anesthetized cat diminishes the arterial chemoreceptor-induced bradycardia to 7% of control and reduces the arterial baroreflex to 66% of control, the carotid baroreceptor reflex to 66% of control, and cardiac receptor-evoked responses to 70% of control. Conversely, the bradycardia elicited by injecting phenylbiguanide into the right atrium, which activates pulmonary C-fibers including J-receptors, is unaffected by lung inflation. The differential pattern of response is retained after upper thoracic sympathectomy, which limits the efferent pathway for these cardioinhibitory responses to the cardiac vagal efferents (see Fig. 4).

With the exception of the response to pulmonary C-fiber activation, these observations are indicative of CVMs that form a homogenous group of neurons with inputs of varying strength. The vagal bradycardia resulting from pulmonary C-fiber activation does not show a respiratory modulation. One explanation offered for this occurrence is that this input affects a discrete subgroup of the vagal efferent population; this subgroup is distinctive in terms of its pattern of afferent input. Such possibilities can only be assessed with studies on CNS cells, where otherwise subliminal events can be investigated using electrophysiological and pharmacological approaches.

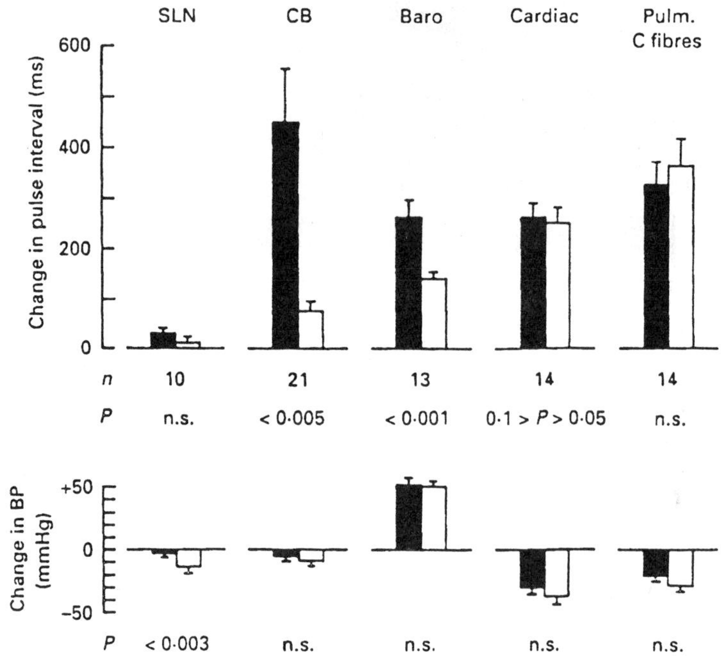

Figure 4. *The effects of inflation of the lungs on the cardioinhibitory responses elicited by electrical stimulation of the superior laryngeal nerves (SLN), and stimulation of the carotid body chemoreceptors (CB; intracarotid sodium cyanide 6.6 ± 0.4 μg Kg^{-1}), of the arterial baroreflex (Baro; increase in blood pressure, 51.0 ± 4.4 mmHg) and of the cardiac receptors (Cardiac; left atrial veratridine, 3.3 ± 0.3 μg Kg^{-1}) and pulmonary C fibres (Pulm. C fibres; right atrial phenylbiguanide, 15.1 ± 0.9 μg Kg^{-1}). All tests carried out during electrical stimulation of the SLNs to inhibit central inspiratory neuronal activity. Filled histograms, excitation of cardioinhibitory responses, the lungs being held at their expiratory volume; open histograms, excitation of cardioinhibitory responses with superimposition of inflation of the lungs. Statistical values refer to comparisons of paired data in filled and open histograms. Reproduced with permission from Daly M de B, Kirkman E: Differential modulation by pulmonary stretch afferents of some reflex cardioinhibitory responses in the cat. J Physiol 417:323, 1989.*

Vagal Motoneurons: Biophysical and Pharmacological Properties

The firing pattern of CVMs, as with all neurons, is dependent on the interplay between ligand- (or neurotransmitter-) activated membrane conductances and intrinsic membrane properties. These factors cannot be analyzed with any precision in vivo, but are resolvable using in vitro preparations of the medulla. In this regard, such data now exist for DVN neurons, but are not available for CVMs specifically. DVN neurons in the guinea pig and rat have similar properties.[35–40] The action potentials resemble those of spinal motoneurons, with the added prominence of an afterdepolarization on the falling phase. This result is enhanced by a calcium current, and these neurons can also generate calcium action potentials when sodium spikes are abolished in the presence of tetrodotoxin (TTX). They are also characterized by a large and prolonged late afterhyperpolarization, partly a consequence of a calcium-dependent K^+-current (I_{AHP}), but supplemented by the transient, slowly inactivating K^+-current I_A that shows repolarization after a period of hyperpolarization.[35,41] These currents persist for long periods, often in excess of 2000 milliseconds and provide a powerful control of vagal neuronal excitability (see Fig. 5). Unlike some NTS neurons, DVN neurons in the rat do not exhibit a marked low threshold and transient calcium current. In the NTS, this current is responsible for a rebound depolarization, which can initiate a burst of action potentials superimposed on a slowly rising membrane potential after a period of hyperpolarization.

In the slice preparation, DVN neurons often exhibit ongoing action potential discharge independent of synaptic activity, and there are indications of "pacemaker" activity.[42] They can be excited by stimulation in either the vicinity of the DVN, within the NTS, or in the tractus solitarius (TS). A recent study, using whole-cell recordings of DVN neurons (Fig. 5) showed in voltage clamp situations the presence of both excitatory postsynaptic potentials (EPSPs) and inhibitory postsynaptic potentials (IPSPs) on perivagal and vagus stimulation as well as ongoing spontaneous EPSPs.[42] These currents were dissected pharmacologically and it was found that the EPSPs are the result of the release of glutamate. This transmitter acts on both N-methyl D-aspartate (NMDA) and non-NMDA receptors (evoked EPSPs). Spontaneous EPSPs are all non-NMDA mediated, while the IPSPs result from the release of γ-aminobutyric acid (GABA), which acts at picrotoxin-sensitive receptors whose effects are mediated by Cl^-. The evoked EPSPs are "gated" with regard to their arrival after an ongoing spike, as would be expected from the above observations. This result correlates well with the in vivo data reviewed for vagal efferent fibers that supply the heart. These fibers have a low discharge rate, both at rest and even when reflexly activated.

Much less is known of the pharmacological properties of these neurons. Acetylcholine, when injected intracellularly, blocks both voltage and calcium-dependent potassium currents in vagal neurons.[36] Further, exogenously applied acetylcholine elicits a nicotine-sensitive depolarization.[43] The actions of noradrenaline on vagal neurons have also been examined in the rat.[38] α_1-mediated depolarizations are observed in 55% of neurons, while in 32% of the cases, hyperpolarization is seen. Interestingly, the α_2 antagonist yohimbine blocks the evoked vagal inhibition that is produced by stimulation within the commissural NTS, and evoked depolarizations are sensitive to prazosin, the α_1 antagonist. The A2 group of brain stem noradrenergic neurons are localized within an area of the medulla that includes the NTS, which suggests that this subset of catecholamine-containing neurons plays a role in vagal control. Whether this occurrence extends to CVMs remains to be resolved.

DVN neurons respond to various neuropeptides when they are applied to the slice preparation. Cholecystokinin excites[39] rat vagal neurons and somatostatin inhibits[40] these neurons. The evoked inhibition is the consequence of an increased K^+ conductance, which results in membrane hyperpolarization. In addition, actions of serotonin,[44] thyrotropin-releasing hormone,[45] oxytocin,[46] and substance P[47] have been observed on DVN neurons.

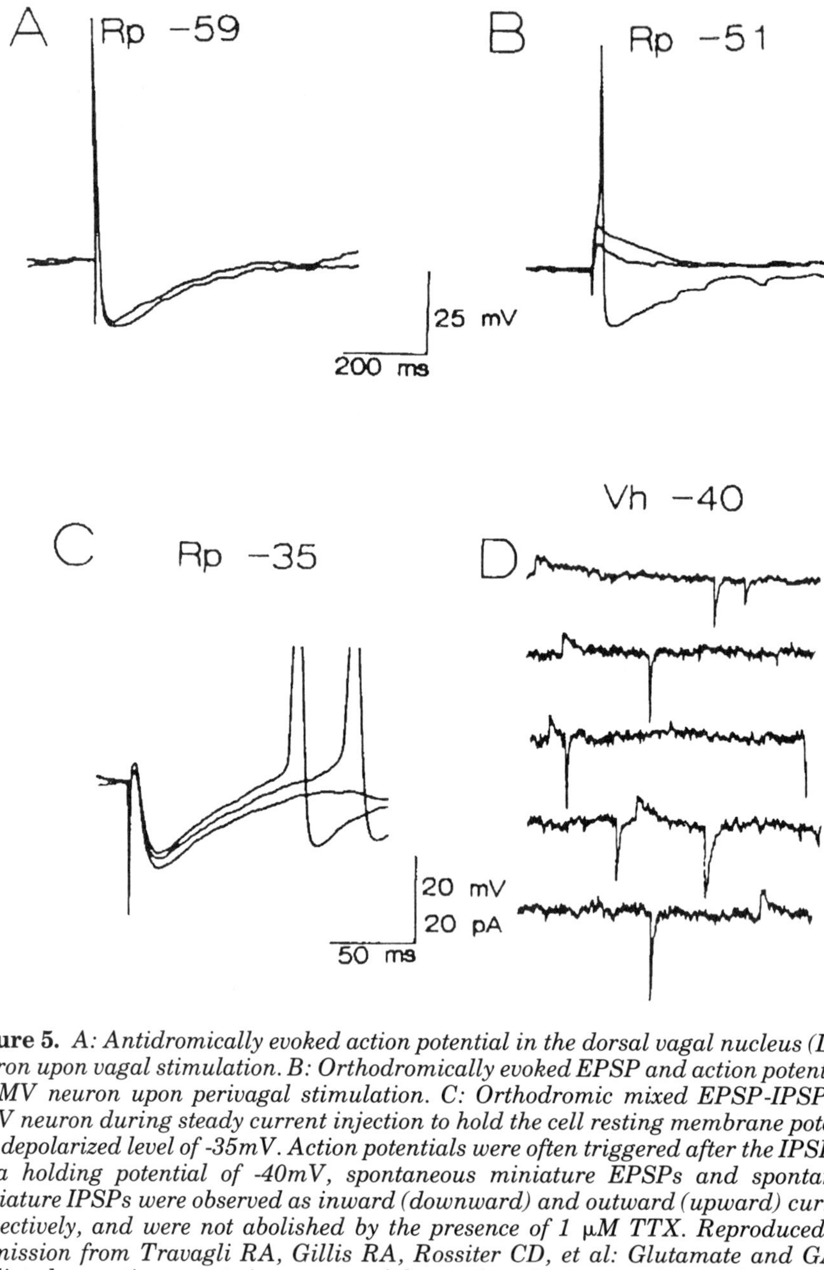

Figure 5. *A: Antidromically evoked action potential in the dorsal vagal nucleus (DMV) neuron upon vagal stimulation. B: Orthodromically evoked EPSP and action potential in a DMV neuron upon perivagal stimulation. C: Orthodromic mixed EPSP-IPSP in a DMV neuron during steady current injection to hold the cell resting membrane potential at a depolarized level of -35mV. Action potentials were often triggered after the IPSPs. D: At a holding potential of -40mV, spontaneous miniature EPSPs and spontaneous miniature IPSPs were observed as inward (downward) and outward (upward) currents, respectively, and were not abolished by the presence of 1 μM TTX. Reproduced with permission from Travagli RA, Gillis RA, Rossiter CD, et al: Glutamate and GABA-mediated synaptic currents in neurons of the rat dorsal motor nucleus of the vagus. Am J Physiol 260:G531–G536, 1991.*

Similar in vitro data are not available for NA vagal neurons, although several recent reports have described the firing patterns of these neurons among other nonvagal neurons of this nucleus[48–50] and, in a few cases, these observations have indicated a potential cardioinhibitory role for a proportion of these neurons.[50] Several reports indicate the pharmacological sensitivity of neurons in the NA that are particularly concerned with heart rate control; these studies have been reviewed elsewhere.

The Physiological Properties of Cardiac Vagal Motoneurons

A series of electrophysiological experiments have been undertaken using antidromic mapping techniques to identify the cell bodies of CVMs in the medulla of the cat.[8,51,52] These CVMs were shown to be restricted to the NA (see Figs. 1, 6A, 6C), although some vagal motoneurons with unmyelinated axons were shown to project through the cervical vagus to the intrathoracic cardiac branches of the vagus from the DVN.[8] In similar studies in the pigeon, CVMs were shown to be restricted to the DVN.[53] Subsequently, the presence of CVMs were shown electrophysiologically in both the DVN and NA in the rabbit.[54] CVMs have also been identified in the NA of the rat.[55] These observations prompted a detailed investigation of the physiological properties of CVMs, and these studies have provided a clear picture of the integrative role that these neurons play in cardiovascular control.

As indicated earlier, information is sparse regarding the properties of vagal efferent fibers supplying the heart, largely because of their low discharge rates under normal experimental situations. Similarly, the majority of CVMs recorded in the initial studies in the cat were either silent or fired with low rates of discharge.[8,51] They were, however, raised to firing threshold by the ionophoresis of excitant amino acids (glutamate or Dl-homocysteate), and this factor allowed a detailed study of their sensitivity to reflex and central inputs.[51,52] As to be expected from earlier observations, CVMs are shown to be powerfully excited by baroreceptor inputs and to exhibit pulse-related discharge when active (Fig. 6B).[52] Their discharge is also modulated in phase with respiratory activity. In the cat, when the animal is artificially ventilated and pneumothoracotomized, this modulation depends largely on inputs related to the central respiratory rhythm.[51] CVMs discharge during stage 1 expiration (postinspiration) and have a variable discharge at the end of expiration, but they are silent during inspiration.[51,56] CVMs of both the DVN and NA in the rabbit display firing characteristics similar to those of the cat, but they display a higher vagal "tone," almost invariably discharging without recourse to the application of excitant amino acids.[54] The physiological properties of the CVMs recorded in the NA and DVN are not obviously different.

The powerful effects of the arterial baroreceptors are confirmed by the sensitivity of CVMs to sinus and aortic nerve stimulation.[52] Marked excitatory influences are shown, but these effects involve the activation of chemoreceptor afferents in addition to baroreceptor inputs. The efficacy of sinus nerve inputs vary considerably with respect to the timing of the stimulus within the respiratory cycle; the effects are largely suppressed during inspiration.[52] The latency of the input to electrical stimulation, and the natural latency of the baroreceptor reflex assessed by the temporal relationship between the sinus nerve afferent volley and the averaged discharge of the CVM over several cardiac cycles, indicate two potential pathways. One is of relatively short latency, while the second pathway is of somewhat longer latency. The former pathway probably represents an action of the monosynaptic pathway between the NTS and vagal neurons of the NA demonstrated by anatomical methods. The longer latency reflects a supramedullary pathway that may involve the pontine parabrachial nucleus and possibly the anterior hypothalamus. These centers have been shown to be involved in the baroreceptor control of both heart rate and peripheral vascular resistance.[1,2]

CVMs in the cat are also shown to be excited by cardiac C-fiber activation, chemoreceptor activation, and superior laryngeal nerve stimulation.[9] Inhibitory

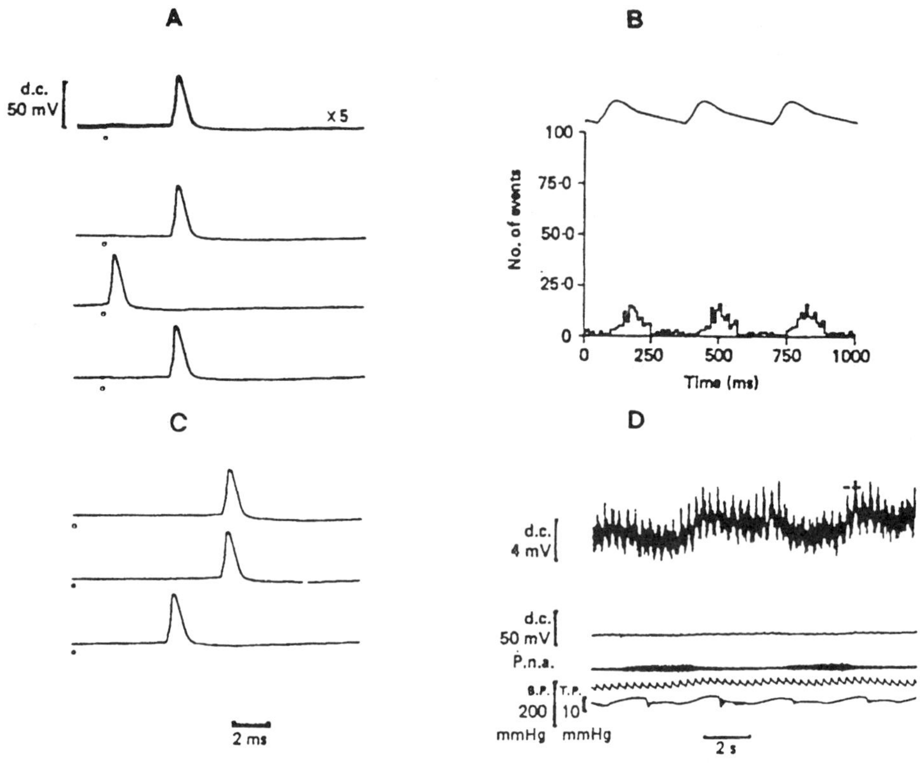

Figure 6. *Intracellular recording from CVM A: Stimulating cervical vagus (0.1 ms, 6 V) at 1 Hz. Five superimposed sweeps. Three consecutive sweeps illustrating the collision of an orthodromic spike, in the middle trace, with the antidromic spike. B: Lower trace: electrocardiogram-(ECG) triggered histogram of ongoing discharge of the CVM identified in A, B, C (110 sweeps, 10-ms bins). Upper trace: femoral arterial wave form averaged over the same time course and triggered from ECG (100 sweeps). C: Stimulation of the cardiac branches of the right vagus (0.1 ms, 3 V). Three consecutive sweeps, collision with orthodromic spike in lower trace. Stimulus marked by (●) in A and C. D: Intracellular recording from a CVM showing respiratory-related changes in membrane potential. The cell stopped firing action potentials 5 min after the cell was penetrated. In each panel traces from above: high and low gain d.c. recordings of membrane potential, phrenic nerve activity, arterial blood pressure, and tracheal pressure. Modified and reproduced with permission from Gilbey MP, Jordan D, Richter DW, et al: Synaptic mechanisms involved in the inspiratory modulation of vagal cardio-inhibitory neurones in the cat. J Physiol 356:65, 1984.*

effects have also been demonstrated. In particular, stimulation within the defense area of the hypothalamus in the cat produces a marked inhibition of the ongoing discharge of CVMs after a relatively short latency (circa eight milliseconds).[9] During the defense reaction, a very profound inhibition of CVM activity results. It is mediated by $GABA_A$ receptors (bicuculline-sensitive). Other studies have shown that the microinjections of bicuculline into the NA increases vagal tone and lowers heart rate.[57] This mechanism is just one of three that contributes to this inhibitory process. The second mechanism results from the profound inhibition that is exerted on NTS neurons during such hypothalamic stimulation (Fig. 7).[58,59] This mechanism is directed especially at those NTS neurons that are excited by baroreceptor inputs and, again, involves a GABAergic synapse mediated via $GABA_A$ receptors,[60] and it arises probably from an intrinsic pool of GABA-containing neurons in the NTS.[61] Hence, during the defense reaction, CVMs are disfacilitated as well as directly inhibited. This mechanism may be

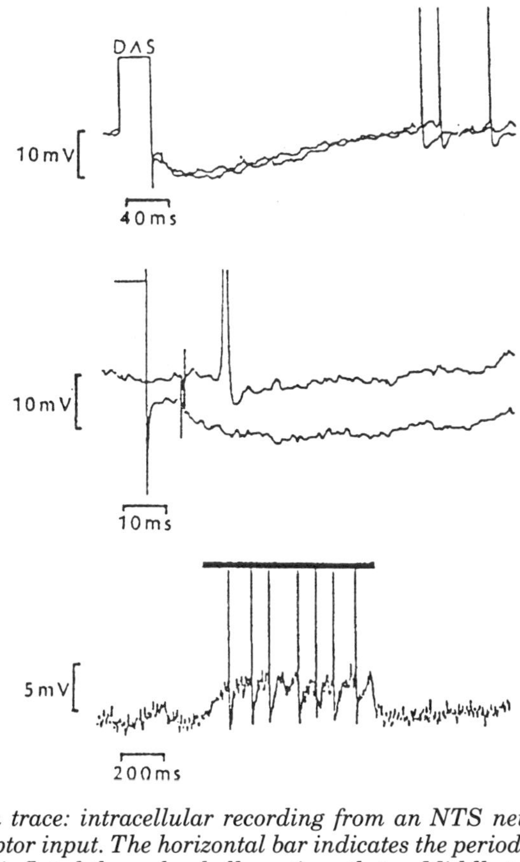

Figure 7. *Bottom trace: intracellular recording from an NTS neuron that received a powerful baroreceptor input. The horizontal bar indicates the period when the ipsilateral carotid sinus was inflated through a balloon-tip catheter. Middle traces: the response of this neuron to electrical stimulation of the sinus nerve alone. The lower of the two traces showing the response after a conditioning stimulus is delivered to the hypothalamic defense area. Note the hyperpolization and absence of the evoked spike response. Upper trace: two superimposed sweeps illustrating the time course of the defense area evoked hyperpolarization. Stimulation to the hypothalamic defense area involved a 30-ms-500 Hz burst of stimuli (DAS).*

engaged by other central inputs, because GABAergic mechanisms in the NTS subserve cerebellar[62] and pontine[63] influences on the circulation. The third mechanism involves the enhanced inspiratory drive that is elicited from the stimulus to the hypothalamus, and this response appears to be an important influence in the regulation of CVM activity.[56]

Respiratory Modulation of Cardiac Vagal Motoneuron Activity

The studies described above have shown that respiration markedly influences the basic discharge pattern of CVMs and their sensitivity to a variety of inputs, both central and reflex. Intracellular recording studies have shown that there are three phases in the membrane potential of CVMs (see Fig. 6D, Fig. 8) in both the cat and rat.[50,56] CVMs are hyperpolarized during inspiration, and are depolarized in postinspiration (Fig. 6D). In expiration, the membrane repolarizes, but it is variably depolarized toward the end of this phase. Indeed, the membrane trajectory of these neurons resembles that of postinspiratory neurons in the cat, which are essential interneurons in the generation of the respiratory rhythm.[64] In the rat, this pattern of discharge is apparent in many cranial motoneurons,[49] including vagal motoneurons, with properties suggestive of a cardioinhibitory function.[50] These observations suggest the hypothesis that the basic rhythms seen in the respiratory motor outputs and the autonomic outflows to the cardiovascular system are generated by a common brain stem cardiorespiratory network.[64] In essence, the identity of a neuron within the network is specified by its connections and CVMs are characterized by their axonal projection to the cardiac parasympathetic ganglia.

Intracellular recordings have also shown that the effects of the arterial baroreceptors can be seen as electrocardiogram- (ECG-) related EPSPs (Fig. 8),

Figure 8. *Upper traces: Dog. Chloralose and morphine. Records of carotid sinus blood pressure, respiratory air flow, and the activity of single cardiac vagal efferent nerve (CVE) are shown. A burst of firing in the CVE was evoked by a baroreceptor stimulus timed so as to occur in the expiratory pause. No firing was evoked when a similar stimulus was given during inspiration. Reproduced with permission from Davidson NS, Goldner S, McCloskey DI: Respiratory modulation of baroreceptor and chemoreceptor reflexes affecting heart-rate and cardiac vagal efferent nerve activity. J Physiol 259:523, 1976. Middle traces: EPSPs evoked by carotid sinus nerve stimulation in a cell depolarized during activation of the baroreceptors. Membrane potential was hyperpolarized with 4-nA dc current and the stimulus intensities adjusted so that EPSPs were subthreshold for action potential generation. Two sweeps during inspiration (left) and expiration (middle), one with the lungs inflated and the other with the lungs deflated, are superimposed. Phrenic nerve activity (PNA) is displayed below. Right, two sweeps superimposed from left and right columns; resting membrane potential - 56mV. HRP-filled electrode. Modified with permission from Mifflin SW, Spyer KM, Withington-Wray DJ: Baroreceptor inputs to the nucleus tractus solitarius in the cat: Postsynaptic actions and the influence of respiration. J Physiol 399:349, 1988. Lower traces: Respiratory modulation of pulse-rhythmic EPSPs recording in a cell in which IPSPs have been reserved previously by Cl^- injection (3nA for 5 min). Further details in text. Traces from above: high and low gain dc recordings of membrane potential, phrenic nerve activity (P.n.a.), femoral arterial blood pressure (B.P.), and tracheal pressure (T.P.). Reproduced with permission from Gilbey MP, Jordan D, Richter DW, et al: Synaptic mechanisms involved in the inspiratory modulation of vagal cardio-inhibitory neurones in the cat. J Physiol 356:65, 1984.*

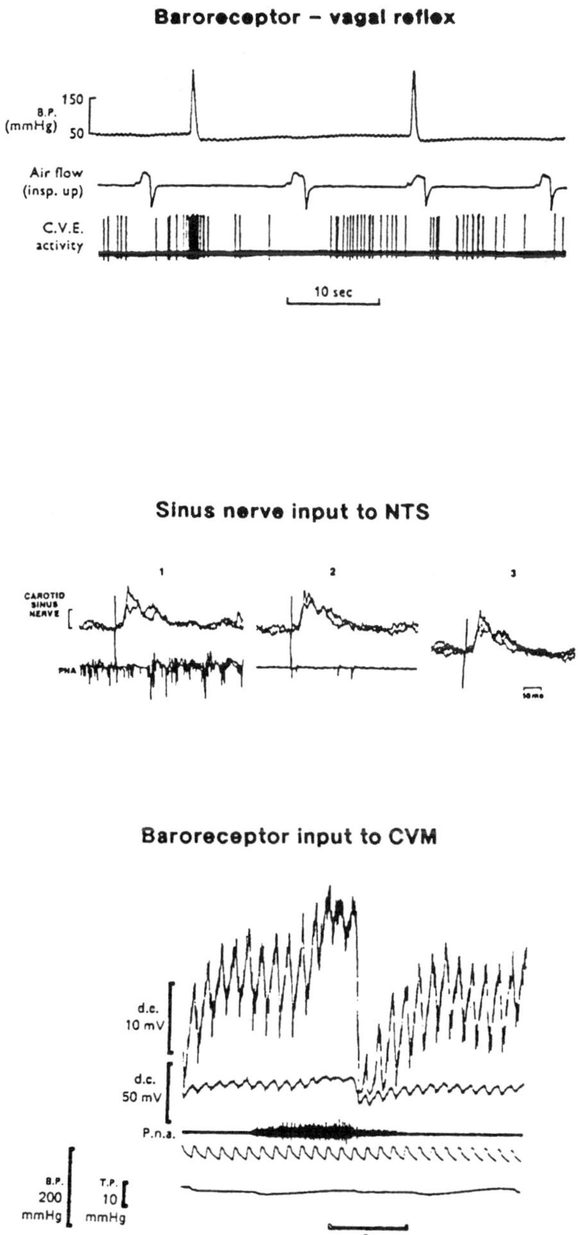

Figure 8. *(see legend on p. 58)*

the magnitude of which vary through the respiratory cycle.[56] In artificially ventilated animals with inflation desynchronized from central respiratory activity, the EPSPs of baroreceptor origin are reduced during inspiration (the period of phrenic nerve discharge) when the membrane is hyperpolarized. This "shunting" is sufficient to explain both the inspiratory refractiveness of the baroreceptor-vagal reflex (Fig. 8) and the respiratory modulation of other inputs to CVMs (see Fig. 9). During inspiration, CVMs are hyperpolarized by a Cl^--dependent mechanism. The hyperpolarizing IPSP can be reversed to a depolarizing wave by either the passage of hyperpolarizing current or the injection of Cl^- into the neuron (Fig. 8). The synaptic action does not appear to be mediated by GABA because it is not antagonized by the ionophoretic application of bicuculline. Its effect can be eliminated, however, by the ionophoresis of atropine, a muscarinic antagonist. This observation explains at least part of the respiratory modulation of CVM activity, but leaves unexplained the action of an input related to lung inflation (see Figs. 8, 9). The intracellular recordings from CVMs have failed to reveal influences of lung inflation, although lung inflation exerts marked effects on the efficacy of many reflex inputs to CVMs, as described above and elsewhere.

One explanation for this discrepancy is that reflex inputs are "gated" at the level of the NTS, where both respiratory and cardiovascular afferents converge.[65] When this suggestion has been tested directly, it has proved negative.[58] NTS neurons that receive baroreceptor inputs and are excited by sinus nerve, vagal, and superior laryngeal inputs (in various combinations) are observed in different phases of the respiratory cycle and in conditions of inflated or deflated lungs. The magnitude of evoked EPSPs remain with the normal level of variability, and show no consistent effect of respiratory state (Fig. 8). Similar results have been obtained for those NTS neurons responding to arterial chemoreceptor inputs. Presumably, the level of interaction must be at a site, as yet unknown, between the NTS and the vagal motoneurons of the NA.

The observations that have been made in CVMs of the cat and rat, with support from studies in the rabbit, regarding the central mechanism eliciting inspiratory suppression of CVM activity appear to be applicable to man also. Several laboratories have described a central action of atropine and other muscarinic cholinergic antagonists in abolishing or reducing sinus arrhythmia.[66] The site of action of these low doses of muscarinic antagonists is not resolved in the human studies, but by analogy an action at the NA would seem reasonable.

Conclusions

The data presented in this chapter support the contention that CVMs form an essential integrative focus in the CNS control of circulation. Figure 9 illustrates certain central and reflex inputs that affect the activity of CVMs. The effectiveness of any input is determined by the excitability of the CVM, which is, itself, a product of its synaptic input and intrinsic membrane properties. The

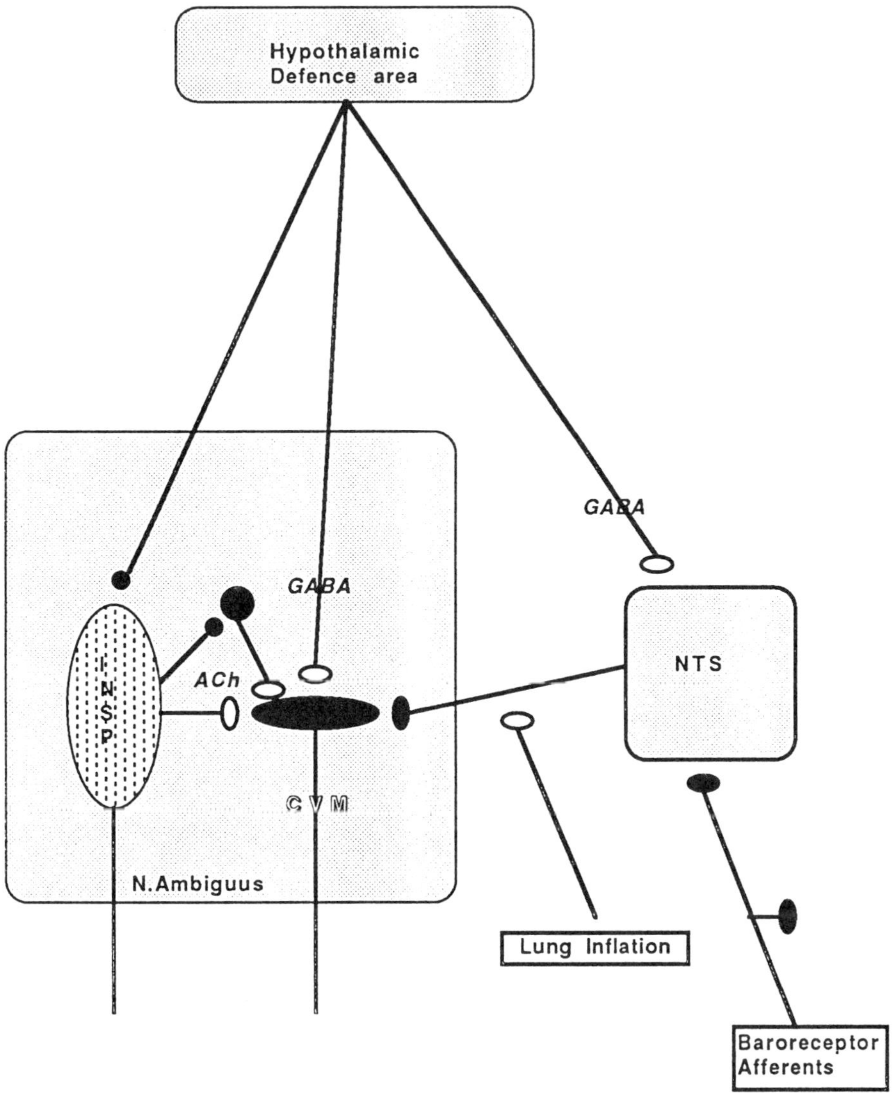

Figure 9. *Diagrams illustrating the control exerted on vagal cardioinhibitory neurons (CVM) by baroreceptor afferent input, inspiratory neurons (I), and the hypothalamic defense area. The influence of lung stretch inputs is also illustrated. Excitatory inputs are shown as ●; inhibitory inputs as o; ACh, as acetylcholine; and GABA as γ-aminobutyric acid. Further details are in the text.*

growing knowledge of the biophysical properties of CVMs and their pharmacology may enhance the understanding of the physiological processes that lead to state-dependent changes in heart rate. They may also provide a convenient experimental tool with which to unravel the complexities of central cardiovascular control and its modification in pathological situations.

References

1. Spyer KM: The central nervous organization of reflex circulatory control. In AD Loewy, KM Spyer (eds): Central Regulation of Autonomic Functions. New York, NY, Oxford University Press, 1990, p. 168.
2. Loewy AD, Spyer KM: Vagal preganglionic neurons. In AD Loewy, KM Spyer (eds): Central Regulation of Autonomic Functions. New York, NY, Oxford University Press, 1990, p. 68.
3. Getz B, Sirnes T: The localisation within the dorsal motor vagal nucleus. J Comp Neurol 90:90, 1949.
4. Mitchell GAG, Warwick R: The dorsal vagal nucleus. Acta Anat 25:371, 1955.
5. Bunzl-Federn E: Der centrale ursprung des nervus vagus. Psychiat Neurol 5:1, 1899.
6. Kosaka K: Über die Vaguskerne des hundes. Neurol CBL 28:406, 1909.
7. Chiarugi E, Mollica A: Contributo alla localizzazione del centro vagale cardio-inibitore. Archivio di Fisiologia 54:Fasc. IV: 249, 1954.
8. McAllen RM, Spyer KM: The location of cardiac vagal preganglionic motoneurons in the medulla of the cat. J Physiol 258:187, 1976.
9. Jordan D, Spyer KM: Central neural mechanisms mediating respiratory–cardiovascular interactions. In EW Taylor (ed): Neurobiology of the Cardiorespiratory System. Manchester, Manchester University Press, 1987 p. 322.
10. Kalia M: Brain stem localisation of vagal preganglionic neurons. J Aut Nerv Syst 3:451,1981.
11. Todo K, Yamamoto T, Satomi H, et al: Origins of vagal preganglionic fibres to the sino-atrial and atrio-ventricular nodes regions in the cat heart as studied by the horseradish peroxidase method. Brain Res 130:545, 1977.
12. Bennett JA, Kidd C, Latif AB, et al: A horseradish peroxidase study of vagal motoneurones with axons in cardiac and pulmonary branches of the cat and dog. Quart J Exp Physiol 66:145, 1981.
13. Nosaka S, Yamamoto T, Yasunaga K: Localisation of vagal cardioinhibitory preganglionic neurones within rat brain stem. J Comp Neurol 186:79, 1979.
14. Miselis RR, Rogers WT, Schwaber JS, et al: Localisation of cardiomotor neurones in the anaesthetised rat; cholera-toxin HRP conjugate and pseudorabies labelling. J Physiol 416:63P, 1989.
15. Bieger D, Hopkins DA: Viscerotopic representation of the upper alimentary tract in the medulla oblongata in the rat; the nucleus ambiguus. J Comp Neurol 262:546, 1987.
16. Deuchars J: *Investigations into the organisation and morphology of vagal preganglionic neurones and the anatomical identification of some of their synaptic inputs.* London, University of London, 1992, Thesis.
17. McLean JH, Hopkins DA: Ultrastructure of the dorsal motor nucleus of the vagus nerve in monkey with a comparison of synaptology in monkey and cat. J Comp Neurol 231:162, 1985.
18. McLean JH, Hopkins DA: Ultrastructural studies of the nucleus ambiguus in cat and monkey following injections of HRP into the vagus nerve. J Neurocytol 14:961, 1985.
19. Deuchars J, Izzo PN: Demonstration of a monosynaptic pathway from the nucleus tractus solitarius to regions of the ventrolateral medulla with specific reference to vagal motoneurones in the nucleus ambiguus of the anaesthetised cat. J Physiol 438:80P, 1991.
20. Kunze DL: Reflex discharge patterns of cardiac vagal efferent fibres. J Physiol 222:1, 1972.
21. Green JH: Cardiac vagal efferent activity in the cat. J Physiol 149:47–49, 1959.
22. Marguth H, Raule W, Schaeffer H: Aktionsströme in zentrifugale Herznerven. Pflügers Arch 54:224, 1951.
23. Okada H, Okamoto K, Nishida I: The activity of the cardioregulatory and abdominal sympathetic nerves during swallowing. Jpn J Physiol 11:44, 1961.

24. Okada K, Okamoto K, Nishida I: The activity of the cardioregulatory and abdominal sympathetic nerves in the cat in the Bainbridge reflex. Jpn J Physiol 11:520, 1961.
25. Iriuchijima J, Kumada M: Efferent cardiac vagal discharge of the dog in response to electrical stimulation of sensory nerves. Jpn J Physiol 13:599, 1963.
26. Iriuchijima J, Kumada M: Activity in single vagal efferent fibres to the heart. Jpn J Physiol 14:479, 1965.
27. Jewett DL: Activity of single efferent fibres in the cervical vagus nerve of the dog, with special reference to possible cardioinhibitory fibres. J Physiol 175:321, 1964.
28. Katona P, Poitras J, Barnett U, et al: Cardiac vagal efferent activity and heart period in the carotid sinus reflex. Am J Physiol 218:1030, 1970.
29. Katona PG, Lipson D, Dauchot PJ: Opposing central and peripheral effects of atropine on parasympathetic cardiovascular control. Am J Physiol 232:146, 1977.
30. Davidson NS, Goldner S, McCloskey DI: Respiratory modulation of baroreceptor and chemoreceptor reflexes affecting heart-rate and cardiac vagal efferent nerve activity. J Physiol 259:523, 1976.
31. Lopes OU, Palmer JF: Proposed respiratory "gating" mechanism for cardiac slowing. Nature 264:454, 1976.
32. Neil E, Palmer JF: Effects of spontaneous respiration on the latency of reflex cardiac chronotropic responses to baroreceptor stimulation. J Physiol 247:16, 1975.
33. Daly M de B: Interactions between respiration and circulation. In NS Cherniack, JG Widdicombe (eds): Handbook of Physiology. The Respiratory System II. Bethesada, MD, American Physiological Society, 1985, pp. 529–594.
34. Daly M de B, Kirkman E: Differential modulation by pulmonary stretch afferents of some reflex cardioinhibitory responses in the cat. J Physiol 417:323, 1989.
35. Yarom Y, Sugimari M, Llinas R: Ionic currents and firing patterns of mammalian motoneurons in vitro. Neuroscience 16:719, 1985.
36. Yarom Y, Brecha O, Werman R: Intracellular injection of acetylcholine blocks various potassium conductances in vagal motoneurones. Neuroscience 16:739, 1985.
37. Champagnat J, Denavit-Saubie M, Grant K, et al: Organisation of synaptic transmission in the mammalian solitary complex studied in vitro. J Physiol 381:551, 1986.
38. Fukuda A, Minami T, Nabekura J, et al: The effects of noradrenaline on neurones in the rat dorsal motor nucleus of the vagus in vitro. J Physiol 393:213, 1987.
39. Plata-Salaman C, Fukuda A, Oomura Y, et al: Effects of sulphated cholecystokinin octapeptide (CCK-8) on the dorsal motor nucleus of the vagus. Brain Res Bull 21:839, 1988.
40. Nabekura J, Mizuno Y, Oomura Y: Inhibitory effect of somatostatin on vagal motoneurons in the rat brain stem in vitro. Am J Physiol 256:C155, 1989.
41. Brooks PA: Actions of 5-hydroxytryptamine on dorsal vagal motoneurones of the rat in vitro. J Physiol 438:131P, 1991.
42. Travagli RA, Gillis RA, Rossiter CD, et al: Glutamate and GABA-mediated synaptic currents in neurons of the rat dorsal motor nucleus of the vagus. Am J Physiol 260:G531, 1991.
43. Ito C, Fukuda A, Nabekura J, et al: Acetylcholine causes nicotinic depolarisation in rat dorsal motor nucleus of the vagus in vitro. Brain Res 503:44, 1989.
44. Glaum SR, Brooks PA, Murphy SM, et al: Activation of 5-HT_3 receptors causes pre- and postsynaptic effects in the nucleus tractus solitarius (NTS) of the rat in vitro. J Physiol 438:253P, 1991.
45. McCann MJ, Roger RC: Thyrotropin-releasing hormone effects on identified neurons of the dorsal vagal complex. J Auton Nerv Syst 26:107, 1981.
46. Charpak S, Armstrong WE, Mühlethaler M, et al: Stimulatory action of oxytocin on neurones of the dorsal motor nucleus of the vagus nerve. Brain Res 300:83, 1984.
47. Plata-Salomon CW, Fukuda A, Minarin T, et al: Substance P effects on the dorsal motor nucleus of the vagus. Brain Res Bull 23:149, 1989.

48. Schwarzacher SW, Wilhelm Z, Anders K, et al: The medullary respiratory network in the rat. J Physiol 435:631, 1991.
49. Zheng Y, Barillot JC, Bianchi AL: Patterns of membrane potentials and distributions of the medullary respiratory neurons in the decerebrate rate. Brain Res 546:261, 1991.
50. Parkes MJ, Lara Munoz JP, Izzo PN, et al: Projections of neurones with respiratory-related discharge in the medulla of the anaesthetised rat. J Physiol 446:429, 1992.
51. McAllen RM, Spyer KM: Two types of vagal preganglionic motoneurones projecting to the heart and lungs. J Physiol 282:353, 1978.
52. McAllen RM, Spyer KM: The baroreceptor input to cardiac vagal motoneurones. J Physiol 282:365, 1978.
53. Schwaber JS, Cohen DH: Field potential and single unit analyses of the avian dorsal motor nucleus of the vagus and criteria for identifying vagal cardiac cells of origin. Brain Res 147:79, 1978.
54. Jordan D, Khalid MEM, Schneiderman N, et al: The location and properties of preganglionic vagal cardiomotor neurones in the rabbit. Pflügers Arch 395:244, 1982.
55. Nosaka S, Yamamoto T, Tamai S: Vagal cardiac preganglionic neurons: Distribution, cell types and reflex discharge. Am J Physiol 243:R92, 1982.
56. Gilbey MP, Jordan D, Richter DW, et al: Synaptic mechanisms involved in the inspiratory modulation of vagal cardio-inhibitory neurones in the cat. J Physiol 356:65, 1984.
57. DiMicco JA, Gale K, Hamilton BL, et al: GABA receptor control of parasympathetic outflow to heart: Characterization and brainstem location. Science 204:1106, 1979.
58. Mifflin SW, Spyer KM, Withington-Wray DJ: Baroreceptor inputs to the nucleus tractus solitarius in the cat: Modulation by the hypothalmus. J Physiol 399:369, 1988.
59. Mifflin SW, Spyer KM, Withington-Wray DJ: Baroreceptor inputs to the nucleus tractus solitarius in the cat: Postsynaptic actions and the influence of respiration. J Physiol 399:349, 1988.
60. Jordan DJ, Mifflin SW, Spyer KM: Hypothalamic inhibition of neurones in the nucleus tractus solitarius of the cat is GABA mediated. J Physiol 399:389, 1988.
61. Izzo PN, Sykes RM, Spyer KM: γ-amino butyric acid immunoreactive structures in the nucleus tractus solitarious: A light and electron microscopic study. Brain Res 591:69–79, 1992.
62. Paton JFR, Spyer KM: Brainstem regions mediating the cardiovascular responses elicited from the posterior cerebellar cortex in the rabbit. J Physiol 427:533, 1990.
63. Paton JFR, Silva-Carvalho L, Thompson CS, et al: Nucleus tractus solitarius as mediator of evoked parabrachial cardiovascular responses in the decerebrate rabbit. J Physiol 428:693, 1991.
64. Richter DW, Spyer KM: Cardiorespiratory control. In AD Loewy, KM Spyer (eds): Central Regulation of Autonomic Functions. New York, NY, Oxford University Press, 1990, p. 189.
65. Potter EK: Inspiratory inhibition of vagal responses to baroreceptor and chemoreceptor stimuli in the dog. J Physiol 316:177, 1981.
66. Katona PG, Lipson D, Dauchot PJ: Opposing central and peripheral effects of atropine on parasympathetic cardiac control. Am J Physiol 232:H146, 1990.

CHAPTER 5

Cardiorespiratory Integration

D.I. McCloskey

Cardiac Vagal Fibers and Their Discharge

The cardiac branch of the vagus contains both afferent and efferent fibers, mainly of the small myelinated and unmyelinated types.[1–4] In 1964, Jewett[5] reported a study in anesthetized dogs in which he recorded the neural activities of fibers in the central end of the cut cervical vagus nerve, and classified these fibers into seven functional types, related to their likely physiological roles. Two groups of fibers were classified as cardioinhibitory. The major group ("Type I") comprised tonically active fibers, whose discharge was strongly pulse-modulated and in which activity was completely, or almost completely, abolished during the inspiratory phase of breathing. These fibers increased and decreased their firing in response to various reflex stimuli in directions appropriate to evoked changes in heart rate. Importantly, the behavior of a small group of efferent fibers recorded from the right cardiac branches of the vagus nerve was, in all respects, similar to that of the larger group of Type I fibers dissected from the cervical vagus. A second, smaller group of fibers ("Type V"), also considered to be cardioinhibitory, was described as well and was, in all respects, similar to the large Type I group, except that the Type V group exhibited little or no resting discharge. None of the other groups of efferent fibers described behaved in a manner consistent with the cardiovascular responses known to be mediated through the vagus. Furthermore, activity recorded from sympathetic nerves in the cardiac branch of the stellate ganglion varied in directions opposite to that of the vagal cardioinhibitory groups in response to cardiovascular and respiratory disturbances. Hence, the vagal cardioinhibitory groups cannot be considered to include aberrant sympathetic fibers. Figure 1 depicts some of the characteristic properties of the vagal cardioinhibitory fibers, including their respiratory and pulse modulation, and contrasts them with those of cardiac and vasoconstrictor sympathetic nerves.[6]

From *Vagal Control of the Heart: Experimental Basis and Clinical Implications* edited by MN Levy, PJ Schwartz © 1994, Futura Publishing Co. Inc., Armonk, NY.

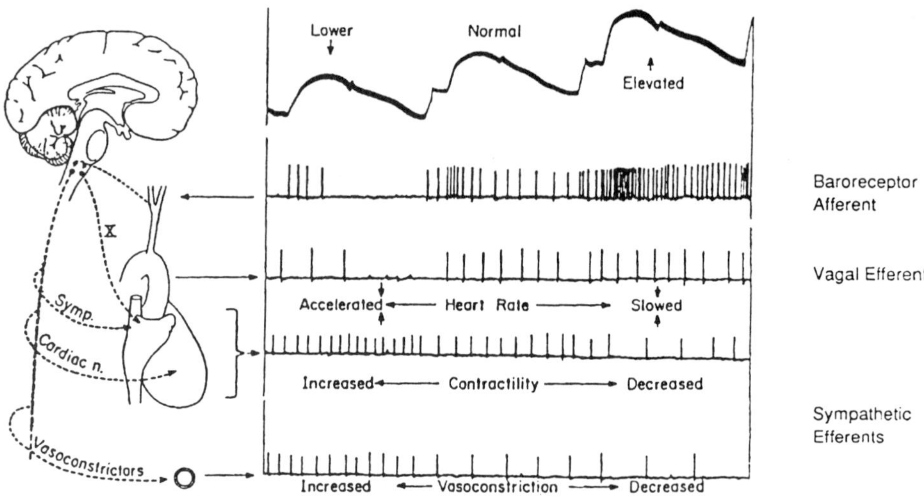

Figure 1. *Diagrammatic representation of characteristic neural firing patterns of arterial baroreceptor afferents, cardiac vagal efferents, and cardiac and vasoconstrictor sympathetic efferents. Reproduced with permission from Spyer KM: Neural mechanisms involved in cardiovascular control during affective behaviour. Trends Neurosci 12:506, 1989.*

Pulse modulation of cardiac vagal efferent firing is marked. Because of the silence of most vagal fibers during the inspiratory phase of breathing, it is usually not apparent that the modulation continues at this time. It has been shown, however, that if the excitability of ca rdiac vagal motoneurons (CVMs) is enhanced by direct effects of local iontophoresis of excitatory amino acids, there remains a prominent pulse modulation and an excitation from electrical stimulation of the carotid sinus nerve (Fig. 2).[7]

A feature to emerge from Jewett's study[5] is that all vagal fibers that he classified as cardioinhibitory increase and decrease their discharge with rises and falls in blood pressure, a behavior that is consistent with all of them receiving an excitatory input from arterial baroreceptors. Put another way, this feature implies no cardioinhibitory vagal input from sources that are not convergent upon the pathways activated by baroreceptors. There are, of course, many reports of inputs from receptors other than baroreceptors that alter the discharge of CVMs. For instance, arterial chemoreceptors and pulmonary stretch receptors would be two sources of inputs of this kind (see Ch. 4).[8,9] On the basis of the observations above, however, these other sources of input must be considered as convergent upon pathways activated by the arterial baroreceptors. It is of interest that the cardiac vagal discharge evoked in response to a brief baroreceptor stimulus continues well beyond the duration of that stimulus.[10,11] Furthermore, there is marked adaptation of the response of CVMs to intermittent or sustained baroreceptor inputs.[10]

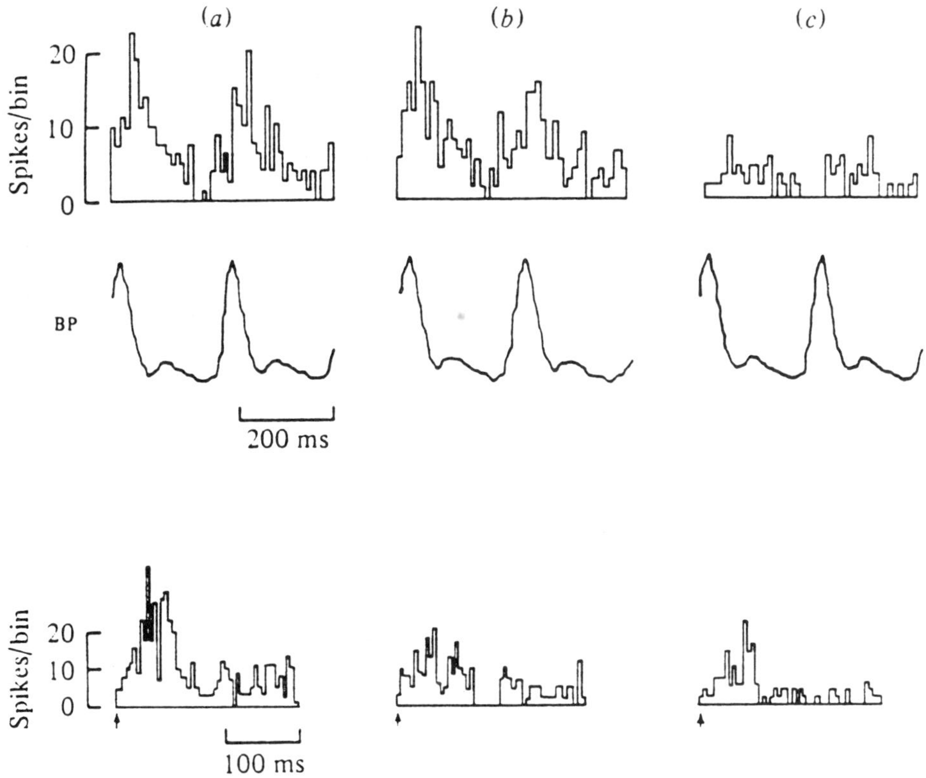

Figure 2. *Cardiac rhythm of a CVM and its response to electrical stimulation of the carotid sinus nerve. Traces, from above: Pulse-triggered histograms of vagal motoneuronal firing; femoral pulse wave on same time scale; and, histograms of vagal motoneuronal firing in response to sinus nerve stimuli at the arrows. a: analyzed throughout the respiratory cycle; b: in expiration only; and c: in inspiration only. Unit firing enhanced in all conditions by local iontophoresis of an excitant amino acid. Reproduced with permission from McAllen RM, Spyer KM: The baroreceptor input to cardiac vagal motoneurones. J Physiol (Lond) 282:365, 1978.*

Respiratory Modulation and Sinus Arrhythmia

Respiratory modulation of cardiac vagal discharge has long been recognized as one of the latter's major distinguishing features.[9] One of the earliest electrophysiological studies on vagal efferent firing was that performed in 1936 by Rijlant,[12] who noted in recordings made in anesthetized dogs that respiratory sinus arrhythmia persisted during paralysis, with the tachycardia in phase with continuously recorded phrenic nerve activity—itself a measure of the animals' continuing central inspiratory drive—and out of phase with recorded vagal neural activity. During inspiration, vagal discharge fell silent.

Whether or not the respiratory rhythm of vagal discharge is necessary or sufficient to account for sinus arrhythmia has long been debated. Bainbridge,[13] for example, proposed in 1920 that "each inspiration increases the diastolic filling of the heart and gives rise to reflex acceleration of the heart rate." The experiments of Linden and his colleagues, however, indicate that any increase in heart rate evoked by increased filling of left or right atria, with consequent stimulation of receptors in these chambers, is mediated by sympathetic excitation rather than vagal withdrawal.[14] Sympathetic innervation of the heart is not essential for sinus arrhythmia to occur,[15–17] although this does not rule out its participation. Local stretch of the sinoatrial (SA) node is another nonvagal mechanism often proposed as the basis of sinus arrhythmia. Supporters of this mechanism can point to the changes in the rate of spontaneous pacemaker depolarization[18] and the tachycardia[19,20] that occur with stretch of the pacemaker tissue. The key observation indicating that neither of these nonvagal mechanisms is of central importance to the genesis of respiratory sinus arrhythmia, however, is that, under normal conditions, sinus arrhythmia depends on the integrity of the vagus nerves.[17,21–23]

Once it is concluded that normal respiratory sinus arrhythmia is critically dependent upon the integrity of the vagus nerves, the question still remains concerning the mechanism by which the respiratory rhythm is imposed upon vagal discharge. One major category of mechanisms would be one in which the rhythm is imposed reflexly. Arterial blood pressure, PCO_2, and pH all fluctuate throughout the respiratory cycle, and lung volume changes. All these factors can be expected to alter the activation of potent cardiorespiratory reflexes known to affect heart rate through the vagus nerves.[9] As was pointed out above, however, respiratory sinus arrhythmia remains prominent in a totally paralyzed animal in which such modulations of reflex input would be absent[13,21,24]; therefore, respiratory patterning of a reflex input cannot be essential for imposing the vagal rhythm.

Respiratory Modulation of Reflex Stimuli

A more important factor in the genesis of sinus arrhythmia seems to be that the effectiveness of reflex inputs varies throughout the respiratory cycle. Koepchen and his colleagues[25,26] were the first to show that brief, similar, arterial baroreceptor stimuli given at different phases of the respiratory cycle are not equally effective in evoking reflex bradycardia. Stimuli delivered in the expiratory phase of breathing (period of expiratory air flow or the expiratory pause) reflexly induce bradycardia, but stimuli delivered in the inspiratory phase do not.[25,26] This observation has been repeated many times,[5,9,24,27–30] and the effect is demonstrable by delivering baroreceptor stimuli through the application of brief periods of negative pressure around the neck in human subjects (Fig. 3).[31]

There has long been debate about the physiological mechanisms underlying the respiratory modulation of reflex effectiveness. Some have drawn attention to central mechanisms dependent upon the overflow of impulses from the respiratory centers to the vagal excitatory pathways, while others have

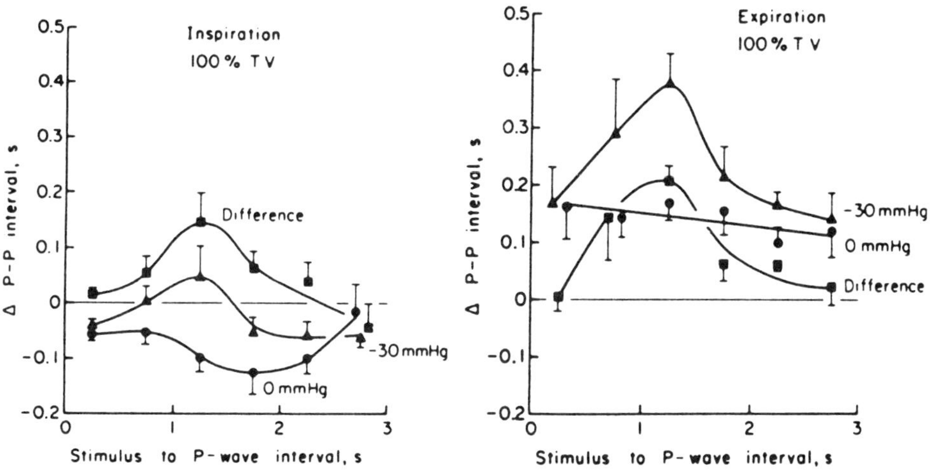

Figure 3. *Effects on changes in P-P (P-wave) interval of stimulating carotid baroreceptors (neck suction, −30 mm Hg: ▲) for 0.6 s during early inspiration (left) and during expiration (right). Averaged P-P intervals for six normal human subjects. Spontaneous changes provoked by inspiration without baroreceptor stimulation (0 mm Hg: ●); changes in pulse interval after neck suction applied in early inspiration; and, net response to baroreceptor stimulation (difference: ■) calculated by subtracting responses without neck suction from responses with neck suction. TV, tidal volume. Reproduced from the Journal of Clinical Investigation, Eckberg D, Orshan CR: Respiratory and baroreceptor reflex interactions in man. 1977, 59:780, by copyright permission of the American Society of Clinical Investigation.*

emphasized the importance of phasic vagal inhibition occurring through afferent nerves excited by lung inflation.

It is now known that both mechanisms are effective, and that either one can impose the respiratory modulation.[8,9,24,30] During normal breathing, the centrally generated inspiratory drive and inflation of the lungs proceed together. These events can be readily separated, however, if the experimental animal is paralyzed. Then, central respiratory cycling continues without accompanying movement, and can be monitored by recording neural activity in a phrenic nerve. The lungs can be inflated or deflated as required, in desired relation to the central respiratory cycling.

Figure 4 shows results from an experiment in which these maneuvers were performed in an anesthetized and paralyzed dog to demonstrate the basis of respiratory modulation of effectiveness of reflex activation of the cardiac vagus. All the recordings illustrated in Figure 4 were obtained during periods in which the respiratory pump was temporarily halted, and the animal was immobile except when its lungs were inflated by the experimenters. Brief baroreceptor stimuli, which consisted of pulses of pressure in the carotid sinus, were delivered in different temporal relations to ongoing central neural, or pulmonary, events. As Figure 4 illustrates, these stimuli evoke prompt falls in heart rate if delivered in the expiratory phase of the central respiratory cycle, and when the animal is immobile. (These prompt falls in heart rate are known to be mediated by the vagus, as they are abolished by atropine.[24])

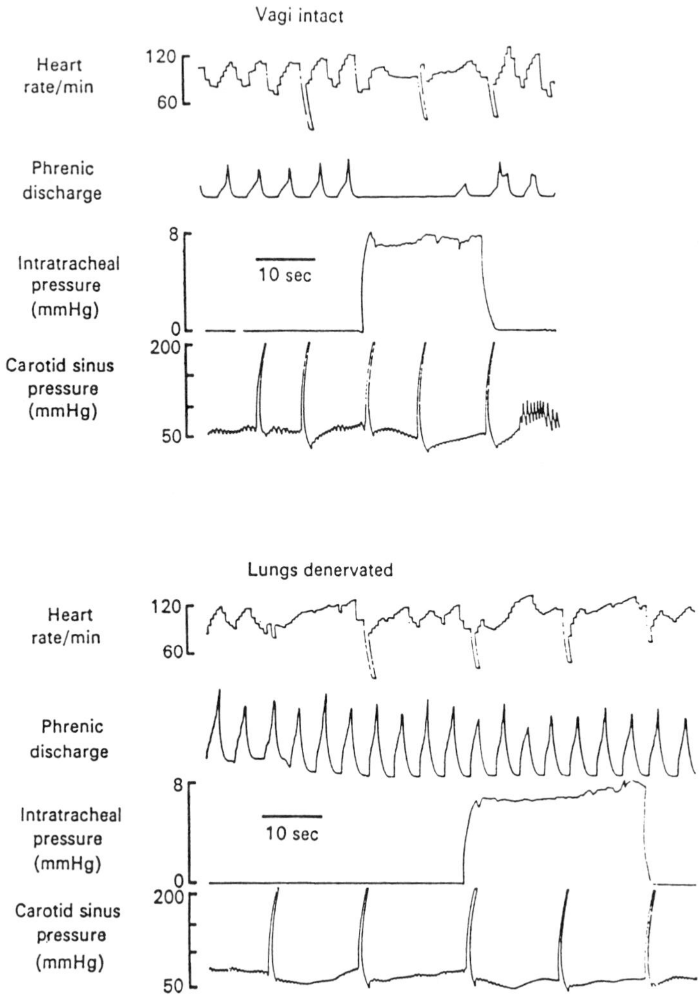

Figure 4. *Dog, anesthetized with chloralose and paralyzed with D-tubocurarine. Upper and lower panels show heart rate, integrated phrenic discharge, intratracheal pressure, and carotid sinus blood pressure, recorded during periods of temporary cessation of artificial ventilation. The effects of baroreceptor stimuli (pulses of intracarotid pressure) on heart rate are seen. When the vagi are intact (upper panel), baroreceptor stimuli evoke bradycardia except when delivered during periods of inspiration (first of the stimuli shown) or while the lungs are expanding in response to a rise in intratracheal pressure (third stimulus). After denervation of the lungs (lower panel), the stimuli remain ineffective during periods of central inspiratory activity (first stimulus), but now evoke a large bradycardia when delivered while the lungs are expanding in response to a rise in intratracheal pressure. Reproduced with permission from Gandevia SC, McCloskey DI, Potter EK: Inhibition of baroreceptor and chemoreceptor reflexes on heart rate by afferents from the lungs. J Physiol (Lond) 276:369, 1978.*

The same stimuli fail to evoke the vagally-mediated bradycardia, however, if delivered when the central inspiratory phase is in progress (even if the lungs are immobile at their relaxation point) or when the lungs are being inflated (even if the central respiratory cycle is not in its inspiratory phase). Therefore, either central inspiratory activity (alone) or lung inflation (alone) is sufficient to block the reflex. Of course, in normal circumstances, these conditions occur together, and so the respiratory-phased effect is doubly assured.

The centrally generated inhibitory mechanism is powerful. Since direct recordings of medullary vagal motoneurons indicate that they receive excitatory inputs from arterial baroreceptors throughout the respiratory cycle,[4] it appears that the inspiratory-phased reduction of reflex effectiveness is not wholly dependent on a gating out of the sensory inputs at an earlier stage in the reflex pathway. Direct recordings at the level of baroreceptor and other reflex inputs into the nucleus tractus solitarius (NTS) reveal no modification of postsynaptic potentials in response to lung inflations or central inspiratory activity. These findings indicate that the respiratory influences on the baroreceptor-vagal reflex occur beyond this point in the pathway.[32] CVMs discharge spontaneously only in expiration and the direct depolarizing action of locally applied excitatory amino acids is more potent in expiration.[4] Also, iontophoresis of atropine on CVMs increases their firing during inspiration (when they are usually silent), while having little effect on their discharge in the expiratory phase. These results suggest that the locally applied atropine blocks a phasic inspiratory input.[32,33] Furthermore, CVMs are located in the medulla close to the lateral group of inspiratory neurons.[34] All these findings point to the likelihood of a direct input that arises from medullary inhibitory neurons and that acts directly at the membrane of the CVMs.

The modulation of reflex effectiveness by lung inflation is clearly based upon excitation of pulmonary afferents, as the modulation is abolished by denervation of the lung (Fig. 4).[24] This inhibitory influence is sensitive to the rate of lung inflation, and it decays with time even when lung inflation is held steady (Fig. 4).[24] It is likely that the effect is based on the pulmonary stretch receptors.[24] Unlike the inhibitory influence exerted by centrally generated inspiratory neural activity, which usually silences vagal firing entirely throughout inspiration, the effect based on pulmonary afferents inhibits reflexly-evoked vagal firing without inhibiting tonic vagal discharge.[11] Potter[11] has proposed that this behavior could be accounted for if the pulmonary afferents exerted their inhibitory effects at a point much earlier in the baroreceptor-vagal reflex pathway. Although later work[35] has not supported her suggestion that this earlier point might be in the nucleus tractus solitarius (NTS), an effect between that point and the CVMs still seems likely. On the basis of studies on sympathetically-mediated effects, it seems that this later point in the pathway occurs beyond the point where the reflex decussates into its vagal and sympathetic limbs.[33]

To this point, the behavior of the baroreceptor to the vagal reflex pathway has been the focus of attention. Such emphasis is reasonable because of the evidence cited earlier that stated that all CVMs probably receive excitatory inputs from the arterial baroreceptors. There are many more sources, however, of input to the CVMs than those from baroreceptors and from the respiratory phase-linked sources outlined above. Some of these sources from within the central nervous system (CNS) itself are likely to be important in modifying vagal firing to suit complex behavioral patterns, and these are reviewed elsewhere (see Ch. 4).[6,8]

Other reflex inputs that can activate CVMs include both those from the arterial chemoreceptors and those of largely trigeminal origin, such as the oculocardiac reflex and the diving reflex.[9,36–39] All of these inputs have been demonstrated to be subject to the same modulations in effectiveness through the respiratory cycle as the baroreceptor reflex. Again, both centrally generated inspiratory inputs and reflex inputs activated by lung inflation are responsible, and either can be effective alone.[39] Indeed, all reflex inputs that excite CVMs appear to be subject to respiratory mechanisms based on modulation through both centrally generated signals and signals from pulmonary afferent nerves (Fig. 5).

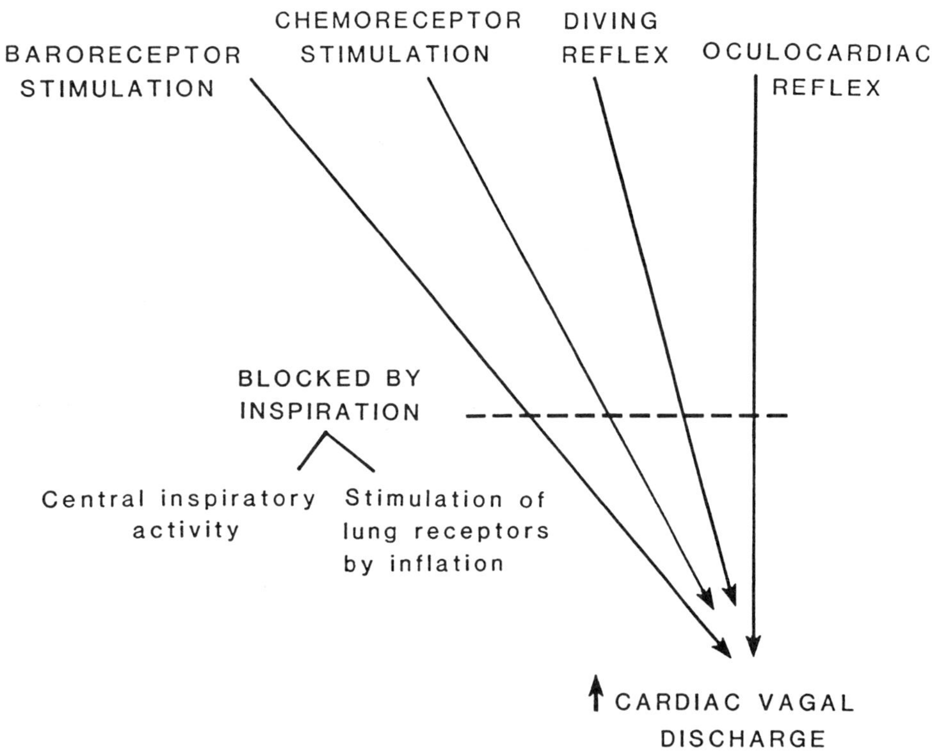

Figure 5. *Summary of respiratory effects on reflexes that activate cardiac vagal efferent nerves.*

Functional Significance of Patterns of Vagal Efferent Nerve Discharge

Clearly, the overall dependence of cardiac vagal discharge on baroreceptor inputs reflects the important role the baroreceptor-cardiodepressor reflex plays in the short-term regulation of arterial pressure. The arterial pulse modulation of vagal discharge occurs because the powerful baroreceptor input itself is strongly pulse-modulated.

The respiratory interactions with the vagal excitatory reflexes are more complex, and are probably best understood in terms of oxygen conservation and delivery. Like the arterial baroreceptor inputs, those from the arterial chemoreceptors are also strongly excitatory to the CVMs, and these excitatory effects are strongly modulated by breathing.[9,24] The chemoreceptors also stimulate respiration; that is, brief chemoreceptor stimuli delivered during the inspiratory phase of breathing stimulates inspiration,[27,40] although they fail to stimulate cardiac vagal nerves.[11,24,27] Thus, if the chemoreceptors are stimulated, and a normal breathing response occurs, that breathing response itself inhibits activation of cardiac vagal nerves. Breathing increases, and the heart can accelerate. At the same time, peripheral vasodilatation occurs as a secondary response to the increased ventilation.[9] All of these responses are consistent with enhancement of oxygen delivery. Chemoreceptor stimulus (in physiological circumstances, probably hypoxia) evokes increased ventilation, tachycardia, and vasodilatation. When the breathing response to chemoreceptor stimulation either fails or is in some way inhibited, however, the secondary effects of increased breathing are lost. In these circumstances, the chemoreceptor stimulus gains access to the CVMs without respiratory-linked inhibition, and bradycardia occurs.[11,24,27] At the same time, peripheral vasoconstriction is prominent.[9] This set of responses is consistent with oxygen conservation. In this case, chemoreceptor stimulus (probably hypoxia) evokes bradycardia and constriction of peripheral vascular beds.

One could postulate that the respiratory modulation of cardiac vagal discharge evolved to ensure appropriate linkages of neural respiratory and cardiovascular control systems and that such linkages enable coordinated function in order to deliver or conserve oxygen appropriately.

This mechanism then manifests itself in other ways in other circumstances. Figure 6, for example, shows how a single level of cardiac vagal motoneuronal tone might be affected at different levels of breathing. During normal breathing, the central inspiratory cycling with its consequent lung inflations periodically interrupts the steady vagal excitatory state, and the result is a bursting of vagal discharge in phase with expiration, and hence sinus arrhythmia occurs. It is noted that, on this model, there is no requirement for the excitatory inputs to the CVMs (baroreceptor, chemoreceptor, and so on) to change with breathing in order for sinus arrhythmia to result. In addition to this process, if the reflex inputs are themselves modulated by

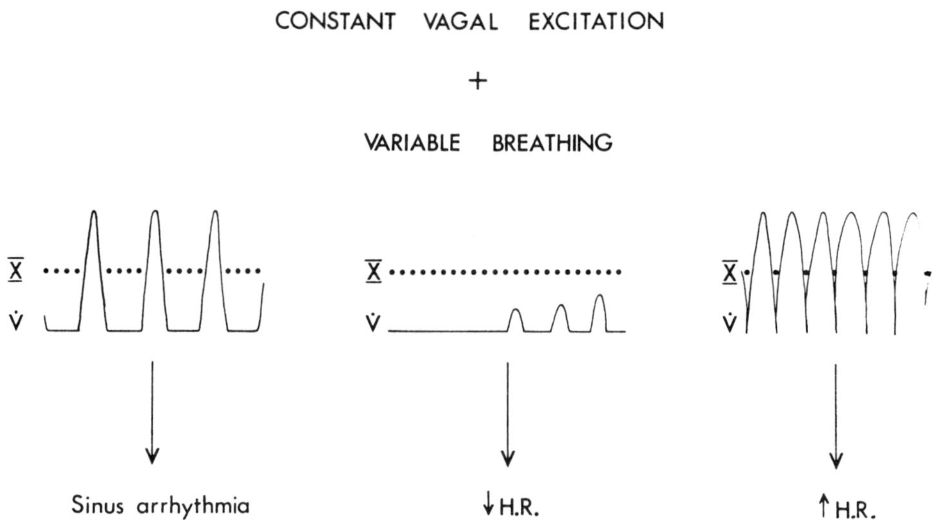

Figure 6. *A diagram summarizing interactions between cardiac vagal discharge and breathing. The dotted line, marked X, represents the firing of cardiac vagal efferent nerves. The lines marked V̇ represent breathing, with inspiration upwards. H.R.: heart rate. In this example, a constant level of vagal excitation is considered. See text.*

breathing, sinus arrhythmia still results. If breathing is depressed or inhibited, the periodic interruption of vagal discharge is removed, and some bradycardia occurs. Of course, if a cardiac vagal stimulus is present at the same time, as would occur with breath-hold diving for example, the effects of removal of respiratory-linked vagal inhibition are further enhanced. Finally, if breathing is increased, even if the background excitation of vagal motoneurons remains unchanged, more frequent and more powerful inhibition of vagal discharge is brought into play, with consequent tachycardia. Voluntary hyperventilation and the hyperpnea of exercise are two common conditions in which this mechanism of cardioacceleration is expected to come into play.

There are immediate potential applications of these findings in the clinic. The clinician wishing to terminate a patient's bout of supraventricular tachycardia is likely to evoke a greater and more sustained increment of discharge in cardiac vagal nerves either by carotid sinus massage or by instructing the patient to hold his or her breath during the maneuver. Similarly, the bradycardia that occurs because of either a simple vaso-vagal faint or excessive vagal discharge induced by ocular or laryngeal surgery can be expected to be offset by an increase in voluntary or artificial ventilation.

References

1. Agostini E, Chinnock JE, Daly M de B, et al: Functional and histological studies of the vagus nerve and its branches to the heart, lungs and abdominal viscera. J Physiol (Lond) 135:182, 1957.

2. Middleton S, Middleton HH, Grundfest H: Spike potentials and cardiac affects of mammalian vagus nerve. Am J Physiol 162:553, 1950.
3. Daly M de B, Evans DHL: Functional and histological changes in the vagus nerve of the cat after degenerative section at various levels. J Physiol (Lond) 120:579, 1953.
4. McAllen RM, Spyer KM: The location of cardiac vagal preganglionic motoneurones in the medulla of the cat. J Physiol (Lond) 258:187, 1976.
5. Jewett DL: Activity of single efferent fibres in the cervical vagus of the dog, with special reference to possible cardioinhibitory fibres. J Physiol (Lond) 175:321, 1964.
6. Spyer KM: Neural mechanisms involved in cardiovascular control during affective behaviour. Trends Neurosci 12:506, 1989.
7. McAllen RM, Spyer KM: The baroreceptor input to cardiac vagal motoneurones. J Physiol (Lond) 282:365, 1978.
8. Spyer KM: Neural organization and control of the baroreceptor reflex. Rev Physiol Biochem Pharmacol 88:23, 1981.
9. Daly M de B: Interactions between respiration and circulation. In Handbook of Physiology. Section 3: The Respiratory System. Part II—Control of Breathing. Bethesda, MD, American Physiological Society, 1986, p. 529.
10. Potter EK: Adaptation of cardiac vagal responses to baroreceptor stimuli in the dog. J Physiol (Lond) 329:411, 1982.
11. Potter EK: Inspiratory inhibition of vagal responses to baroreceptor and chemoreceptor stimuli in the dog. J Physiol (Lond) 316:177, 1981.
12. Rijlant P: L'arrythmic cardiaque respiratoire. Comptes rendu de la societi de Biologie 123:997, 1936.
13. Bainbridge FA: The relation between respiration and the pulse rate. J Physiol (Lond) 54:192, 1920.
14. Linden RJ: Function of cardiac receptors. Circulation 48:463, 1973.
15. Angell-James JE, Daly M de B: The effects of artificial lung inflation on reflexly induced bradycardia associated with apnoea in the dog. J Physiol (Lond) 274:349, 1978.
16. Anrep GV, Pascual W, Rossler E: Respiratory variations of the heart rate. I. The reflex mechanism of the respiratory arrhythmia. Proc R Soc Lond (Biol) 119:119, 1936.
17. Hamlin RL, Smith CR, Smetzer DL: Sinus arrhythmia in the dog. Am J Physiol 210:321, 1966.
18. Lange G, Lu HH, Chang A, et al: Effects of stretch on isolated cat sinoatrial node. Am J Physiol 211:1192, 1967.
19. Keatinge WR: The effect of increased filling pressure on rhythmicity and atrioventricular conduction in isolated hearts. J Physiol (Lond) 149:193, 1959.
20. Pathak CL: Alternative mechanism of cardiac acceleration in Bainbridge's infusion experiments. Am J Physiol 197:441, 1959.
21. Anrep GV, Pascual W, Rossler E: Respiratory variations of the heart rate. II. The central mechanism of the respiratory arrhythmia and the interactions between the central and the reflex mechanisms. Proc R Soc Lond (Biol) 119:218, 1936.
22. Katona PG, Jih F: Respiratory sinus arrhythmia: Noninvasive measure of parasympathetic cardiac control. J Appl Physiol 39:801, 1975.
23. Levy MN, DeGeest H, Zieske H: Effects of respiratory center activity on the heart. Circ Res 18:67, 1966.
24. Gandevia SC, McCloskey DI, Potter EK: Inhibition of baroreceptor and chemoreceptor reflexes on heart rate by afferents from the lungs. J Physiol (Lond) 276:369, 1978.
25. Koepchen HP, Lux HD, Wagner PH: Untersuchungen über Zeitbedarf und zentrale Verarbeitung des pressoreceptor ischen Herzreflexes. Pflügers Arch 273:413, 1961.
26. Koepchen HP, Wagner PH, Lux HD, et al: Über die Zusammenhange zwischen zentralen Erregbarekit refelctorischem Tonus and Atemrhythmus bei der nervosen steverung der Herzfrequenz. Pflügers Arch 273:443, 1961.

27. Haymet BT, McCloskey DI: Baroreceptor and chemoreceptor influences on heart rate during the respiratory cycle in the dog. J Physiol (Lond) 245:699, 1975.
28. Davidson NS, Goldner S, McCloskey DI: Respiratory modulation of baroreceptor and chemoreceptor reflexes affecting heart rate and cardiac vagal efferent nerve activity. J Physiol (Lond) 259:523, 1976.
29. Neil E, Palmer JF: Effects of spontaneous respiration on the latency of reflex cardiac chronotropic responses to baroreceptor stimulation. J Physiol (Lond) 247:16, 1975.
30. Lopes OU, Palmer JF: Proposed respiratory 'gating' mechanism for cardiac slowing. Nature 264:454, 1976.
31. Eckberg D, Orshan CR: Respiratory and baroreceptor reflex interactions in man. J Clin Invest 59:780, 1977.
32. Garcia M, Jordan D, Spyer K: Studies on the properties of cardiac vagal neurones. Neurosci Lett I(suppl):S16, 1978.
33. Spyer KM: Central nervous integration of cardiovascular control. J Exp Biol 100:109, 1982.
34. McAllen RM, Spyer KM: The location of cardiac vagal preganglionic motoneurones in the cat. J Physiol (Lond) 258:198, 1976.
35. Mifflin SW, Spyer KM, Writhington-Wray DJ: Baroreceptor inputs to the nucleus tractus solitarius in the cat: Postsynaptic actions and the influence of respiration. J Physiol (Lond) 399:349, 1988.
36. Daly M de B, Ward J, Wood LM: Modification by lung inflation of the vascular responses from the carotid body chemoreceptors and other receptors in dogs. J Physiol (Lond) 378:13, 1986.
37. Aschner B: Über einen bischer noch nicht beschriebenen reflex vom auge auf Kreislaug und atmung. Wien Klin Wochenschr 21:1529, 1908.
38. Daly M de B, Elsner R, Angell-James JE: Cardiorespiratory control by carotid chemoreceptors during experimental dives in the seal. Am J Physiol 232:H508, 1977.
39. Gandevia SC, McCloskey DI, Potter EK: Reflex bradycardia occurring in response to diving, vasopharyngeal stimulation and ocular pressure, and its modification by respiration and swallowing. J Physiol (Lond) 276:383, 1978.
40. Black AMS, Torrance RW: Respiratory oscillations in chemoreceptor discharge in control of breathing. Respir Physiol 13:221, 1971.

CHAPTER 6

Cardiac Vagal Efferent Nerve Activity

P.J. Schwartz, D. Cerati

A series of experimental and clinical studies, largely discussed in Chs. 29, 32, and 34, have called attention to the consequences of augmented vagal efferent activity. These findings, in turn, are forcing a reappraisal of the knowledge of cardiac vagal activity.

The relationship between vagal activity and cardiac events can be investigated by one of the following methods:

1. indirect markers of vagal activity, such as heart rate variability or baroreflex sensitivity (these measures actually illustrate the result of the summation of vagal and sympathetic influences on the sinus node, and this summation represents vagal activity primarily, but not exclusively);
2. interruption of neural traffic by vagotomy (this procedure eliminates both efferent and afferent vagal traffic);
3. prevention of muscarinic receptor activation by atropine;
4. electrical activation of the cervical vagus (the vagus has to be decentralized prior to stimulation in order to observe only the effect of efferent activation); and
5. recording of neural activity from the cervical vagus or from the cardiac branch of the vagus.

This chapter discusses the technique for recording cardiac vagal efferent activity and the implications derived from these studies.

Vagal Neural Activity

In 1964, Jewett[1] reported a study, performed in anesthetized dogs, that affected much of the subsequent research about vagal neural activity. Due to its importance, the study deserves careful evaluation and analysis of its limitations.

Jewett classified the neural activity of efferent fibers recorded from the cervical vagus into seven functional types, related to what appeared to be their more likely physiological role. Among the recorded fibers, some were probably bronchoconstrictor fibers, and others were motor fibers that innervated the larynx. Two groups of fibers were classified as cardioinhibitory. The major group (Type I) comprised tonically active fibers, whose discharge generally had a cardiac rhythm (thus showing a significant pulse modulation) and whose activity was almost completely suppressed during inspiration. These fibers increased or decreased their firing in response to various reflex stimuli as demonstrated by the appropriate heart rate response. Importantly, the behavior of a small (n = 4) group of efferent fibers recorded from the right cardiac branch of the vagus nerve was in all respects similar to that of the larger group of Type I fibers dissected from the cervical vagus. Jewett also described a second, smaller group of fibers (Type V) that he considered to be cardioinhibitory, except that they exhibited little or no resting discharge. None of the other groups of efferent fibers that he studied behaved in a manner consistent with the cardiovascular responses known to be mediated through the vagus.

Despite the meritorious attempt to identify fibers directed toward the heart among the several different types of vagal efferent fibers running in the cervical vagus, Jewett's study did not overcome the limitation inherent in recording from fibers whose actual target (lungs, heart, stomach, or gut) remained undetermined. This limitation is addressed by recording directly from the cardiac branch of the vagus. Following the initial observations by Iriuchijima and Kumada[2] and by Jewett[1] on a few cardiac fibers, the study that provided the first qualitative and quantitative analysis of the discharge pattern of the contingent of vagal fibers entering the heart was the one published in 1972 by Kunze.[3] After her study, the claim that one is recording with certainty the activity of cardiac-bound vagal fibers when the recording actually takes place from the cervical vagus should be accepted very cautiously. Recordings from the cervical vagus allow the identification of fibers with a pattern of discharge that indicates a baroreceptive input, but the final destination of these fibers remains unproven.

Another important consideration necessary for the evaluation of neural recordings pertains to the number of active fibers that are being recorded. Most studies are based on multifiber recordings, largely because of the significant difficulty in obtaining either single fiber activity or small multifiber preparations with a good signal-to-noise ratio. A small multifiber preparation is one that contains two to three well-identifiable fibers. As scientific journals still publish multifiber recordings or what is usually called "integrated activity," it is fair to call attention to the potential pitfalls of this method. Recording from multifiber preparations or from the whole nerve may be misleading, because the neural activity is quantified not by direct count of individual action potentials (spikes) but by counting whatever passes through a window discriminator within a selected voltage range. This method has been seriously criticized by two careful quantitative analyses.[4,5] Andresen and Yang have concluded that "interactions among spike trains . . . lead to serious underestimation of activity levels" and that "interpretation of results of multifiber or whole nerve recordings whether analyzed with integrative, time-averaging, or spike-counting techniques need to be viewed with caution."[5]

To obtain a recording from vagal fibers directed to the heart, the best anatomical approach is the one depicted in Figure 1. The cardiac branch of the right vagus is traced to the heart as it passes under the azygos vein, and is cut at its entrance in the right atrium. With this method, the recording includes only efferent fibers. It is usually performed by placing small bundles of the nerve across a bipolar platinum electrode and by subsequent splitting of these small bundles under a light microscope. It is a good precaution to ablate the

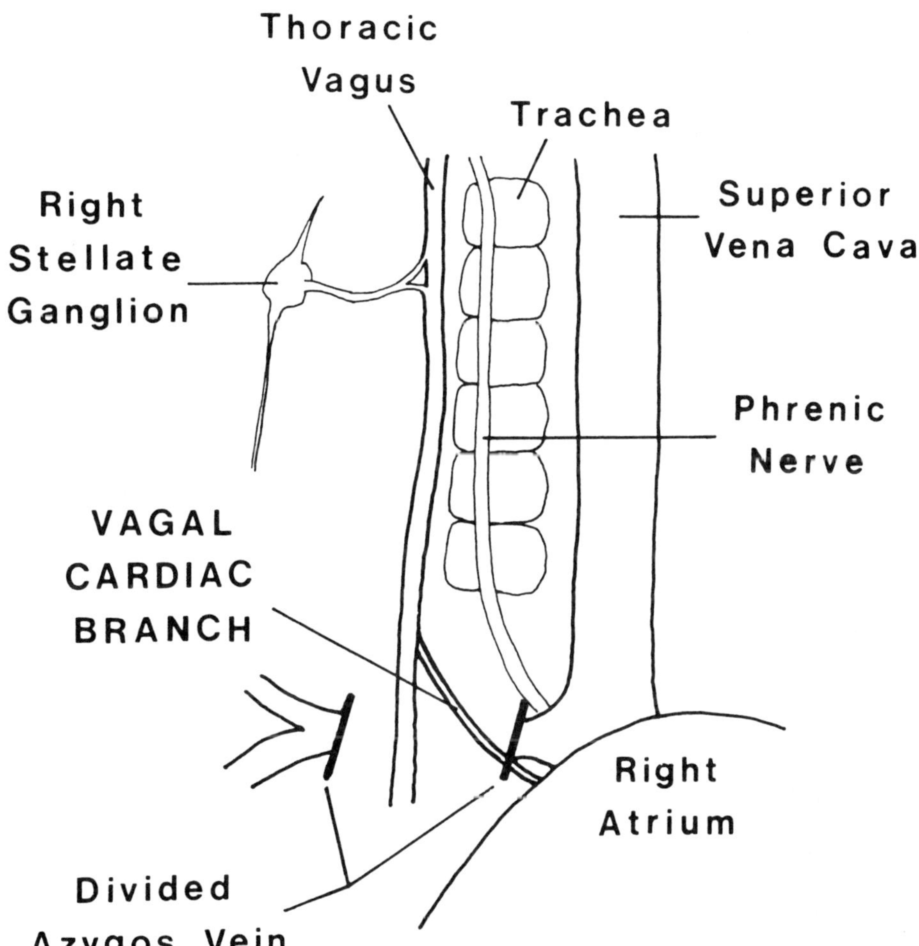

Figure 1. *Schematic drawing of the feline right cardiac nerves as seen from the ventral aspect. The azygos vein is cut to expose the cardiac branch of the vagus nerve as it enters the right atrium. Reproduced with permission from Cerati D, Schwartz PJ: Single cardiac vagal fiber activity, acute myocardial ischemia, and risk for sudden death. Circ Res 69:1389–1401, 1991.*

right stellate ganglion, because some sympathetic fibers run in the cardiac branch of the vagus in proximity with vagal fibers (see below).

An example of the activity of a single cardiac vagal efferent fiber, recorded from the cardiac branch of the right vagus (Fig. 1), and of its modulation by the level of arterial blood pressure is shown in Figure 2.[6] This fiber has a cardiac rhythm which, although very distinctive, is not always evident in vagal efferent fibers. It is also active under control conditions with a systolic blood pressure of 110 mm Hg, and it remains active when blood pressure is lowered. By examining Figure 2, it is evident that, when the quality of the neural recording is good, there is no need for methods such as "integrated activity," "spike analyzers," or "window discriminators," since they all belie poor quality of recordings. The approach of single fiber recording is technically demanding, but it provides safe and reliable quantitative answers.

Modulation of Vagal Activity

Jewett's study[1] implied that all vagal fibers considered to be cardioinhibitory would increase and decrease their discharge with rises and falls in blood pressure, respectively, a behavior consistent with all of them receiving an excitatory input from arterial baroreceptors. It follows that all cardioinhibitory vagal input is from sources that converge on the pathways activated by baroreceptors. Arterial chemoreceptors and pulmonary stretch receptors, however, can alter the discharge of cardiac vagal motoneurons and receive inputs from receptors other than baroreceptors.[7] On the basis of the observations by Jewett, these other sources of input were considered to converge on pathways activated by the arterial baroreceptors. Even though this concept may be largely correct, the assumption by Jewett that *all* cardiac-bound fibers had to behave as the Types I and V fibers described earlier creates a bias. As discussed below, this may or may not bc the case.

A relevant example is provided by a study on the relationship between acute myocardial ischemia and vagal efferent activity.[6] Figure 3 shows the time course of the mean discharge of eight cardiac vagal fibers during a one-hour coronary artery occlusion. It is evident that vagal efferent activity remains at increased levels despite a rather marked decrease in mean arterial blood pressure. This finding implies that input other than the baroreceptive ones can act on efferent vagal fibers.

The relationship between augmented blood pressure and vagal efferent activity is not impervious to modulation from other reflexogenic areas. Schwartz et al[8] demonstrated that activation of afferent cardiac sympathetic fibers,[9] achieved either by electrical or chemical stimulation, has the potential to inhibit tonic vagal efferent discharge, as illustrated in Figures 4 and 5. This "cardio-cardiac sympatho-vagal reflex" represents a neural circuit important from a pathophysiological point of view, because of the activation of cardiac sympathetic afferent fibers during acute myocardial ischemia.[9] Furthermore, the interference exerted by sympathetic afferents on vagal efferents takes place also during

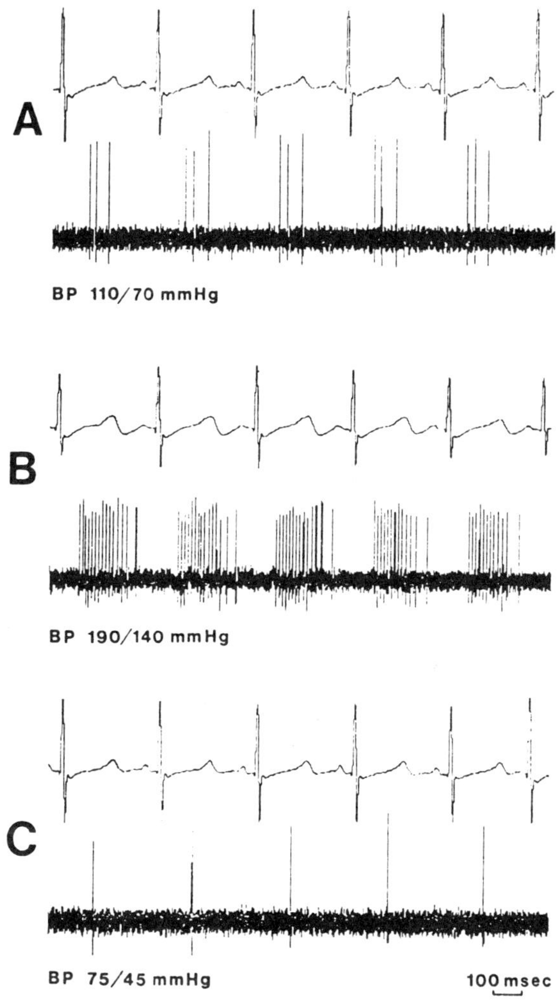

Figure 2. *Tracings showing activity of a single cardiac vagal efferent fiber at three different levels of arterial blood pressure. In each panel, the upper trace shows the electrocardiogram and the lower trace shows the electroneurogram. A: At the resting level of blood pressure, a pulse-synchronous activity, with three impulses in each burst, was present. B: When blood pressure was raised by phenylephrine, the activity of the fiber increased markedly. The activity was still synchronous with the cardiac cycle, but it started 60 msec earlier, and each burst showed more impulses. C: When blood pressure was reduced by bleeding, the activity of the fiber decreased. The activity was still synchronous with the cardiac cycle, but only one impulse per cycle was present. Reproduced with permission from Cerati D, Schwartz PJ: Single cardiac vagal fiber activity, acute myocardial ischemia, and risk for sudden death. Circ Res 69:1389–1401, 1991.*

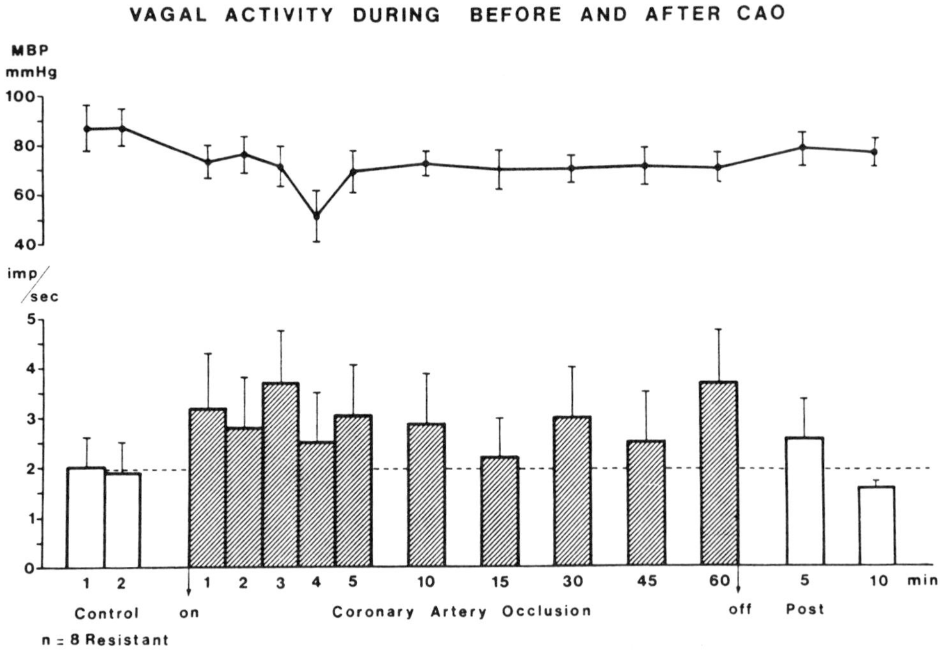

Figure 3. *Analysis of the mean discharge of cardiac vagal fibers in resistant cats before, during, and 5 and 10 min after release of coronary artery occlusion. Data are expressed as imp/sec and averaged every minute. Upper trace: mean blood pressure (MBP). Lower trace: histograms of cardiac vagal activity. Reproduced with permission from Cerati D, Schwartz PJ: Single cardiac vagal fiber activity, acute myocardial ischemia, and risk for sudden death. Circ Res 69:1389–1401, 1991.*

baroreceptor-mediated reflex vagal increase in response to a blood pressure elevation, as clearly illustrated in Figure 6.

Figure 6, derived from an experiment in a chloralose anesthetized cat, contains several important features that are relevant to the present discussion of the characteristics of cardiac vagal efferent activity and are worth a detailed analysis. The first feature is the two single fibers, one vagal and one sympathetic, dissected from the same cardiac branch of the right vagus during the same experiment.[8] This method demonstrated that both vagal and sympathetic efferent fibers travel together in this branch, usually referred to as the cardiac vagus. In this experiment, when the right stellate ganglion was ablated, the activity of the sympathetic fiber disappeared completely, giving final proof of its origin. The second feature is that the single vagal fiber was silent at the resting level of blood pressure, as predicted by Kunze's study,[3] and began to fire—with a cardiac rhythm—only when the blood pressure was elevated by a stenosis of the descending aorta. When the sympathetic afferent cardiac nerves were stimulated at the same level of elevated arterial pressure, a clear reduction of the vagal activity occurred. Thus, this experiment pro-

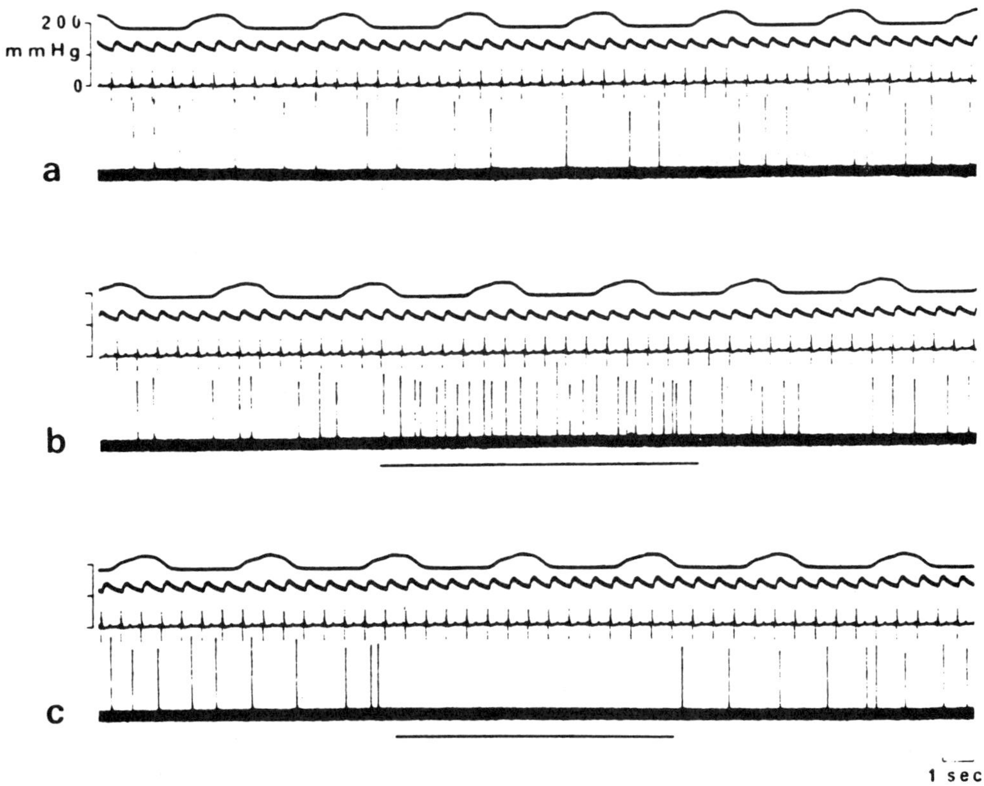

Figure 4. *Effects of electrical stimulation on the neural discharge of a single efferent cardiac vagal fiber in a decerebrate, anesthetized cat. A: Spontaneous activity. B: Electrical stimulation (5 V, 1.5 msec, 30 Hz) of the cut central end of the left cervical vagus. C: Electrical stimulation (10 V, 1.5 msec, 30 Hz) of the cut central end of the left inferior cardiac nerve. The tracings in each section are (from top to bottom): respiration (positive-pressure inflation is an upward deflection), systemic arterial blood pressure, electrocardiogram, and neural activity. Reproduced with permission from Schwartz PJ, Pagani M, Lombardi F, et al: A cardio-cardiac sympatho-vagal reflex in the cat. Circ Res 32:215–220, 1973.*

vided the first direct evidence that a classic baroreceptive reflex (illustrated by the immediate vagal discharge in response to the increase in blood pressure) can be blunted by concurrent activation of cardiac sympathetic afferents.

The final feature illustrated in Figure 6 is the opposite behavior of a cardiac sympathetic efferent fiber. This fiber is already active at a relatively low arterial pressure and is inhibited during the rise in blood pressure, but resumes firing when, at the same level of blood pressure, sympathetic afferents are stimulated. Also of note in Figure 6 is the opposite behavior when, at release of the aortic stenosis, blood pressure falls. The vagal fiber is

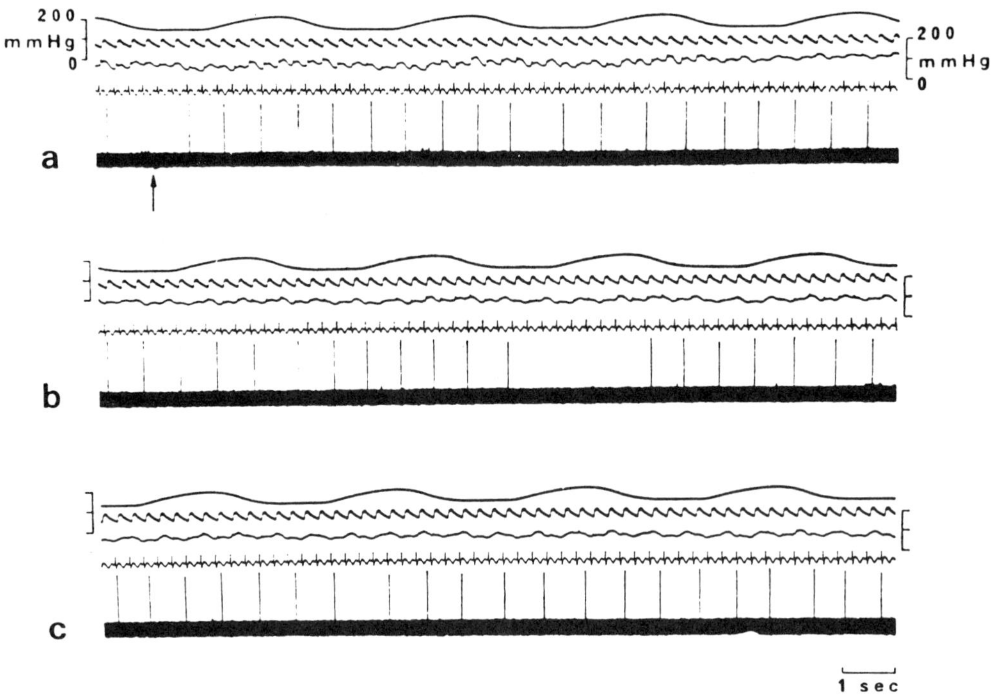

Figure 5. *Effects of intracoronary injection of veratridine on the activity of a single efferent cardiac vagal fiber in an intact, anesthetized cat. At the arrow, 4 μg of veratroidine was injected into the inflow tract of the coronary pump. The time necessary for the drug to reach the main coronary artery was estimated to be about 19 sec. The neural discharge was briefly abolished 21 sec after injection. The continuous tracings (a–c) are (from top to bottom): respiration, systemic arterial blood pressure, electrocardiogram, and neural activity. Reproduced with permission from Schwartz PJ, Pagani M, Lombardi F, et al: A cardio-cardiac sympatho-vagal reflex in the cat. Circ Res 32: 215–220, 1973.*

completely silenced, whereas the sympathetic fiber has an impressive rebound in activity.

The concept of the modulation of baroreceptive reflexes by cardiac sympathetic afferent activity, as proposed in 1973,[8] was subsequently supported by two lines of evidence. The first confirmation was the demonstration that selective removal, by dorsal root section, of the tonic cardiac sympathetic afferent traffic resulted in a potentiation of the reflex bradycardia that follows an increase in blood pressure.[10] The second confirmation was the demonstration, illustrated in Figure 7, that the number of vagal impulses directed toward the sinus node, at the same level of elevated blood pressure, became considerably higher after removal of the left stellate ganglion.[6] When taken all together, these data indicate clearly that both resting and reflex vagal efferent activities are under a tonic restraint exerted by cardiac afferent sympathetic activity.

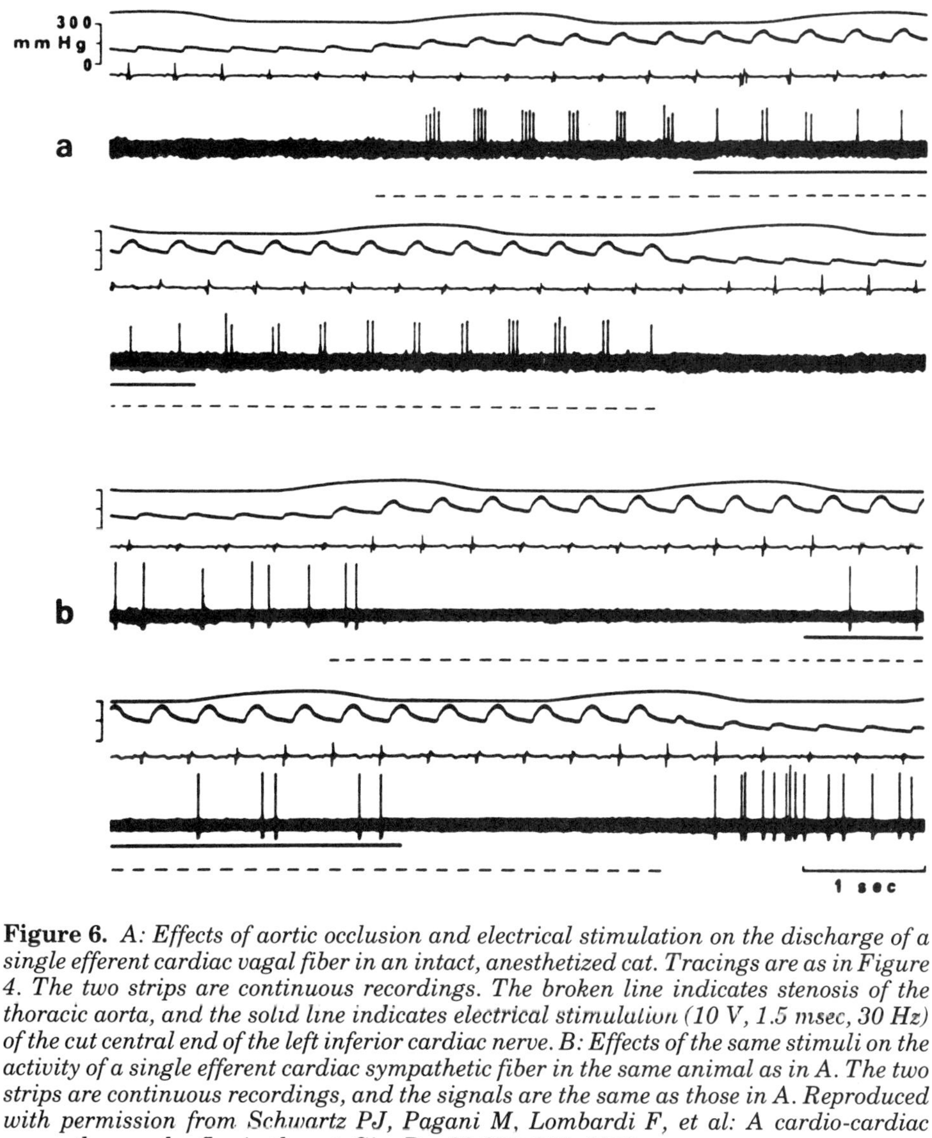

Figure 6. *A: Effects of aortic occlusion and electrical stimulation on the discharge of a single efferent cardiac vagal fiber in an intact, anesthetized cat. Tracings are as in Figure 4. The two strips are continuous recordings. The broken line indicates stenosis of the thoracic aorta, and the solid line indicates electrical stimulation (10 V, 1.5 msec, 30 Hz) of the cut central end of the left inferior cardiac nerve. B: Effects of the same stimuli on the activity of a single efferent cardiac sympathetic fiber in the same animal as in A. The two strips are continuous recordings, and the signals are the same as those in A. Reproduced with permission from Schwartz PJ, Pagani M, Lombardi F, et al: A cardio-cardiac sympatho-vagal reflex in the cat. Circ Res 32:215–220, 1973.*

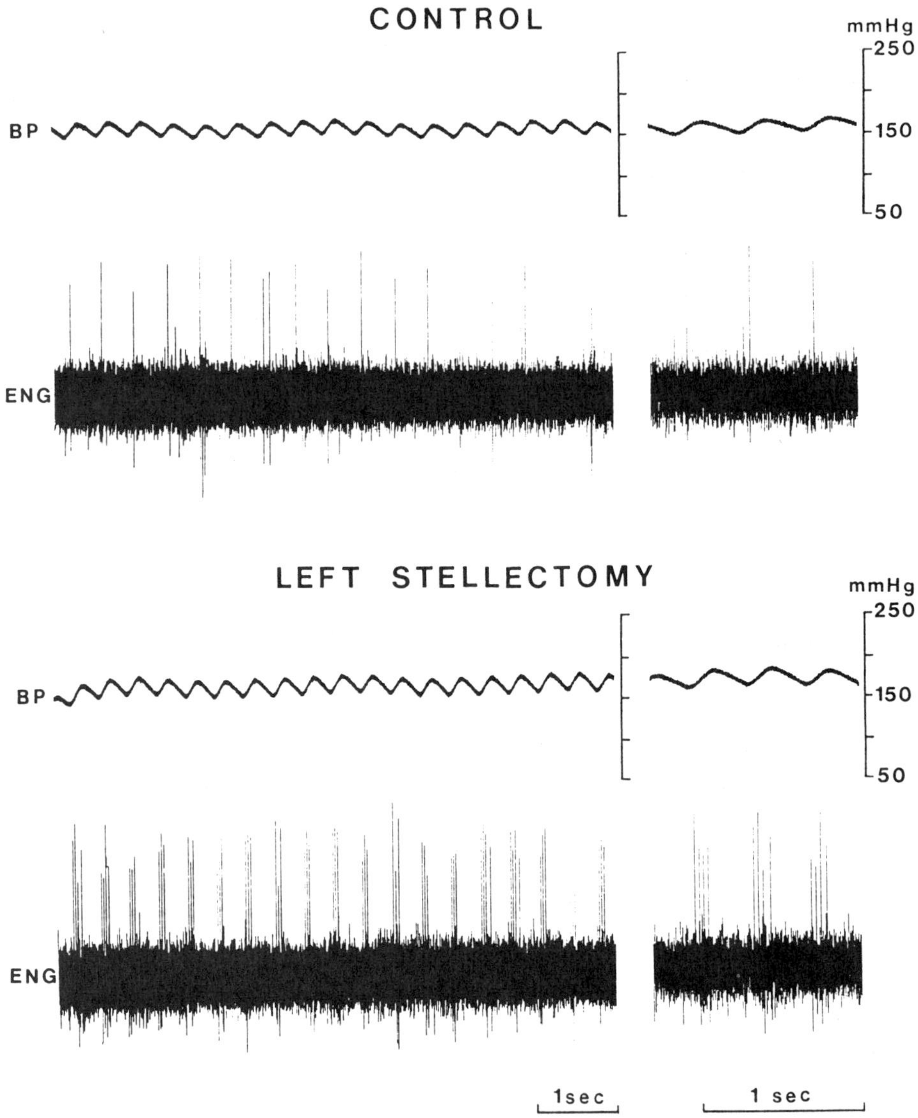

Figure 7. *Tracings showing activity of a single cardiac vagal efferent fiber, at the same blood pressure levels induced by phenylephrine before and after left stellectomy. The fiber shows a pulse-synchronous activity. In each panel, the upper trace shows the blood pressure, the lower trace shows the electroneurogram. Reproduced with permission from Cerati D, Schwartz PJ: Single cardiac vagal fiber activity, acute myocardial ischemia, and risk for sudden death. Circ Res 69:1389–1401, 1991.*

Conclusions

Changes in cardiac vagal efferent activity are often inferred by changes in heart rate. These inferences, however, may be incorrect. The information derived by the most currently used markers of vagal activity, such as heart rate variability and baroreflex sensitivity, should be matched whenever possible by the occurrence of concordant changes in cardiac vagal efferent activity. Also, the study of how and to what extent a given stimulus or intervention may affect the vagal control of the heart requires the direct demonstration of specific changes in neural activity. This finding can be accurately determined by directly recording vagal activity in either single fibers or in small multifiber preparations.

References

1. Jewett DL: Activity of single efferent fibers in the cervical vagus of the dog, with special reference to possible cardioinhibitory fibers. J Physiol 175:321, 1964.
2. Iriuchijima J, Kumada M: Efferent cardiac vagal discharge of the dog in response to electrical stimulation of sensory nerves. J Physiol 13:599, 1963.
3. Kunze DL: Reflex discharge patterns of cardiac vagal efferent fibers. J Physiol (Lond) 222:1, 1972.
4. Hopp FA, Seagard JL, Kampine JP: Comparison of four methods of averaging nerve activity. Am J Physiol 251:R700, 1986.
5. Andresen MD, Yang M: Interaction among unitary spike trains: implications for whole nerve measurements. Am J Physiol 256:R997, 1989.
6. Cerati D, Schwartz PJ: Single cardiac vagal fiber activity, acute myocardial ischemia, and risk for sudden death. Circ Res 69:1389, 1991.
7. Spyer KM: Neural organization and control of the baroreceptor reflex. Rev Physiol Biochem Pharmacol 88:23, 1981.
8. Schwartz PJ, Pagani M, Lombardi F, et al: A cardio-cardiac sympatho-vagal reflex in the cat. Circ Res 32:215, 1973.
9. Malliani A, Recordati G, Schwartz PJ: Nervous activity of afferent cardiac sympathetic fibers with atrial and ventricular endings. J Physiol (Lond) 229:457, 1973.
10. Gnecchi-Ruscone T, Lombardi F, Malfatto G, et al: Attenuation of baroceptive mechanisms by cardiovascular sympathetic afferent fibers. Am J Physiol 253:H787, 1987.

PART II

Biochemistry of the Vagal Control System

CHAPTER 7

Biochemistry and Pharmacology of the Cardiac Muscarinic Receptors

W.R. Roeske, H.I. Yamamura

The parasympathetic nervous system exerts important regulatory control over heart rate and myocardial contractility.[1] The negative chronotropic and inotropic effects of vagal stimulation or acetylcholine (ACh) infusion on atrial tissue has been established in intact animal, isolated heart, and muscle bath preparations.[1–8] Similar effects of vagal stimulation or ACh infusion on ventricular performance have also been demonstrated.[1,2,5] These effects, however, are blocked by atropine in both atrial and ventricular tissues. The receptor for the postganglionic vagal innervation has been classified as muscarinic cholinergic.[1]

Biochemical studies of these cardiac muscarinic receptors (mAChRs) permit correlation of physiological studies with receptor affinities and densities and aid the discovery of drug mechanisms at the receptor level. Initial attempts to characterize the mAChRs of the heart included stimulation of guanylyl cyclase by muscarinic agents[9,10] and measurement of ACh, the native neurotransmitter, and choline acetyltransferase (ChAT), the biosynthetic enzyme.[11,12] These measurements, however, have been complicated by the presence of cardiac parasympathetic ganglia containing cholinergic nicotinic nerve endings.

A direct ligand-binding receptor assay for cardiac mAChRs avoids the limitations of the previous methods. The first attempts to directly measure receptors with radioligands occurred in the 1960s when [^{3}H] atropine and [^{3}H] propranolol were used to label muscarinic uptake sites in the intestinal smooth muscle and adrenergic uptake sites in atria.[13,14] These pioneering experiments demonstrated that radioisotopically-labelled hormones or toxins could be used to directly make such measurements. The technology of this measurement required a molecule that had both high specific activity and high affinity so that a very small portion of the total cellular tissue (sometimes less than 1–10,000th of total tissue) could be measured. The technique also had to be

From *Vagal Control of the Heart: Experimental Basis and Clinical Implications* edited by MN Levy, PJ Schwartz © 1994, Futura Publishing Co. Inc., Armonk, NY.

Table 1.
Radioligand-Binding Studies of Muscarinic Cholinergic Receptors[a]

Receptor Selectivity	*Radioligand*	*K_d (nM)*[b]	*Reference*[c]
Nonselective Antagonist	[^{3}H](−)Quinuclidinyl benzilate	0.02–0.06	(15,16)
	[^{3}H](−)-N-methyl-QNB	0.1–0.4	(17,18)
	[^{3}H](−)-N-methylscopolamine	0.15–0.30	(19)
	[^{3}H](+)Benzetimide	0.4	(20)
	[^{3}H]Propylbenzilylcholine mustard	10–20[d]	(21)
M_1-selective Antagonist	[^{3}H]Pirenzepine	4–10	(22)
M_2-selective Antagonist	[^{3}H]AF-DX 116	20	(23)
Nonselective Agonists	[^{3}H](+) Cis-methyldioxolane	1–2	(24)
	[^{3}H]Oxotremorine-M	1–2	(25)

[a]Only the frequently used radioligands are listed.

[b]K_d values were obtained from the literature, which vary between laboratories depending on the species of animals, tissues, and the assay conditions used. If more than one binding site was found for a radioligand, only the K_d values for the high-affinity sites are given in the table.

[c]References are the papers that have described the pharmacological characteristics of the radioligand with feasible methods.

[d]Reversible binding followed by irreversible alkylation of the receptors.

Modified with permission from Vickroy TW, Watson M, Yamamura HI, et al: Muscarinic cholinergic receptor binding: Utilization in drug research. In RA O'Brien (ed): Receptor Binding and Drug Research. New York, NY, Marcel Dekker Inc, 1986, p. 300. Courtesy of Marcel Dekker, Inc.

highly efficient in separating bound from free ligands. Furthermore, the assay needed low, nonspecific backgrounds so that it would be possible to clearly demonstrate the separated ligand-receptor complex. Table 1 presents summaries of radioligand-binding studies of mAChRs. The application of these assays to the heart are discussed below.

Shortly after the first demonstration of central nervous system (CNS) mAChRs and of ileal smooth muscle mAChRs by the [^{3}H]quinuclidinyl benzilate assay, the ligand was applied to the demonstration of cardiac mAChRs.[15] As indicated in Table 1, the advent of subtype-specific radioligands has more recently appeared. Furthermore, ligands such as [^{3}H](−)N-methyl-QNB, which have better kinetic properties, are hydrophilic, and do not penetrate membranes under normal physiological conditions, have been used.[17,18] In order to further advance the biochemistry and molecular biology of cardiac mAChRs, several chapters in this book employ the direct measurement of cardiac mAChRs by ligand-binding methods. This chapter presents some of the methods used in evaluating the biochemistry of mAChRs, lessons learned from the biochemical measurement of cardiac mAChRs, pharmacological characterization of cardioselective (M_2) muscarinic antagonists, biochemical measurements on cloned mAChRs, and new directions in this area.

Methods for Measurement

The use of the filtration technique in the measurement of mAChRs has been recently reviewed.[26–28] Table 1 summarizes some of the initial characterizations of muscarinic cholinergic radioligands.

[^{3}H](−)QNB-Binding Assay

Yamamura and Snyder initially introduced the nonselective antagonist [^{3}H](±)quinuclidinyl benzilate in 1974.[16] This initial publication, while widely cited, used a ligand that was both racemic and of low-specific activity. Major advances in the assay rapidly followed the introduction of a ligand of higher-specific activity. The first detailed cardiac mAChR measurements using [^{3}H]QNB were published in 1978.[15] This article described conditions for the measurement of binding that have been successfully applied in the cardiac receptor biochemistry field. The ligand used in this study was also racemic. Consequently, it was extremely important to choose low concentrations of the radioligand since, at higher concentrations (about 100fold higher), the second stereoisomer begins to bind. More recently, the single stereoisomer [^{3}H](−)MQNB became available. Higher concentrations of the radioligand can now be used without the complications that are due to interference from the second isomer. These concentrations can be useful for evaluating competition curves since it is possible to occupy essentially 100% of the receptors with [^{3}H](−)QNB at a concentration three times the dissociation constant (K_d) before displacement with the unlabelled drug.

The widespread use of [^{3}H](−)QNB as a muscarinic antagonist of choice reveals several desirable properties:

1. commercial availability;
2. excellent stability and resistance to biotransformation;
3. high-specific activity for muscarinic sites in all tissues that results in an excellent signal-to-noise ratio (specific- to nonspecific-binding ratio) often in excess of 10;
4. a relatively slow dissociation rate for the ligand-receptor complex that allows highly reproducible separation of the bound from free ligand in the filtration machine; and
5. high and relatively uniform affinity for all mAChRs (since it is nonselective).

Several precautions using [^{3}H](−)QNB should be noted. The disadvantage of a slow rate of complex formation (association) requires a long association time. In order to have adequate equilibrium conditions, approximately five times the association half-time (T one half)[29] must be used. Nonequilibrium conditions have also been examined, but this approach is not generally practical.[30] Alterations of greater than 10% in free concentration can sometimes be observed in cardiac tissues and in other tissues with low overall mAChR density.

An important consideration is whether all sites should be measured or whether only the externalized membrane sites should be measured. This issue can be resolved by the comparison of tertiary compounds such as [^{3}H]($-$)QNB with quarternary compounds such as [^{3}H]($-$)N-methyl-QNB.[17,18] Previously, comparisons between the use of [^{3}H]($-$)N-methyl-scopolamine and [^{3}H]($-$)QNB have been done in classic studies in heart cells by Galper et al.[31,32] These investigators showed that an analysis of internalization as opposed to downregulation can be addressed using these ligands.

[^{3}H]Pirenzepine-Binding Assay

Competition curves using pirenzepine (PZ) firmly established the concept of pharmacologically unique mAChR subtypes.[33,34] Our laboratory introduced [^{3}H]pirenzepine ([^{3}H]PZ)[23,35] as a useful radioligand to measure the high-affinity PZ-binding sites in selected tissues. Radioligand-binding studies with [^{3}H]PZ revealed marked degrees of heterogeneity among the [^{3}H]($-$)QNB-binding sites. This approach was subsequently correlated with the identification of unique receptors by molecular biological techniques.[36] This subject is discussed further in Ch. 8. A particularly useful demonstration of the subtype selectivity was done in an initial comparison by Watson et al[35] in which it was demonstrated that [^{3}H]PZ-binding could be identified in the heart. This finding is often ignored when it is stated that the mAChRs in the heart are uniformly of the M_2 subtype. The location of these high-affinity PZ-binding sites remains controversial, but this issue is probably a feature of the complexity of the cardiac tissue. Thus, high-affinity PZ-binding most likely is associated with the M_1 receptors or possibly the M_0 or M_4 receptors that can be localized in nerve cells, ganglionic cells, smooth muscle cells, and other cells that are a part of the cardiac homogenates. [^{3}H]PZ is an effective ligand, although not as easily measured as [^{3}H]($-$)QNB. Glass fiber filters bind a high proportion of [^{3}H]PZ; thus, it is extremely important to pretreat the filters with a cationic polymer polyethyleneimine (PEI). In addition, stability of high-affinity PZ-binding is not always demonstrable and should be carefully monitored in experiments where tissue homogenates or soluble preparations are stored for prolonged periods of time, even if temperatures are low. Such an experiment certainly must be done if the temperatures for the assay are greater than 30°C.

[^{3}H]AF-DX 116-Binding Assay

Recent studies that indicated that PZ was selective for subtypes of the mAChRs in the brain (M_1) subsequently led to the concept that the radioligand {11[[2-[(diethylamino)methyl]-1-piperidinyl]acetyl]-5,11-dihydro-6H-pyrido-[(2,3-b)][(1,4)]benzodiazepine-6-one} (AF-DX 116) was a member of a family of cardioselective muscarinic antagonists.[37] The two compounds are structurally related but demonstrate opposite receptor selectivity as seen in the inhibition of vagally-induced bradycardia (atria) compared with the presence of pressor responses (ganglia) in the pithed rat. Such functional data were correlated with selectivity in antagonist-binding studies. These studies showed that AF-DX 116 had novel muscarinic-binding properties and identified a high-affinity population of sites in the heart. [^{3}H]AF-DX 116 was also used to characterize the cardiac mAChRs that label the dominant subset of the total receptors in the heart.[23] These receptors showed pharmacological characteristics of the M_2 type. A small but significant population of M_2 receptors in the brain was also identified.

Advantages of using [^{3}H]AF-DX 116 include subtype selectivity and the identification of the unique high-affinity quality of AF-DX 116 as separate from the high-affinity PZ subtype. One disadvantage of using [^{3}H]AF-DX 116 is an affinity that is low and, thus, difficult for application in a filtration assay. Thus, use of lower temperatures is often essential in the assay conditions. Another disadvantage is the instability of [^{3}H]AF-DX 116 in room air. Consequently, the general applicability of [^{3}H]AF-DX 116-binding to identification of cardiac mAChR has been somewhat limited. Nonetheless, a useful application of this technique has occurred in studies in the rat brain in which quantitative autoradiography of the M_2 mAChRs using the [^{3}H]AF-DX 116 as a label showed a unique regional distribution separable from both the nonselective compounds such as [^{3}H](−)QNB and selective compounds such as [^{3}H]PZ.[38] Newer generations of subtype-selective M_2 muscarinic antagonists will probably be needed in order to facilitate the biochemical measurements of the cardiac mAChRs.

[^{3}H](+)Cis-Methyldioxolane-Binding Assay

[^{3}H](+)Cis-Methyldioxolane (CD) is a potent muscarinic agonist.[39] Our laboratory has pioneered the use of this prototype compound for direct muscarinic agonist radioligand-binding.[24,40-42] The technical complexities inherent in studies of agonist-binding, however, are extreme. Consequently, the use of an agonist ligand to label the binding sites should be undertaken cautiously. Vickroy et al[42] described a reproducible method for using PEI to measure [^{3}H](+)CD-binding. The use of a low ionic strength buffer containing 1 to 5 mM Mg^{++} promotes a stable high-affinity state. In tissues such as the heart, which have high proportions of high-affinity agonist states, as much as 10% of the total number of muscarinic sites can be measured. Using this assay, it has been shown that there are subtypes of mAChRs that have high and low affinity for selective antagonists such as PZ and AF-DX 116. The measurement of these agonist-binding sites are extremely sensitive to ACh and other endogenous factors such as the guanine nucleotides and ions. Consequently, membranes are generally washed and preincubated. The agonist CD adheres to many surfaces including glass and plastic; therefore, a variety of precautionary steps must be taken.[26,42]

Lessons from the Biochemical Measurement of Cardiac Muscarinic Receptors

Locations and Numbers

The biochemical characteristics of the $[^3H](-)$QNB receptor complex allow for the determination of the receptor density since it is possible to demonstrate a saturable population of receptor sites. The determination of both the high-affinity K_d and the maximum-binding (B_{max}) are readily obtainable from cardiac homogenates. The regional distribution of mAChRs in the rabbit heart (Table 2) establishes the general concept that atrial tissue contains six to nine times more mAChRs than the ventricular tissues. These data are consistent with the relative influence of vagal stimulation and ACh infusion on atrial versus ventricular performance.[2–5]

One study also showed that the number of receptors differed in rabbit, rat, and guinea pig hearts. The guinea pig heart contained 178 ± 13 fmol/mg protein, the rat heart contained 144 ± 13 fmol/mg protein, and the rabbit heart contained 57.2 ± 4.3 fmol/mg protein.[15] The distribution of mAChRs in the human heart is an important question. Table 3 indicates specific $[^3H](-)$QNB binding in 25 cardiac regions of six human hearts examined at autopsy.[43] This study was normalized to present the data as a percent of the left atrial membrane values, since the results of tissues obtained from autopsies were highly variable. Nonetheless, the general concept that atria have higher concentrations of mAChRs than ventricles is clearly seen. Increased densities of mAChRs in putative regions of conduction tissues can also be seen. These findings have been more recently confirmed using better samples and techniques.[44] Studies that examined mAChR distribution in other species have also been published.[45–47] In these studies, the general concept that the atria have more receptors than the ventricles can also be seen.

Table 2.
Regional Distribution of Muscarinic Cholinergic Receptors in Rabbit Heart[a]

Region	*Receptor Density*	*Percentage of Total Cardiac Receptors*
Left Ventricle	37.4 ± 7.6	28.9 ± 2.22
Right Ventricle	52.7 ± 10.2	15.2 ± 1.01
Ventricular Septum	58.1 ± 6.5	$21.7 \pm .74$
Right Atrium	200.0 ± 13.5	17.8 ± 1.32
Left Atrium	302.4 ± 30.9	16.4 ± 2.86

[a] $[^3H]$QNB receptor densities, B_{max}, and percentage of total cardiac receptors. Values listed are from Scatchard plots determined on regions of each of five rabbit hearts and are means ±SEM (fmol/mg protein). Modified with permission from Fields JZ, Roeske WR, Morkin E, et al: Cardiac muscarinic cholinergic receptors: Biochemical identification and characterization. J Biol Chem 253:3251, 1978.

Table 3.
Regional Distribution of Muscarinic Receptors in Human Heart[a]

Region	*Specific [^{3}H](-)QNB Bound (% of Average Left Atrial Value[a])*	*Rank Order*
Left Atrium		
Left Atrial Appendage	112 ± 7	3
Left Atrial Free Wall	88 ± 7	8
Right Atrium		
Right Atrial Appendage	126 ± 15	1
Right Atrial Free Wall	94 ± 14	6
Right Atrial Superior Portion	93 ± 19	7
Intra-atrial Septum		
Muscular Septum	121 ± 17	2
Left Ventricle		
Posterior Wall, Epicardial	44 ± 8	11–13
Posterior Wall, Endocardial	25 ± 4	20
Posterior Papillary Muscle	44 ± 6	11–13
Apex, Epicardial	52 ± 8	9
Apex, Endocardial	37 ± 7	17
Anterior Papillary Muscle	32 ± 10	19
Right Ventricle		
Free Wall	50 ± 8	10
Papillary Muscles	33 ± 9	18
Ventricular Septum		
Right Side	42 ± 6	16
Left Side	44 ± 9	11–13
Center	43.5 ± 8	14–15
Conduction System		
Sinus Node	101 ± 17	5
AV Node	110 ± 20	4
Left Bundle, With Muscle	43 ± 5	14–15
Vessels		
Aorta	2.9 ± 0.8	23
Pulmonary Artery	2.8 ± 0.9	24
Coronary Artery	2.7 ± 2.3	25
Superior Vena Cava	19 ± 8	21
Valves		
Mitral	8 ± 4	22

[a]Values represent the mean±SEM for 25 regions of 6 human hearts taken at autopsy from patients who died of noncardiac causes. Modified with permission from Roeske WR, Yamamura HI: Muscarinic cholinergic receptor regulation. In HI Yamamura, RW Olsen, E Usdin (eds): Psychopharmacology and Biochemistry of Neurotransmitter Receptors. New York, NY, Elsevier North-Holland, 1980, p. 101.

Agonist Affinity States of the Receptor

Agonist states of the mAChR were detected shortly after the introduction of antagonist ligands.[43,48,49] At that time, the effect of guanine nucleotides had been demonstrated in several laboratories.[50–52] These initial observations linked the mAChRs to the family of G-protein coupled receptors. Molecular biological techniques have since confirmed and established these initial observations as being pivotal in the correct classification of the mAChR as a member of the family of G-protein coupled receptors with seven transmembrane signals. A complex literature has emerged that describes the super high-, high-, and low-affinity states for muscarinic agonists in cardiac homogenates and in other tissue homogenates. The advent of molecular biology has not eliminated the problem of agonist affinity states, even with the simple identification of specific molecules with specific affinity states for agonists. Thus, it appears that agonist affinity states are also present for each cloned mAChR and may relate to different degrees of complex formation within the binding sites or with other molecules involved in coupling. Such a proposal was advanced in 1980[43] that was based on the model of Rodbell[53] and Jakobs.[54] Accordingly, the mAChR represented an inhibitory nucleotide complex which was operationally defined, while the β-adrenergic receptor represented a stimulatory nucleotide complex. The number of factors involved in the complex included the two receptors, two agonists, two nucleotide-binding proteins, sodium, magnesium, and the binding site of adenylate cyclase.[43] It was postulated that nine reaction components could be complexed in many ways. Accordingly, the multiple states of the agonist-binding site were proposed to depend on different combinations of these factors. Recent studies with cloned receptors and in reconstitution systems have clearly identified the importance of the G-protein α-subunit and its ability to alter muscarinic agonist affinity. Nonetheless, the role of ions and the presence of guanosine triphosphate (GTP) can be shown even in subtype-selective studies.[55–57]

Antagonist Affinity States of the Receptor

The mAChR antagonist heterogeneity has been resolved through the identification of five mAChR subtypes.[36,58-64] The concept that antagonist affinity is different for cardiac tissue than that for other tissues can usually be resolved with this concept. It is not always appreciated, however, that in low ionic strength buffers which contain high concentrations of magnesium, antagonist affinity states can be demonstrated for single types of mAChRs.[65] This phenomenon can be avoided by using physiological buffers.

Receptor Regulation

Early studies of upregulation and downregulation measuring saturation isotherms from whole tissue homogenates showed interesting and clinically relevant interactions with drugs such as tricyclic antidepressants, antipsychotic neuroleptics, and clinically used antiarrhythmic compounds.[15,66,67] Such changes have been shown in animal models that underwent cardiac transplantation, received 6-hydroxy-dopamine treatment, and experienced chronic cholinesterase inhibition.[47,68]

Alterations in Diseases

Cardiac diseases have not, to this time, been associated with changes in cardiac mAChRs. The 46% decrease of mAChRs in the caudate nucleus, however, is characteristic of Huntington's disease.[69] Changes in the hippocampus and in certain regions of the cerebral cortex have led to a mAChR hypothesis in Alzheimer's disease.[70] Human mAChRs have been detected using positron emission tomography based on the use of a ligand similar to QNB. Thus, it is possible that, with further advances, differences in receptor density may be detected for specific diseases.

Alterations in Development

The influence of ACh on spontaneous atrial rate in the fetal mouse heart in organ culture at various ages was first demonstrated by Wildenthal in 1973.[71] All hearts respond to ACh by developing bradycardia and, at higher concentrations, they demonstrate sinus arrest. The cholinergic response in the 13- to 14-day fetal heart is much less than that in older ages and the response appears to have a relationship to developmental state. We demonstrated a dose-dependent response by ACh in the presence of 1 μM physostigmine to block the cholinesterase and ACh breakdown.[72,73] Thus, at the same concentration of ACh (1 μM), the heart rate response improves from 44% inhibition in the 13- to 14-day fetal mouse heart to 75% inhibition in the 21- to 22-day fetal mouse heart. The increased sensitivity that occurs between these two stages correlates with the increasing density of [^{3}H](−)QNB sites in this period of development. This work was extended into the neonatal period in a study with selective ligands. Comparing [^{3}H](−)QNB with [^{3}H]PZ, it was shown that the cardiac receptor development in the heart was of a different subtype than that predominantly developing in the brain.[74]

Drug Interactions

One of the most useful aspects of the biochemical determination of mAChRs is the rapid determination of direct interaction between the drug of interest and the mAChR measured by radioligand-binding techniques.[15] Table 4 presents the relative potencies of drugs in reducing [^{3}H](−)QNB-binding in rabbit heart homogenates. These data demonstrate the pharmacological specificity of a mAChR. For example, the stereoisomers of dexetimide are more than 2000fold separable. Both ACh and other muscarinic agonists are effective in inhibiting binding. Hill coefficients for antagonists are near one, while the Hill coefficients for agonists are shallow. Nicotinic cholinergic drugs such as

Table 4.
Relative Potencies of Drugs in Reducing [^{3}H]QNB-Binding in Rabbit Heart Homogenates

Drug	K_i(μM)
Muscarinic	
3-Quinuclidinyl benzilate	0.000036
p-OH-QNB	0.00070
Atropine	0.00105
Oxotremorine	0.144
Acetylcholine (physostigmine 1 μM)	0.490
Carbamylcholine	0.528
Dexetimide	0.00069
Levetimide	1.45
Nicotinic[a]	
Benzylquinonium	0.1
Decamethonium	2.15
d-Tubocurarine	4.31
Choline Uptake Inhibitor	
Hemicholinium-3	3.43
Neuroleptics	
Chlorpromazine	0.17
Droperidol	1.57
Spiroperidol	3.22
Haloperidol	27.6
Cardioactive[b]	
Atropine	0.00105
Imipramine	0.173
Quinidine	2.04
Xylocaine	18.2
Procainamide	47.8

[a]Nicotinic agents that were ineffective were α-bungarotoxin at 5.0 μM, hexamethonium at 10.0 μM, and nicotine at 100.0 μM.

[b]Cardioactive agents that were ineffective were: propanolol and ouabain at 100.0 μM and dopamine, norepinephrine, phenylephrine, taurine, histamine, and levo-alprenolol at 10 μM. Other agents that were ineffective at 10 μM were γ-amino butyric acid, glycine, picrotoxin, bicuculline, physostigmine, phenelzine, choline, deanol, and 2,4-dinitrophenol. Modified with permission from Fields JZ, Roeske WR, Morkin E, et al: Cardiac muscarinic cholinergic receptors: Biochemical identification and characterization. J Biol Chem 253:3251, 1978.

α-bungarotoxin and nicotine do not inhibit the cardiac mAChR. Most classical noncholinergic drugs have little or no effect on the cardiac mAChR; however, some agents such as benzilquinonium, decamethonium, and curare show considerable potency in the micromolar range on the mAChRs of the rabbit heart. The nonselectivity of these agents has been subsequently confirmed in several studies. The actions of neuroleptics as cardioactive drugs have also been studied and many commonly used drugs have been found to be active at the mAChRs. Interestingly, ouabain, a cardiac glycoside, does not have any direct effect on the cardiac mAChR, thus supporting the concept that the vagal effect of ouabain is indirect by acting through the CNS. Commonly used antiarrhythmic agents such as quinidine, lidocaine, and procainamide have K_i values that are in the range of 2.0, 18, and 48 μM, respectively. The tricyclic antidepressant imipramine and many of the antipsychotic and neuroleptic drugs are effective inhibitors of QNB-binding. Thus, chlorpromazine, droperidol, spiroperidol, and haloperidol have K_i values of 0.17, 1.57, 3.2, and 28 μM, respectively. This work has been subsequently confirmed and, more recently, has been extended to the cloned mAChR types.

Subtypes of Muscarinic Receptors

Perhaps the most important lesson learned from ligand-binding is the establishment of a firm, scientific, and biochemical basis for the discovery of mAChR subtypes through the use of molecular biological techniques. Characteristics for putative mAChR types have been proposed.[49] Evidence included differential antagonist-binding based on labelled PZ between regions rich in the M_2 receptors, such as the heart, and regions rich in the M_1 receptors, such as the cerebral cortex, the hippocampus, and corpus striatum. Differential drug affinity was demonstrated by PZ, AF-DX 116, and the weak partial agonist, McN-A-343. The linkage to adenyl cyclase was seen predominantly for the putative M_2 receptor, while the linkage for the phosphoinositol response was seen predominantly for the putative M_1 receptor. Each of these responses was identified using biochemical assays. In Chapter 8, the basis for the initial cloning of the mAChR and the subsequent distinction between the five subtypes of receptors are delineated. This subject has also been reviewed in Mei et al.[36]

Pharmacological Characterization of Cardioselective Muscarinic Antagonists

The field of mAChR subtypes stemmed in large part from the availability of the selective antagonist PZ.[33,34] Cardioselective muscarinic antagonists, however, have only been recognized for about 10 years. The first symposium that directly addressed the issue of cardioselective muscarinic antagonists was the 36th Annual Fall Meeting of the American Society for Pharmacology and Experimental Therapeutics, Boston, Mass, August 22, 1985 (chaired by A. Giachetti and U. Mittman).[37] Selective cardiac muscarinic antagonists were also recently reviewed.[36]

PZ was the first anticholinergic agent that discriminated between two distinct subtypes of mAChRs that were subsequently named the M_1 and M_2 receptor subtypes.[33] Further analysis of structural activity and structural selectivity relationships for a large number of tricyclic analogs synthesized and made available at the Karl Thomae Corporation resulted in the discovery of AF-DX 116, which appeared to have an opposite receptor selectivity.[75,76] The selectivity was obtained by modifying the side chain rather than changing the tricyclic portion of the molecule. Initial characterization in both functional and biochemical studies showed classical M_2 receptor selectivity compared to the M_1 receptor selectivity.[37] These observations were extensively confirmed by others. As seen in Table 5, AF-DX 116 selectivity for the five cloned mAChRs is still maintained, although the affinity to the M_4 subtype is very close to the M_2 value. These results explain a portion of the controversy that exists in the literature regarding the selectivity of AF-DX 116 in tissues containing mixtures of receptors. The selectivity for AF-DX 116 has also been confirmed by the use of the radiolabelled compounds.

The alkaloid himbacine has been shown to be cardioselective in pharmacological experiments.[79,80] The degree of selectivity has been modest. Difficulties in the analysis of the selectivity of himbacine are also explained by the mixtures of the M_2 and other mAChRs seen in both the CNS and in peripheral tissues.

Methoctramine has also been recently advanced as a cardioselective compound. Based on the pharmacological studies of Melchiorri and others,[81–84] methoctramine appears to act at more than one site and demonstrates allosteric activity. An additional allosteric compound (gallamine) has also been recognized as M_2 selective. The use of allosteric drugs for receptor subtype classification, however, should be discouraged since their binding is not a simple interaction between a drug and a receptor.

While the classical approach for pharmacological studies has been the direct comparison of atrial responses with either ileal responses or other physiological preparations, the information in Table 5 indicates that the use of the cloned receptors should prove valuable in rapidly screening potential

Table 5.

Comparison of pA_2 Values from the Literature[a] with pK_i Values from Inhibition Constants Derived from Ligand/[^{3}H](-)MQNB Competition Studies on Intact Murine Fibroblast Cell-(B82) Lines for the Rat m1, m2, m3, m4, and m5 Genes

Ligand		*m1* *LK3-3*[b]	*m2* *M2LKB2-2*[c]	*m3* *M3LKB1-2*	*m4* *M4LKB1-5*	*m5* *M5LKB6-4*
Atropine	pK_i	9.29	9.00	9.28	9.66	9.43
	pA_2	9.4–9.7	8.8–9.0	8.8–9.8		
4-DAMP	pK_i	8.92	8.21	9.19	9.15	8.92
	pA_2	8.7–9.1	7.5–7.9	8.5		
HHSiD	pK_i	7.85	6.71	7.99	7.69	7.37
	pA_2	7.4	6.5–6.7	7.7–7.9		
Pirenze-pine	pK_i	7.89	6.38	6.72	7.07	7.06
	pA_2	7.8–8.0	6.2–6.8	6.4–6.7		
AF-DX 116	pK_i	6.27	7.04	5.95	6.57	5.66
	pA_2	5.9–6.4	6.7–7.0	5.3–6.1		

[a]See Mei L, Roeske WR, Yamamura HI[36] for primary references for the functional data (pA_2 values).

[b]Data from Mei L, et al.[77]

[c]Data from Lai J, et al,[62] except for 4-DAMP and HHSiD, which are from Kashihara K, et al.[78]

antagonists for their selectivity. Accordingly, as seen in Table 5, the affinity of antagonists for specific receptors is within the ranges obtained from physiological preparations. These results can be obtained by radioligand-binding experiments using intact cells under physiological conditions that mimic the conditions of the physiological preparations used to obtain the Schild plots that yield the functional measures of antagonist affinities.

Biochemical Measurements Derived from Cloned Muscarinic Receptors

Structure-Function Relationships

The resolution of mAChR heterogeneity by the methods of molecular pharmacology resulted in the identification of five genes for the mAChRs. The pharmacological characterization of cholinergic receptors with muscarinic antagonist, however, has clearly identified only three or possibly four types of receptors.[36] Based on the classical description of the biochemical characteristics of the mAChR and pharmacological studies with PZ and AF-DX 116, the principal cardiac mAChR type has been identified as M_2 and the type of gene expressed for this receptor has been identified as the m_2. Major efforts to characterize the subtypes of receptors have been implemented that attempt to link the pharmacological heterogeneity with the biochemical heterogeneity. Studies are still underway. Biochemical characteristics of the M_2 receptor include 466 amino acids that have been identified in the porcine, rat, or human species.[58,59,85,86] The messenger RNAs detected in Northern blots are 6.5 Kb in the porcine species,[87] but only 5.2 Kb in humans.[86] In addition to the expected location in the heart,[85,87] messenger RNA for the rat M_2 has also been found in the medulla pons[85] and in the small and large intestines, trachea, and urinary bladder.[87] Beyond providing a basis for understanding the biochemical characteristics of mAChRs, the methods of molecular biology can provide useful models for the study of receptor structure-function relationships.

In this connection, the polymerase chain reaction (PCR), which was originally developed by Saiki et al,[88] was used to amplify the rat m_2 mAChR gene. Following amplification, the polymerase reactions were examined by electrophoresis on 1.2% agarose gels. The DNA sequences were cloned into the pGem7. The sequences (Fig. 1) were determined by the dideoxy chain termination method.[89] The sequences were then excised in a recombinant plasmid and cloned into the eukaryotic expression vector, pIIβAPr-1-neo (a gift from Dr. Lionel Kettes, Stanford University), which has a SalI-HindIII-BamHI polylinker downstream from the human β-actin promoter.[90] Recombination was then achieved by directional cloning. The recombinant plasmid was transfected into the murine fibroblast cell-line B82 by the calcium phosphate precipitation method[91] and the transfected cells were selected for the expression of neomycin resistance. Clones that were propagated in selective medium continuously for at least one month were chosen for further studies. These

A

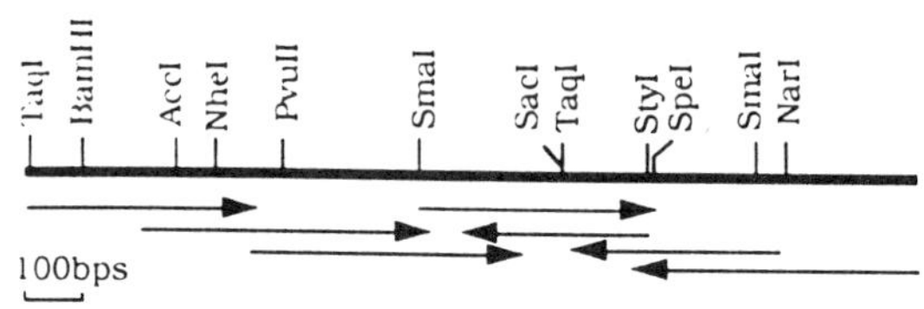

B

```
ATGAATAACTCAACAAACTCCTCGAACAATGGCTTGGCTATTACCAGTCCTTACAAGACA   60
M  N  N  S  T  N  S  S  N  N  G  L  A  I  T  S  P  Y  K  T
TTTGAAGTGGTATTTATTGTCCTTGTGGCTGGATCCCTCAGTCTGGTGACCATCATTGGG  120
F  E  V  V  F  I  V  L  V  A  G  S  L  S  L  V  T  I  I  G
AACATTCTGGTCATGGTTTCCATTAAAGTCAACCGCCACCTTCAGACTGTCAACAATTAC  180
N  I  L  V  M  V  S  I  K  V  N  R  H  L  Q  T  V  N  N  Y
TTCTTGTTCAGCCTGGCCTGTGCTGACCTCATCATAGGTGTTTTCTCCATGAACTTGTAT  240
F  L  F  S  L  A  C  A  D  L  I  I  G  V  F  S  M  N  L  Y
ACCCTCTACACTGTGATTGGCTACTGGCCTTTGGGACCTGTAGTATGTGACCTTTGGCTA  300
T  L  Y  T  V  I  G  Y  W  P  L  G  P  V  V  C  D  L  W  L
GCATTGGACTATGTTGTCAGCAATGCCTCCGTTATGAATCTCCTCATCATCAGCTTTGAT  360
A  L  D  Y  V  V  S  N  A  S  V  M  N  L  L  I  I  S  F  D
AGATACTTCTGTGTCACGAAACCTCTGACCTACCCAGTTAAGCGGACCACAAAAATGGCA  420
R  Y  F  C  V  T  K  P  L  T  Y  P  V  K  R  T  T  K  M  A
GGCATGATGATTGCAGCTGCGTGGGTCCTTTCCTTCATCCTCTGGGCCCCAGCCATTCTC  480
G  M  M  I  A  A  A  W  V  L  S  F  I  L  W  A  P  A  I  L
TTCTGGCAGTTCATCGTAGGGGTGAGGACTGTGGAGGATGGGGAGTGCTATATTCAGTTC  540
F  W  Q  F  I  V  G  V  R  T  V  E  D  G  E  C  Y  I  Q  F
TTTTCCAATGCGGCCGTCACCTTCGGCACTGCCATTGCAGCTTTCTATCTGCCTGTCATC  600
F  S  N  A  A  V  T  F  G  T  A  I  A  A  F  Y  L  P  V  I
ATCATGACTGTGCTCTATTGGCATATATCCCGGGCAAGCAAGAGTAGAATAAAGAAGGAA  660
I  M  T  V  L  Y  W  H  I  S  R  A  S  K  S  R  I  K  K  E
AAGAAGGAACCTGTGGCCAACCAAGACCCAGTATCTCCGAGTCTGGTGCAAGGAAGAATT  720
K  K  E  P  V  A  N  Q  D  P  V  S  P  S  L  V  Q  G  R  I
GTAAAGCCAAACAATAACAATATGCCTGGTGGTGATGGCGGCCTGGAACACAACAAGATC  780
V  K  P  N  N  N  N  M  P  G  G  D  G  G  L  E  H  N  K  I
CAGAATGGCAAGGCTCCACGGGACGGCGTGACTGAAAACTGTGTTCAGGGGGAGGAGAAA  840
Q  N  G  K  A  P  R  D  G  V  T  E  N  C  V  Q  G  E  E  K
GAGAGCTCCAATGATTCGACGTCAGTCAGTGCTGTGGCCTCCAATATGAGAGATGATGAG  900
E  S  S  N  D  S  T  S  V  S  A  V  A  S  N  M  R  D  D  E
ATAACCCAGGATGAAAACACAGTTTCCACTTCGCTGGGCCACTCCAGAGATGACAACTCT  960
I  T  Q  D  E  N  T  V  S  T  S  L  G  H  S  R  D  D  N  S
AAGCAAACATGCATCAAAATTGTCACCAAGGCCCAAAAGGGTGATGTGTACACCCCAACG 1020
K  Q  T  C  I  K  I  V  T  K  A  Q  K  G  D  V  Y  T  P  T
AGTACCACTGTAGAACTAGTTGGGTCGTCGGGTCAGAATGGGGATGAAAAGCAGAACATT 1080
S  T  T  V  E  L  V  G  S  S  G  Q  N  G  D  E  K  Q  N  I
GTAGCCCGCAAAATCGTGAAGATGACCAAGCAGCCTGCCAAAAAGAAGCCTCCACCATCC 1140
V  A  R  K  I  V  K  M  T  K  Q  P  A  K  K  K  P  P  P  S
CGGGAAAAGAAAGTGACCAGGACAATCTTGGCTATCCTGTTGGCTTTCATCATAACGTGG 1200
R  E  K  K  V  T  R  T  I  L  A  I  L  L  A  F  I  I  T  W
GCGCCATACAATGTCATGGTGCTCATCAATACTTTCTGTGCACCCTGCATCCCCAATACA 1260
A  P  Y  N  V  M  V  L  I  N  T  F  C  A  P  C  I  P  N  T
GTATGGACAATTGGCTACTGGCTCTGTTACATCAATAGCACCATCAATCCGGCCTGCTAT 1320
V  W  T  I  G  Y  W  L  C  Y  I  N  S  T  I  N  P  A  C  Y
GCGCTTTGTAATGCCACCTTCAAAAAGACTTTTAAGCACCTCCTCATGTGTCATTACAAG 1380
A  L  C  N  A  T  F  K  K  T  F  K  H  L  L  M  C  H  Y  K
AACATAGGCGCTACACGGTGA                                        1401
N  I  G  A  T  R  *
```

Figure 1. *The coding region of the rat M_2 gene amplified from the rat genomic DNA by polymerase chain reaction (PCR). A: Restriction analysis. B: Nucleotide sequence and deduced amino acid sequence. Arrows denote origin, direction, and extent of sequence determination. Asterisks represent termination of the open reading frame. Reprinted with permission from Life Sci, 47, Lai J, Bloom JW, Yamamura HI, et al: Amplification of the rat m2 muscarinic receptor gene by the polymerase chain reaction: Functional expression of the M2 muscarinic receptor, 1990, Pergamon Press Ltd.*

clones were subsequently maintained in a nonselecting growth medium.[62] Consequently, a model for the continuous expression of the cardiac mAChR was achieved in a transfected cell-line. This process led to the use of radioligand-binding assays using the ligand [^{3}H](−)MQNB with intact cells in culture. Furthermore, inositol lipid hydrolysis could be performed by a method modified frorn Berridge et al.[92] Adenosine 3′,5′-cyclic phosphate (cyclic AMP) formation studies could also be performed on intact cells using a method of detection modified from Gilman.[93] The results of these studies indicated that the transfection of the m_2 gene into B82 cells gave rise to cells that expressed a high level of binding for the nonselective muscarinic antagonist. The M_2 type that was characteristic of this binding was clearly shown by the rank order of potency for the antagonists: himbacine, AF-DX 116, and methoctramine had high affinity for these receptors, while PZ had low affinity.[36] Since stable transfection of the rat M_1 receptor in the same native cell-line (B82) had been previously demonstrated, a comparative study could be done in which it was shown that the ratio of affinities was compatible with the concept that the cell system (M2LKB2–2 cells) expressed the M_2 receptor. The pharmacological definition of the M_2 type was based on the rank order of potency of AF-DX 116>PZ as well as selectivity for PZ and AF-DX 116 for the receptors (Fig. 2; Table 5). There are differences in the comparison between the above results

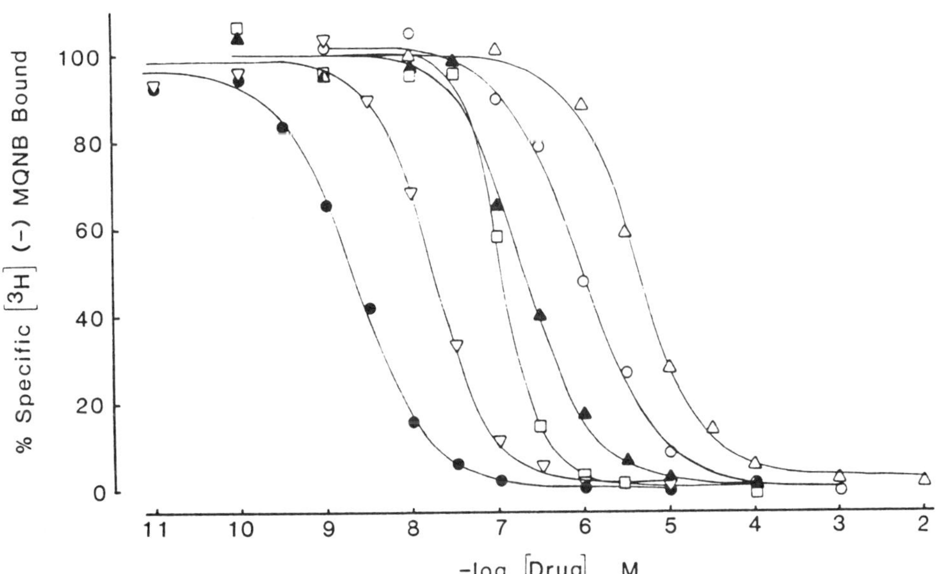

Figure 2. *Inhibition curves from ligand/[^{3}H](−)MQNB competition studies on M_2LKB2–2 cells. The IC_{50} values and Hill coefficients (in parentheses) were 2.1 nM (0.99) for atropine (closed circle); 17.5 nM (1.3) for himbacine (reverse open triangle); 117 nM (1.9) for methoctramine (open square); 202 nM (1.1) for AF-DX 116 (closed triangle); 941 nM (0.96) for pirenzepine (PZ) (open circle); and 4.2 μM (1.2) for carbachol (CCH) (open triangle). Data are representative of three independent determinations that are summarized in Lai J, et al.[62]Reprinted with permission from Life Sci, 47, Lai J, Bloom JW, Yamamura HI, et al: Amplification of the rat m2 muscarinic receptor gene by the polymerase chain reaction: Functional expression of the M2 muscarinic receptor, 1990, Pergamon Press Ltd.*

derived from the intact system, which has physiological buffers, and the results of other studies using membrane-binding assays. For example, the K_i values for AF-DX 116 for receptors expressed from the porcine m_2 gene and the human m_2 gene were 700 nM[94] and 186 nM,[84] respectively. In contrast, PZ showed a 30fold difference in both the above system as well as that of others studies.

Carbachol (CCh) inhibited [^{3}H]($-$)MQNB-binding to cells with a K_i value of 2.0 μM. Unlike the results obtained in cardiac homogenates, the Hill coefficient for this inhibition was steep. The adenylate cyclase system was shown to be inversely coupled to this response. Thus, 10 μM of CCh inhibited forskolin-stimulated cyclic AMP formation by 55% (Fig. 3). This response was also blocked by pertussis toxin (PTX) at a concentration of 1 ng/ml, which showed that these receptors are coupled through a PTX-sensitive G-protein in

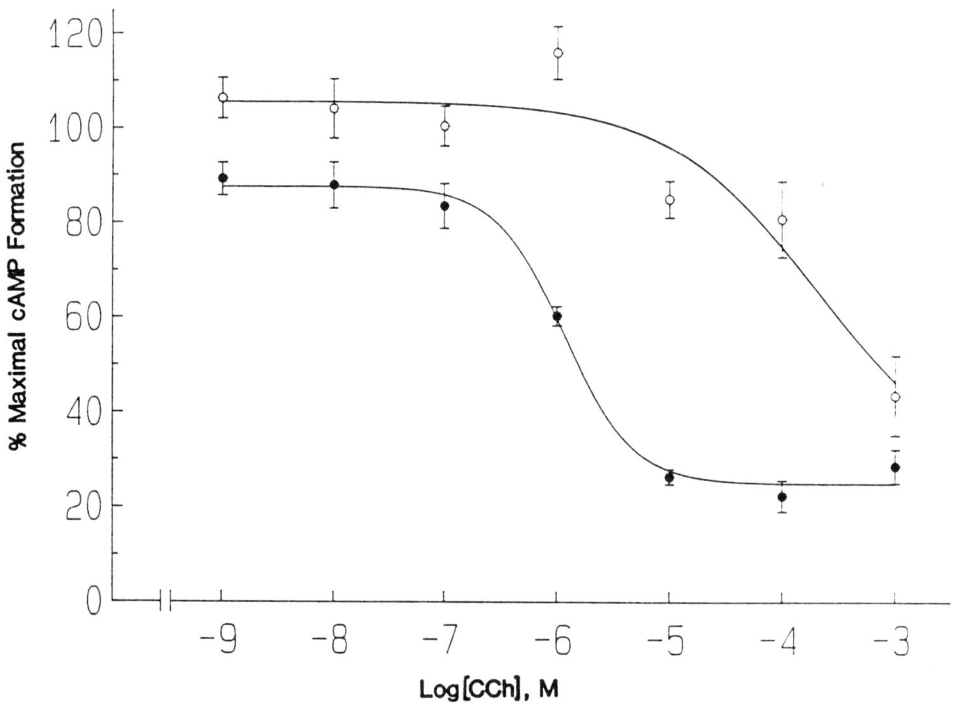

Figure 3. *Inhibition of forskolin-stimulated adenosine 3′5′cyclic phosphate (cyclic AMP) formation by CCh (closed circle) or CCh in the presence of 1 μM atropine (open circle) in the M_2LKB2–2 cells. The dose effect of CCh on cyclic AMP concentration in the presence or absence of atropine in these cells stimulated with 100 μM forskolin is presented as a percentage of the maximal stimulated cyclic AMP content in the cells. The EC_{50} value of CCh in inhibiting cyclic AMP formation by forskolin was 1.2 μM ($n=8$). The maximum reversal of 75% of the forskolin-stimulated cyclic AMP content was observed. Error bars represent ± standard error of the mean of the data points. Methods are described in Lai J, et al.[96] Reproduced with permission from Lai J, Waite SL, Bloom JW, et al: The m2 muscarinic acetylcholine receptors are coupled to multiple signaling pathways via pertussis toxin sensitive guanine regulatory proteins. J Pharm Exp Ther 258:938, 1991. Copyright © American Society of Pharmacology and Experimental Therapeutics.*

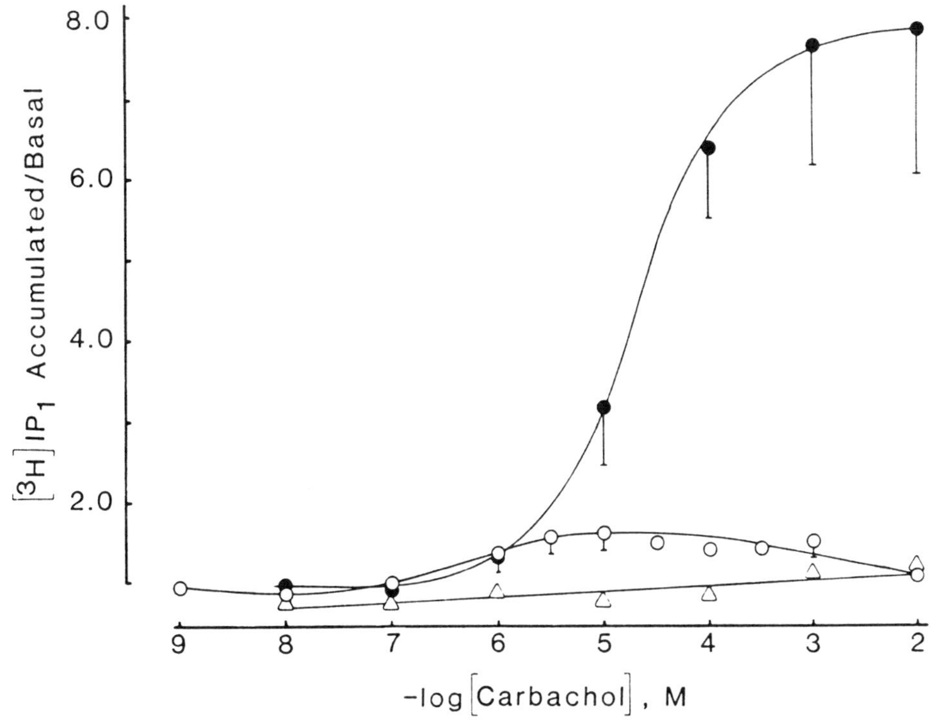

Figure 4. *The effect of CCh on the stimulation of [^{3}H]IP$_1$ formation in LK3–3 cells (closed circles) that express the muscarinic M$_1$ receptor compared with M$_2$LKB2–2 cells (open circles) that express the M$_2$ mAChR and with M$_2$LKB2–2 cells (open triangle) in the presence of 1 μM atropine. Data points represent the mean ± standard error of the mean of three determinations expressed as ratios of the total [^{3}H]IP$_1$ accumulated divided by basal [^{3}H]IP$_1$ accumulated. The EC$_{50}$ value for CCh in stimulating [^{3}H]IP$_1$ formation in the LK33 cells was 15.8 μM, while the EC$_{50}$ value for CCh in stimulating [^{3}H]IP$_1$ formation in the M$_2$LKB2–2 cells was 0.6 μM. Reprinted with permission from Life Sci, 47, Lai J, Bloom JW, Yamamura HI, et al: Amplification of the rat m2 muscarinic receptor gene by the polymerase chain reaction: Functional expression of the M2 muscarinic receptor, 1990, Pergamon Press Ltd.*

this system (Fig. 5). Interestingly, CCh was shown to stimulate phosphoinositol (IP) hydrolysis in these cells (Fig. 4). The response was extremely small compared with responses obtained in a family of cells expressing the M$_1$ receptor. The clinical or scientific relevance of this small response is unclear; it may represent an important mechanism for receptor coupling, but this response was also linked via a PTX-sensitive G-protein (Fig. 6).

Coupling in the Cloned Muscarinic Receptors

It has been proven that the M$_2$ ACh receptor can be coupled to multiple signaling pathways via PTX-sensitive guanine nucleotide regulatory proteins.

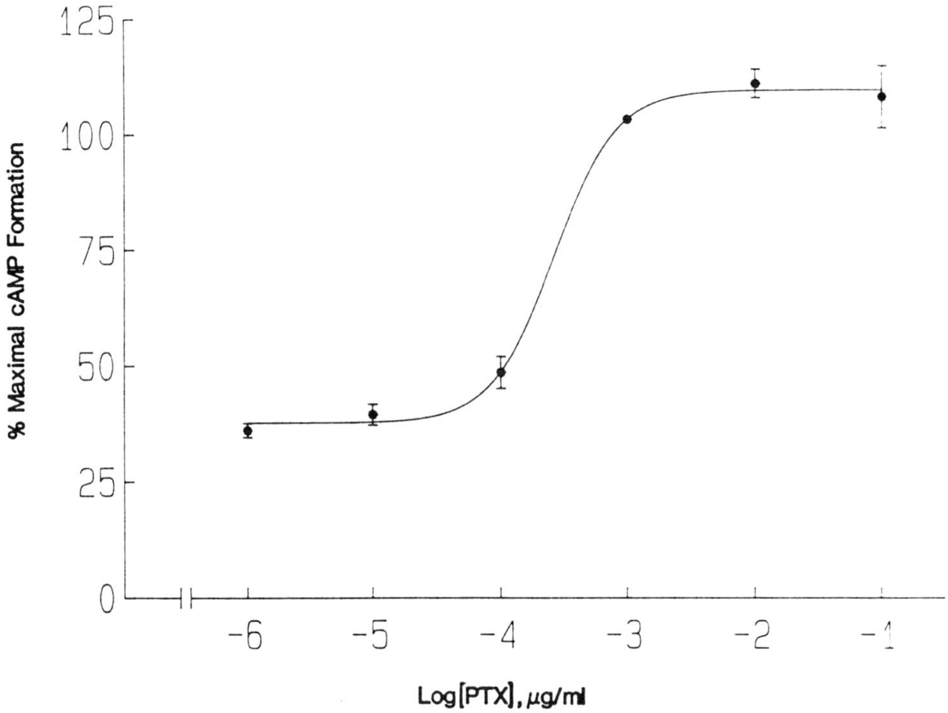

Figure 5. *The dose effect of PTX on CCh-induced (10 μM) inhibition of forskolin-stimulated cyclic AMP formation. The stimulated cyclic AMP level by 100 μM forskolin (9.4 to 14.4 pmol per million cells) was taken as 100%. Maximal inhibition of forskolin-stimulated cyclic AMP formation was attained at 10 μM CCh at a plateau value of 25 to 30% of the forskolin-stimulated cyclic AMP content, which remained in the absence of PTX. The inhibitory effect of CCh was reversed by increasing doses of PTX so that, at 1 ng/ml of PTX, the maximal stimulatory effect of 100 μM forskolin was totally restored in the presence of CCh. The IC_{50} value of this PTX effect was 0.26 ng/ml. Data represent the mean ± standard error of the mean from three independent experiments. Reproduced with permission from Lai J, Waite SL, Bloom JW, et al: The m2 muscarinic acetylcholine receptors are coupled to multiple signaling pathways via pertussis toxin sensitive guanine regulatory proteins. J Pharm Exp Ther 258:938, 1991. Copyright © American Society of Pharmacology and Experimental Therapeutics.*

Studies with cloned receptors [64,5] have shown that the M_2 gene is inversely coupled to cyclic AMP, and this response was also shown to be PTX-sensitive. It has also been shown that CCh stimulated IP_1 formation in the cloned mAChR cells.[96] Thus, Figure 4 shows that, in the clone containing the M_1 receptor, the accumulation of IP_1 is as dramatic as expected. In the clone expressing the M_2 receptor, however, there is a very small but significant response as related to the accumulation of IP_1. The dose response curve for inhibition of forskolin-stimulated cyclic AMP formation by CCh is shown in Figure 3. Thus, the EC_{50} value (concentration at which 50% of the functional response is inhibited) of CCh in inhibiting cyclic AMP formation by forskolin is 1.2 μM (n = 8). PTX inhibits the effect of CCh and the IC_{50} value (concentration at which 50% of the biochemical response is inhibited) of the PTX effect is 0.26 ng/ml (Fig. 5). The IC_{50} value for PTX inhibiting the CCh-mediated IP_1 accumulation is 0.14 ng/ml (Fig. 6). There is no effect of PTX on the inhibition of PI hydrolysis by LK3–3 cells up to a concentration of 1 μg/ml of PTX. Consequently, PTX distinguished the G-proteins that coupled the rat M_1 and M_2 receptors to phosphosinositol hydrolysis.

Binding in the Cloned Cells

Binding to cloned mAChRs has been studied in this transfected cell model. Table 5 compares the pharmacological characterization of cholinergic receptors with muscarinic antagonists and the initial studies of binding to selected antagonists. Table 5 compares functional physiological data from the review of pharmacologically-defined $M1_1$, M_2, and M_3[36] with the binding data on selected antagonist and mAChRs cloned in all five mAChRs studied at physiological conditions.[76] There is excellent correlation between the functional studies and the binding data for the M_1, M_2, and M_3 receptors. M_4 and M_5 receptors are included for completeness. No selective compounds, to this point, have been identified specifically for the M_4 and M_5 receptors. Figure 2 illustrates competition curves obtained from the rat m_2 clone. Under physiological conditions, the order of potency characteristic of an M_2 receptor can be identified.

New Directions

Functional regulation in cloned cells is an important area for new investigation. In preliminary data, it has been shown that receptor regulation from agonists and partial agonists can occur and that these studies can be correlated with functional results.[97] This new area of investigation will permit a careful dissection of the mechanism of internalization, downregulation, and desensitization. The use of specific mutants will also permit an understanding of the regional domains of the molecule that are important for different portions of

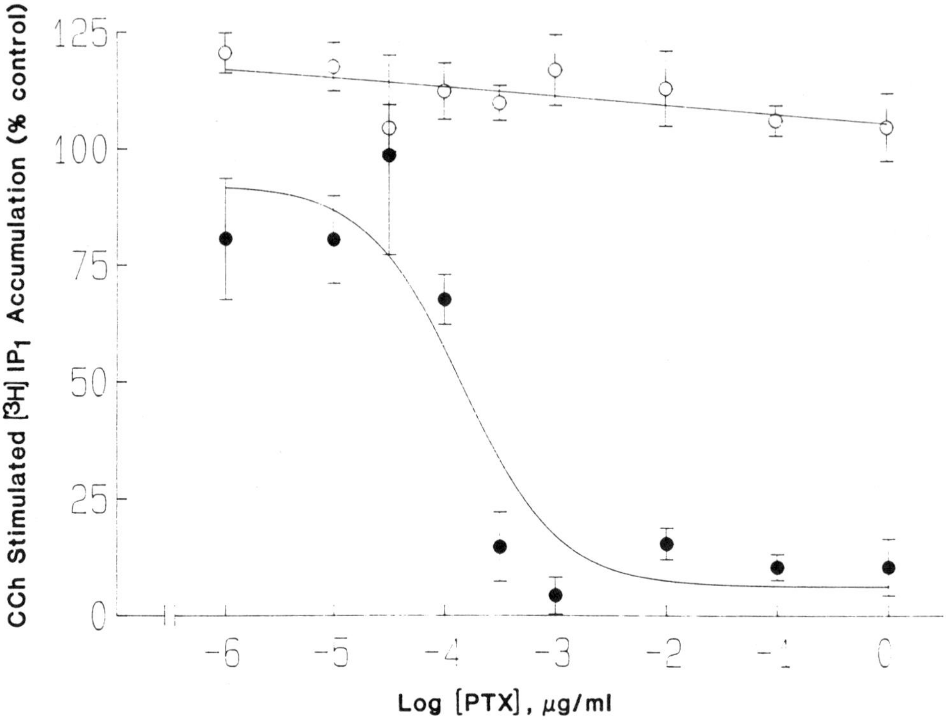

Figure 6. *The dose effect of PTX on CCh-induced (10 µM) hydrolysis of inositol lipids in the LK3–3 cells (open circle) that express the muscarinic M_1 receptor and the M_2LKB2–2 cells (closed circle) that express the cardiac M_2 receptor. Each data point represents the mean ± standard error mean of three determinations of the net [^{3}H]IP$_1$ accumulated expressed as a percentage of the maximal [^{3}H]IP$_1$ accumulated at 10 µM CCh in the absence of PTX. The IC_{50} value for PTX in inhibiting CCh-mediated [^{3}H]IP$_1$ accumulation in the M_2LKB2–2 cells was 0.14 ng/ml. PTX had no effect on the stimulation of PI hydrolysis in the LK3–3 cells by CCh, up to the concentration of 1 µg/ml of PTX. Reproduced with permission from Lai J, Waite SL, Bloom JW, et al: The m2 muscarinic acetylcholine receptors are coupled to multiple signaling pathways via pertussis toxin sensitive guanine regulatory proteins. J Pharm Exp Ther 258:938, 1991. Copyright © American Society of Pharmacology and Experimental Therapeutics.*

this complex reaction. Table 6 presents an alignment of sequences of the five rat mAChRs.

Vagal control of the heart has stimulated extensive research by scientists throughout the world. The biochemical characterization of cardiac mAChRs has permitted the careful correlation of functional studies with specific properties of the cardiac mAChR. Subtle differences in cardiac and CNS mAChRs have led to the M_1/M_2 receptor hypothesis that has formed the basis for an explosion of mAChR molecular biology. The new cloned mAChRs and the use of chimeras and site-directed mutants will permit a more careful dissection of the receptor effector coupling mechanisms and the determinants of drug specificity. This information will lead to new understanding of the role of cardiac muscarinic receptors and their role in vagal control.

Table 6.
Alignment of Sequences of Five Rat Muscarinic Receptor Genes[a]

```
Rat-M4    M----NNFTPVNG----------------------------------------SSANQSV   16
Rat-M2    M----NN----ST----------------------------------------NSSNNGL   12
Rat-M1    M----NT----SVPP--------------------------------------AVSPNIT   14
Rat-M3    MTLHSNS----TTSPLFPNISSSWVHSPSEAGLPLGTVTQLGSYNISQETGNFSSNDTSS   56
Rat-M5    MEGESYN----ESTV--------------------------------------NGTPVNH   18
          *

                        ____________I_____________           _________
Rat-M4    RLVTAAHNHLETVEMVFIATVTGSLSLVTVVGNILVMLSIKVNRQLQTVNNYFLFSLGCA
Rat-M2    AITSP----YKTFEVVFIVLVAGSLSLVTIIGNILVMVSIKVNRHLQTVNNYFLFSLACA   68
Rat-M1    VLAPG----KGPWQVAFIGITTGLLSLATVTGNLLVLISFKVNTELKTVNNYFLLSLACA   70
Rat-M3    DPLGG----HTIWQVVFIAFLTGFLALVTIIGNILVIVAFKVNKQLKTVNNYFLLSLACA  112
Rat-M5    QALER----HGLWEVITIAVVTAVVSLMTIVGNVLVMISFKVNSQLKTVNNYYLLSLACA   74
                           *        * *  ** **    ***  * ***** * ** **

          ___II_________               __________III_________
Rat-M4    DLIIGAFSMNLYTLYIIKGYWPLGAVVCDLWLALDYVVSNASVMNLLIISFDRYFCVTKP  136
Rat-M2    DLIIGVFSMNLYTLYTVIGYWPLGPVVCDLWLALDYVVSNASVMNLLIISFDRYFCVTKP  128
Rat-M1    DLIIGTFSMNLYTTYLLMGHWALGTLACDLWLALDYVASNASVMNLLLISFDRYFSVTRP  130
Rat-M3    DLIIGVISMNLFTTYIIMNRWALGNLACDLWLSIDYVASNASVMNLLVISFDRYFSITRP  172
Rat-M5    DLIIGIFSMNLYTTYILMGRWVLGSLACDLWLALDYVASNASVMNLLVISFDRYFSITRP  134
          *****  **** * *     * **   *****  *** ********* *******  * *
```

(continued)

Table 6.
Alignment of Sequences of Five Rat Muscarinic Receptor Genes[a] *(Continued)*

```
                   ___________IV__________                ____
Rat-M4   LTYPARRTTKMAGLMIAAAWVLSFVLWAPAILFWQFVVGKRTVPDNQCFIQFLSNPAVTF   196
Rat-M2   LTYPVKRTTKMAGMMIAAAWVLSFILWAPAILFWQFIVGVRTVEDGECYIQFFSNAAVTF   188
Rat-M1   LSYRAKRTPRRAALMIGLAWLVSFVLWAPAILFWQYLVGERTVLAGQCYIQFLSQPIITF   190
Rat-M3   LTYRAKRTTKRRGVMIGLAWVISFVLWAPAILFWQYFVGKRTVPPGECFIQFLSEPTITF   232
Rat-M5   LTYRAKRTPKRAGIMIGLAWLVSFILWAPAILCWQYLVGKRTVPPDECQIQFLSEPTITF   194
         * *   **      **  **  ** ******* **  ** ***    * *** *    **

         _______V__________
Rat-M4   GTAIAAFYLPVVIMTVLYIHISLASRSRVHKHRPEGPKEKKAKTLAFL-KSPLMKPSIKK   255
Rat-M2   TTAIAAFYLPVIIMTVLYWHISRASKSRIKKEKKEPVANQDPVSPSLV-QGRIVKPNNNN   247
Rat-M1   GTAMAAFYLPVTVMCTLYWRIYRETENRARELAALQGSETPGKGGGSS-SS-----SERS   244
Rat-M3   GTAIAAFYMPVTIMTILYWRIYKETEKRTKELAGLQASGTEAEAENFVHPTGSSRSCSSY   292
Rat-M5   GTAIAAFYIPVSVMTILYCRIYRETEKRTKDLADLQGSDSVAEAKKREPAQRTLLRSFFS   254
         *** **** **  *  **  *      *

Rat-M4   PPPGGASREELRNGKL-----EEAPPPALPPPPRPVPDKDTSNE-------SSSGSATON   303
Rat-M2   MPGGDGGLE-HNKIQN-----GKAPRDGVTENCVQGEEKESSND-------STSVSAV--   292
Rat-M1   QPGAEGSPE-SPPGRC-----CRCCRAPRLLQAYSWKEEEEEDE-------GSMESLT--   289
Rat-M3   ELQQQGVKR-SSRRKYGRCHFWFTTKSWKPSAEQMDQDHSSSDSWNNNDAAASLENSA--   349
Rat-M5   CPRPSLAQR-ERNQAS-----WSSSRRSTSTTGKTTQATDLSADWEKAEQVTTCSSYP--   306

Rat-M4   TKERPPTELSTAEAT------TPALPAPTLQP---RTLNPASKWSK--------------   340
Rat-M2   -----ASNMRDDEIT------QDENTVSTSLG---HSRDDNSKQTC--------------   324
Rat-M1   -----SSE-GEEPGS------EVVIKMPMVDS---EAQAP--------------------   314
Rat-M3   -----SSD-EEDIGSETRAIYSIVLKLPGHSSILNSTKLPSSDNLQVSNEDLGTVDVERN   403
Rat-M5   -----SSE-DEAKPT-TDPVFQMVYKSEAKES---PGKESNTQETKETVVNTRTENSDYD   356
```

```
                                                                  VI
Rat-M4   ------------------------IQIVTK-----QTGNEC---VTAIEIVPAT---PAG   365
Rat-M2   ------------------------IKIVTK----AQKGDVYTPTSTTVELVGSS---GQN   353
Rat-M1   ----------------------------TK-----QPPKSS---PNTVKRPTKK---GRD   335
Rat-M3   AHKLQAQKSMGDGDNCQKDFTKLPIQLESAVDTG-KTSDTN---SSADKTTATLPLSFKE   459
Rat-M5   TPKYFLSPAAAHRLKSQK-CVAYKFRLVVKADGT-QETNNG---CRKVKIMPCSFPVSKD   411

                                                  __________VI__________
Rat-M4   MR-PAANVARKFASIARNQVRKKRQMAARERKVTRTIFAILLAFILTWTPYNVMVLVNTF   424
Rat-M2   GD-EKQNIVARKIVKMTKQPAKKKPPPSREKKVTRTILAILLAFIITWAPYNVMVLINTF   412
Rat-M1   RG-GKGQKPRGKEQLA----KRKTFSLVKEKKAARTLSAILLAFILTWTPYNIMVLVSTF   390
Rat-M3   ATLAKRFALKTRSQIT----KRKRMSLIKEKKAAQTLSAILLAFIITWTPYNIMVLVNTF   515
Rat-M5   PS-TKGPDPNLSHQMT----KRKRMVLVKERKAAQTLSAILLAFIITWTPYNIMVLVSTF   466
                                 *      * *   *  ******* ** *** ***  **

                  ________VII_____________
Rat-M4   CQSCIPETVWSIGYWLCYVNSTINPACYALCNATFKKTFRHLLLCQ--------------   470
Rat-M2   CAPCIPNTVWTIGYWLCYINSTINPACYALCNATFKKTFKHLLMCH--------------   458
Rat-M1   CKDCVPETLWELGYWLCYVNSTVNPMCYALCNKAFRDTFRLLLLCRWDKRRWRKIPKRPG   450
Rat-M3   CDSCIPKTYWNLGYWLCYINSTVNPVCYALCNKTFRTTFKTLLLCQCDKRKRRKQQYQQR   575
Rat-M5   CDKCVPVTLWHLGYWLCYVNSTINPICYALCNRTFRKTFKLLLLCRWKKKKVEEKLYWQG   526
         *  * * * *  ****** *** ** ******  *  **  ** *

Rat-M4   --YRNIGTA---------R   478
Rat-M2   --YKNIGAT---------R   466
Rat-M1   SVHRTPSRQ---------C   460
Rat-M3   Q-----SVIFHKRVPEQAL   589
Rat-M5   N-----SKL---------P   531
```

[a]The deduced amino acid sequences of the five rat muscarinic receptors have been taken from Lai J, et al,[62] Kashihara K, et al,[78] and Lai J, et al.[98] The 156 sites that are conserved are indicated by astericks. The regions of transmembrane segments are indicated by Roman numerals based on Probst WC, et al.[99]

References

1. Higgins CB, Vatner SF, Braunwald E: Parasympathetic control of the heart. Pharmacol Rev 25:119, 1973.
2. Priola DV, Spurgeon HA, Geis WP: Intrinsic innervation of canine heart: Functional study. Circ Res 40:50, 1977.
3. Priola DV, Fulton RL: Positive and negative inotropic responses of atria and ventricles to vagosympathetic stimulation in isovolumic canine heart. Circ Res 25:265, 1969.
4. Buccino RA, Sonnenblick EH, Cooper T, et al: Direct positive inotropic effect of acetylcholine on myocardium: Evidence for multiple cholinergic receptors in heart. Circ Res 19:1097, 1966.
5. Levy MN, Zieske H: Comparison of cardiac effects of vagus nerve stimulation and of acetylcholine infusions. Am J Physiol 216:89, 1969.
6. DeGeest H, Levy MN, Zieske H, et al: Depression of ventricular contractility by stimulation of vagus nerves. Circ Res 17:222, 1965.
7. Furchgott RF, Sleator W, DeGubareff T: Effects of acetylcholine and epinephrine on the contractile strength and action potential of electrically driven guinea pig atria. J Pharmacol Exp Ther 129:405, 1960.
8. Friedman WF, Buccino RA, Sonnenblick EH, et al: Effects of frequency of contraction and ionic environment of responses of heart muscle to acetylcholine. Circ Res 21:573, 1967.
9. Lee TP, Kuo JF, Greengard P: Role of muscarinic cholinergic receptors in regulation of guanosine 3′-5′-cyclic monophosphate content in mammalian brain, heart-muscle and intestinal smooth muscle. Proc Natl Acad Sci USA 69:3287, 1972.
10. Gardner RM, Allen DO: Regulation of cyclic nucleotide levels and glycogen-phosphorylase activity by acetylcholine and epinephrine in perfused rat hearts. J Pharmacol Exp Ther 197:412, 1976.
11. Brown OM: Cat heart acetylcholine: Structural proof and distribution. Am J Physiol 231:781, 1976.
12. Roskoski R Jr, Schmid PG, Mayer HE, et al: In vitro acetylcholine biosynthesis in normal and failing guinea-pig hearts. Circ Res 36:547, 1975.
13. Paton WD, Rang HP: The uptake of atropine and related drugs by intestinal smooth muscle of the guinea pig in relation to acetylcholine receptors. Proc R Soc Lond (Biol) Ser B 163:1, 1965.
14. Potter LT: Uptake of propranolol by isolated guinea-pig atria. J Pharmacol Exp Ther 155:91, 1967.
15. Fields JZ, Roeske WR, Morkin E, et al: Cardiac muscarinic cholinergic receptors: Biochemical identification and characterization. J Biol Chem 253:3251, 1978.
16. Yamamura HI, Snyder SH: Muscarinic cholinergic binding in rat brain. Proc Natl Acad Sci USA 71:1725, 1974.
17. Roeske WR, Ehlert FJ, Barritt DS, et al: Recent advances in muscarinic receptor heterogeneity and regulation. In T Segawa, HI Yamamura, K Kuriyama (eds): Molecular Pharmacology of Neurotransmitter Receptors. New York, NY, Raven Press, 1983, p. 15.
18. Serra M, Mei L, Roeske WR, et al: The intact human neuroblastoma cells (SH-SY5Y) exhibits high-affinity [^{3}H]pirenzepine binding associated with hydrolysis of phosphatidylinositols. J Neurochem 50:1513, 1988.
19. Hulme EC, Birdsall NJM, Burgen ASV, et al: The binding of antagonists to brain muscarinic receptors. Mol Pharmacol 14:737, 1978.
20. Beld AJ, Ariens EJ: Stereospecificity as a tool in attempts to localize and isolate muscarinic receptors. II. Binding of (+)−benzetimide, (−)−benzetimide, and atropine to a fraction from bovine tracheal smooth muscle and to bovine caudate nucleus. Eur J Pharmacol 25:203, 1974.

21. Birdsall NJM, Hulme EC: Biochemical studies on muscarinic acetylcholine receptors. J Neurochem 27:7, 1976.
22. Watson M, Roeske WR, Yamamura HI: [^{3}H]pirenzepine selectively identifies a high affinity population of muscarinic cholinergic receptors in the rat cerebral cortex. Life Sci 31:2019, 1982.
23. Wang J-X, Roeske WR, Gulya K, et al: [^{3}H] AF-DX 116 labels subsets of muscarinic cholinergic receptors in rat brain and heart. Life Sci 41:1751, 1987.
24. Ehlert FJ, Dumont Y, Roeske WR, et al: Muscarinic receptor binding in the rat brain using the agonist, [^{3}H]-cis-methyldioxolane. Life Sci 26:961, 1980.
25. Birdsall NJM, Burgen ASV, Hulme EC: The binding of agonists to brain muscarinic receptors. Mol Pharmacol 14:723, 1978.
26. Vickroy TW, Watson M, Yamamura HI, et al: Muscarinic cholinergic receptor binding: Utilization in drug research. In RA O'Brien (ed): Receptor Binding and Drug Research. New York, NY, Marcel Dekker Inc, 1986, p. 297.
27. Ehlert FJ, Roeske WR, Yamamura HI: Muscarinic receptor [^{3}H]ligand binding methods. In PJ Marangos, RM Cohen, I Campbell (eds): Brain Receptor Methodologies, Part A. New York, NY, Academic Press, 1984, p. 339.
28. Wang J-X, Yamamura HI, Wang W, et al: The use of the filtration technique in the in vitro radioligand binding assay for the membrane-bound and solubilized receptor. In EC Hulme (ed): Receptor-Ligand Interactions: A Practical Approach. New York, NY, IRL Press, 1992, 213–234.
29. Motulsky HJ, Mahan LC: The kinetics of competitive radioligand binding predicted by the law of mass action. Mol Pharmacol 25:1, 1984.
30. Ehlert FJ, Roeske WR, Yamamura HI: Mathematical analysis of the kinetics of competitive inhibition in neurotransmitter receptor binding assays. Mol Pharmacol 19:367, 1981.
31. Galper JB, Smith TW: Properties of muscarinic acetylcholine receptors in heart cell cultures. Proc Natl Acad Sci USA 75:5831, 1978.
32. Galper JB, Dziekan L, O'Hara DS, et al: The biphasic response of muscarinic cholinergic receptors in cultured heart cells to agonists. J Biol Chem 257:10344, 1982.
33. Hammer R, Berrie CP, Birdsall NJM, et al: Pirenzepine distinguishes between different subclasses of muscarinic receptors. Nature 283:90, 1980.
34. Hammer R, Giachetti A: Muscarinic receptor subtypes: M_1 and M_2 biochemical and functional characterization. Life Sci 31:2291, 1982.
35. Watson M, Yamamura HI, Roeske WR: A unique regulatory profile and regional distribution of [^{3}H]pirenzepine binding in the rat brain provides evidence for distinct M_1 and M_2 muscarinic receptor subtypes. Life Sci 32:3001, 1983.
36. Mei L, Roeske WR, Yamamura HI: Molecular pharmacology of muscarinic receptor heterogeneity. Life Sci 45:1831, 1991.
37. Giachetti A, Mittmann U, Brown JH, et al: Cardioselective muscarinic antagonists. Fed Proc 46:2523, 1987.
38. Wang J-X, Roeske WR, Hawkins KN, et al: Quantitative autoradiography of M_2 muscarinic receptors in the rat brain identified by using a selective radioligand [^{3}H]AF-DX 116. Brain Res 477:322, 1989.
39. Chang KJ, Deth RC, Triggle DJ: Structural parameters determining cholinergic and anticholinergic activities in a series of 1,3-dioxolanes. J Med Chem 15:243, 1972.
40. Ehlert FJ, Yamamura HI, Triggle DJ, et al: The influence of guanyl-5′-yl imidodiphosphate and sodium chloride on the binding of the muscarinic agonist, [^{3}H]cis methyldioxolane. Eur J Pharmacol 61:317, 1980.
41. Vickroy TW, Yamamura HI, Roeske WR: Differential regulation of high affinity agonist binding to muscarinic sites in the rat heart, cerebellum, and cerebral cortex. Biochem Biophys Res Comm 116:284, 1983.
42. Vickroy TW, Roeske WR, Yamamura HI: Pharmacological differences between the

high-affinity muscarinic agonist binding states of the rat heart and cerebral cortex labelled with [^{3}H](+)cis-methyldioxolane. J Pharm Exp Ther 229:747, 1984.
43. Roeske WR, Yamamura HI: Muscarinic cholinergic receptor regulation. In HI Yamamura, RW Olsen, E Usdin (eds): Psychopharmacology and Biochemistry of Neurotransmitter Receptors. New York, NY, Elsevier North-Holland, 1980, p. 101.
44. Deighton NM, Motomera S, Borquez D, et al: Muscarinic cholinoceptors in the human heart: Demonstration, subclassification, and distribution. Naunyn-Schmiedeberg's Arch Pharmacol 341:14, 1990.
45. Wei JW, Sulakhe PV: Agonist-antagonist interactions with rat atrial muscarinic cholinergic receptor sites: Differential regulation by guanine nucleotides. Gen Pharmacol 10:263, 1979.
46. Wei JW, Sulakhe PV: Regional and subcellular-distribution of myocardial muscarinic cholinergic receptors. Eur J Pharmacol 52:235, 1978.
47. Yamada S, Yamamura HI, Roeske WR: Alterations in cardiac autonomic receptors following 6-hydroxydopamine treatment in rats. Mol Pharmacol 18:185, 1980.
48. Ehlert FJ, Roeske WR, Yamamura HI: The muscarinic receptor: Regulation by guanine nucleotides, ions, and N-ethylmaleimide. Fed Poc 40:153, 1981.
49. Vickroy TW, Watson M, Yamamura HI, et al: Agonist binding to multiple muscarinic receptors. Fed Proc 43:2785, 1984.
50. Rosenberger LB, Roeske WR, Yamamura H: The regulation of muscarinic cholinergic receptors by guanine nucleotides in cardiac tissue. Eur J Pharmacol 56:179, 1979.
51. Berrie CP, Birdsall NJM, Burgen ASV, et al: Guanine nucleotides modulate muscarinic receptor binding in the heart. Biochem Biophys Res Commun 87:1000, 1979.
52. Rosenberger LB, Yamamura HI, Roeske WR: Cardiac muscarinic cholinergic receptor binding is regulated by NaCl and guanyl nucleotides. J Biol Chem 255:820, 1980.
53. Rodbell M: The role of hormone receptors and GTP-regulatory proteins in membrane transduction. Nature 284:17, 1980.
54. Jakobs KH: Inhibition of adenylate cyclase by hormones and neurotransmitters. Mol Cell Endocrinol 16:147, 1979.
55. Watson M, Yamamura HI, Roeske WR: [^{3}H]pirenzepine and [^{3}H](−)quinuclidinyl benzilate binding to rat cerebral cortical and cardiac muscarinic cholinergic sites: I. Characterization and regulation of agonist binding to putative muscarinic subtypes. J Pharm Exp Ther 237:411, 1986.
56. Watson M, Roeske WR, Yamamura HI: [^{3}H]Pirenzepine and [^{3}H](−)quinuclidinyl benzilate binding to rat cerebral cortical and cardiac muscarinic cholinergic sites: II. Characterization and regulation of antagonist binding to putative muscarinic subtypes. J Pharm Exp Ther 237:419, 1986.
57. Wang J-X, Mei L, Yamamura HI, et al: Solubilization with digitonin alters the kinetics of pirenzepine binding to muscarinic receptors from rat forebrain and heart. J Pharm Exp Ther 242:981, 1987.
58. Bonner TI, Buckley NJ, Young AC, et al: Identification of a family of muscarinic acetylcholine receptor genes. Science 237:527, 1987.
59. Peralta EG, Winslow JW, Peterson GL, et al: Primary structure and biochemical properties of an M_2 muscarinic receptor. Science 236:600, 1987.
60. Kubo T, Fukuda K, Mikami A, et al: Cloning, sequencing and expression of complementary DNA encoding the muscarinic acetylcholine receptor. Nature 323:411, 1986.
61. Kubo T, Maeda A, Sugimoto K, et al: Primary structure of porcine cardiac muscarinic acetylcholine receptor deduced from the cDNA sequence. FEBS Lett 209:367, 1986.
62. Lai J, Bloom JW, Yamamura HI, et al: Amplification of the rat M2 muscarinic receptor gene by the polymerase chain reaction: Functional expression of the M2 muscarinic receptor. Life Sci 47:1001, 1990.

63. Lai J, Mei L, Roeske WR, et al: The cloned murine m1 muscarinic receptor is associated with the hydrolysis of phosphatidylinositols in transfected murine B82 cells. Life Sci 42:2489, 1988.
64. Ashkenazi A, Winslow JW, Peralta EG, et al: An M2 muscarinic receptor subtype coupled to both adenylyl cyclase and phosphoinositide turnover. Science 238:672, 1987.
65. Ehlert FJ, Roeske WR, Yamamura HI: Striatal muscarinic receptors: Regulation by dopaminergic agonists. Life Sci 28:2441, 1981.
66. Snyder SH, Yamamura HI: Antidepressants and the muscarinic acetylcholine receptor. Arch Gen Psych 34:236, 1977.
67. Snyder SH, Banerjee SP, Yamamura HI, et al: Drugs, neurotransmitters, and schizophrenia. Science 184:1243, 1974.
68. Schwab BW, Hand H, Costa LB, et al: Reduced muscarinic receptor binding in tissues of rats tolerant to the insecticide disulfoton. Neurotoxicology 4:635, 1981.
69. Enna SJ, Bird ED, Bennett JP Jr, et al: Huntington's Chorea: Changes in neurotransmitter receptors in brain. N Engl J Med 294:1305, 1976.
70. Reisine TD, Yamamura HI, Bird ED, et al: Presynaptic and postsynaptic neurochemical alterations in Alzheimer's disease. Brain Res 159:477, 1978.
71. Wildenthal K: Maturation of responsiveness to cardioactive drugs: Differential effects of acetylcholine, norepinephrine, theophylline, tyramine, glucagon, and dibutyryl cyclic AMP on atrial rate in hearts of fetal mice. J Clin Invest 52:2250, 1973.
72. Roeske WR, Yamamura HI: Maturation of mammalian myocardial muscarinic cholinergic receptors. Life Sci 23:127, 1978.
73. Roeske WR, Wildenthal K: Responsiveness to drugs and hormones in the murine model of cardiac ontogenesis. Pharmacol Ther 14:55, 1981.
74. Evans RA, Watson M, Yamamura HI, et al: Differential ontogeny of putative M_1 and M_2 muscarinic receptor binding sites in the murine cerebral cortex and heart. J Pharm Exp Ther 235:612, 1985.
75. Hammer R, Giraldo E, Schiavi GB, et al: Binding profile of a novel cardioselective muscarinic receptor antagonist, AF-DX 116, to membranes of peripheral tissues and brain in the rat. Life Sci 38:1657, 1986.
76. Giachetti A, Micheletti R, Montagna E: Cardioselective profile of AF-DX 116, a muscarinic M_2 receptor antagonist. Life Sci 38:1663, 1986.
77. Mei L, Lai J, Yamamura HI, et al: The relationship between agonist states of the M1 muscarinic receptor and the hydrolysis of inositol lipids in transfected murine fibroblast cells (B82) expressing different receptor densities. J Pharmacol Exp Ther 251:90, 1989.
78. Kashihara K, Varga EV, Waite SL, et al: Cloning of the rat M3, M4 and M5 muscarinic acetylcholine receptor genes by the polymerase chain reaction (PCR) and the pharmacological characterization of the expressed genes. Life Sci 51:955, 1992.
79. Eglen PM, Montogomery WW, Dainty IA, et al: The interaction of methoctramine and himbacine at atrial, smooth muscle and endothelial muscarinic receptors in vitro. Br J Pharmacol 95:1031, 1988.
80. Anwar-ul S, Gilani H, Cobbin LB: The cardiac-selectivity of himbacine: A muscarinic receptor antagonist. Naunyn-Schmiedeberg's Arch Pharmacol 332:16, 1986.
81. Melchiorre C, Angeli P, Lambrecht G, et al: Antimuscarinic action of methoctramine, a new cardioselective M_2 muscarinic receptor antagonist alone and in combination with atropine. Eur J Pharmacol 144:117, 1987.
82. van Charldorp KJ, Davidesko D, van Zwieten PA: Selectivity of methoctramine for muscarinic receptor in porcine cerebral arteries. Eur J Pharmacol 150:197, 1988.
83. Lambrecht G, Gmelin G, Moser U, et al: Selectivity profiles of antagonists at muscarinic receptor subtypes. Naunyn-Schmiedeberg's Arch Pharmacol 337:R92, 1988.
84. Buckley NJ, Bonner TI, Buckley CM, et al: Antagonist binding properties of 5

cloned muscarinic receptors expressed in CHO-K1 cells. Mol Pharmacol 35:469, 1989.

85. Gocayne J, Robinson DA, Fitzgerald MG, et al: Primary structure of rat cardiac β-adrenergic and muscarinc cholinergic receptors obtained by automated DNA sequence analysis: Further evidence for a multigene family. Proc Natl Acad Sci USA 84:8296, 1987.
86. Peralta EG, Ashkenazi A, Winslow JW, et al: Distinct primary structures, ligand-binding properties and tissue-specific expression of four human muscarinic acetylcholine receptors. EMBO J 6:3023, 1987.
87. Maeda A, Kubo T, Mishina M, et al: Tissue distribution of mRNAs encoding muscarinic acetylcholine receptor subtypes. FEBS Lett 239:339, 1988.
88. Saiki RK, Scharf S, Faloona F, et al: Primer-directed enzymatic amplification of DNA with a thermostable DNA polymerase. Science 230:1350, 1985.
89. Sanger F, Nicklen S, Coulson AR: DNA sequencing with chain-terminating inhibitors. Proc Natl Acad Sci USA 74:5463, 1977.
90. Gunning P, Leavitt J, Muscat G, et al: A human β-actin expression vector system directs high-level accumulation of antisense transcripts. Proc Natl Acad Sci USA 84:4831, 1987.
91. Graham F, Van Der Eb A: A new technique for the assay of infectivity of human adenovirus 5 DNA. Virology 52:456, 1973.
92. Berridge MJ, Downes CP, Hanley MR: Lithium amplifies agonist-dependent phosphatidylinositol responses in brain and salivary glands. Biochem J 206:587, 1982.
93. Gilman AG: A protein binding assay for adenosine 3′,5′ cyclic monophosphate. Proc Natl Acad Sci USA 67:305, 1970.
94. Akiba I, Kubo T, Maeda A, et al: Primary structure of porcine muscarinic acetylcholine receptor III and antagonist binding studies. FEBS Lett 235:257, 1988.
95. Peralta EG, Ashkenazi A, Winslow JW, et al: Differential regulation of PI hydrolysis and adenylyl cyclase by muscarinic receptor subtypes. Nature 334:434, 1988.
96. Lai J, Waite SL, Bloom JW, et al: The m2 muscarinic acetylcholine receptors are coupled to multiple signaling pathways via pertussis toxin sensitive guanine regulatory proteins. J Pharmacol Exp Ther 258:938, 1991.
97. Wei H, Roeske WR, Lai J, et al: Pharmacological characterization of a novel muscarinic partial agonist, YM796, in transfected cells expressing the m1 or m2 muscarinic receptor gene. Life Sci 50:355, 1991.
98. Lai J, Smith TL, Mei L, et al: The molecular properties of the M_1 muscarinic receptor and its regulation of cytosolic calcium in a eukaryotic gene expression system. In S Kito, T Segawa, R Olsen, et al (eds): Neuroreceptor Mechanisms in Brain. New York, NY, Plenum Press, 1991, p. 313.
99. Probst WC, Snyder LA, Schuster DI, et al: Sequence alignment of the G-protein coupled receptor superfamily. DNA and Cell Biology 11:1, 1992.

CHAPTER 8

Molecular Biology of the Muscarinic Receptors

M. Schimerlik

With the availability of highly purified muscarinic receptor (mAChR) preparations from both heart atria[1] and brain,[2] experiments were initiated to clone and sequence the genes coding for the DNA sequence of those mAChRs. Deduction of the amino acid sequence of the protein from the DNA sequence then allows for predictions of the secondary structure and topology of the protein. By transfecting the genes into cells that do not normally express mAChRs, but do contain the complement of proteins that are involved in mAChR-mediated signal transduction, interaction between mAChRs and their respective physiological effector systems can be examined. Finally, the amino acid sequence of mAChRs can be modified using the technique of site-directed mutagenesis in order to study the relationship between structure and function for individual amino acids or for various regions of the protein. This chapter summarizes the rapid growth progress in these areas over the last five years.

Cloning of the Muscarinic Receptor Gene Family

The cloning of the gene coding for a mAChR was first reported by Numa et al.[3] The strategy employed in this process is outlined in Figure 1. In this study, the purified porcine brain mAChR was treated with the protease trypsin in order to prepare peptides that were then fractionated by high-pressure liquid chromatography. The amino acid sequence of the peptides was determined and the oligodeoxynucleotide probes containing all possible DNA sequences predicted from the amino acid sequence were synthesized. The DNA probes were used to screen a complementary DNA (cDNA) library prepared from poly A^+ RNA isolated from porcine brain cerebrum. The cDNA clones isolated by this procedure were then sequenced and used as probes to rescreen the same cDNA

From *Vagal Control of the Heart: Experimental Basis and Clinical Implications* edited by MN Levy, PJ Schwartz

Purified mAChR

↓ trypsin digest

polypeptide purification and sequencing

Amino acid sequence data

↓

Design Oligodeoxynucleotide Probes

↓

Screen cDNA or genomic DNA Libraries

↓

Sequence the DNA of Isolated Clones

↓

Deduce the Amino Acid Sequence of the Protein

Figure 1. *Approach used to clone genes coding for mAChRs.*

library. This action permitted identification of additional clones and led to eventual determination of the complete DNA sequence coding for the receptor protein. Deduction of the amino acid sequence from the DNA sequence showed that the gene coded for a protein of 460 amino acids.

A similar strategy was used to clone the gene for the porcine atrial mAChR.[4] A comparison of the amino acid sequences of these two proteins showed that, although similar, the proteins were clearly distinct. This finding indicated that at least two different subtypes of mAChRs were encoded by different genes. Assuming that amino acid sequences common to both receptor subtypes may also be present in as yet unidentified subtypes, oligodeoxynucleotide probes coding for a conserved amino acid sequence were employed to screen both human and rat cDNA as well as genomic libraries. As a result of these experiments,[5–7] three additional mAChR subtypes were identified; a total of five distinct mAChRs have been discovered to date. The properties of the five subtypes are summarized in Table 1.

Table 1.
Muscarinic Receptor Subtypes

Subtype	*Number of Amino Acids*	*Molecular Weight*[1]	*Physiological Effector Systems*	*Location*
m1	460	51387	Stimulation of phospholipase C, A_2, D Release of intracellular calcium	brain, exocrine glands
m2	466	51681	Inhibition of adenylyl cyclase Activation of atrial K^+_{AcCh} channels Weakly coupled to phospholipase C, D	brain, atria, smooth muscle
m3	590	66085	Stimulation of phospholipases C, A_2, D Release of intracellular calcium	exocrine glands
m4	479	53014	Inhibition of adenylyl cyclase Weakly coupled to stimulation of phospholipase C, D	brain
m5	532	60120	Stimulation of phospholipase C, A_2 Release of intracellular calcium	brain

[1]Does not include carbohydrate.

Muscarinic Receptor Structure

The amino acid sequence of mAChR proteins can be analyzed by a technique called hydropathy analysis,[8] in which an average of relative hydrophobicity (based on water/organic solvent partition data or some other parameter of relative polarity) is calculated for each protein segment of defined length throughout the complete protein sequence. In this manner, hydrophobic regions of the protein that are of sufficient length to correspond to membrane-spanning domains and hydrophilic regions most likely to be located on either the internal or external side of the membrane can be identified. Such an analysis is shown in Figure 2 for the porcine atrial mAChR; however, all five subtypes show similar profiles. These data suggest that the mAChR has seven membrane-spanning regions or transmembrane (TM) segments.

Comparisons of amino acid sequence data and hydropathic analysis of mAChRs with other TM proteins such as rhodopsin,[9] which also couple to physiological effector systems through guanine nucleotide-binding proteins (G-proteins), suggests a similar structural motif consisting of seven TM segments. Another protein belonging to this gene family is bacteriorhodopsin,

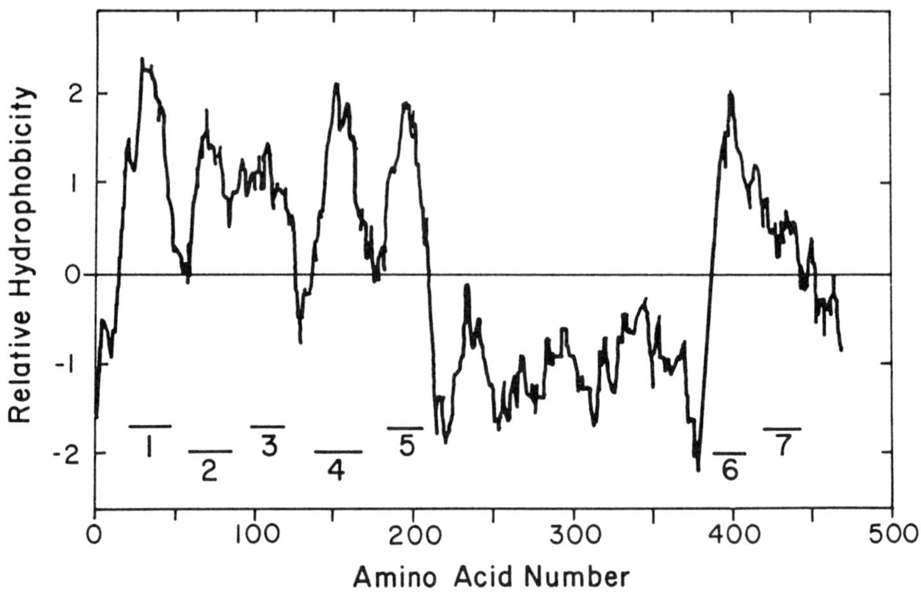

Figure 2. *Hydropathy plot of porcine m2 mAChR. Relative hydropathy is plotted versus amino acid number using the method of Kyte and Doolittle[8] with average hydropathy computed over a 19 amino acid window. The bars indicate putative transmembrane sequences (TM) numbered 1 to 7 from the amino to carboxyl terminus of the protein.*

a light-driven proton pump found in the halophilic bacteria *Halobacterium halobium*. Since bacteriorhodopsin is available in large quantities and occurs naturally as two-dimensional crystals, it has been possible to obtain both biochemical data and structural information about this protein to a resolution of about 3.5Å from high-resolution electron cryo-microscopy studies.[10]

Application of the results of the bacteriorhodopsin model system to the mAChR suggests several common structural and topological features (Fig. 3). First, the amino terminus is located extracellularly and, because there are an odd number of TM segments, the carboxyl terminus is believed to be located on the cytoplasmic side of the membrane. By analogy with bacteriorhodopsin, the seven TM segments of the mAChR are thought to have helical secondary structures, with the helices slightly tilted off the vertical axis with respect to each other. Fourier transform analysis of the periodicity of conserved α-helical residues in the TM sequences suggests that the sides of the helices facing the hydrophilic interior space of the protein are more highly conserved than those facing the membrane.[11,12] These results support two concepts: one, that the helices are amphipathic and two, the side of the helix that interacts with membrane lipids tolerates greater variability. There are four conserved extracellular cysteine residues: one each in extracellular loops 2-3 and 4-5, and two in extracellular loop 6-7. The importance of extracellular cysteines in the binding of adrenergic ligands has been shown,[13] and sequence analysis of m1

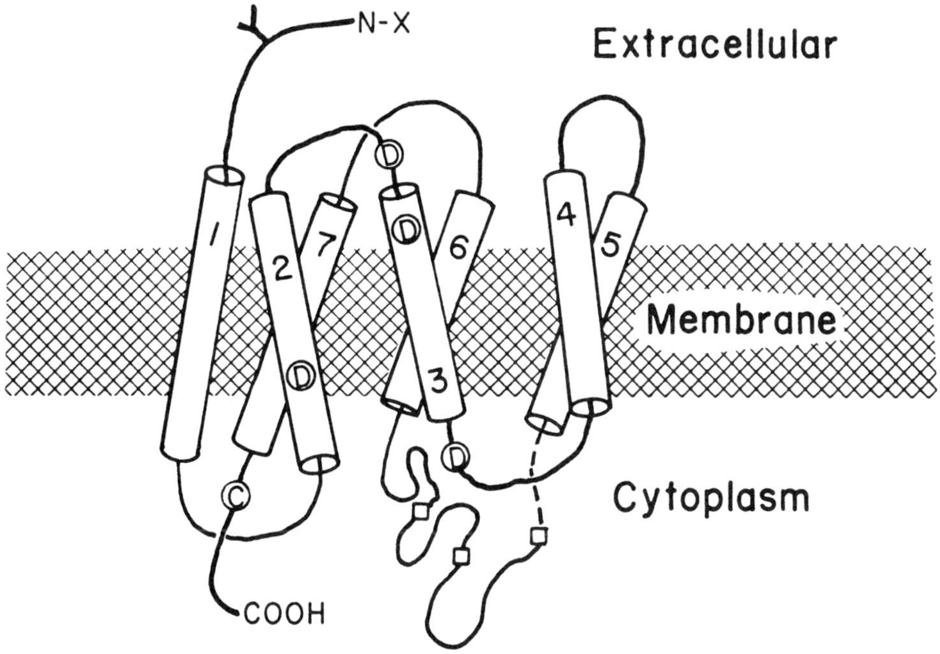

Figure 3. *Predicted mAChR structure and topology. By analogy to the high-resolution structure of bacteriorhodopsin,[10] the seven TM helices, shown as cylinders, are slightly tilted with respect to each other. The branched structure near the amino terminus represents a potential site for N-linked glycosylation. The amino terminus is blocked by the unknown group (X) and a cysteine (C) residue near the carboxyl terminus represents a potential site for palmitoylation. Conserved aspartate residues (D) are shown in TM2 and 3 and the squares in intracellular loop 5-6 represent potential phosphorylation sites. The dashed line representing the first 15 to 20 amino acids at the amino terminus of loop 5-6 signify that this region of the protein is a major determinant of G-protein selectivity.*

mAChRs[14] has demonstrated a disulfide bond between the cysteines in extracellular loops 2-3 and 4-5. Peptide mapping studies also suggest a disulfide bond between the two cysteines in extracellular loop 6-7,[12] but the evidence is not yet definitive. Potential extracellular sites for attachment of sugars to asparagine amide nitrogens, identified from the consensus sequence asparagine–any amino acid–serine or threonine, can also be found in the amino acid sequence in agreement with biochemical studies[15] that show that mAChRs are glycoproteins.

Alignment of the amino acid sequences of the five muscarinic subtypes and other G-protein-linked receptors shows that there is a high degree of sequence similarity. The highest amino acid correspondence occurs in the seven TM regions and intracellular loops 1-2 and 3-4, with weaker agreement at the amino and carboxyl termini. The large intracellular loop 5-6 appears to be distinct for each muscarinic subtype and, in general, this region shows very little amino acid identity among individual G-protein-linked receptors.

Coupling to Physiological Effector Systems

Once the genes for the five muscarinic subtypes are cloned, they can be transfected into cell-lines that do not normally contain mAChRs. Alternatively, messenger RNA (mRNA) can be synthesized in vitro and injected into *Xenopus* oocytes, which then translates the mRNA to active protein. While eliminating interference from endogenous mAChRs, this procedure suffers from the disadvantage that the physiological effector systems and G-proteins in the transfected cell-lines are not normally coupled to mAChRs. Results may therefore vary somewhat, depending on the cell-line used.

As shown in Figure 4, muscarinic signal transduction is mediated by G-proteins.[16–18] In the absence of the G-protein, the receptor binds agonists with low affinity. Transient association of the G-protein with the mAChR promotes

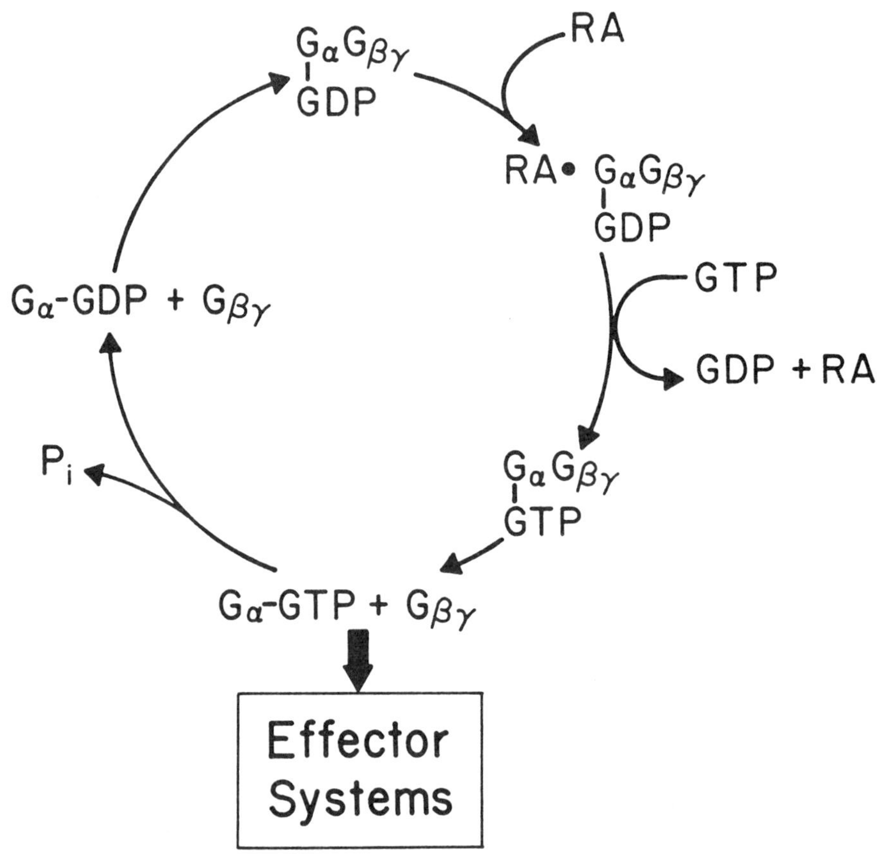

Figure 4. *G-proteins mediate mAChR signal transduction. The receptor agonist complex (RA) binds to the heterotrimeric G-protein catalyzing the exchange of a bound GDP for GTP. The binding of GTP causes dissociation of the receptor agonist complex followed by dissociation of the G-protein into Gα-GTP and Gβγ subunits. These subunits stimulate or inhibit physiological effector systems. The response is terminated by hydrolysis of GTP followed by subunit reassociation.*

high-affinity agonist-binding and the exchange of guanosine diphosphate (GDP) for guanosine triphosphate (GTP) at the α subunit of the heterotrimeric G-protein. The binding of GTP results in the dissociation of the agonist receptor complex from the G-protein, which then dissociates into α and βγ subunits. The subunits can activate or inhibit different physiological effector systems in a parallel signalling process. The response is terminated by the hydrolysis of GTP to GDP by the GTPase activity of the α subunit. This process is followed by reassociation of G-protein subunits so as to form the holoprotein with GDP bound to the α subunit. Physiological effector systems coupled to mAChRs that are regulated by G-proteins include adenylyl cyclase (AC), inhibited by G_i; phospholipase C (PLC), activated by G_q and G_{11}; inward recifying atrial potassium channels, activated by G_i; calcium channels, stimulated by G_o, and both phospholipase A_2 (PLA_2) and phospholipase D stimulated by as yet unknown G-proteins. With the exception of AC, which is inhibited by $G_{i\beta\gamma}$ subunits in vitro, most of the above systems appear to be regulated by the G-protein α subunits. Since there have been at least 16 distinct G_α subunit genes identified, four G_β subunit genes and four G_γ subunit genes cloned to date as well as multiple genes for effectors such as PLC, it can be seen that the explicit determination of which G-protein isotype activates a given effector protein can be formidable.

Transfection of mAChRs into A9L cells[19] showed that the m1 and m3, but not the m2 and m4, subtypes coupled to G-proteins activated phospholipid-signalling pathways. This process included stimulation of PLA_2, which resulted in an increase in cellular arachidonic acid, and PLC. The latter enzyme catalyzed the hydrolysis of phosphatidylinositol 4,5 bisphosphate to yield diacylglycerol, an activator of protein kinase C, and inositol 1,4,5, trisphosphate (IP_3), which released calcium from intracellular compartments. The increase in intracellular calcium activated the calcium-dependent potassium channels and hyperpolarized the cell membranes.[20] m2 mAChRs transfected into Chinese hamster ovary cells (CHO cells) activated distinct G-proteins that either stimulated PLC or inhibited AC. The m2 subtype however, appeared to interact preferentially with the G-protein that mediated the inhibition of AC.[21]

In human embryonic kidney cells, m1 and m3 subtypes efficiently stimulated PLC while the m2 and m4 subtypes were more tightly coupled to the inhibition of AC.[22] Different G-protein-linked receptors in the same cell may couple to the same physiological effector system via different G-proteins, as seen in the use of CHO cells.[23] Stimulation of PLC was uncoupled from endogenous thrombin and cholecystokinin (CCK) receptors, or transfected m1, m2 and m3 mAChRs by pertussis toxin (PTX) catalyzed adenosine diphosphate-(ADP-) ribosylation of endogenous G-proteins in CHO cells. Both thrombin receptors and m2 mAChRs were completely uncoupled at high PTX concentrations, whereas m1 and m3 mAChRs showed a plateau corresponding to about half of the maximal effect. CCK receptor stimulation of PLC was unaffected by PTX treatment. These different receptors were thus coupled to PLC as follows: m2 mAChRs and thrombin receptors by a pertussin toxin-sensitive G-protein; CCK receptors by a PTX-insensitive G-protein; and m1 and m3 mAChRs by both types of G-protein. Further discrimination in effector coupling was observed between the m1 and m3 subtypes[24] in CHO cells, where the m1 mAChR showed a greater stimulation of PLC than m3 and was also coupled to increases in intracellular adenosine 3′5′-cyclic phosphate (cyclic AMP) levels, which were unaffected by the m3 subtype.

Agonist-binding to m2 and m4 subtypes expressed in NG108-15 neuroblastoma x glioma cells were shown to inhibit neuronal calcium currents.[25] Activation of m1 and m3 subtypes,[26] however, stimulated PLC and intracellular calcium release, activated calcium-dependent potassium channels, and inhibited m-currents (a type of voltage-dependent potassium current that is regulated by mAChRs). m5 responses were studied in both CHO cells[27] and murine L cells.[28] In both systems, agonists increased intracellular calcium levels by activation of PLC, while in the CHO cells, PLA_2 was also activated. The effects of PLA_2 were attributed to a combination of increased protein kinase C activity, as a result of diacylglycerol formation, and entry of extracellular calcium into the cell. Coupling of mAChR subtypes to phospholipase D in a human embryonic kidney cell-line[29] showed that the m1 and m3 receptors coupled more efficiently to this effector than the m2 and m4 subtypes although all four subtypes stimulated enzyme activity. The mAChR subtypes (m1, m3, m5) that were coupled to stimulation of PLC were capable of acting as oncogenes in NIH 3T3 cells continually exposed to a muscarinic agonist,[30] although the explicit biochemical pathways involved in cellular transformation remain to be determined. *Xenopus* oocytes injected with mRNA coding for the m3 mAChR were used to study the temporal and spacial patterns of intracellular calcium release.[31] Regenerative spiral waves of calcium release were observed and, in order to model wave propagation and annihilation, it was assumed that the oocyte cytosol behaved as an excitable medium. In summary (see Table 1), the m1, m3, and m5 subtypes appear to couple selectively to G-proteins that activate phospholipases and release intracellular calcium, while the m2 and m4 subtypes interact most efficiently with G-proteins that are coupled to and inhibit AC.

Clonal cell-lines have also been used to examine the antagonist-binding properties of muscarinic subtypes.[32] Of the ligands studied, the greatest subtype selectivities were shown by pirenzepine (PZ) (m1), methoctramine (m2), and hexahydrosiladifenidol (m3). Selective ligands for the m4 and m5 subtypes have not yet been identified.

Muscarinic Receptor Mutants

The roles of specific amino acids or regions of the mAChR subtypes in the binding of ligands and the coupling to G-proteins that act as signal transducers have been explored either by making specific mutations in an amino acid residue, by removing portions of the protein by deletions of the DNA sequence coding for that region, or by constructing chimeric receptors. These three methods are explored below.

One approach used to construct mutant receptors[33] is shown in Figure 5. In this example, DNA coding for the mAChR is cloned into a vector for the bacteriophage M13. The phage are then grown in an *Escherichia coli* strain that is deficient in both uracil N-glycosylase, a repair enzyme that normally

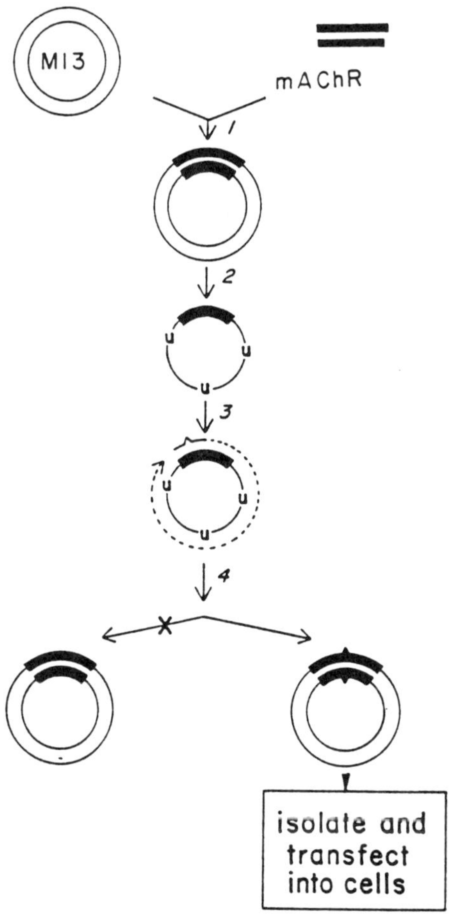

Figure 5. *Construction of mutant mAChRs. Using the procedure developed by Kunkel et al,*[33] *the gene coding for the receptor is cloned into a plasmid of double-stranded M13 DNA (step 1). The plasmid is used to transform an E coli strain lacking dUTPase and uracil N-glycosylase, and single-stranded uracil containing DNA is isolated from the phage (step 2). A mutagenic primer is used to synthesize the second DNA strand in vitro (step 3) followed by transformation of an E coli strain that contains the normal complement of repair enzymes (step 4). This process favors selection of bacteria containing the mutant receptor since the wild type DNA, which contains uracil, is degraded. The gene coding for the mutant is then isolated by restriction enzyme cleavage and inserted into a vector for transfection into cells.*

removes uracil misincorporated into DNA, and dUTPase, an enzyme that hydrolyzes dUTP. As a result, the single-stranded phage DNA contains multiple substitutions of uracil for thymine. A mutagenic primer is then used for enzymatic synthesis of the cDNA strand in the presence of the four 2′-deoxynucleotide triphosphates. The duplex DNA is used to transform a second *E coli* strain that contains a normal complement of repair enzymes. When the bacteriophage are produced from this host, there is strong selective pressure against production of DNA from the uracil-containing parent strand, which is degraded, and in favor of production from the mutant DNA strand, which contains no uracil. The bacterial clones are then screened either by sequencing phase DNA or by performing restriction analysis of bacterial DNA to identify mutants. After confirming the mutation by DNA sequencing, the gene coding for the mutant receptor is isolated by restriction enzyme digestion and cloned into the appropriate vector for transfection into cells.

Extensive studies of the β-adrenergic receptor (β-AR) structure by site-directed mutagenesis[13] suggested that the anionic side chains of aspartate residues occurring near the top of TM3 may act as counterions for positively charged amine ligands. Mutagenesis of these aspartate residues individually to asparagine[34] in m1 mAChRs indicated that one or both of these residues may be important in the binding of the quarternary ammonium group of muscarinic agonists. The largest reduction in ligand affinity was found for the mutant aspartate in TM3 (aspartate 105). This residue was more deeply embedded within the membrane-spanning segment, in agreement with protein sequencing studies[14] that indicated that this residue was covalently modified by the site-directed affinity label, propylbenzilylcholine mustard. The binding site for acetylcholine (ACh), therefore appears to be located within the TM regions of the receptor near the extracellular surface of the membrane. A second interesting result of these experiments is that mutagenesis of the aspartates at the bottom of TM2 and TM3 reduced coupling as a result of stimulation of PLC.

The importance of asparagine-linked glycosylation in expression and function of the m3 subtype was examined by site-directed mutagenesis.[35] Asparagine residues at putative extracellular glycosylation sites were altered to either aspartate or glutamine, and the mutant receptors were expressed in CHO cells. That the receptor was not glycosylated in these mutants was verified biochemically. A comparison of the properties of the mutant receptors with those of the wild type protein indicated that glycosylation was not required for either receptor expression at the cell surface, ligand-binding, or coupling to physiological responses.

Additional sites for potential posttranscriptional modification include the amino terminus, known from protein sequencing studies to be blocked, and a cysteine residue near the carboxyl terminus, shown to be palmitoylated in the β-AR.[36] Intracellular loop 5-6 contains several potential sites for phosphorylation by protein kinases and may therefore be important in downregulation of mAChRs. Deletion of 123 of the 156 amino acids of loop 5-6 of the mouse m1 mAChR had no effect on either the ligand-binding properties or the coupling to PLC in Y1 adrenal carcinoma cells.[37] No effect was observed on short-term internalization of receptor-binding sites in the presence of an agonist. Long-term loss of binding sites from the cell surface, however, was only 25% for the mutant, compared to a 60% reduction for wild type m1 mAChRs. This region of the protein, therefore, may be important in the long-term regulation of receptor expression by agonists at the cell surface.

As an alternative to specifically mutating single amino acids, hybrid receptors, or chimeras, can be constructed in which a region of one subtype replaces the corresponding domain of the protein in a second muscarinic subtype or closely related G-protein-linked receptor. This process was first executed by Numa and colleagues,[38] who showed that switching the 5-6 loop and part of the carboxyl terminus of TM5 between m1 and m2 mAChRs changed their coupling to physiological effector systems. The m2 receptor containing the 5-6 loop from the m1 receptor coupled like an m1 subtype, and the m1 receptor containing the 5-6 loop from the m2 receptor behaved as the m2 subtype. Similar studies using A9 L cells[39] and *Xenopus* oocytes[40] in which portions of the 5-6 loop were interchanged between m2 and m3 mAChR subtypes further localized the predominant region for G-protein specificity to the amino terminal 15-20 amino acids in intracellular loop 5-6. Replacement of the intracellular 5-6 loop of the dopamine D_2 receptor with the corresponding region of the m1 mAChR produced a protein that increased intracellular calcium in response to dopaminergic agonists[41] in CHO cells. Replacement of both intracellular loop 3-4 and the amino terminal of intracellular loop 5-6 in the m1 mAChR subtype with the corresponding amino acids from the β-AR resulted in a chimeric receptor that gave a β-AR-like response by activating AC upon addition of muscarinic agonists.[42] Thus, intracellular loop 5-6, particularly the amino terminal segment, appears to be a major determinant of receptor G-protein specificity.

Receptor Localization

With the clones and amino acid sequences known for the five mAChR subtypes, receptor distribution could then be mapped either by in situ hybridization to mRNA,[5] by Northern analysis of tissue mRNA samples,[6] or by subtype-specific antibodies raised against unique receptor amino acid sequences.[43,44] The results of these experiments indicate that all five subtypes are found in the brain (different subtypes are localized to different brain regions) with m5 being the least abundant. The atria show expression of only the m2 subtype, which is also abundant in smooth muscle. The m1 and m3 subtypes are also abundant in exocrine glands. These results (summarized in Table 1), in combination with Northern analysis of mRNA from several different cell-lines, show that expression of receptor subtypes appears to be specific (generally, two subtypes or less) for a particular tissue or cell-line.

Summary and Conclusions

Knowledge of mAChR molecular biology has been increasing at a very rapid pace over the past five years. With the successful cloning of the genes for the five receptor subtypes, it has been possible to deduce their amino acid sequence, to determine their ligand-binding properties, and to delineate their specificity of coupling to physiological effector systems. The tissue distribution of the subtypes has been determined and detailed analysis of the roles of receptor domains in ligand-binding and interaction with G-proteins has begun. Several questions remain to be answered. Are there more, as yet undiscovered, mAChR subtypes? Why is there an apparent redundancy in interaction with effector systems (m1, m3, and m5 appear to couple to the same effectors as do m2 and m4)? Are there additional factors, such as different regulatory mechanisms or undiscovered effector systems, that necessitate multiple subtypes? Which G-protein and effector isotypes couple to each mAChR subtype? Can high-resolution structural data be obtained for wild type mAChRs and mutants? These problems should provide challenging and exciting topics for future research in mAChR molecular biology.

References

1. Peterson GL, Herron GS, Yamaki M, et al: Purification of the muscarinic receptor from porcine atria. Proc Natl Acad Sci USA 81:4993, 1984.
2. Haga K, Haga T: Purification of the muscarinic acetylcholine receptor from porcine brain. J Biol Chem 260:7927, 1985.
3. Kubo T, Fukuda K, Mikami A, et al: Cloning, sequencing and expression of complementary DNA encoding the muscarinic acetylcholine receptor. Nature (London) 323:411, 1986.
4. Peralta EG, Winslow JW, Peterson GL, et al: Primary structure and biochemical properties of an M_2 muscarinic receptor. Science 236:600, 1987.
5. Bonner TI, Buckley NJ, Young AL, et al: Identification of a family of muscarinic acetylcholine receptor genes. Science 237:527, 1987.
6. Peralta EG, Ashkenazi A, Winslow JW, et al: Distinct primary structures, ligand binding properties and tissue specific expression of four human muscarinic acetylcholine receptors. EMBO J 6:3923, 1987.
7. Bonner TI, Young AC, Brann MR, et al: Cloning and expression of the human and rat m5 muscarinic acetylcholine receptor genes. Neuron 1:403, 1988.
8. Kyte J, Doolittle R: A simple method for displaying the hydropathic character of a protein. J Mol Biol 157:105, 1982.
9. Dratz EA, Hargrave PA: The structure of rhodopsin and the rod outer segment disc membrane. Trends Biochem Sci 8:128, 1983.
10. Henderson R, Baldwin JM, Ceska TA, et al: Model for the structure of bacteriorhodopsin based on high-resolution electron cryo-microscopy. J Mol Biol 213:899, 1990.
11. Donnelly D, Johnson MS, Blundell TL, et al: An analysis of the periodicity of conserved residues in sequence alignments of G-protein coupled receptors. Implications for the three-dimensional structure. FEBS Lett 251:109, 1989.
12. Hulme EC, Kurtenbach E, Curtis CAM: Muscarinic acetylcholine receptors: Structure and function. Biochem Soc Trans 19:133, 1991.
13. Dixon RAF, Sigal IS, Strader CD: Structure-function analysis of the β-adrenergic receptor. Cold Spring Harbor Symp on Quant Biol 53:487, 1988.
14. Kurtenbach E, Curtis CAM, Pedder EK, et al: Muscarinic acetylcholine receptors. Peptide sequencing identifies residues involved in antagonist binding and disulfide bond formation. J Biol Chem 265:13702, 1990.
15. Herron GS, Schimerlik MI: Glycoprotein properties of solubilized atrial muscarinic receptors. J Neurochem 41:1414, 1983.
16. Birnbaumer L: G proteins in signal transduction. Ann Rev Pharmacol Toxicol 30:675, 1990.
17. Simon MI, Strathmann MP, Gautam N: Diversity of G proteins in signal transduction. Science 252:802, 1991.
18. Bourne HR, Sanders DA and McCormick F: The GTPase superfamily: Conserved structure and molecular mechanism. Nature (London) 349:117, 1991.
19. Conklin B, Brann MR, Buckley NJ, et al: Stimulation of arachidonic acid release and inhibition of mitogenesis by cloned genes for muscarinic receptor subtypes stably expressed in A9 L cells. Proc Natl Acad Sci USA 85:8698, 1988.
20. Jones SVP, Barker JL, Buckley NJ, et al: Cloned muscarinic receptor subtypes

expressed in A9 L cells differ in their coupling to electrical responses. Molec Pharmacol 34:421, 1988.

21. Ashkenazi A, Winslow JW, Peralta EG, et al: An M2 muscarinic receptor subtype coupled to both adenylyl cyclase and phosphoinositide turnover. Science 238:672, 1987.
22. Peralta EG, Ashkenazi A, Winslow JW, et al: Differential regulation of PI hydrolysis and adenylyl cyclase by muscarinic receptor subtypes. Nature (London) 334:434, 1988.
23. Ashkenazi A, Peralta EG, Winslow JW, et al: Functionally distinct G proteins selectively couple different receptors to PI hydrolysis in the same cell. Cell 56:487, 1989.
24. Buck MA, Fraser CM: Muscarinic acetylcholine receptor subtypes which selectively couple to phospholipase C: Pharmacological and biochemical properties. Biochem Biophys Res Comm 173:666, 1990.
25. Higashida H, Hashii M, Fukuda K, et al: Selective coupling of different muscarinic acetylcholine receptors to neuronal calcium currents in DNA-transfected cells. Proc R Soc Lond Biol 242:68, 1990.
26. Fukuda K, Higashida H, Kubo T, et al: Selective coupling with K^+ currents of muscarinic acetylcholine receptor subtypes in NG108-15 cells. Nature (London) 335:355, 1988.
27. Felder CC, Dieter P, Kinsella J, et al: A transfected m_5 muscarinic acetylcholine receptor stimulates phospholipase A_2 by inducing both calcium influx and activation of protein kinase C. J Pharmacol Exp Ther 255:1140, 1990.
28. Liao C-F, Schilling WP, Birnbaumer M, et al: Cellular responses to stimulation of the m5 muscarinic acetylcholine receptor as seen in murine L cells. J Biol Chem 265:11273, 1990.
29. Sandmann J, Peralta EG, Wurtman RJ: Coupling of transfected muscarinic acetylcholine receptor subtypes to phospholipase D. J Biol Chem 266:6031, 1991.
30. Gutkind JS, Novotny EA, Brann MR, et al: Muscarinic acetylcholine receptor subtypes as agonist-dependent oncogenes. Proc Natl Acad Sci USA 88:4703, 1991.
31. Lechleiter J, Girard S, Peralta E, et al: Spiral calcium wave propagation and annihilation in *Xenopus laevis* oocytes. Science 252:123, 1991.
32. Buckley NJ, Bonner TI, Buckley CM, et al: Antagonist binding properties of five cloned muscarinic receptors expressed in CHO-K1 cells. Molec Pharmacol 35:469, 1989.
33. Kunkel TA, Roberts JD, Zakour RA: Rapid and efficient site specific mutagenesis without phenotypic selection. Methods Enzymol 154:367, 1987.
34. Fraser CM, Wang C-D, Robinson DA, et al: Site directed mutagenesis of m_1 muscarinic acetylcholine receptors: Conserved aspartic acids play important roles in receptor function. Molec Pharmacol 36:840, 1989.
35. van Koppen CJ, Nathanson NM: Site-directed mutagenesis of the m2 muscarinic acetylcholine receptor. Analysis of the role of N-glycosylation in receptor expression and function. J Biol Chem 265:20887, 1990.
36. O'Dowd BF, Hnatowich M, Caron MG, et al: Palmitoylation of the human β_2-adrenergic receptor. J Biol Chem 264:7564, 1989.
37. Shapiro RA, Nathanson NM: Deletion analysis of the mouse m1 muscarinic acetylcholine receptor: Effects on phosphoinositide metabolism and down-regulation. Biochemistry 28:8946, 1989.
38. Kubo T, Bujo H, Akiba I, et al: Location of a region of the muscarinic acetylcholine receptor involved in selective effector coupling. FEBS Lett 241:119, 1988.
39. Wess J, Bonner TI, Dörje F, et al: Delineation of muscarinic receptor domains conferring selectivity of coupling to guanine nucleotide-binding proteins and second messengers. Molec Pharmacol 38:517, 1990.
40. Lechleiter J, Hellmiss R, Duerson K, et al: Distinct sequence elements control the specificity of G protein activation by muscarinic acetylcholine receptor subtypes. EMBO J 9:4381, 1990.

41. England BP, Ackerman MS, Barrett RW: A chimeric D_2 dopamine/m1 muscarinic receptor with D_2 binding specificity mobilizes intracellular calcium in response to dopamine. FEBS Lett 279:87, 1991.
42. Wong SK-F, Parker EM, Ross EM: Chimeric muscarinic cholinergic: β-adrenergic receptors that activate G_s in response to muscarinic agonists. J Biol Chem 265:6219, 1990.
43. Levey AI, Stormann TM, Brann MR: Bacterial expression of human muscarinic receptor fusion proteins and generation of subtype-specific antisera. FEBS Lett 275:65, 1990.
44. Wall SJ, Yasuda RP, Hory F, et al: Production of antisera selection for m1 muscarinic receptors using fusion proteins: Distribution of m1 receptors in rat brain. Molec Pharmacol 39:643, 1991.

CHAPTER 9

Coupling of G-Proteins to Cardiac Ion Channels

A.M. Brown

Perspective

In order to describe the role of guanine nucleotide-binding proteins (G-proteins) in vagal control of the heart, this chapter presents a hypothesis in which these proteins provide the regulatory basis for the synergistic or antagonistic effects on heart rate that are produced by stimulation of the cardiac vagus and sympathetic nerves (Fig. 1). One of the most classical observations of regulatory physiology is that vagal slowing of heart rate is much greater when the sympathetic nerves are active (synergism) and sympathetic quickening is reduced when the vagi are active (antagonism). The neurotransmitters acetylcholine (ACh) and norepinephrine (NE) mimic the neural effects[1,2] which are, in reality, opposite sides of the same coin. The allosteric effects of two G-proteins, G_0 and G_s, on the pacemaker I_f channels present in the sinoatrial (SA) node pacemaker cells of the heart can account for the above observation. Since these particular G-proteins have been studied extensively and may be important in cardiac vagal control, this chapter also applies the hypothesis to the effects of the proteins G_i or G_k on the atrial K^+[ACh] channel.

How G-Proteins Couple Receptors to Ion Channels

A diagram of the three elements in the response pathway of a cardiac cell to an autonomic neurotransmitter is shown in Figure 2. The receptors compose

This work was supported in part by National Institutes of Health Grant HL36930.

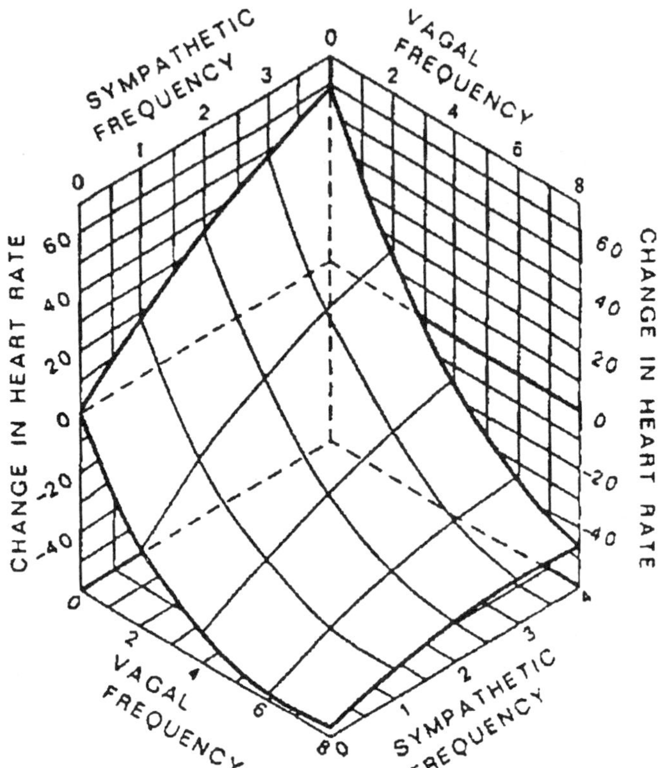

Figure 1. *Changes in heart rate produced by various combinations of vagal and sympathetic nerve stimulation. Vagal inhibition is much greater when the sympathetics are active. Sympathetic stimulation is much less when the vagi are active. The former exemplifies synergism, the latter antagonism. Reproduced with permission from Levy MN, Zieske H Jr: Autonomic control of cardiac pacemaker activity and atrioventricular transmission. J Appl Physiol 27:465–470, 1969.*

a family that has a motif of seven α-helical transmembrane (TM) segments and three cytoplasmic loops, the third of which is thought to interact with G-proteins.[3] The heterotrimeric αβγ, signal-transducing G-proteins are classified as another superfamily with as many as 15 different α subunits,[4] several different β subunits, and at least two different γ subunits. The voltage-sensitive Na^+, K^+, and Ca^{2+} channels, which are targets for G-proteins, are yet another family.[5] Nothing is known, however, about the molecular structure of the channels that are directly gated by heterotrimeric G-proteins; such channels include the muscarinic atrial K^+ (K^+[ACh]) channel,[6] a variety of K^+ channels in neurons,[7] the ATP-sensitive K^+ (K^+_{ATP}) channel,[8,9] and the I_f channel.[10,11] Much more is known about the coupling among these elements, with the biochemistry of G-protein activation being especially well understood.

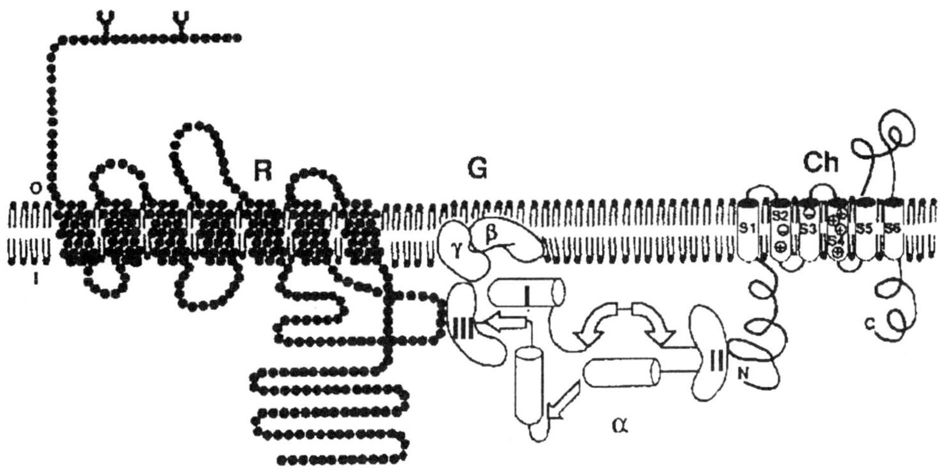

Figure 2. *Receptor-G-protein-ionic channel complex. The G-protein-coupled system is vectorial; information flows from receptor to signal-transducing G-protein to ionic channel. The topography of each element is based on models derived from primary amino acid sequences. R: G-protein receptor; G: heterotrimeric G-protein; Ch: ion channel; N: amino terminus of ion channel; and C: carboxy terminus of ion channel. The third cytoplasmic loop in the receptor is thought to be especially important. For G-proteins the α subunit is thought to mediate effector activation. Domains I, II, and III are proposed to interact with βγ subunits, ionic channel, and receptor, respectively. The region between the arrows forms a pocket in which the guanine nucleotides GDP or GTP lie. Voltage-gated ionic channels have a basic motif of six TM segments, one of which, S4, may be a positively-charged voltage sensor. They also have consensus sequences for phosphorylation by cyclic AMP-dependent protein kinase A (PKA) (not shown). Initially, cytoplasmic second messengers were thought to be the sole pathway between the G-protein and the ionic channel. Reproduced with permission from Brown AM: Regulation of heartbeat by G protein-coupled ion channels. Am J Physiol 259:H1621–1628, 1990.*

The G-Protein Switch

Signal transduction is thought to be mediated by G-proteins on the following basis. The G-protein is activated when guanosine triphosphate (GTP) is bound to it, presumably by dissociating into α-GTP and βγ. In the absence of receptor agonist, bound GTP is hydrolyzed at approximately .01/seconds, whereas the off rate for guanosine diphosphate (GDP) is approximately .1/seconds.[12] Consequently, the G-protein is mostly GDP-bound and inactive. The agonist opens up the GTP-binding site and the off rate for GDP increases by approximately 10-fold. Hence, the G-protein may now be active for about 50% or more of the time during agonist occupancy of the receptor. Since the activated G-protein has this well-defined lifetime, it may be thought of as a three-way switch: empty, GTP-bound, and GDP-bound.[13]

Indirect Coupling

The pathways by which information flows from the receptor to the G-protein to the ionic channel may be direct or indirect (Fig. 3). The G-protein coupling to ionic channels was initially thought to be entirely indirect via cytoplasmic second messengers such as adenosine 3',5'-cyclic phosphate (cyclic AMP) or cyclic guanosine monophosphate (cGMP) (Fig. 3). One of the most thoroughly studied signalling pathways consists of information flowing from agonist-occupied β-adrenergic receptors (β-AR) to Ca^{2+} channels via the G-protein G_s, which stimulates adenylyl cyclase (AC). As a result, the cyclic AMP levels increase, cyclic AMP-dependent protein kinase A (PKA) is activated, cardiac Ca^{2+} channels are phosphorylated, and Ca^{2+} currents become greater.[14–16] Other important, but less well-defined, pathways use the pertussis toxin (PTX)-sensitive G_i-proteins or the G-protein G_p. These G-proteins often couple receptors to phospholipase C (PLC), stimulation of which leads to the production of diacylglycerol (DAG) and inositol triphosphate (IP_3). DAG activates protein kinase C, which phosphorylates ionic channels at residues other than those phosphorylated by PKA.[17] IP_3 is know to activate sarcoplasmic or endoplasmic reticulum channels that release Ca^{2+}[11] and it may act

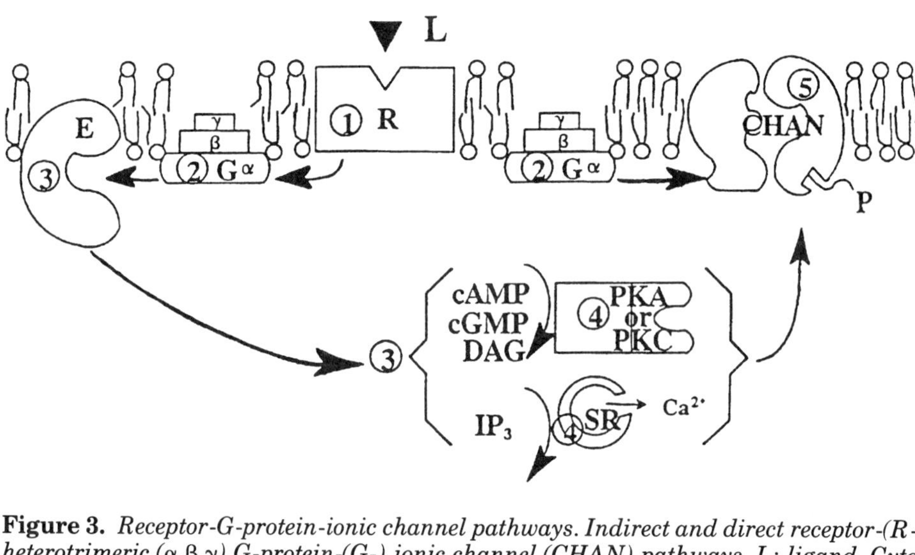

Figure 3. *Receptor-G-protein-ionic channel pathways. Indirect and direct receptor-(R-) heterotrimeric (α,β,γ) G-protein-(G-) ionic channel (CHAN) pathways. L: ligand. Cytoplasmic, indirect pathways have AC, cGMP phosphodiesterase, PLC, and PLA_2 as G-protein effectors (E). Cytoplasmic messenger replays to channels include: 1: cyclic AMP (cAMP), protein kinase A (PKA), and ion channel phosphorylation; 2: cGMP and cGMP-gated ion channel; 3: diacylglycerol (DAG), protein kinase C (PKC), and ion channel phosphorylation; 4: inositol 1,4,5-trisphosphate (IP_3), Ca^{2+}-release channel in sarcoplasmic reticulum (SR), and Ca^{2+}; and 5: CHAN: ion channel. For direct pathways, G-proteins act within the membrane on ionic channels. Reproduced with permission from Brown AM: Regulation of heartbeat by G protein-coupled ion channels. Am J Physiol 259:H1621–1628, 1990.*

directly on plasmalemmal ionic channels. Ca^{2+} may act on ionic channels directly or indirectly via Ca^{2+}-activated kinases, including Ca^{2+}-calmodulin kinase. It also appears that G-proteins may couple receptors to phospholipase A2 (PLA_2) and, ultimately, to ionic channels. Lipoxygenase metabolites of arachidonic acid, a product of phospholipase action on phospholipids, have been implicated in the activation of a K^+ channel in *Aplysia*[18] and in the atrial K^+[ACh] channel.[19]

Direct Coupling

Direct coupling between a G-protein and an ionic channel seemed most likely to be demonstrated for an atrial muscarinic M_2 receptor and a K^+[ACh] channel. The experimental results pointing to this possibility were the following:

1. the latency after ACh application was about 100 milliseconds,[20–23] which was much longer than the latency at the nicotinic ACh receptor (1 millisecond) where the receptor and the ionic channel were the same protein;
2. the occupation of the receptor by the agonist was not the rate-limiting step[24]; and
3. possible second messengers such as cGMP,[24–26] cyclic AMP,[24,26] and Ca^{2+}[26] were ruled out. Subsequently, it was shown that when ACh was applied outside a cell-attached patch of membrane, it could not activate K^+ channels, whereas ACh in the patch pipette could activate these channels.[27]

From binding studies, it was known that muscarinic M_2 receptors were linked to G-proteins in the heart and that PTX substrates were present in atrial tissues.[28–31] The link with electrophysiology was established when a block by PTX of muscarinic effects on inwardly-rectifying whole-cell current and resting membrane potential were shown together with a requirement for intracellular GTP.[32–34] In addition, the nonhydrolyzable GTP analog, Gpp(NH)p, disconnected the currents from ACh control.[35] These experiments were complicated by the fact that a non-PTX-sensitive phosphoinositide pathway[36] was also present in atrial cells and may have contributed inward current to the whole-cell current or membrane potential measurements.[37]

A revealing set of experiments showed that GTPγS applied to the cytoplasmic face of an inside-out (I-O) membrane patch activated a specific set of inwardly-rectifying, single K^+ channel currents that were the same as those activated by ACh and did so in a Mg^{2+}-dependent manner.[38,39] The particular G-proteins involved to this point had not been specified nor had a membrane-associated G-protein effect, such as protein kinase C activation, been excluded. In the author's experiments, specific G-proteins purified from natural membranes were applied to I-O patches for observation of their effects. These experiments established that a G-protein, probably G_i-3, when preactivated with GTPγS, activated single channel K^+[ACh] currents in the absence of any substrate. Moreover, the activation, just like physiological activation by ACh, was simply due to an increase in opening frequency. In addition, testing was done to determine whether protein kinase C activation could be involved.[40,41] The effects discussed above occurred in the presence of AMP-PNP, and phorbol ester had no effect in the presence of ATP. Phosphorylation by protein kinase C could, therefore, be excluded. Picomolar concentrations of the preactivated G-proteins stimulated K^+[ACh] channels, whereas nanomolar concentrations of GTPγS were required to activate the responsible endogenous G-protein.

Role of G-Protein Subunits

Adenosine diphosphate-ribosylation with PTX blocked muscarinic activation and the response was reconstituted by unactivated G_i-3 in the presence of GTP. Thus, endogenous G_k cannot be tightly coupled to the muscarinic receptor (mAChR), because adenosine diphosphate-ribosylation with PTX would, in this case, have led to permanent loss of receptor-G-protein-K^+ channel coupling. Nor can the endogenous G_k be tightly coupled to the K^+[ACh] channel, because exogenous G_i^*-3 or α_i^*-3 activated the channel. While GTP plus the unactivated trimeric G_i-3 stimulated K^+[ACh] channels in the presence of agonist and PTX, GTP plus βγ could not reconstitute the response and this finding, together with the fact that α_i^*-3 and holo G_i^*-3 were equipotent, indicated that α_i^*-3 mediated the effect. While it was originally proposed that βγ was responsible, it is now agreed that α subunits may produce the response.[19,42] βγ subunits activated PLA_2,[19] and arachidonic acid and its 5'-lipoxygenase metabolites[43] activated these same atrial K^+ channels. This mechanism was not operative, however, in muscarinic or purinergic stimulation of K^+[ACh] channels, because eicosanoid pathway blockers had no effect on the agonist-induced responses.[19,43] Furthermore, there were inconsistencies between the observations of Kurachi et al[43] and Kim et al[19] regarding the postulated mediation of βγ effects via arachidonic acid release. The most noteworthy was that the effects of arachidonic acid and its metabolites observed by Kurachi et al[43] required the presence of GTP, whereas the βγ effects reported by Kim et al[19] occurred in its absence.[44] Recently, it has been shown that bromphenacyl bromide, which blocked entry of arachidonic acid to downstream metabolism, had effects on ionic channels.[45] Nordihydroguiaretic acid, which blocks 5'-lipoxygenase pathways, also had nonspecific effects.[45] Furthermore, biochemical evidence for a 5'-lipoxygenase pathway was lacking in heart muscle.[46]

In most cases where it has been investigated, effects of βγ have been shown to be inhibitory through a mass action effect on the α subunit,[47,48] although in the case of retinal PLA_2, a direct stimulatory effect for βγ subunits has been proposed.[49] Evidence for βγ mediation of the pheromone receptor response in *Saccharomyces cerevisiae* has been summarized by Bourne.[13] In the retina, the concentrations of βγ were in the micromolar range, i.e., ca. 10^6-fold higher than those needed to obtain an effect with α_i-3 on K^+ channels[41,50] or on AC.[51] In the atrial K^+ channel experiments, nanomolar βγ was used. The βγ activator results were complicated, however, because the zwitterionic detergent CHAPS used in the experiments of Clapham and collaborators[42,44] could by itself activate atrial K^+ channels[52,53] as well as other ionic channels.[52] It is known that ionic detergents may act upon Na^+ channels and other membrane proteins including PLA_2.[52]

The idea that βγ subunits may be stimulatory to atrial K^+ channels has also been challenged by experiments that show that βγ subunits, including the same ones used by Logothetis et al,[42,44] inhibited these channels.[55] In some of these experiments, the detergent Lubrol was used to suspend the βγ subunits. While care was taken to avoid any direct inhibitory effects of Lubrol, these effects can never be ruled out completely. More convincing were the observations that the same results occurred (i.e., inhibition of muscarinic atrial K^+ channels) when hydrophilic βγ of transducin was used without the use of detergents. Moreover, βγ was found to be more potent as an inhibitor of channels in the absence of agonist;[55] this finding suggested that βγ subunits have, as one role, the suppression of agonist-independent background noise, and it supported the idea that the inhibitory effect was physiologically relevant.

The experiments to this point have dealt mainly with reconstitution of the K^+[ACh] response. To probe further functional aspects, a monoclonal antibody was used that bound to α but not to βγ subunits. Monoclonal antibody 4A bound to α_T and α_i-3 and was shown to block the light-induced transition of rhodopsin to metarhodopsin II.[56,57] The results showed that monoclonal antibody 4A blocked the muscarinic M_2 receptor effect and, furthermore, the block was irreversible only if endogenous G-protein was activated. Only two conclusions were possible: one, that βγ was liberated at a time when the mAChR effect was blocked or two, that αGTPβγ and βγ were equipotent, which was not the case. Neither result was consistent with a role for βγ in muscarinic M_2 receptor activation of K^+[ACh].[58]

While recombinant α_i-3, activated either by GTPγS or AlF^{4-}, did stimulate the K^+ channel and thus removed any doubt as to the structural identity of the α subunit of G_k,[59,60] the other recombinant forms of α_i proved to be equipotent when tested for effects on atrial K^+ channels.[60] This result, led to the testing of the native versions, that were contaminated by each other at <5%. Native GTPγS-activated α_i-1 (α_i^*-1) and α_i-2 (α_i^*-2) were prepared from purified bovine brain G_i-1 and human erythrocyte G_i-2 as described earlier for α_i^*-3 and were tested for effects on atrial K^+ channels. The native type 1 and type 2 molecules were active at the same low concentrations as α_i^*-3 and, therefore, the results from the recombinant forms of the α_i molecules were valid.[60] Thus, at least with respect to atrial K^+ channel regulation, types 1, 2 and 3 of the G_i's are G_k isoforms.

Interaction Between the $G_i\alpha$ Subunit and K^+[ACh] Channel

Little is known about the site of protein-protein interaction at which the α subunit activates the K^+ channel. Based on the assumption that an inactivating particle kept the K^+[ACh] channel closed, several protein-modifying agents, including trypsin, papain, glyoxal, and phenylglyoxal, that remove Na^+-channel inactivation were tested. Of the agents tested, only trypsin activated muscarinic K^+ channels, and it did so irreversibly. Trypsin activation produced single-channel currents in which inward rectification, single-channel conductance, mean open time, and burst duration were indistinguishable from muscarinic activation. Trypsin was effective in the absence of muscarinic agonist or intracellular Mg^{2+} and guanosine 5'-triphosphate (GTP). Heat-denatured trypsin was ineffective and trypsin inhibitor blocked the effect. Since trypsin was known to inactivate G-proteins, the effect probably occurred on the K^+ channel or a structure closely associated with it. Trypsin cleaves proteins at lysine or arginine residues, and the arginine-specific reagents glyoxal and phenylglyoxal did not activate K^+ channels. The hypothesis is that trypsin disrupted an inhibitory gating mechanism that normally held the channel closed in the absence of activated G_k. The inhibitory gate was physically distinct from the gate that mediated bursting and contained at least one trypsin cleavage point located at a lysine residue accessible from the cytoplasmic surface of the cell membrane. The inhibitory subunit is, therefore, analogous to the γ subunit of cGMP PDE.[9]

Dual G-Protein Coupling and Biphasic Responses

G-protein coupling was both direct and indirect for voltage-gated Ca^{2+} and Na^+ channels, and the pathway components were β-AR, G_s, AC, and Ca^{2+} or NA^+ channels.[61–63] Since direct responses, as exemplified by atrial K^+[ACh] currents, occurred within 1 second[64] and indirect responses took longer,[65] it was predicted that dual pathways might produce a biphasic response when the receptor was activated by agonist. The required rapid application of agonist was achieved by using a concentration clamp method.[64] The prediction was confirmed for the response of cardiac Ca^{2+} and Na^+ channels to β-adrenergic agonists.[64,66] The possibility that two types of β-receptors were involved was ruled out; only the β_1-receptor mediates the response in guinea pig ventricular myocytes.[64] The results on dual G-protein-ionic channel pathways and the interpretation of them are as follows:

1. $G_s\alpha$ has AC, Ca^{2+}, and Na^+ channels as effectors;
2. $G_s\alpha$ acts on these channels by direct and indirect pathways;
3. β-adrenergic agonists have biphasic (fast, direct; slow, indirect) effects on these channels; and
4. the fast pathway for β-adrenergic agonists may mediate inotropic regulation. The proposed pathways are shown in Figure 4.

Dual direct and indirect effects of G_s on Ca^{2+} channels may have other implications.[63] As noted, it is not clear whether G_s is required for the effects of

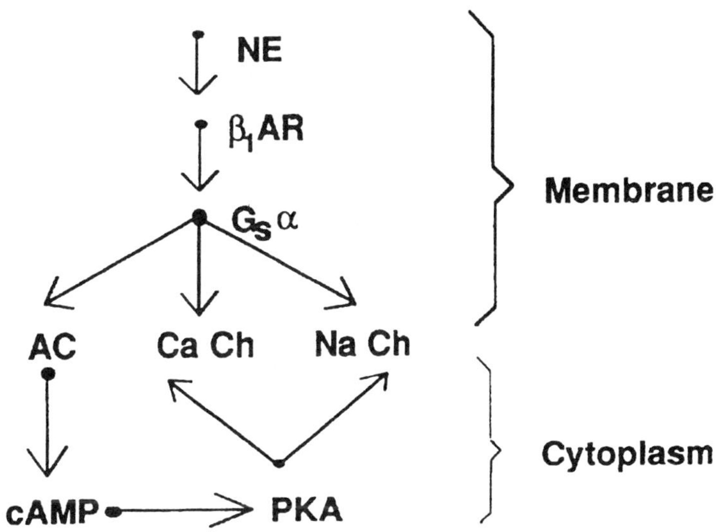

Figure 4. *Dual G-protein pathways to Ca^{2+} and Na^+ channels. NE: norepinephrine; β_1AR: β_1-adrenoreceptor; AC: adenylyl cyclase; $G_S\alpha$: stimulator of AC acting through its α-subunit; cAMP: adenosine 3′,5′-cyclic monophosphate; and PKA: protein kinase A. Reproduced with permission from Brown AM: Regulation of heartbeat by G protein-coupled ion channels. Am J Physiol 259:H1621–1628, 1990.*

protein kinase (PK) phosphorylation of Ca^{2+} channels or whether the latter is required for G_s effects. A similar statement applies to Na^+ channels.

Hartzell et al[67] have recently claimed that β-AR are coupled to Ca^{2+} channels by the cytoplasmic pathway alone, because they are unable to demonstrate a fast response to the β-agonist isoproterenol. Evidence of membrane-delimited and cytoplasmic pathways between G_s and cardiac Ca^{2+} channels, however, has been obtained by Pelzer et al[68] and Cavalié et al.[69] In these experiments, the cytoplasmic pathways were blocked and guanine nucleotide-dependent, isoproterenol-activated increases in Ca^{2+} currents were demonstrated. Moreover, Bean (personal communication) has observed the biphasic response in rat cardiac myoctyes and Kozlowski et al,[70] using flash-activated hydrolysis of caged GTPγS, have shown fast and slow responses in guinea pig cardiac myocytes.

Direct G-Protein Coupling to Ion Channels in Cardiac Pacemakers

The interpretation of the fast effects on Ca^{2+} channels discussed in the previous section is that the direct pathway is important for second-to-second or beat-to-beat regulation of heart rate by the nervous system.[64] All of the experiments concerning this point, however, used atrial or ventricular cardiac myocytes, not cardiac pacemaker cells. A necessary precondition for the direct coupling hypothesis of beat-to-beat regulation would be that G-proteins directly regulate ionic channels in SA pacemaker cells. These cells have a very complicated set of ionic currents, but the most interesting is the hyperpolarization-activated current I_f. This current is thought to be essential for pacemaker activity and is more sensitive to ACh than K^+[ACh] currents.

This problem was examined with the same strategy that had proved useful for K^+[ACh] channels; namely, an attempt to record I_f currents from excised I-O membrane patches. The great strength of this approach is that when care is taken to identify access problems, the ambiguities of whole-cell perfusion are avoided. It proved possible to record I_f currents under such conditions.[71] It was then found that preactivated G_s^* or its α_s^* subunit stimulated hyperpolarization-activated pacemaker current (I_f) channels in I-O membrane patches excised from SA cells under substrate-free conditions.[72] The preactivated G-proteins, G_o^* and G_i^*, or their respective α subunits, α_o^* and α_i^*, inhibited I_f channels, with G_o^* being more potent. Inhibitory G-protein effects predominated when endogenous G-proteins were activated by GTPγS. An unexpected result was that G_o^* and G_s^*, or their preactivated α subunits acted noncompetitively and simultaneously on the same I_f channels. This finding demonstrated for the first time that different isolated G-protein α subunits produce allosteric changes in a single effector. In turn, allosteric changes in I_f channels may provide a molecular explanation for that classical observation of regulatory biology, the synergistic effects of muscarinic and β-adrenergic agonists on heart rate. Note that the argument for allosteric regulation of I_f channels is unchanged even if there are membrane intermediates between the G-proteins and the I_f channels. G_o and G_s also interact at the level of AC, but the effects are competitive and would not explain the above effects. The results and conclusions may be summarized as follows:

1. $G_o\alpha$ mediates muscarinic cholinergic effects and $G_s\alpha$ mediates β-adrenergic effects on I_f channels, with $G_o\alpha$ effects predominanting;
2. $G_o^*\alpha$ and $G_s^*\alpha$ act irreversibly on I_f channels; and
3. I_f channels have allosteric sites for $G_o\alpha$ and $G_s\alpha$.

The allosteric actions explain the synergistic or antagonistic effects of sequential stimulation of the cardiac vagal and sympathetic nerves. This would be the predominant effect, although the nonlinear, current-voltage relationship of I_f could play a small role as well. A further cautionary note is that a deactivating, outward K^+ current and a Ca^{2+} current[73,74] may also contribute to pacemaker cell currents.

Acknowledgments: I thank M. Anderson and J. Breedlove for their secretarial assistance in the preparation of this chapter.

References

1. Carrier GO, Bishop VS: The interaction of acetylcholine and norepinephrine on heart rate. J Pharmacol Exp Ther 180:31, 1972.
2. Levy MN, Martin PJ: Neural control of the heart. In RM Berne, N Sperelakis (eds): Handbook of Physiology (Section 2: the Cardiovascular System) Vol 1. Bethesda, MD, American Physiological Society, 1979, pp. 581–620.
3. Lefkowitz RJ, Caron MG: Adrenergic receptors: Models for the study of receptors coupled to guanine nucleotide regulatory proteins. J Biol Chem 263:4993, 1988.
4. Lochrie MA, Simon MI: G protein multiplicity in eukaryotic signal transduction systems. Biochemistry 27:4957, 1988.
5. Numa S, Noda M: Molecular structure of sodium channels. Ann NY Acad Sci 479:338, 1986.
6. Brown AM, Birnbaumer L: Ionic channels and their regulation by G protein subunits. Annu Rev Physiol 52:197, 1990.
7. VanDongen AMJ, Codina J, Olate J, et al: Newly identified brain potassium channels gated by the guanine nucleotide binding protein, G_o. Science 242:1433, 1988.
8. Noma A: ATP-regulated K^+ channels in cardiac muscle. Nature 305:147, 1983.
9. Kirsch GE, Brown AM: Trypsin activation of atrial muscarinic K^+ channels. Am J Physiol 257:H334, 1989.
10. DiFrancesco D, Tromba C: Muscarinic control of the hyperpolarization-activated current i_f in rabbit sino-atrial node myocytes. J Physiol (Lond) 405:493, 1988.
11. Dolphin AC: G protein modulation of calcium currents in neurons. Annu Rev Physiol 52:243, 1990.
12. Gilman AG: G proteins: Transducers of receptor-generated signals. Annu Rev Biochem 56:615, 1987.
13. Stryer L, Bourne HR: G-proteins: A family of signal transducers. Annu Rev Cell Biol 2:391, 1986.
14. Kameyama M, Hescheler J, Hofmann F, et al: Modulation of Ca current during the phosphorylation cycle in the guinea pig heart. Pflügers Arch 407:123, 1986.
15. Reuter H: Calcium channel modulation by neurotransmitters, enzymes and drugs. Nature 301:569, 1983.
16. Trautwein W, Hescheler J: Regulation of cardiac L-type calcium current by phosphorylation and G proteins. Annu Rev Physiol 52:257, 1990.
17. Brown DA: G proteins and potassium currents in neurons. Annu Rev Physiol 52:215, 1990.
18. Piomelli D, Volterra A, Dale N, et al: Lipoxygenase metabolites of arachidonic acid as second messengers for presynaptic inhibition of aplysia sensory neurons. Nature 328:38, 1987.
19. Kim D, Lewis DL, Graziadei L, et al: G-protein $\beta\gamma$-subunits activate the cardiac muscarinic K^+ channel via phospholipase A_2. Nature 337:557, 1989.
20. Purves RV: Function of muscarinic and nicotinic acetylcholine receptors. Nature 261:151, 1976.
21. Glitsch HG, Pott L: Effects of acetylcholine and parasympathetic nerve stimulation on membrane potential in quiescent guinea-pig atria. J Physiol (Lond) 279:655, 1978.
22. Hartzell H: Distribution of muscarinic acetylcholine receptors and presynaptic nerve terminals in amphibian heart. J Cell Biol 86:6, 1980.
23. Osterrieder W, Yang Q-F, Trautwein W: Mode of action of acetylcholine on the rabbit SA node cell. In LN Bouman, HT Jongsma (eds): Cardiac Rate and Rhythm. Boston, MA, Martinus Nijhoff, 1982, p. 485–505.
24. Nargeot J, Nerbonne JM, Engels J, et al: Time course of the increase in the myocardial slow inward current after a photochemically generated concentration jump of intracellular cAMP. Proc Natl Acad Sci USA 80:2395, 1983.

25. Nawrath H: Does cyclic GMP mediate the negative inotropic effect of acetylcholine in the heart? Nature 267:72, 1977.
26. Trautwein W, Taniguchi J, Noma A: The effect of intracellular cyclic nucleotides and calcium on the action potential and acetylcholine response of isolated cardiac cells. Pflügers Arch 392:307, 1982.
27. Soejima M, Noma A: Mode of regulation of the ACh-sensitive K-channel by the muscarinic receptor in rabbit atrial cells. Pflügers Arch 400:424, 1984.
28. Rosenberger LB, Roeske WR, Yamamura HI: The regulation of muscarinic cholinergic receptors by guanine nucleotides in cardiac tissue. Eur J Pharmacol 56:179, 1979.
29. Hazeki O, Ui M: Modification by islet-activating protein of receptor-mediated regulation of cAMP accumulation in isolated rat heart cells. J Biol Chem 256:2856, 1981.
30. Kurose H, Ui M: Functional uncoupling of muscarinic receptors from adenylate cyclase in rat cardiac membranes by the active component of islet-activating protein, pertussis toxin. J Cyclic Nucleotide Protein Phosphor Res 9:305, 1983.
31. Halvorsen SW, Nathanson NM: Ontogenesis of physiological responsiveness and guanine nucleotide sensitivity of cardiac muscarinic receptors during chick embryonic development. Biochemistry 23:5813, 1984.
32. Pfaffinger PJ, Martin JM, Hunter DD, et al: GTP-binding proteins couple cardiac muscarinic receptors to a K channel. Nature 317:536, 1985.
33. Endoh M, Manyama M, Tajima T: Attenuation of muscarinic cholinergic inhibition by islet-activating protein in the heart. Am J Physiol 249:H309, 1985.
34. Sirota S, Tsuji Y, Pappano A: Pertussis toxin blocks muscarinic hyperpolarization and action potential shortening in chick atrium. Fed Proc 44:729, 1985.
35. Breitwieser GE, Szabo G: Uncoupling of cardiac muscarinic and β-adrenergic receptors from ion channels by a guanine nucleotide analogue. Nature 317:538, 1985.
36. Brown JH, Brown SL: Agonists differentiate muscarinic receptors that inhibit cyclic AMP formation from those that stimulate phosphoinositide metabolism. J Biol Chem 259:3777, 1984.
37. Tajima T, Tsuji Y, Brown JH, et al: Pertussis toxin-insensitive phosphoinositide hydrolysis, membrane depolarization, and positive inotropic effect of carbachol in chick atria. Circ Res 61:436, 1987.
38. Kurachi Y, Nakajima T, Sugimoto T: On the mechanism of activation of muscarinic K^+ channels by adenosine in isolated atrial cells: Involvement of GTP-binding proteins. Pflügers Arch 407:264, 1986.
39. Kurachi Y, Nakajima T, Sugimoto T: Acetylcholine activation of K^+ channels in cell-free membrance of atrial cells. Am J Physiol 251:H681, 1986.
40. Yatani A, Codina J, Brown AM, et al: Direct activation of mammalian atrial muscarinic potassium channels by GTP regulatory protein G_k. Science 235:207, 1987.
41. Codina J, Yatani A, Grenet D, et al: The alpha subunit of the GTP binding protein G_k opens atrial potassium channels. Science 236:442, 1987.
42. Logothetis DE, Kim D, Northup JK, et al: Specificity of action of guanine nucleotide-binding regulatory protein subunits on the cardiac muscarinic K^+ channel. Proc Natl Acad Sci USA 85:5814, 1988.
43. Kurachi Y, Ito H, Sugimoto T, et al: Arachidonic acid metabolites as intracellular modulators of the G protein-gated cardiac K^+ channel. Nature 337:555, 1989.
44. Logothetis DE, Kurachi Y, Galper J, et al: The βγ subunits of GTP-binding proteins activate the muscarinic K^+ channel in heart. Nature 325:321, 1987.
45. Yatani A, Okabe K, Birnbaumer L, et al: Detergents, dimeric Gβγ dimers, and eicosanoid pathways to muscarinic atrial K^+ channels. Am J Physiol 258:H1507, 1990.
46. Hohl CM, Rosen R: The role of arachidonic acid in rat heart cell metabolism. Biochem Biophys Acta 921:356, 1987.

47. Katada T, Bokoch GM, Northup JK, et al: The inhibitory guanine nucleotide-binding regulatory component of adenylate cyclase. Properties and function of the purified protein. J Biol Chem 259:3568, 1984.
48. Katada T, Bokoch GM, Smigel MD, et al: The inhibitory guanine nucleotide-binding regulatory component of adenylate cyclase. Subunit dissociation and the inhibition of adenylate cyclase in S49 lymphoma cyc- and wild type membranes. J Biol Chem 259:3586, 1984.
49. Jelsema CL, Axelrod J: Stimulation of phospholipase A2 activity in bovine rod outer segments by the beta-gamma subunits of transducin and its inhibition by the alpha subunit. Proc Natl Acad Sci USA 84:3623, 1987.
50. Codina J, Grenet D, Yatani A, et al: Hormonal regulation of pituitary GH_3 cell K^+ channels by G_k is mediated by its alpha subunit. FEBS Lett 216:104, 1987.
51. Northup JK, Smigel MD, Sternweis PC, et al: The subunits of the stimulatory regulatory component of adenylate cyclase. Resolution of the activated 45,000-Dalton α subunit. J Biol Chem 258:11369, 1983.
52. Kirsch GE, Yatani A, Codina J, et al: α subunit of G_k activates atrial K^+ channels of chick, rat and guinea pig. Am J Physiol 23:H1200, 1988.
53. Cerbai E, Klöckner U, Isenberg G: The α subunit of the GTP binding protein activates muscarinic potassium channels of the atrium. Science 240:1782, 1988.
54. Pind S, Kuksis A: Solubilization and assay of phospholipase A2 activity from rat jejunal brush-border membranes. Biochem Biophys Acta 938:211, 1988.
55. Okabe K, Yatani A, Evans T, et al: βγ dimers of G proteins inhibit atrial muscarinic K^+ channels. J Biol Chem 265:12854, 1990.
56. Hamm HE, Deretic D, Hofmann KP, et al: Mechanism of action of monoclonal antibodies that block the light activation of the guanyl nucleotide-binding protein, transducin. J Biol Chem 262:10831, 1987.
57. Deretic D, Hamm HE: Topographic analysis of antigenic determinations recognized by monoclonal antibodies to the photoreceptor guanyl nucleotide binding protein, transducin. J Biol Chem 262:10839, 1988.
58. Yatani A, Hamm HE, Codina J, et al: A monoclonal antibody to the α subunit of G_k blocks muscarinic activation of atrial K^+ channels. Science 241:828, 1988
59. Mattera R, Yatani A, Kirsch GE, et al: Recombinant α_i-3 subunit of G protein activates G_k-gated K^+ channels. J Biol Chem 264(1):465, 1989.
60. Yatani A, Mattera R, Codina J, et al: The G protein-gated atrial K^+ channel is stimulated by three distinct $G_i\alpha$-subunits. Nature 336:680, 1988.
61. Schubert B, VanDongen AMJ, Kirsch GE, et al: β-adrenergic inhibition of cardiac sodium channels by dual G protein pathways. Science 245:516, 1989.
62. Yatani A, Codina J, Imoto Y, et al: A G protein directly regulates mammalian cardiac calcium channels. Science 238:1288, 1987.
63. Yatani A, Imoto Y, Codina J, et al: The stimulatory G protein of adenylyl cyclase, G_s, also stimulates dihydropyridine-sensitive Ca^{2+} channels. J Biol Chem 263(20):9887, 1988.
64. Yatani A, Broown AM: Rapid β-adrenergic modulation of cardiac calcium channel currents by a fast G protein pathway. Science 245:71, 1989.
65. Powell T, Twist V: Isoprenaline stimulation of cyclic AMP production by isolated cells from adult rate myocardium. Biochem Biophys Res Commun 72:1218, 1976.
66. Schubert B, VanDongen AMJ, Kirsch G, et al: Inhibition of cardiac Na^+ currents by isoproterenol. Am J Physiol 258:H977, 1990.
67. Hartzell HC, Méry P-F, Fischmeister R, et al: Sympathetic regulation of cardiac calcium current is due exclusively to cAMP-dependent phosphorylation. Nature 351:573, 1991.
68. Pelzer S, Shuba YM, Tatsuya A, et al: Membrane-delimited stimulation of heart cell calcium current by β-adrenergic signal-transducing G_s protein. Am J Physiol 259:H264, 1990.
69. Cavalié A, Allen TJA, Trautwein W: Role of the GTP-binding protein G_s in the β-adrenergic modulation of cardiac Ca channels. Pflügers Arch 419:433, 1991.

70. Kozlowski RZ, Twist VW, Brown AM, et al: Flash photolysis of intracellular caged GTPγS increases L-type Ca^{2+} currents in cardiac myocytes. Am J Physiol 261:H1665, 1991.
71. Yatani A, Brown AM: Regulation of the cardiac pacemaker current I_f in excised membranes from sinoatrial node cells. Am J Physiol 258:H1947, 1990.
72. Yatani A, Okabe K, Codina J, et al: Heart rate regulation by G proteins acting on the cardiac pacemaker channel. Science 249:1163, 1990.
73. Campbell GD, Edwards FR, Hirst GDS, et al: Effects of vagal stimulation and applied acetylcholine on pacemaker potentials in the guinea pig heart. J Physiol (Lond) 415:57, 1989.
74. Shibata EF, Giles W, Pollack GH: Threshold effects of acetylcholine on primary pacemaker cells of the rabbit sino-atrial node. Proc R Soc Lond (Biol) 223:355, 1985.

CHAPTER 10

Acetylcholine Synthesis and Release in the Heart

K. Löffelholz, R. Lindmar

The first proof of the chemical mediation of neuronal activity was obtained in 1921 by Otto Loewi using the isolated heart preparation.[1] Stimulation of the vagus nerve of a frog heart caused the release of a substance, which Loewi called "Vagusstoff," from the tissue into the medium. A few years later, Loewi and Navratil identified this substance as acetylcholine (ACh).[2] Biosynthesis of ACh follows the equation:

$$\text{Acetyl-CoA} + \text{Choline} \rightleftharpoons \text{ACh} + \text{CoA.}$$

The reaction is catalyzed by the enzyme choline acetyltransferase (ChAT; EC 2.3.1.6), the apparent K_m values being 5 to 20 μM for acetylcoenzyme A (acetyl-CoA) and 0.3 to 1.2 mM for choline.[3] Although the reaction is reversible, its equilibrium is markedly shifted to the right (K_{eq} 12.3).[4]

ACh can also be synthesized by the mitochondrial enzyme carnitine acetyltransferase (CarAT; EC 2.3.1.7), which can acetylate both its natural substrate carnitine and choline. Even though the K_m value of CarAT for choline (8.7 mM)[5] is higher than that of the ChAT, the possibility of a synthesis of ACh catalyzed by CarAT has to be considered for each tissue and for each in vitro or in vivo condition.

Presence of Acetylcholine, Choline Acetyltransferase, and Carnitine Acetyltransferase Activities in Heart Tissue

Preganglionic and Postganglionic Distribution

ACh and ChAT activity are present in both the intrinsic parasympathetic ganglia and in the parasympathetic postganglionic fibers of the "autonomic

The original experimental work of the authors was supported by the Deutsche Forschungsgemeinschaft.

groundplexus" (see Ch. 1). After bilateral cervical vagotomy in rats, the activity of the ChAT was lowered by only 30% in the atria and was unchanged in the ventricles.[6] This finding indicates that ganglionic ChAT activity is restricted to the atria and, even in this region, ChAT activity is dominated by the postganglionic localization of the enzyme. It is, therefore, not surprising that heart transplantation did not appreciably alter the ACh content of the rat heart.[7] Morphological studies demonstrated that, indeed, the predominant location of cardiac ganglia are the atria, especially the subepicardial connective tissue of the posterior aspect (see Ch. 2). In mammals, ventricular ganglion cells are absent or, more precisely, were not consistently observed.[8–10] The conclusion that most of the cardiac ACh is synthesized in postganglionic neurons is supported by release experiments. When the vagus nerves (preganglionic fibers) were stimulated, blockade of ganglionic transmission by (+)-tubocurarine diminished the release of [^{3}H]-ACh to less than 5% in rabbit atria and to 12% in chicken hearts.[11,12] The remaining tubocurarine-resistant release was even further reduced by muscarinic receptor blockade of isolated chicken hearts.[13]

The above considerations indicate that the distribution of ACh and the activity of ChAT in various regions of mammalian hearts reflect the density of postganglionic rather than of preganglionic neurons.

Regional Distribution of Acetylcholine, Choline Acetyltransferase, and Carnitine Acetyltransferase Activities

The highest ACh content and ChAT activity were found in the sinus node and the lowest values of these substances were found in the left ventricle.[14–17] Biochemical results indicate that the innervation density of the left ventricle is one tenth of that of the sinus node. This value correlates well with morphologically described differences in innervation densities.[9]

Figure 1 shows that the ACh content and the ChAT activity of the rat heart gradually decline in the following order: right atrium > left atrium > right ventricle > left ventricle.[18] The same order was found for the ACh contents of cat and rabbit hearts.[14,19] Only in the guinea pig heart were the ACh content and ChAT activity lower in the left atrium than in the right ventricle (Fig. 1).[15,16] In contrast to the ChAT activity, CarAT activities are higher in the ventricles than in the atria of rat and guinea pig hearts (Fig. 1). Thus, a significant contribution of the CarAT activity to the biosynthesis of ACh under normal conditions is very unlikely, a failure that might be due to the low affinity of this enzyme for choline (see above). When high concentrations of choline, however, are present, e.g., when enzyme activities are measured in homogenates of ventricular tissue, biosynthesis of ACh may be catalyzed by both ChAT and CarAT, as the activity (V_{max}) of CarAT is remarkably high in the ventricles (Fig. 1). This occurrence may explain why, in some earlier work, the difference in "ChAT activities" between atria and ventricles was rather low.[20] Correct measurements of ChAT and CarAT

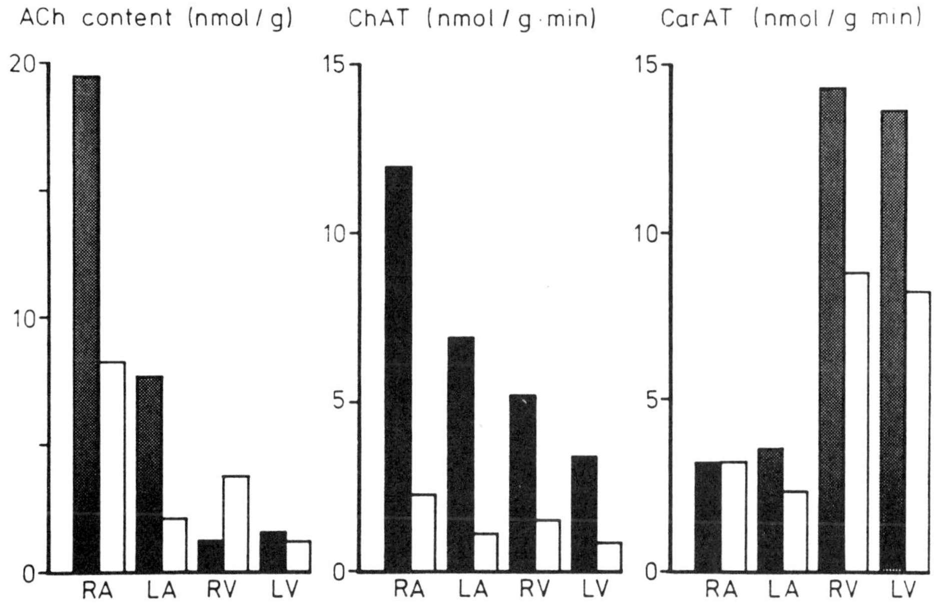

Figure 1. *Regional distribution of ACh, ChAT, and CarAT activities in mammalian hearts. RA: right atrium; LA: left atrium; RV: right ventricle; and LV: left ventricle. Columns indicate ACh content (nmol per g wet weight). ChAT or CarAT activity were expressed as rate of ACh formation from choline (nmol/g min). In rat and guinea pig hearts (closed and open columns), the ACh contents were determined by Lund et al*[18] *and Brown et al*[15]*; ChAT activities were determined by Slavikova and Tuček*[17] *and Schmid et al*[16]*; and CarAT activities were determined by Slavikova and Tuček*[17] *and Roskoski et al.*[65] *Presented are mean values.*

activities were obtained by using specific enzyme inhibitors, bromoacetylcholine to inhibit ChAT and bromoacetylcarnitine to inhibit CarAT.[17] In this study, bromoacetylcholine-sensitive synthesis of ACh was considered to reflect the activity of ChAT.

There are significant species differences in the ACh contents, first, among mammalian atria and, second, between mammalian and avian hearts. Both ACh content and ChAT activity of the right atrium are much higher in the rat than in the guinea pig (Fig. 1). The sparse innervation of the ventricles, however, was unequivocally reported for all mammalian species.[9] In contrast, the avian ventricles exhibit a relatively dense cholinergic innervation.[9] In the ventricles of chickens, but not in mammals (see above), the presence of ganglia is a consistent feature. This peculiarity, which has been found not only morphologically but also in biochemical and pharmacological investigations, appears to be responsible for the fact that the overall ACh contents of chicken, duck, and pigeon hearts are significantly higher (8.3; 10.3; 11.5 nmol/g) than those of mouse, guinea pig, rabbit, rat, and cat hearts (1.1; 2.1; 2.2; 5.6; 6.4 nmol/g).[21–23] Likewise, ACh release from the perfused Langendorff preparation of the chicken heart evoked by field and vagal stimulation was severalfold higher than that from perfused mammalian hearts.[23] Finally, pharmacological experiments on ventricular slices from chickens and pigeons revealed that avian ventricular muscle was much more sensitive to exogenous ACh and to endogenous ACh released by field stimulation than mammalian ventricles.[24] The functional role of the cholinergic innervation of the ventricles seems to be qualitatively different in avian and mammalian hearts.

Release, Synthesis, and Turnover of Acetylcholine

For the reasons given above, the isolated perfused chicken heart proved to be a useful tool for studying ACh synthesis, release, hydrolysis, and washout.[9,25] We used this preparation to examine the release and resynthesis of ACh and its dependence on choline availability. Repetitive vagal stimulation at a high frequency of 20 Hz for 20 minutes causes an overflow of ACh into the perfusate (Fig. 2). The high initial overflow rapidly declines to a steady state release at about half the initial overflow both in the absence and presence of physostigmine. This time-course has been observed in other peripheral organs, such as the isolated sympathetic ganglion, and it appears to be typical for an ACh release caused by high-frequency stimulation in the autonomic nervous system.[26] Only the plateau release depends on the concomitant neuronal uptake of choline. Thus, hemicholinium-3, an inhibitor of the high-affinity choline uptake (HACU), does not alter the initial release, but blocks resynthesis and the plateau release of ACh (Fig. 2). This finding indicates that the initial output reflects release from a preformed, easily available ACh pool, whereas the plateau is determined by the rate of resynthesis of released ACh. In other words, the rate of resynthesis cannot keep pace with the initial release. In an analogy to very similar observations in the cat superior cervical ganglion, it is likely that the initial ACh release leads to a depletion of the preformed, easily available ACh pool, which may even be reflected by a transient reduction of the total ACh content.[27,28] The depletion that was observed after high-frequency stimulation of the vagus may be functionally relevant and may attenuate the chronotropic response to vagal stimulation.[29]

In the experiment shown by the inset of Figure 2, the amount of ACh released within the 20-minute period of stimulation is almost equivalent to the ACh content (7.5 nmol/g). The rate of ACh resynthesis in the whole chicken heart is 0.3 nmol/g per minute or 4% of the ACh store per minute. The in vivo turnover rates of ACh synthesis in rat and guinea pig hearts revealed similarly high values of 2% to 10% of total store per minute.[18,30,31]

Resynthesis of ACh depends on a supply of the precursor choline, which is transported from the extracellular space into the cholinergic neuron by the hemicholinium-3-sensitive, Na^+-dependent HACU. In the chicken heart, vagal stimulation (20 Hz) for 1 minute caused the release of ACh which, in turn, accelerated the HACU (Fig. 3). The acceleration of HACU followed the ACh release with a time-lag of 1 to 2 minutes.[32] The delayed activation of HACU was shown by both the transient removal of extracellular unlabelled choline

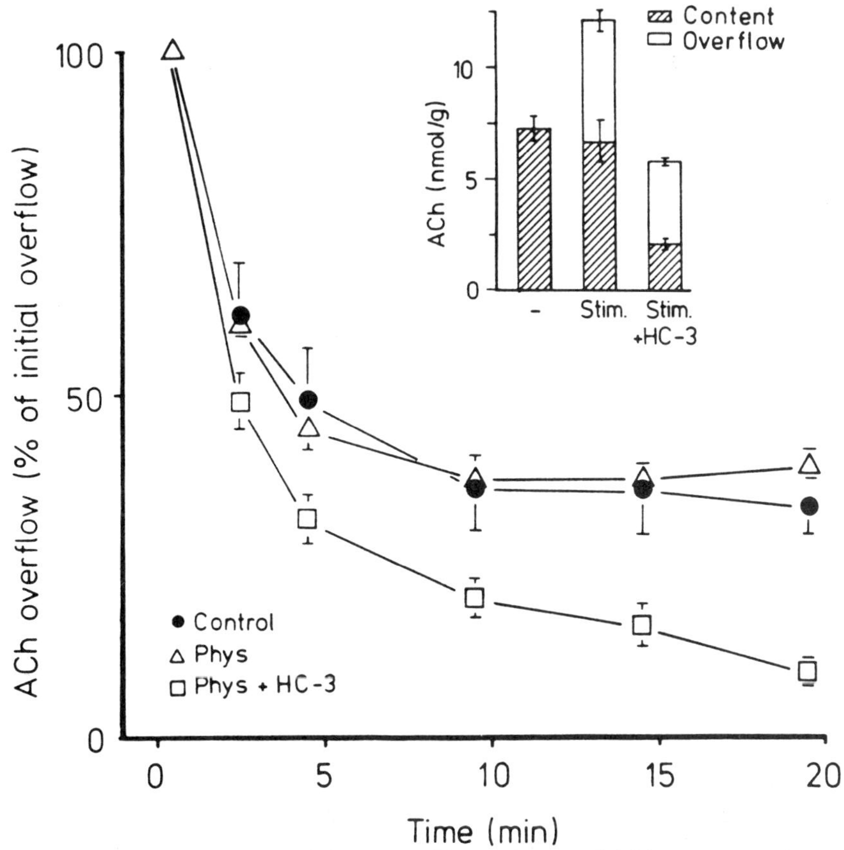

Figure 2. *Effects of vagal stimulation on ACh overflow and ACh content in the isolated perfused chicken heart. Both vagus nerves were stimulated for 20 min at 20 Hz. Ordinate: ACh overflow in percent of "initial overflow" (first min); 100% = 321 ± 90 (N = 8) under control conditions, 584 ± 43 (N = 4) or 657 ± 84 (pmol $g^{-1}min^{-1}$) (N = 4) in the presence of 10^{-6}M physostigmine (Phys) or Phys plus 2 × 10^{-5}M hemicholinium-3 (HC-3), respectively. Abscissa: time of vagal stimulation (min). Inset: ACh content (hatched columns) and total ACh overflow (open columns) without stimulation (first stimulation) and after the 20-min period of vagal stimulation in the presence of Phys (second column) and Phys plus HC-3 (third column). Data shown by second and third columns were obtained by the experiments indicated by open triangles and open squares, respectively. Means ± SEM of 4–8 experiments. Data were taken from Löffelholz et al.*[25]

("negative phase") and by the time-dependent utilization of extracellular [^{14}C]-choline for synthesis of labelled ACh. Utilization was highest (condition d in Fig. 3) when the maximum uptake of extracellular choline was observed.

In principle, under in vivo conditions, extracellular choline for the synthesis of ACh is derived from three sources:

1. free choline in plasma;
2. release from phospholipids; and
3. hydrolysis of released ACh catalyzed by cholinesterase (ChE) activity.

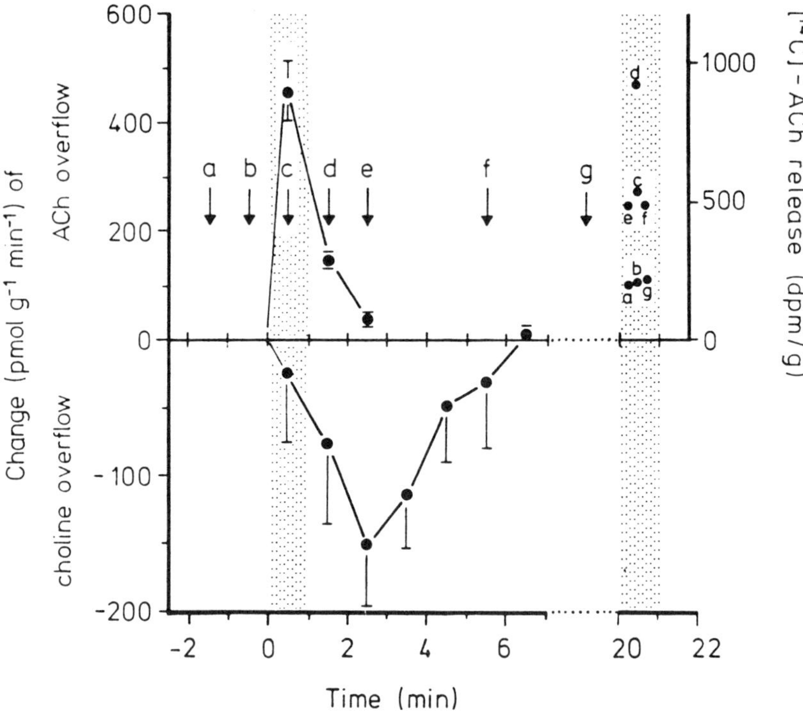

Figure 3. *Activation of neuronal uptake of choline by vagal stimulation in the perfused chicken heart. First experiment: in the presence of 10^{-6}M physostigmine, the efflux of unlabelled ACh or of choline was determined before, during (stippled area at first min), and after vagal stimulation (20 Hz, 1 min). Under resting conditions, the efflux was 64 and 2400 pmol $g^{-1}min^{-1}$. Second experiment: both vagus nerves were stimulated (10 Hz, 1 min; stippled area at zero-time); [^{14}C]-choline was infused for 1 min at seven different times indicated by the arrows a to g. The efficacy of this procedure was studied by measuring the release of [^{14}C]-ACh evoked by a second period of vagal stimulation (10 Hz, 1 min) 20 min after the first one (stippled area). Left ordinate (first experiment): change in efflux of ACh (top) and of choline (bottom) expressed in pmol $g^{-1}min^{-1}$; note that the ACh efflux is enhanced, whereas that of choline is reduced. Right ordinate (second experiment): release of [^{14}C]-ACh in response to the second vagal stimulation at 20 min; note that the height of the release (a–g) markedly depends on the time of [^{14}C]-choline infusion (a–g). Abscissa: time (min) of perfusate collection or of infusion of [^{14}C]-choline into the heart (arrows). It should be mentioned that the data showing choline efflux and arrows showing [^{14}C]-choline infusion should be corrected by 0.5 min (towards opposite directions) due to the dead spaces of the heart and of the perfusion apparatus. When this delay is taken into account, the maximally effective infusion of [^{14}C]-choline (condition d) coincides precisely with the maximum activation of choline uptake (maximum of "negative phase"). For further details see the original study by Lindmar et al.[32]*

In peripheral organs, in contrast to the brain, the plasma choline determines the extracellular choline concentration under in vivo conditions. Free choline in the plasma is maintained at a remarkably constant level of about 10 μM in mammals and in man.[33,34] Thus, the availability of plasma choline in the periphery makes it highly unlikely that synaptic sources, i.e., reuse of choline derived from ACh breakdown and choline released from phospholipids, play a rate-limiting role in the ACh synthesis of the parasympathetic nervous system. The possibility cannot be totally excluded, however, that, in man and chicken, in areas such as the sinus node, with very dense innervation and narrow neuroeffector junctions (<600 Å synaptic width), the synaptic sources may become important, especially at times of vigorous neuronal activity.[9]

The second precursor of ACh biosynthesis is acetyl-CoA, which is produced within the nerve cells. The source of the acetyl groups (e.g., glucose, pyruvate, acetate) has not yet been studied in the heart.

Extracellular Clearance of Released Acetylcholine

In principle, clearance of released ACh from the extracellular space is controlled by hydrolysis catalyzed by both ChE activity and diffusion. The time-limits of ACh inactivation may vary between microseconds in the motor end plate and several seconds in the heart.[35] In this organ, the functional importance of the hydrolysis of ACh has been clearly demonstrated by showing that the rate of ACh hydrolysis markedly affected the so-called phase dependency of cardiac responses to vagal stimulation (see Ch. 11).[36] Hydrolysis is less important, however, for the synaptic clearance in the heart than it is in the motor end plate, where the apparent rate of diffusion is reduced by receptor-binding (buffered diffusion) and the activity of the surface ChE is extremely high.[37] In the heart, a large part of released ACh diffuses over long distances and escapes into the vascular lumen. After a brief period of vagal stimulation (5 seconds) in the isolated perfused heart, the mean extracellular concentration of ACh declined in a multiexponential fashion and reached the 50% level after 2.5 seconds due to both hydrolysis and washout.[35] The decline of the extracellular concentration of ACh plus choline (formed from ACh) was of first order and was characterized by a rate constant of 0.069 s^{-1} and a half-time of 10 seconds. The data clearly demonstrate the importance of both diffusion and hydrolysis in the extracellular clearance of released ACh in the perfused heart. It deserves mention that Otto Loewi (see above) detected ACh in the superfusate of frog hearts in the absence of ChE inhibition.[1]

Presynaptic Modulation of Acetylcholine Release

The concept that presynaptic receptors modulate the release of neurotransmitters is well established and three mechanisms for this release have been proposed. First, transmitter substances may modulate their own release through autoreceptors. Second, these substances may modulate the release of transmitters liberated from adjacent varicosities via heteroreceptors (e.g., in the adrenergic-cholinergic interactions). Finally, transmitter release may be modulated by paracrine factors and by cotransmitters, such as neuropeptides, which are released together with the classical transmitter.

Presynaptic Muscarinic Autoinhibition

ACh may inhibit its own release depending on the synaptic concentration of the transmitter. Presynaptic muscarinic autoinhibition appears to play an important modulatory role in the cardiac ACh release in animals and man. This finding has been studied by exposure of heart preparations to either ACh itself, or to other muscarinic receptor agonists, or to ChE inhibitors.[32,38,39] In the absence of ChE inhibition, muscarinic receptor antagonists markedly increase the release of ACh (Fig. 4). This finding indicates the endogenous presence of autoinhibition.[13,38,40] The presynaptic receptor subtype, M_2 in the mammalian heart, seems to be identical with, or similar to, its postsynaptic counterpart (Fig. 4).[40] Evidence indicates, however, that, in man and chicken, the presynaptic inhibitory autoreceptors may belong to the M_1-subtype, in contrast to the postganglionic receptor, which is M_2 in the human heart and atypical in the chicken heart.[41–44]

Presynaptic α-Adrenergic Inhibition

In the heart, axo-axonal contacts have been observed for the classical opponents in the autonomic nervous system, the adrenergic (sympathetic) and the cholinergic (parasympathetic) terminal fibers both running in the autonomic ground plexus.[45,46] There is good evidence for an inhibitory adrenergic-cholinergic interaction at the presynaptic, postganglionic level in mammalian species. Exogenous ACh inhibits the release of noradrenaline through presynaptic inhibitory muscarinic receptors of the sympathetic terminal nerve fibers.[47,48] Vagal stimulation of the heart has the same effect as exogenous ACh.[11,49,50]

In contrast, an α-adrenoceptor-mediated, postganglionic inhibition of ACh release has not been unequivocally shown for mammalian hearts in general. The most convincing evidence has been obtained in isolated rat atria.[39,51–53] An α_1-subtype appeared to be responsible for this inhibition. Consequently, vagally-induced bradycardia of the rat heart in vivo was attenuated by α_1-adrenoceptor activation.[54] Some indication for such an inhibitory heteroreceptor exists for the rabbit and the guinea pig heart.[55,56] Negative results have been reported, however, for the chicken heart and guinea pig atria.[38,57] Possibly there are species differences.

The picture is even more complicated; in the rat heart in vivo and in vitro, an α_1-receptor-mediated facilitation of the ACh release has been described.[58,59] The conflicting conclusions may be due to methodical problems. The isolated heart contains preganglionic and postganglionic parasympathetic structures, both of which may be equipped with inhibitory and excitatory α-adrenoceptors. Effects observed with adrenoceptor agonists may represent a mixed and variable response, depending on the methodical approach and, consequently, the receptors that are involved in the overall effect.

In conclusion, the evidence for an adrenergic inhibition of ACh release is much less clear than for a cholinergic inhibition of norepinephrine release.[57]

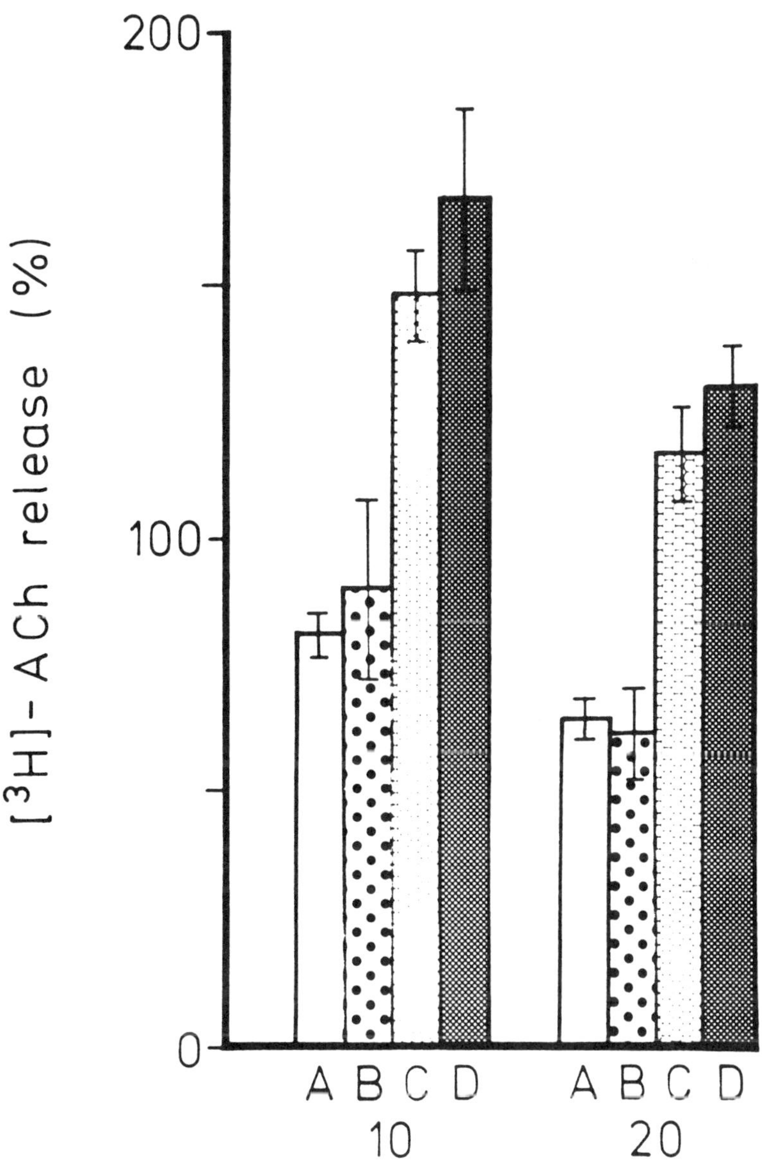

Figure 4. *Increase by pirenzepine and atropine of the evoked release of [^3H]-ACh in the perfused guinea pig heart. ACh was labelled according to Lindmar et al[32] and was released by field stimulation (1 min, 5 Hz) at zero-time (control = 100%, not shown), at 10 and 20 min. Pirenzepine or atropine were added after the first stimulation period. Columns: [^3H]-ACh release in % of control. A: absence of drug; B: 3 × 10^{-8}M pirenzepine; C: 3 × 10^{-7}M pirenzepine; and D: 3 × 10^{-7}M atropine. Means ± SEM of four experiments. Data were taken from Jeck et al.[13]*

Moreover, the functional importance of the inhibitory adrenergic-cholinergic interactions will be even more difficult to assess and to delineate from other interactions that are present along the course of the autonomic nervous system. Sympathetic-parasympathetic cross-communications begin at the central structures involved in cardiovascular control and end at the signal-transduction mechanisms of the innervated cell. It may be concluded that all of these mechanisms more or less contribute to the reciprocal activation of the sympathetic and parasympathetic nervous systems as it is observed in many physiological conditions.

Serotonin and Acetylcholine Release

Serotonin caused bradycardia in isolated perfused rabbit hearts pretreated with reserpine.[60] The effect was mediated by stimulation of excitatory 5-HT_3-receptors. Although these receptors are likely to be ganglionic, a postganglionic location has not been excluded.[61,62]

Neuropeptides and Acetylcholine Release

The effect of neuropeptides, such as somatostatin[63] and neuropeptide Y,[64] on the release of ACh will be the subject of Ch. 18 and, therefore, will not be discussed here.

References

1. Loewi O: Über humorale Übertragbarkeit der Herznervenwirkung. I. Mitteilung. Pflügers Arch Ges Physiol 189:239, 1921.
2. Loewi O, Navratil E: Über humorale Übertragbarkeit der Herznervenwirkung. XI. Mitteilung. Über den Mechanismus der Vaguswirkung von Physostigmin und Ergotamin. Pflügers Arch Ges Physiol 214:689, 1926.
3. Tuček S: Choline acetyltransferase and the synthesis of acetylcholine. In VP Whittaker (ed): The Cholinergic Synapse: Handbook of Experimental Pharmacology. Vol. 86. Berlin, Heidelberg, New York, Springer-Verlag, 1988, p. 125.
4. Pieklik JR, Guynn RW: Equilibrium constants of the reactions of choline acetyltransferase, carnitine acetyltransferase, and acetylcholinesterase under physiological conditions. J Biol Chem 250:4445, 1975.
5. White HL, Wu JC: Choline and carnitine acetyltransferases of heart. Biochemistry 12:841, 1973.
6. Slaviková J, Tuček S: Choline acetyltransferase activity and distribution in rat hearts after bilateral cervical vagotomy. Physiol Bohem 34:217, 1985.
7. Oda RP, Whiteis CA, Schmid PG, et al: Choline and acetylcholine concentration in transplanted rat heart. Am J Physiol 252:H125, 1987.
8. Jacobowitz D: Histochemical studies of the relationship of chromaffin cells and adrenergic nerve fibres to the cardiac ganglia of several species. J Pharmacol Exp Ther 158:227, 1967.
9. Löffelholz K, Pappano AJ: The parasympathetic neuroeffector junction of the heart. Pharmacol Rev 37:1, 1985.
10. Smith RB: Intrinsic innervation of the avian heart. Acta Anat 79:112, 1971.

11. Habermeier-Muth A, Muscholl E: Short- and long-latency muscarinic inhibition of noradrenaline release from rabbit atria induced by vagal stimulation. J Physiol (Lond) 401:277, 1988.
12. Lindmar R, Löffelholz K, Weide W, et al: Evidence for bilateral vagal innervation of postganglionic parasympathetic neurons in chicken heart. J Neural Transm 56:239, 1983.
13. Jeck D, Lindmar R, Löffelholz K, et al: Subtypes of muscarinic receptor on cholinergic nerves and atrial cells of chicken and guinea-pig hearts. Br J Pharmacol 93:357, 1988.
14. Brown OM: Cat heart acetylcholine: Structural proof and distribution. Am J Physiol 231:781, 1976.
15. Brown OM, Salata JJ, Graziani LA: The distribution of acetylcholine and choline in guinea pig heart. Life Sci 36:383, 1985.
16. Schmid PG, Greif BJ, Lund DD, et al: Regional choline acetyltransferase activity in the guinea pig heart. Circ Res 42:657, 1978.
17. Slavikova J, Tuček S: Choline acetyltransferase in the heart of adult rats. Pflügers Arch 392:225, 1982.
18. Lund DD, Oda RP, Pardini BJ, et al: Vagus nerve stimulation alters regional acetylcholine turnover in rat heart. Circ Res 58:372, 1986.
19. Kilbinger H: Gas chromatographic estimation of acetylcholine in the rabbit heart using a nitrogen selective detector. J Neurochem 21:421, 1973.
20. Stanley RL, Conatser J, Dettbarn WD: Acetylcholine, choline acetyltransferase and cholinesterases in the rat heart. Biochem Pharmacol 27:2409, 1978.
21. Nomura A, Yasuda H, Shimono H, et al: Cardiac acetylcholine concentration in the mouse. Life Sci 43:801, 1988.
22. Dieterich HA, Löffelholz K, Pompetzki H: Acetylcholine overflow from isolated perfused hearts of various species in the absence of cholinesterase inhibition. Naunyn-Schmiedeberg's Arch Pharmacol 296:149, 1977.
23. Dieterich HA, Lindmar R, Löffelholz K: The role of choline in the release of acetylcholine in isolated hearts. Naunyn-Schmiedeberg's Arch Pharmacol 301:207, 1978.
24. Bolton TB: Intramural nerves in the ventricular myocardium of the domestic fowl and other animals. Br J Pharmacol Chemother 31:253, 1967.
25. Löffelholz K, Lindmar R, Weide W: Isolated perfused heart and its parasympathetic neuro-effector junction. In I Hanin, AM Goldberg (eds): Model Cholinergic Synapses: Progress in Cholinergic Biology. New York, NY, Raven Press, 1982, p. 95.
26. Birks RI, Fitch SJG: Storage and release of acetylcholine in a sympathetic ganglion. J Physiol (Lond) 240:125, 1974.
27. MacIntosh FC: Synthesis and storage of acetylcholine in nervous tissue. Can J Biochem Physiol 41:2555, 1963.
28. Tuček S: Acetylcholine Synthesis in Neurons. London, GB Chapman and Hall Ltd, 1978, pp. 128–164.
29. Dexter F, Rudy Y, Levy MN: Muscarinic autoreceptors do not modulate kinetics of acetylcholine release in hearts. Am J Physiol (Lond) 256:H1073, 1989.
30. Haubrich DR, Wang PFL, Wedeking PW: Distribution and metabolism of intravenously administered choline [methyl-^{3}H] and synthesis in vivo of acetylcholine in various tissues of guinea pigs. J Pharmacol Exp Ther 193:246, 1975.
31. Brown OM, Salata JJ: In vivo acetylcholine turnover in rat heart. Life Sci 33:213, 1983.
32. Lindmar R, Löffelholz K, Weide W, et al: Neuronal uptake of choline following release of acetylcholine in the perfused heart. J Pharmacol Exp Ther 215:710, 1980.
33. Klein J, Köppen A, Löffelholz K: Small rises in plasma choline reverse the negative arteriovenous difference of brain choline. J Neurochem 55:1231, 1990.
34. Zeisel SH: Dietary choline: Biochemistry, physiology and pharmacology. Ann Rev Nutr 1:95, 1981.
35. Lindmar R, Löffelholz K, Weide W: Interstitial washout and hydrolysis of ace-

tylcholine in the perfused heart. Naunyn- Schmiedeberg's Arch Pharmacol 318:295, 1982.
36. Henning RJ, Masuda Y, Yang T, et al: Rate of acetylcholine hydrolysis affects the phase dependency of cardiac responses to vagal stimulation. Cardiovasc Res 21:169, 1987.
37. Katz RI, Miledi R: The binding of acetylcholine to receptors and its removal from the synaptic cleft. J Physiol (Lond) 231:549, 1973.
38. Löffelholz K, Brehm R, Lindmar R: Hydrolysis, synthesis and release of acetylcholine in the isolated heart. Fed Proc 43:2603, 1984.
39. Wetzel GT, Brown JH: Presynaptic modulation of acetylcholine release from cardiac parasympathetic neurons. Am J Physiol 248:H33, 1985.
40. Bognar IT, Beinhauer B, Kann P, et al: Different muscarinic receptors mediate autoinhibition of acetylcholine release and vagally-induced vasoconstriction in the rat isolated perfused heart. Naunyn-Schmiedeberg's Arch Pharmacol 341:279, 1990.
41. Lindmar R, Löffelholz K, Lambrecht G, et al: Presynaptic autoreceptors in chicken heart exhibit M_1 characteristics. Trends Pharmacol Sci 10(suppl):108, 1989.
42. Pitschner HF, Wellstein A: Dose-response curves of pirenzepine in man in relation to M_1- and M_2-cholinoceptor occupancy. Naunyn-Schmiedeberg's Arch Pharmacol 338:207, 1988.
43. Wellstein A, Pitschner HF: Complex dose-response curves of atropine in man explained by different functions of M_1- and M_2-cholinoceptors. Naunyn-Schmiedeberg's Arch Pharmacol 338:19, 1988.
44. Tietz H, Lindmar R, Löffelholz K, et al: High affinity pirenzepine receptors in chicken atria are different from M_1 type. Trends Pharmacol Sci 10(suppl):107, 1989.
45. Ehinger B, Falck B, Sporrong B: Possible axo-axonal synapses between peripheral adrenergic and cholinergic nerve terminals. Z Zellfschg 107:508, 1970.
46. Thoenen H, Tranzer JP: Chemical sympathectomy by selective destruction of adrenergic nerve endings with 6-hydroxydopamine. Naunyn-Schmiedeberg's Arch Pharmacol 261:271, 1968.
47. Levy MN, Blattberg B: Effect of vagal stimulation on the overflow of norepinephrine into the coronary sinus during cardiac sympathetic nerve stimulation in the dog. Circ Res 38:81, 1976.
48. Löffelholz K, Muscholl E: A muscarinic inhibition of the noradrenaline release evoked by postganglionic sympathetic nerve stimulation. Naunyn-Schmiedeberg's Arch Pharmacol 265:1, 1969.
49. Löffelholz K, Muscholl E: Inhibition by parasympathetic nerve stimulation of the release of the adrenergic transmitter. Naunyn-Schmiedeberg's Arch Pharmacol 267:181, 1970.
50. Muscholl E, Muth A: The effect of physostigmine on the vagally induced muscarinic inhibition of noradrenaline release from the isolated perfused rabbit atria. Naunyn-Schmiedeberg's Arch Pharmacol 320:760, 1982.
51. Benkirane S, Arbilla S, Langer SZ: Phenylethylamine-induced release of noradrenaline fails to stimulate α_1-adrenoceptors modulating [^{3}H]-acetylcholine release in rat atria, but activates α_2-adrenoceptors modulating [^{3}H]-serotonin release in the hippocampus. Naunyn-Schmiedeberg's Arch Pharmacol 334:149, 1986.
52. McDonough PM, Wetzel GT, Brown JH: Further characterization of the presynaptic alpha-1 receptor modulating [^{3}H]ACh release from rat atria. J Pharmacol Exp Ther 238:612, 1986.
53. Wetzel GT, Goldstein D, Brown JH: Acetylcholine release from rat atria can be regulated through an α_1-adrenergic receptor. Circ Res 56:763, 1985.
54. McGrattan PA, Brown JH, Brown OM: Parasympathetic effects on in vivo rat heart can be regulated through an α_1-adrenergic receptor. Circ Res 60:465, 1987.
55. Starke K: Alpha sympathomimetic inhibition of adrenergic and cholinergic transmission in the rabbit heart. Naunyn-Schmiedeberg's Arch Pharmacol 274:18, 1972.

56. Loiacono RE, Story DF: Effect of α-adrenoceptor agonists and antagonists on cholinergic transmission in guinea-pig isolated heart. Naunyn-Schmiedeberg's Arch Pharmacol 334:40, 1986.
57. Manabe N, Foldes FF, Töröcsik A, et al: Presynaptic interaction between vagal and sympathetic innervation in the heart: Modulation of acetylcholine and noradrenaline release. J Auton Nerv Syst 32:233, 1991.
58. Flavahan NA, McGrath JC: α_1-Adrenoceptor activation can increase heart rate directly or decrease it indirectly through parasympathetic activation. Br J Pharmacol 77:319, 1982.
59. Bognar IT, Baretti R, Fischer S, et al: Alpha-adrenoceptor mediated facilitation of acetylcholine release in the rat perfused heart. J Pharmacol Exp Ther 254:702, 1990.
60. Fozard JR: Neuronal 5-HT receptors in the periphery. Neuropharmacol 23:1473, 1984.
61. Akasu H, Hasuo H, Tokimasa T: Activation of 5-HT_3 receptor subtypes causes rapid excitation of rabbit parasympathetic neurones. Br J Pharmacol 91:453, 1987.
62. Saxena PR, Villalon CM: Cardiovascular effects of serotonin agonists and antagonists. J Cardiovasc Pharmacol 15(suppl):S17, 1990.
63. Wiley JW, Uccioli L, Owyang C, et al: Somatostatin stimulates acetylcholine release in the canine heart. Am J Physiol 257:H483, 1989.
64. Potter E: Presynaptic inhibition of cardiac vagal postganglionic nerves by neuropeptide Y. Neurosci Letts 83:101, 1987.
65. Roskoski R Jr, Meyer HE, Schmid PG: Choline acetyltransferase activity in guinea-pig heart in vitro. J Neurochem 23:1197, 1974.

CHAPTER 11

Biochemical Basis of Cardiac Sympathetic-Parasympathetic Interaction

J. Neumann, R.C. Gupta, A.M. Watanabe

The primary aim of this chapter is to review briefly the biochemical basis for the inhibitory effects of the muscarinic cholinergic system on the facilitatory influence exerted by the sympathetic nerves on the heart.

Physiological Effects of Acetylcholine

The physiological effects of acetylcholine (ACh) on the heart are well established and are summarized in earlier excellent reviews[1,2] as well as in other chapters in this book. Hence, they will be reiterated only briefly in this chapter.

ACh exerts its negative chronotropic effects by hyperpolarizing the cell membranes and by reducing the rate of diastolic depolarization in sinoatrial (SA) node cells. ACh retards the conduction of impulses through the atrioventricular (AV) node. In atria, ACh shortens action potential duration, hyperpolarizes the cell membranes, and decreases the refractory period. These electrophysiological changes are accompanied by a profound negative inotropic effect. In all species investigated, ACh inhibits atrial contractility. In isolated mammalian ventricles, ACh at low or moderate concentrations usually has little or no inotropic effect. At high concentrations, ACh (1 mM) may have a positive inotropic effect on the mammalian ventricle. In avian ventricles, ACh exerts a strong negative inotropic effect.

In isolated cells, isolated organs, and whole animals, ACh antagonizes the effects of β-adrenoceptor (β-AR) stimulation. The positive chronotropic and inotropic effects of catecholamines or sympathetic nerve stimulation are antagonized in various species and preparations by ACh.

From *Vagal Control of the Heart: Experimental Basis and Clinical Implications* edited by MN Levy, PJ Schwartz © 1994, Futura Publishing Co. Inc., Armonk, NY.

Structure and Classification of Muscarinic Receptors

Classically, muscarinic receptors (mAChRs) have been divided into brain (M_1) and cardiac (M_2) cholinoceptors.[1] This finding from functional studies in humans[3] has been supported by both radioligand-binding studies[1,3] and by cloning and sequencing experiments.[4,5] Myocardial mAChRs exhibit low affinity for pirenzepine (PZ) in binding experiments, and hence they are regarded as the M_2 type.[1]

Functional data (such as negative inotropic effects in atria), biochemical data, and cloning experiments differentiate clearly between the mAChRs in heart and brain. The mAChR from bovine brain was purified by affinity chromatography to homogeneity. It exhibited an apparent molecular weight of about 70 kd and belongs to the M_1 type.[5] The mAChR from bovine atria has also been purified to homogeneity. The apparent molecular weight was 78–90 kd and belongs to the M_2 type.[5] Initially, the M_1 receptor from the brain and subsequently the atrial M_2 receptors were cloned, sequenced, and expressed.[4] Additional mAChRs were identified by low stringency hybridization. These receptors are called m_1-4 or M_1-4.[5] Hence, the functional, binding, and hybridization characteristics are reasonably correlated for cardiac $\hat{M_2}$-cholinoceptors.[4,5]

Intracellular Effectors Coupled to Muscarinic Receptors

Cyclic Guanosine Monophosphate

The role of ACh-induced increases in cardiac cyclic guanosine monophosphate (cGMP) has received considerable attention in the past. Arguments for and against a physiological role of cGMP have been raised and are reviewed elsewhere.[1,2] Some new evidence does support a role for cGMP. In frog myocytes, cGMP apparently stimulates a phosphodiesterase and, hence, reduces adenosine 3′ 5′-cyclic phosphate (cyclic AMP). This process may be responsible for a reduction in calcium current (i_{Ca}).[6] In rat ventricular myocytes, however, cGMP derivatives may activate a cGMP-dependent protein kinase (PK). This kinase may phosphorylate target proteins, such as the calcium channel proteins, and thereby reduce i_{Ca}.[7] These findings seem to indicate that species differences might in part explain earlier discrepancies concerning the physiological importance of cGMP in modulating cardiac contractility.

Adenosine 3′ 5′-Cyclic Phosphate

The importance of cyclic AMP for modulating cardiac contractility is much more firmly established than is that of cGMP. There have been efforts to link the effects of ACh and cyclic AMP in the heart. Activation of cardiac mAChRs clearly inhibits adenylyl cyclase (AC).[8] The inhibition of AC by ACh alone, however, in broken cell preparations is relatively weak (15–25%).[8] That is, even 100-μM ACh is required in order to detect a small inhibition of AC activity. In contrast, the physiological and protein phosphorylation effects occur at much lower concentrations and are usually maximal at 1-μM ACh.[1,9]

It is difficult to understand why ACh alone does not reduce the force of contraction in ventricles but does inhibit AC activity. Patch clamp experiments have shown that ACh activates atrial potassium channels by a direct effect via guanine nucleotide-binding proteins (G-proteins), without changing the cyclic AMP content (see below). This finding suggests that at least the atrial effects of ACh are cyclic AMP-independent.

In addition, several laboratories observed independently that in the presence of agents such as isoproterenol, forskolin, and isobutylmethylxanthine (IBMX) that increase cyclic AMP, the negative inotropic effects of ACh in the mammalian ventricle were not accompanied by changes in cyclic AMP content.[9–11] Isoproterenol acts via cardiac β-ARs, forskolin acts directly on AC, and IBMX is a phosphodiesterase inhibitor, which increases cyclic AMP by inhibiting its degradation. Thus, regardless of which mechanism is used to elevate cyclic AMP, ACh antagonizes that effects and reduces contractility.

As phosphodiesterase inhibitors increase cyclic AMP without affecting AC the fact that their inotropic effects are antagonized by ACh could be regarded as strong evidence that ACh does not act solely by inhibiting AC activity. It has been argued, however, that reductions in cyclic AMP might be confined to the myocytes themselves and, therefore, cyclic AMP reductions may be undetectable in whole hearts, which are comprised of many types of tissues.[12] It has also been argued that reductions in cyclic AMP are confined to subcellular compartments.[13] Indeed, some investigators reported a 40% reduction of cyclic AMP by ACh in isolated myocytes (see George et al[14]). In these studies, however, the incubation conditions for the myocytes were unphysiological in that they included phosphodiesterase inhibitors, which increase the basal cyclic AMP content 10-fold.[14] It remains to be established whether reductions of cyclic AMP are meaningful after the cyclic AMP level had previously been elevated to an unphysiologically high level.

Protein Phosphorylation

As discussed above, some of the effects of ACh may occur independently of changes in cyclic AMP. Such effects might result, for example, from inhibition of AC. As shown in Figure 1, cyclic AMP activates cyclic AMP-dependent PK, and this leads to the phosphorylation and activation of several regulatory proteins in the heart. ACh might act by inhibiting a step in this cascade distal to cyclic AMP generation. There is no evidence, however, that ACh can inhibit PK activity.

Conversely, steps distal to PK are clearly affected by ACh. In perfused

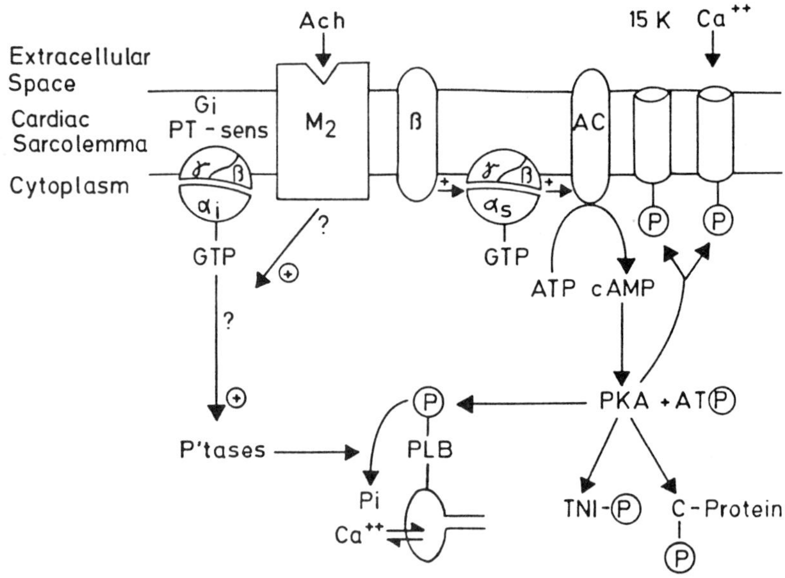

Figure 1. *The regulation of cardiac contractility by phosphorylation and dephosphorylation. Activation of* β*-AR activates adenylate cyclase (AC) activity via a stimulatory guanosine triphosphate-(GTP-) binding protein* (α_S)*. This process leads to the conversion of ATP to cyclic AMP (cAMP). Increased cAMP content stimulates cAMP-dependent protein kinase A (PKA). PKA catalyzes the phosphorylation of various regulatory proteins. In the sarcolemmal membranes, the calcium channels and a 15-kd protein (15 K) are phosphorylated. The phosphorylation of the calcium channel increases the influx of* Ca^{++} *into the cell and enhances the myocardial contractility. Activation of PKA also leads to the phosphorylation of troponin I (TnI), located in the thin filaments, and of C-protein, located in the thick filaments. Furthermore, PKA phosphorylates phospholamban (PLB), a protein in the sarcoplasmic reticulum. Phosphorylation of PLB increases the uptake of* Ca^{++} *into the sarcoplasmic reticulum. Phosphorylation of proteins is reversed by the activity of phosphatases (P'tases); e.g., phosphatase dephosphorylates PLB by releasing inorganic phosphate* (P_I)*. A hypothetical effect of ACh is also indicated. Activation of* M_2*-cholinergic receptors stimulates the activity of phosphatases. In this way, ACh might abolish the catecholamine-induced increases in the phosphate content of the regulatory proteins and thereby reduce cardiac contractility.*

hearts, ACh reduced the phosphorylation state of several regulatory proteins (Fig. 1). In an early study, ACh enhanced the dephosphorylation of troponin I (TnI) that had been phosphorylated by isoproterenol.[15] Similarly, the phosphorylation state of phospholamban (a regulator of sarcoplasmic Ca^{2+} uptake) had been increased by agents such as isoproterenol, forskolin, or IBMX that increase cyclic AMP (Fig. 1). Under such conditions, the phosphorylation state was then greatly reduced by ACh, but the effects on the cyclic AMP content were negligible.[10] Hence, the phosphorylation state of cardiac regulatory proteins can be reduced without reductions in cyclic AMP content.

Protein Dephosphorylation

Dephosphorylation of proteins in the heart can be catalyzed by several phosphatases. Protein phosphatases have been categorized into type 1 and 2.[16] Type 1 phosphatase is inhibited by phosphatase inhibitor-1 and inhibitor-2. The remaining phosphatases are regarded as type 2. Both phosphatases are present in the heart, although type 1 is predominant.[17] Phosphatase inhibitor-1 is a phosphoprotein that inhibits type I phosphatase only if it is phosphorylated by PK.[16] Type 1 phosphatase regulation is physiologically important because it is present in the cytosol and in sarcoplasmic reticulum membranes of the heart and, in vitro, it dephosphorylates and inactivates regulatory proteins such as phospholamban[17] and the enzymes involved in glycogen metabolism.[16]

Muscarinic agonists may exert their effects by modulating phosphatase activities. This hypothesis is supported by experiments in which isoproterenol was shown to inhibit phosphatase activity in membrane vesicles from isolated perfused hearts. This effect of isoproterenol was abolished by additional application of ACh.[17]

The isoproterenol-induced inhibition of phosphatase activity was accompanied by an increased activity of inhibitor-1 in isoproterenol-perfused hearts. The activity of inhibitor-1 was reduced to control levels after addition of both isoproterenol and ACh.[17]

This finding seems to be a general phenomenon, because cyclic AMP increasing agents can stimulate phosphatase inhibitor-1 activity and reduce phosphatase activity in skeletal muscle.[18]

In order to gain insight into the regulation of phosphatase activity, the regulation of phosphatase inhibitor-1 was studied in great detail. In the initial studies, the changes in phosphatase inhibitor-1 activity were regarded as indicative of the phosphorylation state of phosphatase inhibitor-1. Subsequently, the regulation of phosphatase inhibitor-1 was studied more directly.

Extracts enriched in phosphatase inhibitor-1 from [^{32}p]-labelled hearts were prepared. A phosphorylated protein of about 26 kd (Fig. 2) was prominent, indicating that the protein is a good physiological substrate for PK(s). In addition, more radioactive material was immunoprecipitated with antiserum from isoproterenol-stimulated hearts than from nonstimulated hearts, and the signal was greatly attenuated by pretreating the antiserum with authentic phosphatase inhibitor-1 (Fig. 2). This finding strongly suggests that catecholamines increase the phosphorylation state of inhibitor-1, and hence its activity, in vivo.[19]

This result may be important, in view of the species and tissue differences in the expression of phosphatase inhibitor-1. For example, in rat and mouse liver, no phosphatase inhibitor-1 could be detected immunologically,[20] whereas it was present in the rat heart (tissue differences) and in the rabbit liver (species differences). Its lack of expression in rat liver versus its existence in rabbit liver implies different mechanisms for the regulation of phosphatases in

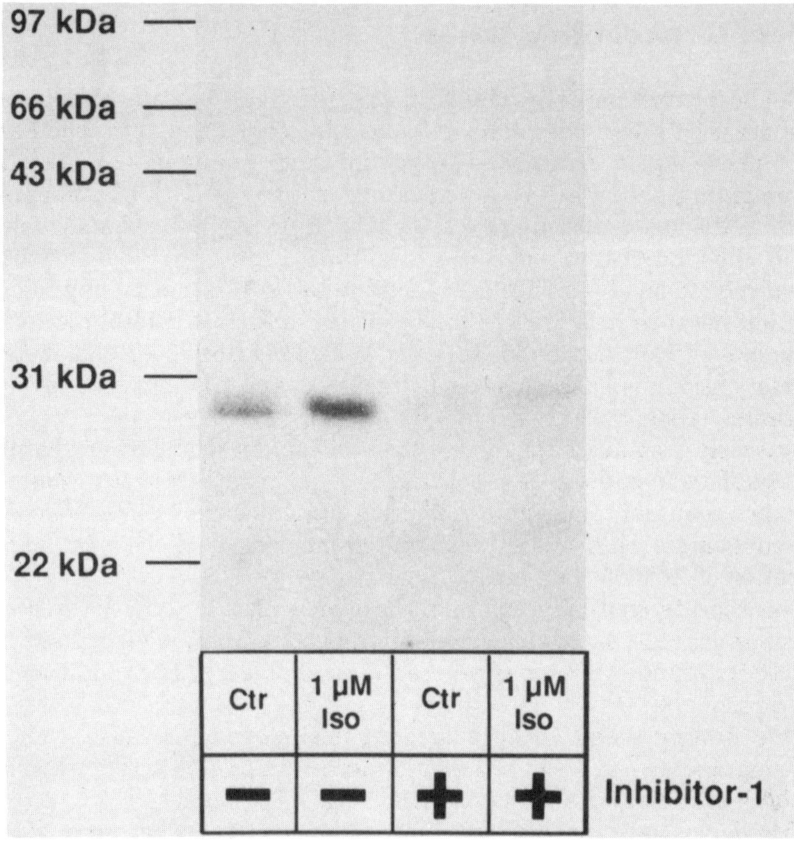

Figure 2. *Autoradiography of an enriched fraction of immunoprecipitated phosphatase inhibitor-1 from an isolated, perfused guinea pig ventricle labelled with [^{32}p]. The ventricle was electrically stimulated (3 Hz) in the absence (Ctr) or presence of 1-μM isoproterenol (Iso). Fractions were immunoprecipitated with native antisera (−) or antiserum pretreated with pure phosphatase inhibitor-1 (+) from skeletal muscle. The results indicate that phosphatase inhibitor-1 is phosphorylated in vivo in the presence of catecholamines. (Unpublished experiments J. Neumann, R. C. Gupta, and A. M. Watanabe.)*

these two species. It also indicates that the regulation of phosphatase in the rat heart is different from that in the rat liver (tissue differences).

From these results, it seems established that cardiac phosphatase inhibitor-1 is phosphorylated in vivo. It is still unclear, however, precisely which PKs regulate the phosphorylation state of phosphate inhibitor-1 and the roles the phosphatases play in this regulation.

The classical assumption from in vitro studies is that phosphatase inhibitor-1 is phosphorylated by PK. In the heart, however, phosphatase inhibitor-1 may also be phosphorylated by cyclic AMP-independent PKs. Cyclic AMP-independent kinases can phosphorylate inhibitor-1-like proteins in various tissues.[21] Therefore, these cyclic AMP-independent kinases might be regulated in an unknown way by β-adrenergic stimulation. Alternatively, the phosphorylation state of inhibitor-1 could be stimulated by inhibition (Fig. 3) of a specific or nonspecific inhibitor-1 phosphatase. Such an inhibition of a specific phosphatase has already been considered as a mechanism for regulating protein phosphorylation, independent of the activation of PKs.[21] Other mechanisms for changes in phosphatase activity, such as translocation of the catalytic subunit of type 1 phosphatase, may also exist.

Hence, by either of these mechanisms, isoproterenol would elevate the phosphorylation state of phosphatase inhibitor-1 which, in turn, inhibits phosphatase type 1. This process would increase the phosphate content of phosphoproteins (regulatory proteins; compare Figs. 1 and 3) by a mechanism other than the direct activation of protein kinase A (PKA) by isoproterenol via increases in cyclic AMP. Hence, the effects of isoproterenol on protein phosphorylation would be amplified by inhibition of phosphatase type 1, mediated via the phosphorylation of phosphatase inhibitor-1.

Regardless of the precise mechanisms by which isoproterenol inhibits phosphatase activity, ACh reduces the isoproterenol-stimulated activity of phosphatase inhibitor-1. This finding could explain the increased phosphatase activity in the presence of ACh (Fig. 3). Whether the actual phosphate content

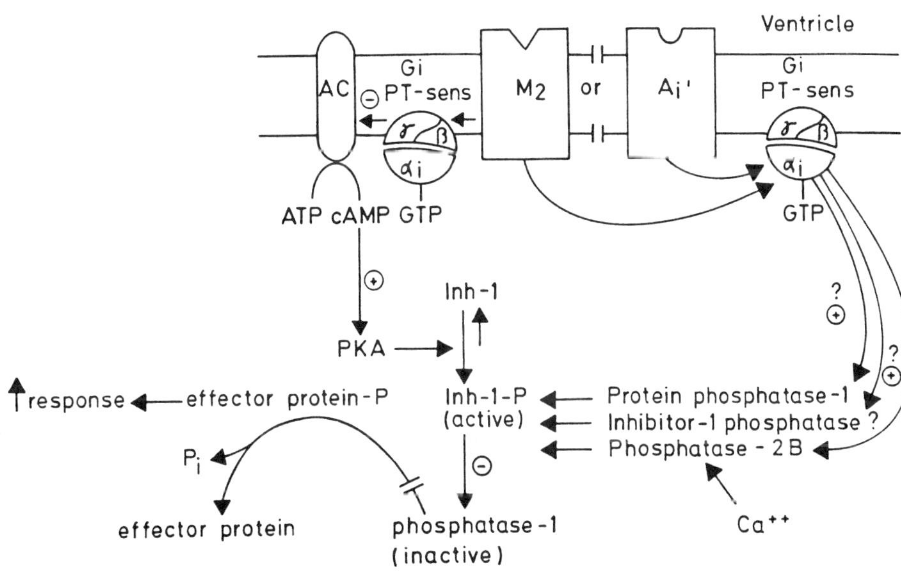

Figure 3. *The regulation of cardiac dephosphorylation. The increase in phosphorylation state of regulatory proteins (see Fig. 1) mediates the positive inotropic effects of compounds that increase cyclic AMP (cAMP). Dephosphorylation reverses these inotropic effects. Regulatory proteins can be dephosphorylated by type 1 phosphatase. Type 1 phosphatase is activated by dephosphorylation of phosphatase inhibitor-1 (Inh-1) and can be achieved via reduced activity of cAMP-dependent protein kinase A (PKA) or via other undefined Inh-1 kinases. Alternatively, phosphorylated Inh-1 might be dephosphorylated by certain phosphatases, some of which are indicated. How these phosphatases are regulated in unknown; they may be activated via M_2-cholinoceptors.*

of phosphatase inhibitor-1 is reduced by ACh is not known. Therefore, one can only speculate about the way in which the activity of phosphatase inhibitor-1 is reduced. One explanation is that ACh reduces the cyclic AMP content and, therefore, less phosphatase inhibitor-1 is phosphorylated by PK. In many intact tissue experiments, however, no change in cyclic AMP is detectable, as discussed above. Compartments of cyclic AMP linked to phosphatase inhibitor-1 may exist. The activation of a specific phosphatase inhibitor-1 phosphatase or phosphatase 2B (calcineurin), however, has also been suggested.[21] Theoretically, type 1 phosphatase would be able to dephosphorylate phosphatase inhibitor-1, and thereby inactivate it (Fig. 3). This reaction, however, needs millimolar concentrations of Mn^{2+}; such concentrations do not exist in vivo. How these phosphatases are linked to the mAChR and whether G-proteins are involved in this linkage are additional questions that merit further study.

Electrophysiological Effects

In atrial preparations, ACh activates the potassium current (i_K) via a G-protein that is sensitive to pertussis toxin (PTX).[22] Whether this effect is mediated via the β and γ subunits[23] or the α subunit of the G-proteins is debatable.[24] i_K is absent in most ventricles.[12] Hence, in the ventricles, i_K is unlikely to mediate the negative inotropic effects of ACh in the presence of isoproterenol. The effect of ACh on SA cells is probably due to a shift of the activation curve of the hyperpolarization-activated current (i_f) toward negative potentials. This effect is sensitive to PTX and is mediated by G-proteins. i_f is mainly a slowly activating inward current carried by Na and K.[25] ACh reduces the isoproterenol-stimulated i_{Ca} in atria and ventricles. This response has been demonstrated in frog myocytes[26] and isolated guinea pig ventricular myocytes.[27] Whether the activity of these ventricular channels is regulated in vivo mainly via phosphorylation and dephosphorylation or via a direct coupling between the M_2-cholinoceptor, G-protein, and ion channel is not known. Dephosphorylation of calcium channels is very important for the ventricular cardiac effects of ACh and it may be regulated via a membrane-bound phosphatase.

Conclusion

ACh affects the heart via M_2-cholinoceptors that are connected to various effectors in different regions of the heart. mAChR agonists interact at more than one level in the cascade of reactions that mediate the intracellular effects of catecholamines. The relative importance of the different effectors that are regulated by M_2-cholinoceptors in evoking the physiological responses to ACh in various portions of the heart remains to be elucidated.

References

1. Löffelholz K, Pappano AJ: The parasympathetic neuroeffector junction of the heart. Pharmacol Rev 37: 1–24, 1985.
2. Lindemann JP, Watanabe AM: Mechanisms of adrenergic and cholinergic regulation of cardiac contractility. In N Sperelakis (ed): Physiology and Pathophysiology of the Heart. Norwell, MA, Kluwer Academic Publishers, 1988, pp. 423–452.
3. Deighton NM, Motomura S, Borquez D, et al: Muscarinic cholinoceptors in the human heart: Demonstration, subclassification, and distribution. Naunyn Schmiedebergs Arch Pharmacol 341: 14–21, 1990.
4. Venter JC, Fraser CM, Kervelage AR, et al: Molecular biology of adrenergic and muscarinic cholinergic receptors. Biochem Pharmacol 38:1197–1208, 1989.
5. Hulme EC, Birdsall NJM, Buckley NJ: Muscarinic receptor subtypes. Annu Rev Pharmacol Toxicol 30:633–673, 1990.
6. Fischmeister R, Hartzell HC: Regulation of calcium current by low-K_m cyclic AMP phosphodiesterases in cardiac cells. Mol Pharmacol 38:426–433, 1990.
7. Mery P-F, Lohmann S, Walter U, et al: Ca^{2+} current is regulated by cyclic GMP-dependent protein kinase in mammalian cardiac myocytes. Proc Natl Acad Sci USA 88:1197–1201, 1991.
8. Watanabe AM, Besch HR: Myocardial adenylate cyclase: Studies on the relationship of activity and purity of sarcolemmal preparation. J Mol Cell Cardiol 7:563–575, 1975.
9. Watanabe AM, Besch HR: Interaction between cyclic adenosine monophosphate and cyclic guanosine monophosphate in guinea pig ventricular myocardium. Circ Res 37:309–317, 1975.
10. Lindemann JP, Watanabe AM: Muscarinic cholinergic inhibition of β-adrenergic stimulation of phospholamban phosphorylation and Ca^{2+} transport in guinea pig ventricles. J Biol Chem 260:13122–13129, 1985.
11. Schmied R, Korth M: Muscarinic receptor stimulation and cyclic AMP-dependent effects in guinea-pig ventricular myocardium. Br J Pharmacol 99:401–407, 1990.
12. Hartzell HC: Regulation of cardiac ion channels by catecholamines, acetylcholine and second messenger systems. Prog Biophys Mol Biol 52:165–247, 1988.
13. Buxton ILO, Brunton LL: Compartments of cyclic AMP and protein kinase in mammalian myocytes. J Biol Chem 258: 10233–10239, 1983.
14. George EF, Romano FD, Dobson JR Jr: Adenosine and acetylcholine reduce isoproterenol-induced protein phosphorylation of rat myocytes. J Mol Cell Cardiol 23:749–764, 1991.
15. England PJ: Studies on the phosphorylation of the inhibitory subunit of troponin during modification of contraction in perfused rat heart. Biochem J 160:295–304, 1976.
16. Cohen P, Cohen PTW: Protein phosphatases come of age. J Biol Chem 264:21435–21438, 1989.
17. Ahmad Z, Green FJ, Subuhi HS, et al: Autonomic regulation of type 1 protein phosphatase in cardiac muscle. J Biol Chem 264:3859–3863, 1989.
18. Foulkes JG, Cohen P, Strada SJ, et al: Antagonistic effects of insulin and β-adrenergic agonists on the activity of protein phosphatase inhibitor-1 in skeletal muscle of perfused rat hemicorpus. J Biol Chem 257:12493–12496, 1982.
19. Neumann J, Gupta RC, Schmitz W, et al: Evidence for isoproterenol-induced phosphorylation of phosphatase inhibitor-1 in the intact heart. Circ Res 69:1450–1457, 1991.
20. MacDougall LK, Campbell DG, Hubbard MJ, et al: Partial structure and hormonal regulation of rabbit liver inhibitor-1: Distribution of inhibitor-1 and inhibitor-2 in rabbit and rat tissues. Biochem Biophys Acta 1010:218–226, 1989.
21. Nemenoff RA, Blackshear PJ, Avruch J: Hormonal regulation of protein dephosphorylation. J Biol Chem 258:9437–9443, 1983.

22. Pfaffinger JP, Martin JM, Hunter DD, et al: GTP binding proteins couple to cardiac muscarinic receptors to K channels. Nature (Lond) 317:536–538, 1985.
23. Logothetis DE, Kurachi Y, Galper J, et al: The βγ subunits of GTP binding proteins activate the muscarinic K^+ channel in heart. Nature (Lond) 325:321–326, 1987.
24. Codina J, Yatani A, Grenet D, et al: The α-subunit of the GTP binding protein G_k opens atrial potassium channels. Science 236:442–445, 1987.
25. DiFrancesco D, Tromba C: Inhibition of the hyperpolarization-activated current induced by acetylcholine in sino-atrial node myocytes. J Physiol (Lond) 405:477–491, 1988.
26. Breitweisser GE, Szabo G: Uncoupling of cardiac muscarinic and β-adrenergic receptors from ion channels by a guanine nucleotide analogue. Nature (Lond) 317:538–540, 1985.
27. Hescheler J, Kameyama M, Trautwein W: On the mechanism of muscarinic inhibition of the cardiac Ca current. Pflügers Arch 407:182–189, 1986.

PART III

Physiological Effects on the Heart

CHAPTER 12

Neural Control of Sinoatrial Pacemaker Activity

J. Jalife, D.C. Michaels

The coordinated contraction of the heart during each cardiac cycle is accomplished by a complex biochemical process that is set in motion by the arrival of an electrical "trigger" (the action potential) at each cardiac muscle cell. Thus, a wave of electrical excitation precedes the wave of muscle contraction during the cardiac cycle. Intuitively, one would predict that the pacemaker lies at the site of earliest electrical activation, and indeed that prediction was verified many years ago.[1,2] While, as is seen later, several cardiac tissues are capable of generating pacemaker activity (at least when isolated), the normal cardiac pacemaker is the structure known as the sinoatrial (SA) node.[3]

The development of increasingly complex techniques for measuring electrical activity from isolated tissues with extracellular electrodes,[4–8] from the whole heart with the electrocardiogram (ECG),[9,10] from cells with intracellular microelectrodes,[11–13] and even from patches of cell membrane containing only a single ionic channel by means of patch clamp electrodes[14,15] has allowed for the accumulation of a large body of information on the electrical phenomena generated by the heart. This frenzy of reductionism has led to the point where one can describe in reasonable detail the workings of an individual pacemaker cell (at least electrically). The way in which multiple pacemaker cells interact to synchronize their activity to give rise to a single pacemaker impulse once each cardiac cycle has, however, only recently been investigated.[16–24] Indeed, what is needed for this next level of understanding is the development of a kind of "population biology" for groups of individual cells. The emergence

This work was supported in part by National Heart, Lung and Blood Institute Grant No. HL-29439 and HL-P01-39707, and National Science Foundation Grant No. DMB-8612771. Additional computational support was provided by the New York State Center for Advanced Technology in Computer Applications and Software Engineering (CASE Center) at Syracuse University and by the Cornell National Supercomputer Facility, Cornell University, that is supported in part by the National Science Foundation, New York State, and IBM Corporation.
From *Vagal Control of the Heart: Experimental Basis and Clinical Implications* edited by MN Levy, PJ Schwartz © 1994, Futura Publishing Co. Inc., Armonk, NY.

of new experimental techniques such as multiple electrode[25] and optical mapping[26,27] and the contributions of studies on dynamical systems theory,[28] topology,[18] and mathematical modelling provide tools for both the elucidation of the nature of beat-to-beat interactions between cells and groups of cells[29,30] and the study of the dynamic influence of the autonomic nervous system on these populations.[31–33]

This present chapter briefly summarizes what is currently known about the electrical workings of individual normal pacemaker cells, and particular attention is paid to those cells comprising the natural pacemaker of the heart. In addition, phase-resetting behavior of cardiac pacemakers and the dynamic interaction of multiple pacemakers and of pacemakers with their surroundings are described. Finally, identification of those areas in which future progress needs to be made in order to fully elucidate the functioning of cardiac pacemakers is attempted.

The Sinoatrial Node

The natural cardiac pacemaker of the mammalian heart is the SA (or sinus) node, which is located on the roof of the right atrium near the insertion of the superior vena cava. It is further bounded on the sides by the crista (sulcus) terminalis and the interatrial septum.[3] In smaller mammals, the SA node is relatively free of muscle tissue, while in larger mammals, it is frequently sandwiched within muscle layers of overlying and underlying atrial muscle.[34] The cells of the SA node proper are considerably smaller than muscle cells, and all exhibit pacemaker activity with a distribution of intrinsic frequencies.[35] The cells are clustered in small groups (as in a cluster of grapes) and embedded in a fibrous matrix of connective tissue.[34,36] In the rabbit, there is a small ($\approx$0.3 mm^2) compact central region to the SA node consisting of several thousand cells in which the dominant pacemaker activity is thought to arise.[35] Cells in this region are the earliest to activate and have the smoothest transition to an upstroke. Cells outside this region have slower intrinsic frequencies and a more abrupt transition to the upstroke phase. These characteristics suggest that these cells are brought to threshold by means of electrotonic currents from cells in the central compact region.

The main outflow tract of the SA node is the crista terminalis. From here, the impulse spreads throughout the atria proper and on to the atrioventricular (AV) node from which it invades the specialized conduction system of the ventricles and finally the ventricles themselves. There is some evidence that there are specialized conducting tracts within the atria that ensure that the impulse reaches the AV node[36]; however, this hypothesis remains controversial.[37]

Pacemaker Mechanisms

A detailed review of the various ionic mechanisms that have been proposed to explain pacemaker activity is well beyond the scope of this chapter. The reader is referred to excellent articles on the subject including those by Giles et al,[38] Irisawa and Giles,[39] DiFrancesco,[40] and Irisawa et al.[41] It is now well established that the heart has its own intrinsic pacemaker mechanisms and that these are, for the most part, confined to specialized cells that make up specialized tissues.[34] While several different cardiac tissues can exhibit pacemaker activity under normal conditions (hereafter referred to as the normal pacemakers), other tissues (including cardiac muscle) can exhibit spontaneous automaticity under abnormal conditions such as stretch, hypoxia, and ischemia. Most of the normal pacemakers exhibit overdrive suppression[42] in which stimuli occurring at a rate faster than the intrinsic rate of the pacemaker lead to a suppression of its rate of impulse formation. The importance of this mechanism in maintaining a hierarchy of pacemaker function is discussed later.

Ionic Mechanisms in the Sinus Node

Although considerable progress has been made in determining the specific ionic currents that occur during the action potentials of the SA cells,[41,43,44] the precise role of each of these currents in the development of diastolic depolarization remains controversial.[40,45] SA node cells typically have resting membrane potentials of about −60 mV[46] and have a variety of ionic channels that mediate specific transmembrane currents (see Fig. 1A).[38] These include:

1. a slow inward current carried by calcium ions (i_{Ca});
2. a delayed-rectifier potassium current (i_K);
3. a fast sodium current (i_{Na}) similar to that of nerve and muscle; and
4. a hyperpolarization-activated current (i_f) that is thought to be similar to the i_f current found in Purkinje fibers.[47]

In addition, there are background currents that are voltage-dependent, but time-independent. There is a significant inward background ("leak") current in the SA nodal cell, which probably corresponds to the sodium background current ($i_{Na,b}$), with relatively small electrogenic contributions of the Na/K pump and the Na/Ca exchanger.[41] The presence of the leak current, together with the relatively high input resistance[48] secondary to the existence of a negligible number of inwardly-rectifying, i_{K1}, channels,[49] is partly responsible for the relatively low maximum diastolic potential (MDP, ~ −60 mV) of the SA nodal cell,[48] as compared with other cell types such as atrial or ventricular myocytes. Moreover, because of the relatively low MDP, the rate of rise of the action potential is very low, which suggests that i_{Na} is inactive or very low, particularly in the center of the node. Indeed, most authors have reported a lack of sensitivity to tetrodotoxin (TTX) in SA nodal cells (for review, see Irisawa et al[41]).

Pacemaker cells differ from nonpacemaker cells in that they exhibit spontaneous depolarization during diastole. In the SA node, this depolarization is brought about by a net flow of inward current across the membrane. The net

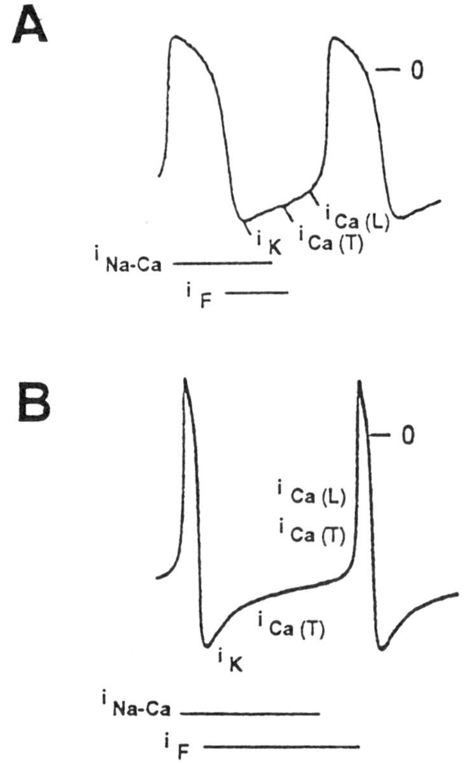

Figure 1. *Role of various ionic currents during diastolic depolarization in pacemaker cells. A: Action potentials from the SA node. Labels indicate contribution of various currents at different phases of diastolic depolarization. B: Recordings from tricuspid valve pacemaker cell. This different pattern of involvement of ionic currents may also be pertinent to pacemaker activity in Purkinje fibers. Modified with permission from Anumonwo JMB, Jalife J: Initiation and modulation of pacemaker activity in cardiac cells. In C Fisch, B Surawicz (eds): Cardiac Electrophysiology and Arrhythmias. New York, NY, Elsevier, 1991, pp. 35–47.*

flow results from an imbalance between specific inward (depolarizing) and outward (repolarizing) currents.[39] Knowledge derived from studies conducted during the last 30 years in isolated tissue preparations[44,50–52] and in single cells[40,45] has led investigators to divide the time-course of slow diastolic depolarization into two major phases: an early phase and a late phase. The proposed mechanisms to explain the ionic bases of the two phases have been nicely summarized by Irisawa et al[41] and by DiFrancesco.[40] Briefly, two major hypotheses have been put forth to explain the first phase: the "i_K decay" hypothesis[41,50] and the "i_f activation" hypothesis.[40]

The proponents of the i_K decay hypothesis postulate that pacemaker depolarization is the result of slow deactivation of the delayed-rectifier current, i_K, which, in the presence of a constant (time-independent) background inward current (perhaps $i_{Na,b}$) causes diastolic depolarization.[39,41] Conversely, DiFrancesco's i_f activation hypothesis is based on the assumption that, upon termination of the action potential, the hyperpolarization-activated current, i_f, also dubbed the "pacemaker current,"[40,53] provides a slowly activating inward component that predominates over the decaying i_K and allows for initiation of the process of slow diastolic depolarization. The major difference with the i_K decay hypothesis is in the premise that the inward component, which eventually outweighs i_K and drives the membrane potential toward less negative levels, is the time-dependent i_f. In favor of the latter, DiFrancesco[40] argues that there is no net inward current at voltages within the pacemaker potential range (~ -60 to -35 mV) of the SA nodal cell. Hence, the only inward current available to initiate diastolic depolarization from the MDP would be i_f because, according to DiFrancesco, i_f activates well within the range of voltages of the pacemaker potential. This issue, however, remains controversial, because other authors have reported that the activation range of i_f is negative to the MDP of the SA nodal cells[54] and that the time-course of this current is much too slow to account for pacemaker activity in these cells.[55,56] Moreover, Hagiwara and Irisawa[56] have demonstrated that the voltage dependence of i_f is modulated by the intracellular concentration of Ca. In fact, they showed that 1 to 3 mM of Mn produces a positive shift in the i_f activation curve. They attributed this shift to a possible increase in intracellular Ca secondary to Mn-induced blockade of Na/Ca exchange.[56] This finding has led some authors to speculate that the differences in the data that have been reported in the literature regarding the role of i_f in SA pacemaker depolarization are the result of differences in experimental conditions,[41] particularly in relation to the concentrations of Ca and other ions.

Unfortunately, a major issue remains unresolved that greatly weakens DiFrancesco's contention that i_f plays a primary role in initiating diastolic depolarization. It has been shown that complete blockade of this current with 2 mM of Cs does not eliminate pacemaker activity[45] of the SA nodal cell (see the section below entitled Atrioventricular Valve Pacemakers). Consequently, at the present time, one cannot escape the conclusion that i_f is not essential for pacemaker activity in the SA node and that this current plays only a modulatory role in the process of slow diastolic depolarization.

The major currents involved in the later phase of pacemaker depolarization appear to be the two components of inward Ca current[41,57] that have been found in cardiac tissues.[58–60] Present evidence indicates that there are at least two types of Ca channel: an early, transient channel that responds to weak depolarizations with a rapidly inactivating Ca current ($i_{Ca,T}$), and another channel mediating a more slowly inactivating current ($i_{Ca,L}$) activated by stronger depolarizations (see Hess[61]). Slow depolarization is initiated by a decrease in K conductance in the presence of inward $i_{Na,b}$, pump, and exchanger currents. Inward $i_{Ca,T}$ is activated by this sequence and it contributes to further diastolic depolarization, bringing the membrane potential to the threshold for $i_{Ca,L}$. The long-lasting $i_{Ca,L}$ current then results in the upstroke of the action potential and the plateau phase. Slow activation of the delayed-rectifier current i_K[51,62–64] during the action potential leads to repolarization by eventually overtaking the inactivating $i_{Ca,L}$. The MDP is then reached and the process of diastolic depolarization begins again (for details, see Irisawa et al[41]).

Pacemaker Activity in the Atrioventricular Node

Normally, the AV node serves as a conducting pathway that transmits the wave of activation from the atria to the specialized ventricular conduction system and then on to the ventricles. Cells located within the AV node, however, generate spontaneous pacemaker activity when either the structure[65–67] or individual cells[63] are isolated. Normally, any such pacemaker activity would be masked by the process of overdrive suppression[42] and only SA pacemaker activity would be manifest. Indeed, if normal SA activity is stopped or blocked, it is possible for a pacemaker in the AV nodal region to take over control of heart rate at a considerably slower frequency.[67] Whatever the role of these pacemakers in the normal heart, they do become manifest on isolation and have ionic mechanisms similar to those for the SA node.[63,68] There may be quantitative differences in the contributions of various currents to this activity, but the overall scheme is thought to be roughly the same.[39]

Atrioventricular Valve Pacemakers

Recent studies have demonstrated the presence of subsidiary pacemaker cells in the leaflets of the atrioventricular valves (AVV).[69–72] It is unclear as yet whether these cells derive from the atria or from the AV node,[73] but when isolated they exhibit stable pacemaker activity at a frequency slower than that of the normal SA node. It would be expected that this activity would be overdrive-suppressed under normal conditions, but it might become manifest under conditions where SA pacemaker activity was absent or blocked. In contrast to SA and AV nodal cells, these cells have more negative resting potentials (≈ -80 mV) and considerably faster upstroke velocities.[71,72,74] The sequence of events and the specific currents involved in slow diastolic depolarization in these cells are similar to those for the two nodal tissues.[75] The more negative resting potential, however, probably accounts for a larger contribution of i_f to the initial depolarization phase.[75] In addition, the $i_{Ca,T}$ current probably activates in the late phase of diastolic depolarization but at a more negative voltage than in the SA nodal cell, and helps to contribute to the more rapid upstroke (Fig. 1B).

Purkinje Fibers

Purkinje fibers form part of the specialized conduction system in the ventricle and, as such, contribute to the coordinated activation of ventricular muscle. Isolated Purkinje fibers exhibit diastolic depolarization that is greatly enhanced by the lowering of extracellular K concentration.[66,76] Whereas this relatively low frequency automaticity is most likely overdrive-suppressed under conditions of normal SA rhythm, it may become manifest when activity from above is absent or blocked. It is also possible that, as with AVV pacemakers, these pacemakers may become manifest under abnormal conditions and give rise to ectopic pacemaker sites.[77–79] The MDPs of these cells are among the most negative of any in the heart (−90 to −100 mV) and the upstroke velocities, which depend on the rapid inward i_{Na}, are among the fastest.[11] The mechanism of pacemaker activity in these cells is similar to that for AVV pacemaker cells. It appears to depend, however, to a much greater extent on the activation of i_f,[80,81] with $i_{Ca,T}$ and $i_{Ca,L}$ only becoming evident at the very end of diastole and during the action potential upstroke.[82,83] Indeed, i_f was first recognized because of its contribution to automaticity in Purkinje fiber cells.[47]

Triggered Activity

Pacemaker activity can be observed under normal conditions for any of the pacemaker tissues listed above, but it is also possible to observe spontaneous activity in cardiac muscle tissue under extreme conditions. In addition, there are other mechanisms whereby single or repetitive impulses can be generated in sites not normally associated with pacemaker activity. One form of abnormal impulse generation is known as triggered activity.[84] The name derives from the fact that this form of automaticity requires an action potential to "trigger" it. The activity results from afterdepolarizations that reach threshold and fire. There are two types of such afterdepolarizations, early[84–86] and delayed.[87–90] They have different ionic mechanisms and respond differently to changes in the basic driving frequency.[91] These impulses can occur as single coupled events or as bursts of repetitive activity, and they have been implicated in various clinical arrhythmias.[92,93]

Depolarization-Induced Automaticity

A final means for inducing automaticity in cardiac tissues is depolarization. In experimental preparations of cardiac muscle and Purkinje fibers, the application of constant depolarizing current gives rise to the development of spontaneous automaticity.[94,95] The fact that automaticity can be induced in this way has led to speculation that the injury currents flowing between normal and ischemic myocardium may give rise to depolarization-induced activity resulting in cardiac arrhythmias.[95,96]

Pacemaker Interactions

As evidenced in the preceding sections, considerable information exists regarding the mechanisms of pacemaker activity within single cells. The heart, however, consists of myriad cells grouped into various types. The way in which these cells interact with one another and with their environment has a major impact on the normal functioning of the heart as an organ. In fact, the cells and the tissues they comprise must react with events in their surroundings to maintain normal cardiac function. This is as true in an electrical sense as it is in the biochemical or mechanical sense.

All cardiac cells are electrically coupled via low-resistance pathways identified as the gap junctions.[35,97–101] These junctions allow for the passage of ions and small molecules, and this action permits the flow of ionic current between cells.[102,103] Thus, electrical activity occurring in one cell influences electrical events in its neighbors. In addition, external stimuli such as vagal[104,105] and sympathetic[106,107] impulses alter the electrical characteristics of the cells and thus alter their behavior.

In the following sections, the dynamic control of SA pacemaker activity by external periodicities is discussed. Particular attention is given to the phase-resetting behavior of cardiac pacemakers as the basis for the development of synchrony in the SA node and for the phasic, reflexly-mediated control of heart rate by the parasympathetic nervous system.

Interactions with External Current Sources

One of the agents that can alter pacemaker activity is external current. While at first glance this factor might seem a very nonphysiological mechanism for the control of pacemaker activity, it has already been noted that constant current can flow between cell populations when one group is tonically depolarized with reference to another.[95] This injury current provides a relatively constant external current source. In addition, the gap junctions connecting cardiac cells provide for the flow of phasic electrotonic currents when the cells are at different potentials as happens when one cell is firing an action potential.[99] The influence of these external currents depends on their duration, intensity and timing, and on the degree of coupling between cells.

CONSTANT CURRENT

Application of constant current to the normal cardiac pacemakers results primarily in a change in their rate of firing.[62,108] Furthermore, as noted above, constant current can even induce pacemaker activity in cells that do not normally exhibit such activity.[96] The mechanism for the influence of constant current on pacemaker activity is quite straightforward. It simply alters the balance of inward and outward currents that controls spontaneous automaticity. Thus, constant depolarizing current increases the frequency of pacemaker cells by further shifting the current balance in a depolarizing direction. The cells depolarize faster, reach threshold faster, and ultimately have a faster frequency. Conversely, hyperpolarizing current retards diastolic depolarization, lengthens the time required to reach threshold, and decreases pacemaker frequency. While the application of constant current would not appear to be a normal physiological mechanism for pacemaker control, it does come into play when some regions are abnormally depolarized (e.g., by ischemia). Furthermore, pacemaker regions such as the SA node are coupled to excitable, nonpacemaker cells such as the atrium. Thus, even under normal conditions, one would expect hyperpolarizing influence from the muscle cells with a more negative resting potential.[34,109] This electrotonic influence of muscle would be expected to lower pacemaker frequency with respect to the frequency that the cells would have in isolation.

PHASE-RESETTING BEHAVIOR OF CARDIAC CELLS

The study of periodically-forced pacemakers dates back to Van der Pol and Van der Mark's relaxation oscillator model of the heart.[110] This model has been a cornerstone in the mathematical analysis of biological oscillators. The concepts of phase resetting and mutual synchrony in excitable pacemaker tissues, however, saw their origin in the elegant but much ignored studies of Fessard.[111,112] Fessard gave a detailed and accurate account of the complex dynamics leading to coordination in the spontaneous discharges of electrically-coupled nerve fibers. According to Fessard's scheme, nerve cells are not only capable of spontaneous discharges, but they are sensitive to the discharges generated by their neighbors, and this sensitivity is phase-dependent.

Subsequently, Segers[113] demonstrated the development of synchrony in cardiac tissue by connecting two segments of spontaneously-beating frog heart through a piece of cotton that had been soaked with Ringer's solution. Segers hypothesized that the mechanism of this synchronization was electrical in nature and that, as previously suggested by Fessard, it was the result of phase-dependent interactions between the respective pacemaker discharges. He tested that hypothesis by studying the effects of brief depolarizing current pulses, applied repetitively, on the activity of a spontaneously beating heart segment. His results clearly showed that when the periodicity of the pulses was slightly slower than that of the heart segment, there was a slowing of the automatic rhythm, which locked in with the rhythm of the pulses. This, he suggested, was brought about by the fact that each pulse somehow produced a postcathodic depression that delayed the onset of the subsequent beat. These changes occurred repetitively because the pulses always fell slightly later than the discharge of the cardiac tissue segment, and thus during its refractory phase. If the same pulses were applied at a slightly faster rhythm than that of the spontaneously beating segment, however, the discharges of the latter were forced to accelerate and its rhythm was entrained in a 1:1 manner by the repetitive stimuli. In this case, the pulses always fell slightly earlier than the cardiac segment's discharge; that is, outside its refractory phase. From all these experiments, Segers[113] concluded that, in fact, synchronization of two pacemakers is the result of a reciprocal and constant control over each other's frequency.

In 1950, Weidmann[114] used microelectrode recording and current application techniques to confirm Fessard's postcathodic depression hypothesis in isolated Purkinje fiber pacemakers. He demonstrated that depolarizing current pulses of relatively brief duration and subthreshold magnitude, applied early in diastole, can slow diastolic depolarization and thus delay the approach to threshold for a subsequent discharge. Hyperpolarizing pulses had the opposite effect.[114]

In 1964, Perkel et al[115] conducted a systematic study of phase resetting and entrainment of neuronal pacemaker cells by excitatory or inhibitory input. These authors devised a mathematical model to determine the response patterns of oscillatory neurons to repetitive synaptic input in the abdominal ganglion of *Aplysia* and the stretch receptor of *Procambarus*. The early predictions of Fessard's[111,112] were borne out by the demonstration in these experiments that the basic condition for entrainment in neurons is the functional dependence of the phase shift on the timing of the input.

More recently, electrically-mediated synchronization of cardiac Purkinje fibers was confirmed by the intracellular microelectrode studies of Jalife and Moe.[77,79] These authors demonstrated that phase resetting and entrainment of a parasystolic pacemaker by the ventricular responses to SA impulses could explain a wide variety of cardiac rhythm disturbances. In 1978, Sano et al[17] showed that phase resetting was also a property of SA pacemaker tissue. Subsequently, Jalife et al[108] presented a detailed experimental study of the phase-resetting behavior of isolated SA nodal pacemaker tissue in response to current pulses scanning the pacemaker cycle. Common to the mechanisms of entrainment of all biological oscillator systems studied thus far in this manner is the fact that the sensitivity of the oscillator's period to the entraining stimulus is a function of the timing of the stimulus.[18]

PHASE-DEPENDENT EFFECTS OF SINGLE PULSES

The overall organizing principle of the heart is that all cells are connected together through gap junctions.[100] This principle implies not only that action potentials can propagate from one cell to another, but also that an action potential in one cell can be transmitted as a subthreshold electrotonic event to another. Previous studies[77] indicated that, in addition to pulse duration and intensity, one of the major features determining the influence of a brief pulse occurring during an oscillatory cycle was its time of occurrence or phase within the cycle. To study the importance of this principle for cardiac function, a variety of experimental[29,30,108,116,117] and theoretical[22,118,119] studies have been performed to investigate the influence of brief current pulses on cardiac pacemaker activity.

As seen in Figure 2,[120] the application of a brief depolarizing current pulse at an early phase in the cycle of a pacemaker leads to a delay in the next spontaneous firing (Fig. 2A). The same pulse, applied at a later time in the cycle (Fig. 2B), accelerates the next spontaneous discharge. The amount of delay or acceleration produced depends on the phase of the stimulus. By scanning the entire cycle with pulses of constant intensity and duration, and observing the change in pacemaker cycle length, it is possible to generate a phase-response curve (PRC) (Fig. 2C), which summarizes the phase-dependent effect (expressed as a phase shift, $\Delta\phi$) of the pulses on cycle length as a function of the stimulus timing (expressed as phase, ϕ). For depolarizing current pulses, early pulses delay the next discharge and later ones accelerate it. As is seen below, this PRC can then be used to predict the limits of entrainment if such pulses are applied repetitively. Phase-dependent effects of brief current pulses

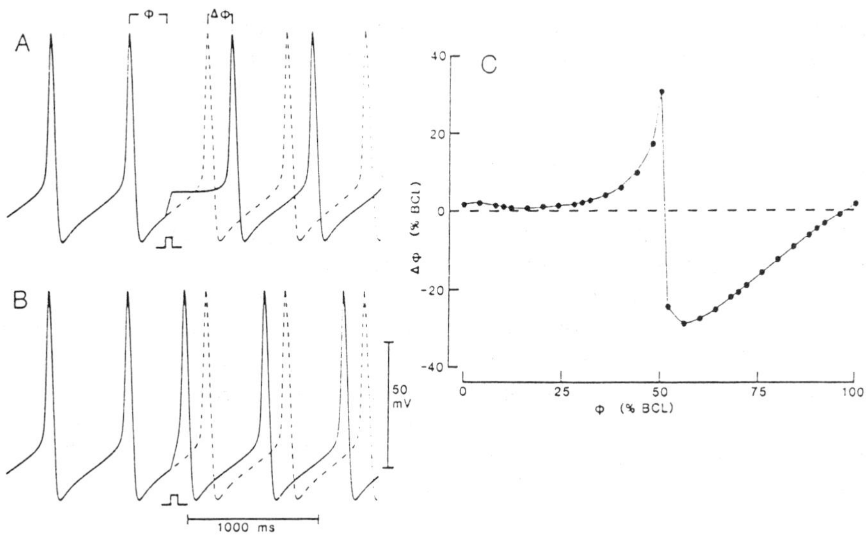

Figure 2. *Phase dependence of the effects of brief depolarizing current pulses on pacemaker activity of a SA cell. Pacemaker is simulated using the model of Yanagihara et al.*[62] *Spontaneous cycle length is adjusted to 610 ms by the application of constant hyperpolarizing current (0.4 μA/cm²). A: A 50-ms current pulse (−0.2 μA/cm²) applied at a phase (ϕ) = 50% of the intrinsic cycle length delays the next spontaneous discharge (phase shift, Δϕ = 34%). Dotted lines indicate pacemaker activity without the presence of perturbation. B: A similar pulse applied at ϕ = 52% shortens the spontaneous cycle (Δϕ = −28%). C: A PRC showing the phase shift as a function of phase for the entire spontaneous cycle, where both are expressed as a percentage of the intrinsic cycle length. Modified with permission from Jalife J, Michaels D: Phase-dependent interactions of cardiac pacemakers as mechanisms of control and synchronization in the heart. In DP Zipes, J Jalife (eds): Cardiac Electrophysiology and Arrhythmias. Orlando, FL, Grune & Stratton Inc, 1985, pp. 109–119.*

have been identified in modelling studies,[22,118,119] in strips of isolated SA node,[20,21,108] in embryonic heart cell aggregates,[29,117] and most recently in enzymatically-dissociated single cells of the SA node.[30] It has been demonstrated that similar effects can be produced by the electrotonic currents flowing between active and quiescent pacemaker cells or as a result of phasic vagal discharges (see below), so phase-dependent effects of single current pulses do have physiological relevance.

Before considering the issue of repetitively applied pulses, there is one more issue of single current pulses that should be presented. Theoretical studies[18] concerning the dynamics of oscillatory systems that can be perturbed in a phase-dependent fashion suggest that, under the right conditions, it should be possible to stop or annihilate pacemaker activity with a single pulse of the proper amplitude, polarity, and timing. Experimental studies in isolated strips of SA node[116] have demonstrated that it is possible to annihilate pacemaker activity with a single current pulse, and these studies have been confirmed in a modelling study[121] and in isolated SA nodal myocytes.[30] The constraints on the system required to demonstrate this phenomenon in the in situ heart make it highly unlikely under normal circumstances. In terms of continued survival of the organism, it is perhaps not surprising that it is difficult to annihilate pacemaker activity.

PHASE-DEPENDENT EFFECTS OF MULTIPLE PULSES

When brief current pulses are applied repetitively, it is possible to entrain a pacemaker to beat at a frequency related to the frequency of perturbation.[22,108,120] As illustrated in Figure 3, this entrainment phenomenon derives directly from the phase dependence of the effect of single pulses. Given a pacemaker with an intrinsic, free-running period (T_{fr}) and a PRC that describes the changes in period as a function of the phase of the stimulus (both expressed as a percentage of T_{fr}), it is possible to predict the behavior of the pacemaker in response to repetitive perturbation. As shown in the middle panel of Figure 3, if the stimulus is applied repetitively such that it always occurs at an early

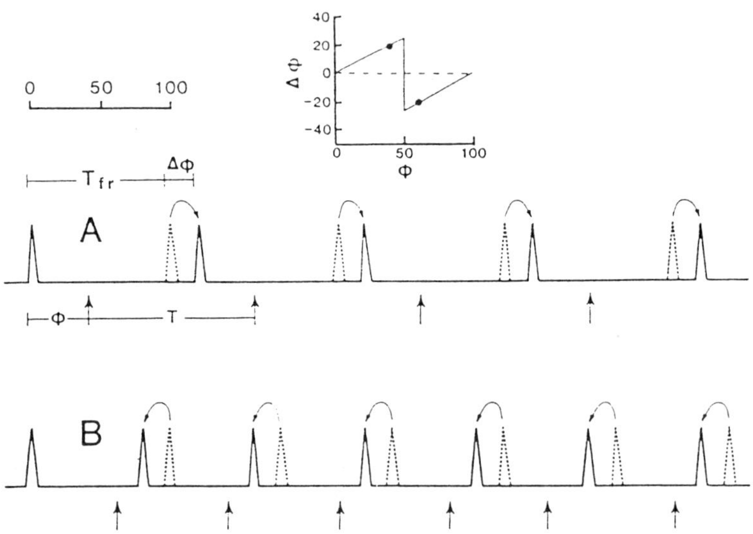

Figure 3. *Entrainment of a single pacemaker with repetitively applied pulses. A pacemaker, whose intrinsic period is T_{FR} and whose PRC is shown at the top of the figure, is subjected to repetitive external stimuli. A: The first stimulus occurs early in the cycle and delays the next spontaneous firing. If subsequent pulses are applied so that they all fall at the same phase of the cycle, the pacemaker is entrained to fire at the frequency of the applied pulses, and its new frequency is slower than its intrinsic frequency. B: Entrainment to a frequency faster than the intrinsic frequency. In this case, the first stimulus occurs late in the spontaneous cycle and advances the next firing. Since subsequent stimuli occur at the same phase of the cycle, entrainment to the external perturbation is again achieved. Modified with permission from Jalife J, Michaels D: Phase-dependent interactions of cardiac pacemakers as mechanisms of control and synchronization in the heart. In DP Zipes, J Jalife (eds): Cardiac Electrophysiology and Arrhythmias. Orlando, FL, Grune & Stratton Inc, 1985, pp. 109–119.*

phase in the cycle, the overall effect is to entrain the pacemaker to fire at a slower frequency (longer period) than it would intrinsically. Conversely, the bottom panel of Figure 3 shows that if the pulses are delivered at a frequency such that they always occur late in the pacemaker cycle, each pulse accelerates the next spontaneous discharge and the overall effect is to entrain the pacemaker to a faster frequency. The limits of this 1:1 (stimulus:response) entrainment behavior are established by the limits (amplitude) of the PRC.[23]

PHASE-RESETTING BEHAVIOR OF SINGLE SINUS NODAL CELLS

The theoretical predictions summarized above have been borne out by recent experimental studies in isolated SA nodal tissue preparations,[20,21,23,77] in pacemaker cell aggregates,[29,117] and in single SA nodal cells.[30] The studies have demonstrated that repetitive application of brief depolarizing current pulses results in 1:1 entrainment, or in simple harmonically-related ratios such as 2:1, 3:2, and 5:4. For example, in the case of the single cell experiments,[30] it has been possible to predict quantitatively the range of entrainment possible with a particular stimulus by constructing the PRC for that stimulus. The derived PRC (see Anumonwo et al[30]) presented in panel A of Figure 4 is obtained by measuring the effects of repetitive depolarizing pulses (duration, 20 milliseconds; strength, 0.17 nA) applied at various stimulus periods to an isolated SA node pacemaker cell whose intrinsic period is relatively constant (within 5%) at about 280 milliseconds. As shown in panel B of Figure 4, this action results in variable phasic relations and entrainment patterns that change in a stepwise manner as the stimulus cycle length is gradually reduced. Thus, the predictions about entrainment from the phase-resetting data are completely confirmed in the single SA node cell.

The phase-resetting behavior of the single SA nodal cell has been analyzed also on the basis of topological theory of one-dimensional limit cycle oscillators.[18,28,119] A common way of analyzing data in this manner is by constructing a "phase-transition curve" (PTC) that plots the new phase (ϕ') after a stimulus as a function of the old phase (ϕ) of the stimulus. In Figure 5, for each data point, the PTC ($\phi'[\phi]$) was calculated using the equation $\phi' = \phi - \Delta\phi$. By iterating the PTC, one may reproduce the entrainment behavior obtained experimentally (see Fig. 4) and make predictions about complex response patterns of the SA nodal pacemaker to the repetitive stimulus. It is important to note that, in the plot of Figure 5, the new phase is a monotonically increasing function of the old phase, which is usually the case for PTCs obtained when stimuli of low amplitude are used.[18] This type of response is known as "type-1" phase resetting, and is usually associated with predictable phase-locking patterns, including Wenckebach periodicity, and the sequences of appearance of these patterns are entirely predicted by the so-called "Farey rule."[28]

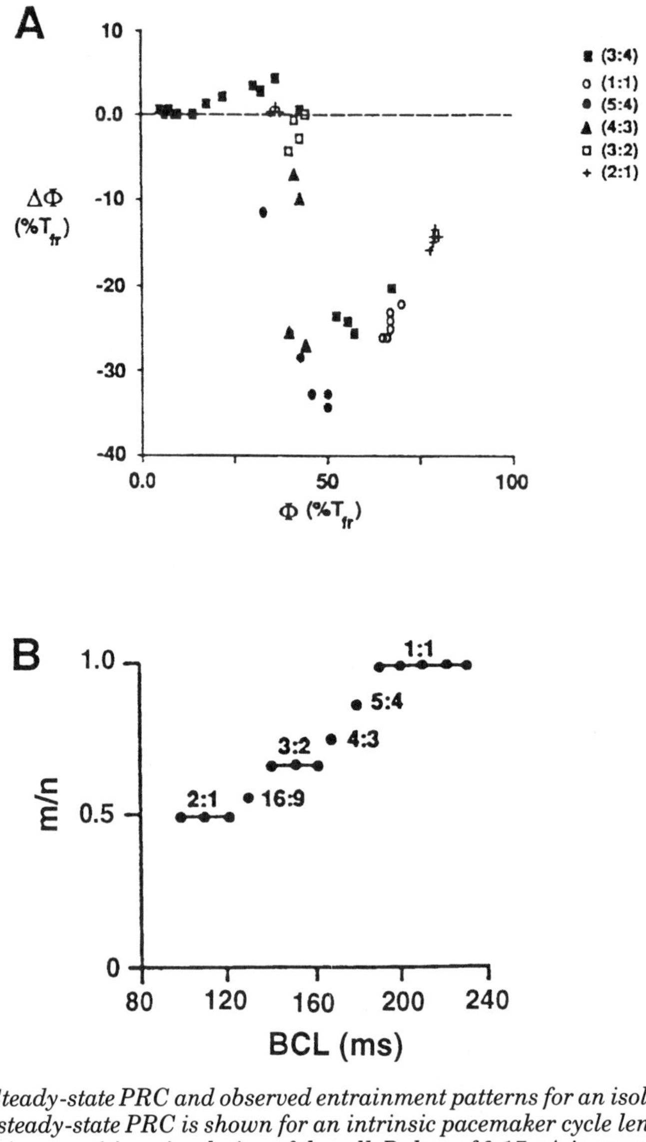

Figure 4. *Steady-state PRC and observed entrainment patterns for an isolated SA nodal cell. A: The steady-state PRC is shown for an intrinsic pacemaker cycle length of 280 ms, obtained during repetitive stimulation of the cell. Pulses of 0.17 nA in strength and 20 ms in duration are used. Phase (ϕ) and phase shift ($\Delta\phi$) are both expressed as percentages of the pacemaker free-running cycle (T_{FR}). Symbols represent the different entrainment patterns obtained during repetitive stimulation. B: The reciprocal of the stimulus:pacemaker discharge pattern, i.e., the entrainment (or activation) ratio (m/n) is plotted against the basic cycle length (BCL). Modified by permission of the American Heart Association, Inc. from Anumonwo JMB, Delmar M, Vinet A, et al: Phase-resetting and entrainment of pacemaker activity in single sinus nodal cells. Circ Res 68:1138–1153, 1991.*

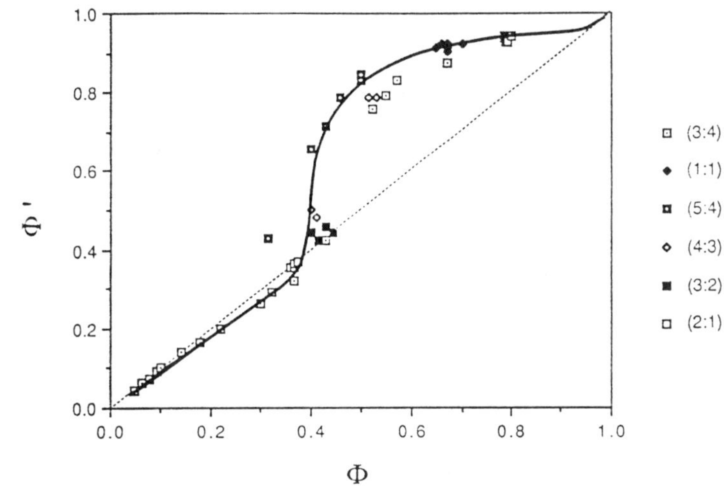

Figure 5. *The PTC from entrainment data of experiments shown in Figure 4. Data are taken from an isolated SA nodal cell during repetitive stimulation. This figure is a plot of new phase (ϕ') versus old phase (ϕ) of data obtained from the experiments shown in Figure 4. Symbols represent the different entrainment patterns. The curve was fitted by eye. Reproduced by permission of the American Heart Association, Inc. from Anumonwo JMB, Delmar M, Vinet A, et al: Phase-resetting and entrainment of pacemaker activity in single sinus nodal cells. Circ Res 68:1138, 1991.*

Pacemaker-to-Pacemaker Interactions and Mutual Entrainment

Due to the fact that pacemakers react in a phase-dependent fashion to external current pulses and that cardiac cells are coupled together through gap junctions that allow for current flow between cells, it is possible for activity in one cell to continuously interact with that of its neighbors. This interaction forms the basis for the synchronization of pacemaker activity within the SA node.[20,22]

As discussed in a previous section, a theory of synchronization involving electrical coupling, phase-related interactions, and mutual entrainment of neighboring cardiac pacemaker centers was formulated and supported by experiments done more than 40 years ago. In fact, even though Fessard's[112] theory of synchronization and Segers'[113] discoveries in the frog heart had been almost forgotten by nerve and cardiac physiologists, the concepts of mutual entrainment and phase-resetting behavior have found widespread application in a variety of biological oscillatory systems. For example, since the early 1960s, it has been known that circadian oscillators are entrained by the daily periodism of the earth.[122] In some cases, pairs of circadian oscillators interact through phase resetting and maintain mutual entrainment.[18] The phenomenon is also found in large groups of yeast cells that interact metabolically and synchronize their glycolytic cycles.[18] The males of certain species of fireflies in Malaysia and New Guinea congregate in large numbers and synchronize their flashing[123] through reciprocal light-flash-induced phase resetting of each individual's period.

Ypey et al[124] used spherical aggregates of embryonic chick heart cells to study synchronization and demonstrated that, when two aggregates of different spontaneous frequencies were manipulated into close apposition, their activities synchronized to a common frequency. This frequency was different from the intrinsic rate of either pacemaker before apposition, and has been attributed to electrotonically-mediated mutual entrainment, secondary to the formation of gap junction channels between aggregates.[125,126]

The bidirectional nature of the connection between cells allows for a process of mutual entrainment based on the mutual phase-dependent interaction of one pacemaker with another.[120] The mechanism of this process is illustrated in Figure 6. Two pacemakers, one fast (F) and one slow (S), are allowed to interact through a common coupling resistance. For this example, it is assumed that both pacemakers had the same PRC, although in reality that need not be the case as long as the PRC for each pacemaker is known. If both pacemakers fire initially at the same time, F will fire next before S. F will thus fire late in the cycle of S and advance its next discharge. S will now fire early in the cycle of F and delay its next discharge. This reciprocal interaction between the two pacemakers will continue with F advancing the discharges of

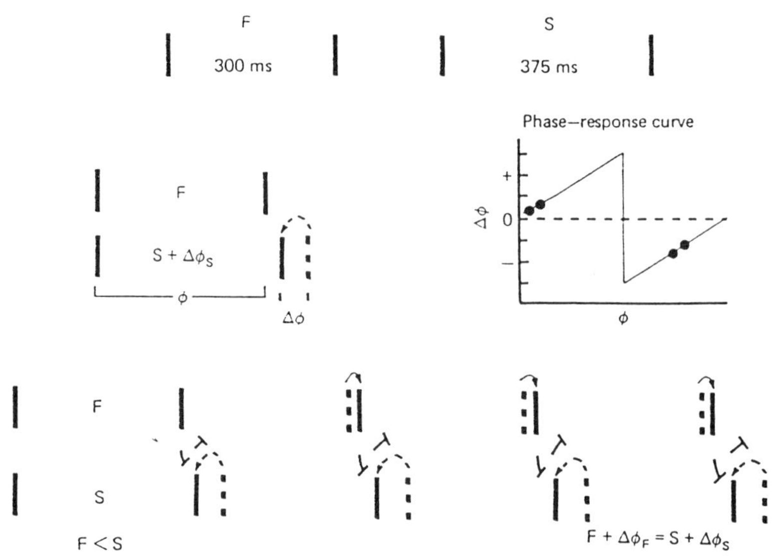

Figure 6. *Mutual entrainment of coupled pacemakers. Two pacemakers, one fast (F) and one slow (S), both having the same PRC, are permitted to interact. If the first firings of both pacemakers occur simultaneously, the next firing of F occurs late in the cycle of S and advances its next discharge. This discharge of S now occurs early in the cycle of F and delays its next discharge. This reciprocal interaction stabilizes and the two pacemakers fire at a common frequency intermediate to the intrinsic frequencies of the two pacemakers. Modified with permission from Jalife J, Michaels D: Phase-dependent interactions of cardiac pacemakers as mechanisms of control and synchronization in the heart. In DP Zipes, J Jalife (eds): Cardiac Electrophysiology and Arrhythmias. Orlando, FL, Grune & Stratton Inc, 1985, pp. 109–119.*

S and S delaying the discharges of F. After a brief interval of stabilization, the two pacemakers will fire at the same common frequency that is somewhere intermediate between their intrinsic frequencies. While they fire at the same common frequency, they cannot fire at the same time. If they did, the phase difference necessary to drive the phase advance and phase delay would be lost.

Mutual entrainment of two pacemaker centers was demonstrated experimentally in strips of SA node placed in a three-chambered bath[20,21] and in pairs of embryonic cardiac cell aggregates.[124,126] In the case of the three-chambered bath experiments,[20] the spontaneously-beating segments of the tissue strip located in the two outer chambers were superfused with normal Tyrode's solution, while the tissue in the central chamber was superfused with sucrose solution containing small amounts of Ca. The sucrose gap separated the tissue in the two outer chambers and prevented the electrical interaction of their pacemaker activity. By connecting an external shunt resistance between the two outer chambers, it was possible to vary the degree of electrical coupling between the two pacemaker centers.

Figure 7 shows the results of such an experiment. In panel A, all three chambers are perfused with Tyrode's solution and there is good electrical coupling between the fast (F) and slow (S) pacemaker centers in the two outer

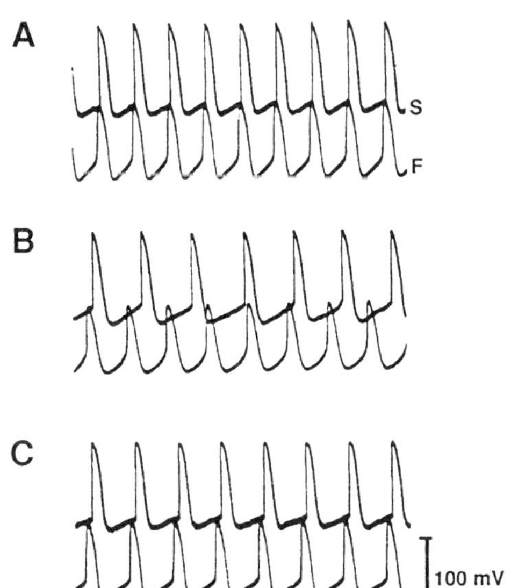

Figure 7. *Sucrose gap experiment demonstrating the effect of electrical coupling on mutual entrainment between two pacemaker sites in an isolated SA nodal strip. Two sites, one fast (F) and the other slow (S), are coupled through a shunt variable resistor. A: Potential recording is carried out while Tyrode's solution is being superfused in all segments. Synchronous discharges of F and S are manifest. B: After 30-min superfusion of the central segment with sucrose (with shunt resistance set at infinity), a loss of synchrony is evident. C: Recorded a few seconds later, the shunt resistance is set at 0 Ω, demonstrating the electrical nature of the synchronization mechanism. Reproduced with permission from Jalife J: Mutual entrainment and electrical coupling as mechanisms for synchronous firing of rabbit sino-atrial pace-maker cells. J Physiol (Lond) 356:221, 1984.*

chambers. Under these conditions, the pacemakers are mutually entrained to a common frequency. Panel B shows the situation 30 minutes after beginning sucrose superfusion of the middle chamber. At this point, it is evident that electrical connection between the two outer chambers has been lost and the two centers fire at their intrinsic frequencies. By adjusting an external shunt resistor to improve electrical coupling between the two outer chambers (panel C), it is possible to re-establish the mutual entrainment of the two pacemaker centers.

Similar results were obtained by using the Yanagihara model[62] to reconstruct the pacemaker action potential from the specific time-and voltage-dependent ionic currents, as illustrated in Figure 8.[22] The frequency of one pacemaker is slowed by applying a constant hyperpolarizing bias current. As seen in panel A, when the resistance between cells is set to a very high value, there is no coupling and, thus, no interaction between the two cells. Both cells fire at their different intrinsic frequencies. As the coupling resistance between cells is lowered (i.e., as coupling between cells is improved; see panels B and C), complex patterns of interaction develop. The patterns depend on the mutual phase-dependent responses of the cells to activation of their neighbors. Finally, when the coupling resistance is lowered to a relatively small value (panel D), the cells mutually entrain to a common frequency intermediate between their intrinsic frequencies.

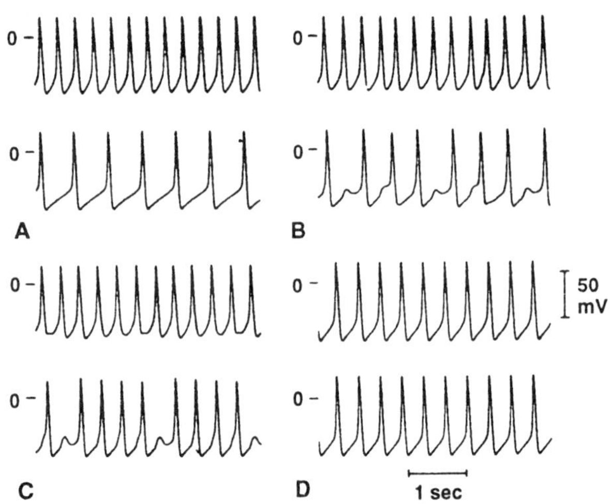

Figure 8. *Mutual entrainment in a model of electrically-coupled pacemakers. Pacemakers are simulated using the model of Yanagihara et al.*[62] *In all panels, constant bias hyperpolarizing current (0.4 μA/cm²) is added to the cell shown in the bottom trace to slow its firing rate. A: The results when there is an extremely large (1 × 10⁶ kΩ) coupling resistance between cells; i.e., they are firing at their intrinsic frequencies. B: Coupling resistance is reduced to 100 kΩ and the cells mutually entrain to a complex 5:3 pattern. C: Further reduction of coupling resistance to 200 kΩ results in an alteration of the pattern of mutual entrainment to 5:4. D: When coupling resistance is reduced to 10 kΩ, cells mutually entrain to a common frequency intermediate between the two intrinsic frequencies. Modified by permission of the American Heart Association, Inc. from Michaels DC, Matyas EP, Jalife J: Dynamic interactions and mutual synchronization of sinoatrial node pacemaker cells. Circ Res 58:706–720, 1986.*

Synchronization of Multiple Pacemakers

The concept of mutual entrainment between two pacemakers can be extended to multiple pacemakers in an attempt to describe their synchronization.[24] Pacemaker cells in the region of the SA pacemaker fire at different intrinsic frequencies when they are enzymatically dissociated.[30,45] How is it that they coordinate their activity to give rise to only one synchronized impulse each cardiac cycle? The traditional view of pacemaker synchronization had been that a master dominant pacemaker cell fires first and all other cells simply follow suit. The concept of phase-dependent interaction just described, however, suggested the hypothesis that pacemaker synchronization could occur through a process of mutual entrainment involving multiple pacemakers.[24] To test this hypothesis, a mathematical model was developed in which a large array of pacemakers with different intrinsic frequencies was coupled through a common coupling resistance. Figure 9 shows the patterns of activity in such an array under conditions where there is either no coupling or good coupling between the cells. With no coupling, cells fire at their preset intrinsic frequencies. When coupling is adjusted to provide reasonable interaction between cells, however, the array develops a "dominant" pacemaker region

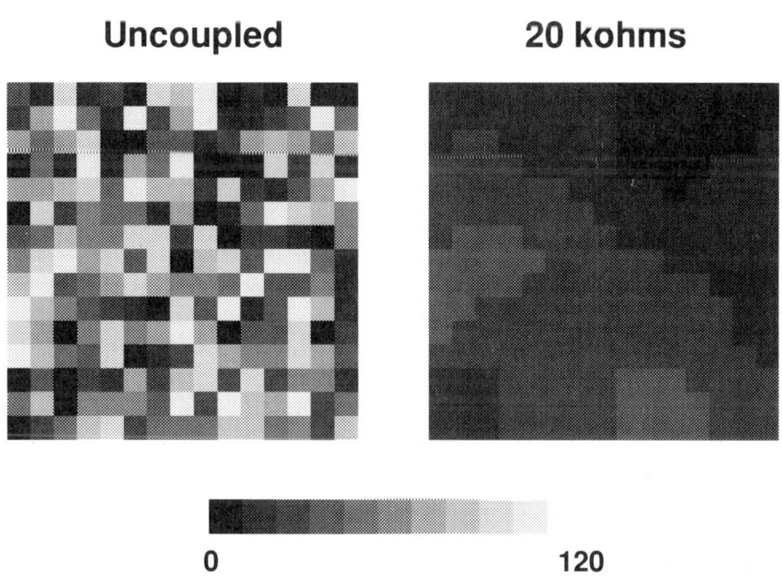

Figure 9. *Mutual entrainment in a randomly distributed array of 225 pacemakers with different intrinsic frequencies. Each cell is randomly assigned 1 of 10 possible intrinsic cycle lengths (ranging from 290 to 390 msec), adjusted by the application of constant bias current. In the absence of electrical coupling (left panel), the activation pattern is indeed random. When coupling resistance between cells is set to 20 kΩ (right panel), pacemakers mutually entrain to a common cycle length of 322 msec. By beat 8, a dominant pacemaker center emerges in the upper right-hand corner. Modified by permission of the American Heart Association, Inc. from Michaels DC, Matyas EP, Jalife J: Mechanisms of sinoatrial pacemaker synchronization: A new hypothesis. Circ Res 61:704–714, 1987.*

with apparent spread of activity in an organized fashion to other cells of the array. This pattern develops in spite of the fact that all cells of the array are pacemaker cells, and it indicates that phase-dependent mutual entrainment can be a mechanism for the synchronization of multiple pacemakers.

Control of Heart Rate by the Autonomic Nervous System

Although it is well established that automaticity in the heart is intrinsic to the various pacemaker tissues, heart rate and rhythm are indeed very much under the control of the autonomic nervous system.[104–106,127] Normally, the parasympathetic (cholinergic) influence is to slow heart rate and conduction and to decrease the force of contraction.[104,128] The sympathetic (adrenergic) nervous system has opposite effects.[107] Both systems exert a tonic influence on the SA pacemaker and the final control of cardiac activity results from the balance between them.[106]

Parasympathetic Effects

Parasympathetic influence on the heart rate is mediated via the vagus nerves. Stimulation of these nerve fibers releases acetylcholine (ACh) in the vicinity of the nerve endings. Muscarinic acetylcholine receptors (mAChRs) on the various cardiac cell types respond to this release most commonly by an increase in cell membrane conductance to K[129,130] through activation of a specific class of cardiac K channels, known as K_{ACh}.[131] In addition, ACh may also decrease i_{Ca} through inhibition of adenosine 3′5′-cyclic phosphate (cyclic AMP) synthesis,[104,132] and it has been suggested that, in the SA node myocyte, ACh inhibits i_f.[53] This latter effect may mediate the negative chronotropic effect of ACh.[40,53] The action of ACh at the cardiac cell membrane is terminated by the acetylcholinesterase-mediated hydrolysis of ACh.[104] Although there is a tonic level of cholinergic activity, various cardiac reflexes, such as the baroreceptor reflex, involve the transient release of ACh in brief bursts.[133,134] Experimental evidence[135–137] indicates that the response to such brief bursts of ACh is phase-dependent, and this finding suggests that repetitive vagal stimuli can entrain the cardiac pacemaker in much the same fashion as brief current pulses.

Figure 10 illustrates the phase dependence of the effects of brief vagal pulses in a strip of SA node.[136] ACh release is produced by field stimulation of nerve endings within the preparation. As seen in Figure 10, there is a progressive increase in the phase-delaying effect of an ACh pulse as it is applied later and later in the spontaneous cycle. The loss of effect toward the end of the cycle is a consequence of the latency between nerve stimulation and hyperpolarization of the pacemaker membrane.[136,137] When the cycle length of the pacemaker is long relative to the duration of the ACh effect, however, it is possible to see pacemaker acceleration with pulses applied early in the cycle.[137–139]

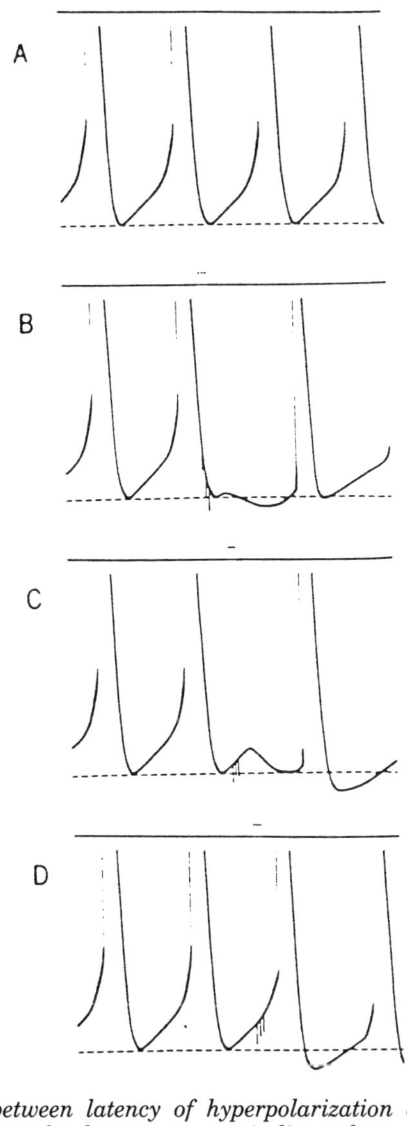

Figure 10. *Relation between latency of hyperpolarization and latent period of the inhibitory effect. In all panels, the upper traces indicate the moment of application of the vagal stimulus. The lower traces are bottom parts of the transmembrane potentials of an SA nodal cell recorded at a high gain. A is the control. In B, C, and D, the vagal trains are applied 475, 325, and 180 msec, respectively, in advance of the next expected discharge. Calibrations are 10 mV (vertical) and 500 msec (horizontal). Reproduced by permission of the American Heart Association, Inc. from Jalife J, Moe GK: Phasic effects of vagal stimulation on pacemaker activity of the isolated sinus node of the young cat. Circ Res 45:595–607, 1979.*

As discussed in a previous section, phase-resetting behavior implies the ability to entrain the pacemaker period by an external periodicity. Several studies have demonstrated that the occurrence of impulse grouping in efferent cardiac vagal fibers results in part from periodic activation by afferent baroreceptor impulses.[133,140] Thus, it seems likely that entrainment and vagus-SA node phase-locking play a significant role in the dynamic regulation of cardiac pacemaker activity by the autonomic nervous system. Since, under most conditions, the effect of brief vagal bursting is usually to delay the next spontaneous discharge, vagally-mediated entrainment usually results in a frequency slower than the intrinsic frequency of the pacemaker.[31,137,141] Since it is possible to have phasic acceleratory effects of vagal stimulation, especially when applied very early in the cycle,[32,137–139] it is possible to get a paradoxical acceleration of pacemaker activity with repetitive application of what is normally thought to be an inhibitory stimulus. Figure 11 illustrates the results of computer simulations in which the effect of ACh pulses applied at a fixed coupling interval to the preceding spontaneous discharge was studied.[138] This simulation mimics the baroreceptor reflex in which the pulse wave produced by ventricular contraction transiently activates the baroreceptors and leads to a

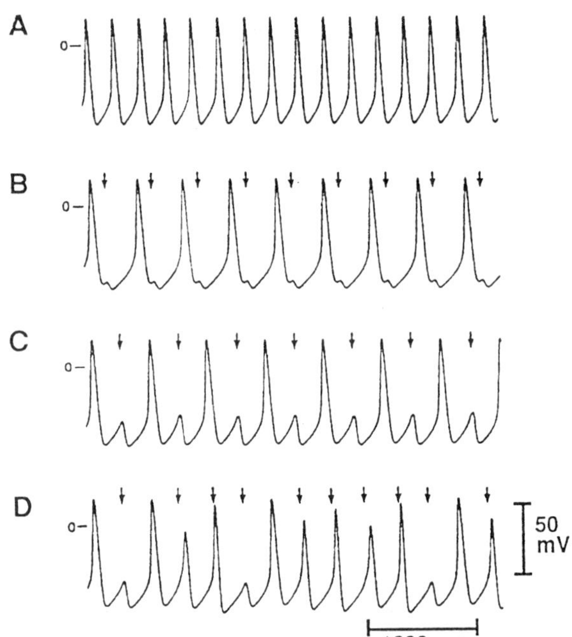

Figure 11. *Simulation demonstrating the effect of vagal pulses (downward arrows) applied at fixed coupling intervals (FCIs) on a simulated pacemaker cell. A: Control pacemaker cycle length is 318 ms. B: ACh pulses (1 × 10^{-6} M; 50-ms duration) are applied at an FCI = 140 ms. C: 260 ms. D: 270 ms. See text for more description. Reproduced by permission of the American Heart Association, Inc. from Michaels DC, Matyas EP, Jalife J: Dynamic interactions and mutual synchronization of sinoatrial node pacemaker cells. Circ Res 58:706–720, 1986.*

brief burst of vagal activity. As shown in Figure 11, as the coupling interval is increased, there is an increase in the delay produced by the ACh pulse (since it arrives at later phases of the spontaneous cycle) and thus the entrainment is to a progressively slower frequency.

When the coupling interval is long enough that some pulses arrive during the latency interval (Fig. 11, panel D), the patterns of entrainment can become quite complex. Indeed, analysis of this complex behavior according to the methods of dynamical systems theory[33] indicates that it is "chaotic" behavior, i.e., behavior that is apparently random, but follows deterministic rules and shows an exquisite sensitivity to initial conditions.

To further analyze the effects of brief ACh pulses in the SA node, simulations were done in a large array of pacemaker cells similar to that described previously.[24] Cells of the array are randomly assigned 1 of 10 possible intrinsic frequencies and are coupled together at a common coupling resistance (Fig. 12, left panel). Once a stable pattern of activity has been achieved, a single ACh pulse is applied to a randomly selected 20% of the cells. This action produces effects (middle panel) similar to those seen with vagal stimulation of the isolated SA node. The next spontaneous discharge is delayed and there is a shift of the "dominant" pacemaker region to another area of the array. In addition, there is a slowing of apparent conduction within the node.

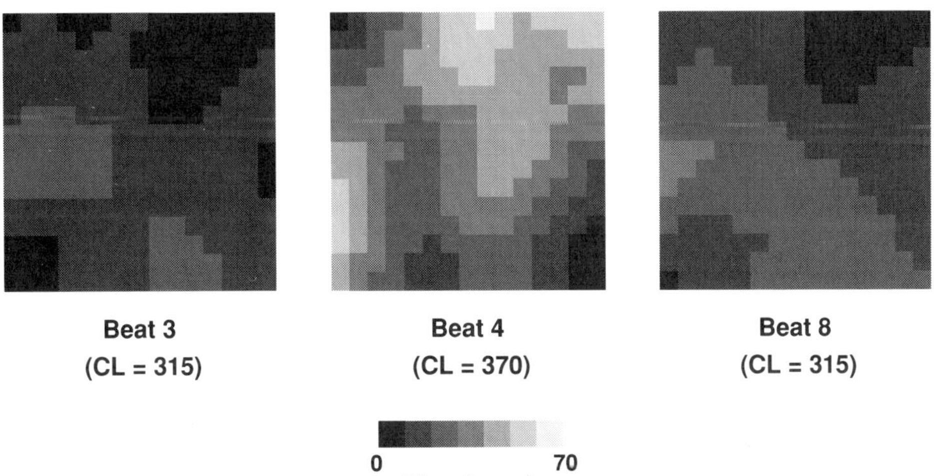

Figure 12. *Pacemaker shift induced in a mutually entrained array by the application of a single ACh pulse. Intrinsic frequencies are distributed as described in the text, and the coupling resistance is set to 20 kΩ. Between beats 3 and 4 (at 750 msec), a single ACh pulse (duration = 100 msec, ACh = 1 × 10^{-6} M) is applied to a randomly selected 20% of the cells. This action produced a shift of the dominant pacemaker region from the upper right to the lower right corner, an increase in the apparent conduction time, and a delay of the next spontaneous discharge of the array. By beat 10, conditions have returned to normal. Modified by permission of the American Heart Association, Inc. from Michaels DC, Matyas EP, Jalife J: Mechanisms of sinoatrial pacemaker synchronization: A new hypothesis. Circ Res 61:704–714, 1987.*

By several beats later (right panel), activity in the array has returned to its control pattern.

In another set of simulations,[33] the influence of repetitively applied ACh pulses in such an array of cells was investigated. ACh (vagal) pulses were applied to a randomly selected 60% of the mutually entrained cells at various vagal cycle lengths. For most of the range of cycle lengths of vagal stimulation, the stimulus:response patterns followed patterns typical of the Farey sequence. Thus, the stimulus:response ratios were simple (1:2, 2:3, 1:1, 2:1). Embedded within this sequence, however, were critical frequencies of vagal stimulation at which complex irregular dynamics could be obtained. Figure 13 shows the irregular dynamics obtained in three cells of the array at one such value of vagal cycle length. Similar patterns of activity have been noted in the case of atrial fibrillation where the SA node is bombarded with rapid, irregular impulses and, at least in the border zone with atrial muscle, develops irregular patterns of activation.[159] The possible physiological role of chaotic dynamics in response to repetitive vagal input remains to be determined, but might be involved with some types of SA arrhythmia.

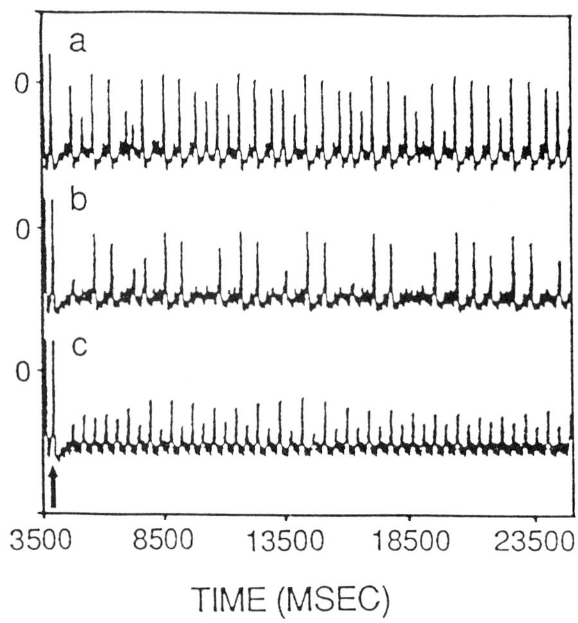

Figure 13. *Irregular ("chaotic") dynamics seen in individual cells of a 15 × 15 array of pacemakers. Beginning at the time indicated by the arrow, ACh pulses are applied repetitively at a constant cycle length of 230 msec to a randomly selected 60% of the cells in the array. The resulting irregular pattern of activation is shown for three selected cells (a, b, c) of the array. Membrane potential is plotted versus time. Reproduced by permission of the American Heart Association, Inc. from Michaels DC, Matyas EP, Jalife J: Mechanisms of sinoatrial pacemaker synchronization: A new hypothesis. Circ Res 61:704–714, 1987.*

Sympathetic Effects

The major effect of sympathetic stimulation on pacemaker activity is to increase the frequency of spontaneous activity. Sympathetic stimulation of the heart is mediated by release of epinephrine and norepinephrine (NE) from adrenergic nerve terminals within the heart and also by the release of epinephrine by the adrenal glands. Activation of β-receptors (β-AR) at the surface of the SA nodal cell activates adenylyl cyclase (AC) and results in an increase in cyclic AMP.[107] The increased cyclic AMP activates protein kinase A (PKA), which phosphorylates membrane proteins and produces increases in $i_{Ca,L}$[142] and i_f.[56,143–145] Recent studies have shown that β-adrenergic stimulation also increases i_K,[146] apparently through changes in protein kinase C (PKC), as well as PKA.[147,148] β-adrenergic agonists increase the SA nodal action potential upstroke velocity, abbreviate the action potential duration, and lead to a positive inotropic effect through an increase in the slope of diastolic depolarization.[39,41] It has been suggested that one of the main roles of i_f in SA pacemaker activity is to mediate the β-adrenergic effects of catecholamines on diastolic depolarization.[149]

The effects of α-adrenergic stimulation on SA pacemaker activity have not been studied in any detail. In Purkinje fibers, α-adrenergic agonists may either increase or decrease automaticity, depending on the experimental circumstances. This finding has led to the idea that perhaps α-adrenergic effects are mediated by changes arising through at least two distinct receptor-effector pathways.[150]

Future Directions

Several questions remain unanswered about the functioning of the SA pacemakers, and these questions can be expected to form the basis of research over the next several years. An issue of interest in regard to the control of pacemaker activity is the way in which the interactions of multiple pacemaker sites contribute to the maintenance of normal pacing activity. Although in most mammals each heart beat is initiated by a single SA nodal pacemaker center,[34] evidence suggests that, at least in some larger mammals, there may be multicentric foci of pacemaker activity.[151] The interaction of these sites and their response to phasic and tonic autonomic input need to be better understood in order to fully elucidate the normal control mechanisms for pacemaker activity.

A second question that deserves particular attention is the way in which a small SA pacemaker is able to stimulate the large excitable mass of the atria without the electrotonic influence of the larger structure stopping pacemaker activity. Initial studies in this regard indicate that the geometry of connections is an important factor.[152] When there is an abrupt change of coupling resistance between a pacemaker and nonpacemaker region, it is difficult to maintain pacing. If a gradient of coupling resistance is established, however, then pacing can be maintained.[152] These simulation results suggest that groups of pacemaker cells and their connections to nonpacemaker cells are organized in such a fashion as to promote propagation from the pacemaker region. It is expected that experimental studies using optical mapping techniques[26,27,153] coupled with further modelling studies will provide insight into this area of interest.

Another topic of interest is whether or not the SA node represents a medium where reentrant arrhythmias[154] can occur. Some clinical studies have suggested that the SA node plays an important role in high atrial tachycardias, and that sustained SA nodal reentrant tachycardia may indeed occur. The issue remains speculative, however, because the diagnosis of SA nodal reentry is based on indirect criteria that do not suffice to ascertain the mechanism of the arrhythmia (see Bonke et al[155]). Experimentally, SA nodal reentry has been demonstrated only for single echo beats.[155–157] This finding may have been the result of technical limitations since, to date, most studies on SA nodal reentry have used intracellular microelectrode recordings that do not provide the spatial resolution required for the demonstration of reentry in cardiac tissues.[158] Mapping the electrical activity with optical methods[26,27,153] may provide excellent resolution to map reentrant excitation in the SA node. In fact, with the help of optical mapping and of realistic computer simulations,[24] it should be possible to demonstrate with great accuracy the mechanism of echo beats and to predict whether or not reentrant tachycardia may indeed be possible in the mammalian SA node.

A final interesting issue is the functioning of pacemaker activity in the presence of extrasystoles or repetitive activity, such as occurs during atrial fibrillation.[159] For many years, it has been thought that activity outside the SA node is capable of fully invading and thus resetting SA activity. Indeed, this principle is the basis of the clinical measure of SA node recovery time, in which a single stimulus is given to the atrium and the time required for the SA node to regain control of heart rate is determined. Some preliminary evidence suggests that instead of an invasion of the SA node, the extrastimuli simply produce a zone of collision that causes a transient exit block of impulses from the SA node.[159] Again, optical mapping experiments that provide high spatial and temporal resolution of activity in the SA node and surrounding atrium should make it possible to address this question directly.

References

1. Lewis T, Oppenheimer A, Oppenheimer BS: The site of origin of the mammalian heart beat: The pacemaker in the dog. Heart 2:147, 1910.

Acknowledgments: The authors wish to thank Dr. Mario Delmar for reading the manuscript and for his helpful comments, and Wanda Coombs for expert assistance in preparing the figures.

2. Wybauw MR: Sur le point d'origine de la systole cardiaque dans l'oreillette droite. Arch Int Physiol 10:78, 1910.
3. Keith A, Flack M: The form and nature of the muscular connections between the primary divisions of the vertebrate heart. J Anat Physiol 41:172, 1907.
4. Kölliker A, Müller H: Nachweis der negativen Schwankung des Muskelstroms am natürlich sich contrahirenden Muskel. Verhandl d phys med Gesellsch i Wurzburg 6:528, 1855.
5. Marey EJ: Des variations électriques des muscles et du coeur en particulier, étudiées au moyen de l'électromètre de M. Lippmann. C R Acad Sci 82:975, 1876.
6. Engelmann TW: Ueber das electrische Verhalten des thätingen Herzen. Pflügers Arch 17:68, 1878.
7. Sanderson JB, Page FJM: On the time relations of the excitatory process in the ventricle of the heart of the frog. J Physiol (Lond) 2:384, 1879.
8. Bayliss WM, Sterling EH: On the electromotive phenomena of the mammalian heart. J Physiol (Lond) 13:407, 1892.
9. Einthoven W: Ein neues Galvanometer. Ann Physiol S4 12:1059, 1903.
10. Einthoven W: Le télécardiogramme. Arch Int Physiol 4:132, 1906.
11. Coraboeuf E, Weidmann S: Potentiel de repos et potentiel d'action du muscle cardiaque mesure a l'aide d'electrodes internes. CR Soc Bio 143:1329, 1949.
12. Draper MH, Weidmann S: Cardiac resting and action potentials recorded with an intracellular electrode. J Physiol (Lond) 115:74, 1951.
13. Trautwein W, Zink K: Uber Membran und Aktionspotentiale einzelner Myokardfasers des Kalt-und Warmblüterherzens. Pflügers Arch 256:68, 1952.
14. Hamill OP, Marty A, Neher E, et al: Improved patch clamp techniques for high resolution current recording from cells and cell-free membrane patches. Pflügers Arch 391:85, 1981.
15. Neher E, Sakmann B: Single channel currents recorded from membrane of denervated frog muscle fibers. Nature 260:779, 1976.
16. Winfree AT: Phase control of neural pacemakers. Science 197: 761, 1977.
17. Sano T, Sawanobori T, Adaniya H: Mechanism of rhythm determination among pacemaker cells of the mammalian sinus node. Am J Physiol 235:H379, 1978.
18. Winfree AT: The Geometry of Biological Time. New York, NY, Springer Verlag, 1980.
19. Jongsma HJ, Tsjernina L, De Bruijne J: The establishment of regular beating in populations of pacemaker heart cells. J Mol Cell Cardiol 15:123, 1983.
20. Jalife J: Mutual entrainment and electrical coupling as mechanisms for synchronous firing of rabbit sino-atrial pace-maker cells. J Physiol (Lond) 356:221, 1984.
21. Delmar M, Jalife J, Michaels DC: Effects of changes in excitability and intracellular coupling on synchronization in the rabbit sino-atrial node. J Physiol (Lond) 370:127, 1986.
22. Michaels DC, Matyas EP, Jalife J: Dynamic interactions and mutual synchronization of sinoatrial node pacemaker cells. Circ Res 58:706, 1986.
23. Jalife J, Michaels D: Phase-dependent interactions of cardiac pacemakers as mechanisms of control and synchronization in the heart. In D Zipes, J Jalife (eds): Cardiac Electrophysiology and Arrhythmias. Orlando, FL, Grune & Stratton Inc, 1985, pp. 109–119.
24. Michaels DC, Matyas EP, Jalife J: Mechanisms of sinoatrial pacemaker synchronization: A new hypothesis. Circ Res 61:704, 1987.
25. Allessie MA, Hoeks APG, Schmitz GML, et al: On-line mapping system for the visualization of the electrical activation of the heart. Int J Card Imaging 2:59, 1986.
26. Salama G, Lombardi R, Elson J: Maps of optical action potentials and NADH fluorescence in intact working hearts. Am J Physiol 252:H384, 1987.
27. Davidenko JM, Kent PF, Chialvo DR, et al: Sustained vortex-like waves in normal isolated ventricular muscle. Proc Natl Acad Sci USA 87:8785, 1990.
28. Glass L, Mackey MC: From Clocks to Chaos: The Rhythms of Life. Princeton, NJ, Princeton University Press, 1988.

29. Guevara MR, Glass L, Shrier A: Phase locking, period-doubling bifurcations, and irregular dynamics in periodically stimulated cardiac cells. Science 214:1350, 1981.
30. Anumonwo JMB, Delmar M, Vinet A, et al: Phase-resetting and entrainment of pacemaker activity in single sinus nodal cells. Circ Res 68:1138, 1991.
31. Reid JVO: The cardiac pacemaker: Effects of regularly spaced nervous input. Am Heart J 78:58, 1969.
32. Levy MN, Martin PJ, Iano TH, et al: Paradoxical effect of vagus nerve stimulation on heart rate in dogs. Circ Res 25:303, 1969.
33. Michaels DC, Chialvo DR, Matyas EP, et al: Chaotic activity in a mathematical model of the vagally driven sinoatrial node. Circ Res 65:1350, 1989.
34. Opthof T: *The Mammalian Sinoatrial Node: A Comparative Morphological and Electrophysiological Study*. Amsterdam, University of Amsterdam, 1986. Thesis.
35. Bleeker WK, MacKaay AJC, Masson-Pevet M, et al: Functional and morphological organization of the rabbit sinus node. Circ Res 46:11, 1980.
36. James TN: The sinus node. Am J Cardiol 40:965, 1977.
37. Meijler F, Janse M: Morphology and electrophysiology of the mammalian atrioventricular node. Physiol Rev 68(2):608, 1988.
38. Giles W, van Ginneken A, Shibata EF: Ionic currents underlying cardiac pacemaker activity: A summary of voltage-clamp data from single cells. In RD Nathan (ed): Cardiac Muscle: The Regulation of Excitation and Contraction. New York, NY, Academic Press Inc, 1986, pp. 1–27.
39. Irisawa H, Giles WR: Sinus and atrioventricular node cells: Cellular electrophysiology. In DP Zipes, J Jalife (eds): Cardiac Electrophysiology: From Cell to Bedside. Philadelphia, PA, WB Saunders, 1990, pp. 95–102.
40. DiFrancesco D: The contribution of the pacemaker current (i_f) to generation of spontaneous activity in rabbit sino-atrial node myocytes. J Physiol (Lond) 434:23, 1991.
41. Irisawa H, Brown HF, Giles WR: Cardiac pacemaking in the sinoatrial node. Physiol Rev 73:197, 1993.
42. Vassalle M: The relationship among cardiac pacemakers. Overdrive suppression. Circ Res 41:269, 1977.
43. Irisawa H: Comparative physiology of cardiac pacemaker mechanisms. Physiol Rev 58:461, 1978.
44. Brown HF: Electrophysiology of the sinoatrial node. Physiol Rev 62:505, 1982.
45. Denyer JC, Brown HF: Pacemaking in rabbit isolated sino-atrial node cells during Cs^+ block of the hyperpolarization activated current i_f. J Physiol (Lond) 429:401, 1990.
46. West TC: Ultramicroelectrode recording from the cardiac pacemaker. J Pharmacol Exp Ther 115:282, 1955.
47. DiFrancesco D: The cardiac hyperpolarizing activated current I_f: Origins and developments. Prog Biophys Mol Biol 46:163, 1985.
48. Denyer JC, Brown HF: Rabbit sino-atrial node cells: Isolation and electrophysiological properties. J Physiol (Lond) 428:405, 1990.
49. Noma A, Nakayama T, Kurachi Y, et al: Resting K conductances in pacemaker and non-pacemaker heart cells of the rabbit. Jpn J Physiol 34:245, 1984.
50. Trautwein W, Kassebaum DG: On the mechanism of the spontaneous impulse generation in the pacemaker of the heart. J Gen Physiol 45:315, 1961.
51. Noma A, Irisawa H: Membrane currents in rabbit sinoatrial node cells as studied by the double microelectrode method. Pflügers Arch 364:45, 1976.
52. Noble D: The surprising heart: A review of recent progress in cardiac physiology. J Physiol (Lond) 353:1, 1984.
53. DiFrancesco D, Tromba C: Muscarinic control of the hyperpolarization-activated current (i_F) induced by acetylcholine in rabbit sinoatrial node myocytes. J Physiol (Lond) 405:493, 1988.
54. Yanagihara K, Irisawa H: Inward current activated during hyperpolarization in rabbit sinoatrial node cells. Pflügers Arch 385:11, 1980.

55. Noma A, Morad M, Irisawa H: Does the pacemaker current generate the diastolic depolarization in the rabbit SA node cells? Pflügers Arch 397:190, 1983.
56. Hagiwara N, Irisawa H: Modulation by intracellular Ca of the hyperpolarization-activated inward current in rabbit single sino-atrial cells. J Physiol (Lond) 409:121, 1989.
57. Doerr T, Denger R, Trautwein W: Calcium currents in single SA nodal cells of the rabbit heart studied with action potential clamp. Pflügers Arch 413:599, 1989.
58. Bean B: Two kinds of calcium channels in canine atrial cells: Differences in kinetics, selectivity, and pharmacology. J Gen Physiol 86:1, 1985.
59. Mitra R, Morad M: Two types of calcium channels in guinea pig ventricular myocytes. Proc Natl Acad Sci USA 93:5340, 1986.
60. Hagiwara N, Irisawa H, Kameyama M: Contribution of two types of calcium currents to the pacemaker potentials of rabbit sino-atrial node cells. J Physiol (Lond) 395:85, 1988.
61. Hess P: Cardiac calcium channels. In DP Zipes, J Jalife (eds): Cardiac Electrophysiology: From Cell to Bedside. Philadelphia, PA, WB Saunders, 1990, pp. 10–17.
62. Yanagihara K, Noma A, Irisawa H: Reconstruction of sino-atrial node pacemaker potential based on the voltage clamp experiments. Jpn J Physiol 30:841, 1980.
63. Nakayama T, Kurachi Y, Noma A, et al: Action potential and membrane currents of single pacemaker cells of the rabbit heart. Pflügers Arch 402:248, 1984.
64. Shibasaki T: Conductance and kinetics of delayed rectifier potassium channels in nodal cells of the rabbit heart. J Physiol (Lond) 387:227, 1987.
65. Paes de Carvalho A, de Almeida DF: Spread of activity through the atrioventricular node. Circ Res 8:801, 1960.
66. Hoffman BF, Cranefield PF: Electrophysiology of the Heart. New York, NY, McGraw-Hill, 1960.
67. Tse W: Evidence for the presence of automatic fibers in the canine atrioventricular node. Am J Physiol 225:716, 1973.
68. Kokubun S, Nishimura M, Noma A, et al: The spontaneous action potential of rabbit atrioventricular node cells. Jpn J Physiol 30:529, 1980.
69. Wit AL, Fenoglio JJ, Wagner BM, et al. Electrophysiological properties of cardiac muscle in the anterior mitral valve leaflet and adjacent atrium in the dog: Possible implications for the genesis of atrial dysrhythmias. Circ Res 32:731, 1973.
70. Makarychev V, Kosharskaya I, Ul'Yaniskii L: Automatic activity of pacemaker cells of the atrioventricular valves in the rabbit heart. Biull Eksp Biol Med 81:646, 1976.
71. Rozanski G, Jalife J: Automatic activity in atrioventricular valve leaflets of rabbit heart. Am J Physiol 250:H397, 1986.
72. Anumonwo JMB: *Ionic Currents Underlying Pacemaker Activity in the Rabbit Tricuspid Valve.* Syracuse, NY, SUNY Health Science Center at Syracuse, 1988. Dissertation.
73. Gross L, Kugel M: Topographic anatomy and histology of the valves in the human heart. Am J Pathol 7:445, 1931.
74. Rozanski GJ: Electrophysiological properties of automatic fibers in rabbit atrioventricular valves. Am J Physiol 253:H720, 1987.
75. Anumonwo JMB, Delmar M, Jalife J: Electrophysiology of single heart cells from the rabbit tricuspid valve. J Physiol (Lond) 425:145, 1990.
76. Noble D, Tsien WR: The kinetic and rectifier properties of the slow potassium current in cardiac Purkinje fibers. J Physiol (Lond) 195:185, 1968.
77. Jalife J, Moe GK: Effects of electrotonic potentials on pacemaker activity of canine Purkinje fibers in relation to parasystole. Circ Res 39:801, 1976.
78. Moe GK, Jalife J, Mueller WJ, et al: A mathematical model of parasystole and its application to clinical arrhythmias. Circulation 56:968, 1977.
79. Jalife J, Moe GK: A biologic model of parasystole. Am J Cardiol 43:761, 1979.
80. DiFrancesco D: A new interpretation of the pacemaker current i_{k2} in Purkinje fibres. J Physiol (Lond) 314:359, 1981.

81. Callewaert G, Carmeliet E, Vereeke J: Single cardiac Purkinje cells: General electrophysiology and voltage clamp analysis of the pacemaker current. J Physiol (Lond) 349:643, 1984.
82. Noble D: Ionic basis of rhythmic activity in the heart. In DP Zipes, J Jalife (eds): Cardiac Electrophysiology and Arrhythmias. Orlando, FL, Grune & Stratton Inc, 1985, pp. 3–11.
83. Tseng G-N, Boyden P: Multiple types of Ca^{2+} currents in single canine Purkinje cells. Circ Res 65:1735, 1989.
84. Cranefield PF: Action potentials, afterpotentials, and arrhythmias. Circ Res 41:415, 1977.
85. Sano T, Sawanobori T: Abnormal automaticity in cardiac Purkinje fibers focally subjected to low external concentrations of calcium. Circ Res 31:158, 1972.
86. Damiano BP, Rosen MR: Effects of pacing on triggered activity induced by early after depolarizations. Circulation 69:1013, 1984.
87. Davis LD: Effects of changes in cycle length on diastolic depolarization produced by ouabain in cardiac Purkinje fibers. Circ Res 32:206, 1973.
88. Ferrier GR, Saunders JH, Mendez C: Cellular mechanism for the generation of ventricular arrhythmias by acetylstrophanthidin. Circ Res 32:600, 1973.
89. Hashimoto K, Moe GK: Transient depolarizations induced by acetylstrophanthidin in specialized tissue of dog atrium and ventricle. Circ Res 32:618, 1973.
90. Rosen MR, Gelband H, Hoffman BF: Correlation between effects of ouabain in the canine electrocardiogram and transmembrane potential of isolated Purkinje fibers. Circulation 47:65, 1973.
91. Wit AL, Rosen MR: Afterdepolarizations and triggered activity. In HA Fozzard, E Haber, RB Jennings, et al (eds): The Heart and the Cardiovascular System. New York, NY, Raven Press, 1986, pp. 1449–1490.
92. Brachmann J, Scherlag BJ, Rosenshtraukh LV, et al: Bradycardia-dependent triggered activity: Relevance to drug-induced multiform ventricular tachycardia. Circulation 68: 846, 1983.
93. Jackman WM, Friday KL, Anderson JL, et al: The long QT syndromes: A critical review, new clinical observations and unifying hypothesis. Prog Cardiovasc Dis 31:115, 1988.
94. Hauswirth O, Noble D, Tsien RW: The mechanism of oscillatory activity at low membrane potentials in cardiac Purkinje fibers. J Physiol (Lond) 200:255, 1969.
95. Katzung BG: Electrically induced automaticity in ventricular myocardium. Life Sci 14:1133, 1974.
96. Katzung BG, Morgenstern J: Effects of extracellular potassium on ventricular automaticity and evidence for a pacemaker current in mammalian ventricular myocardium. Circ Res 40:105, 1977.
97. Barr L, Dewey MM, Berger W: Propagation of action potentials and the structure of the nexus in cardiac muscle. J Gen Physiol 48:797, 1965.
98. Masson-Pévet M, Bleeker WK, Gros D: The plasma membrane of leading pacemaker cells in the rabbit sinus node. Circ Res 45: 621, 1979.
99. Fozzard HA: Conduction of the action potential. In RM Berne, N Sperelakis (eds): Handbook of Physiology. Section 2: The Cardiovascular System-the Heart, Vol. 1. Bethesda, MD, American Physiological Society, 1979, pp. 335–356.
100. De Mello WC: Intercellular communication and junctional permeability. In E Bittar (ed): Membrane Structure and Function. New York, NY, John Wiley and Sons, 1980, pp. 128–170.
101. Anumonwo JMB, Wang H-Z, Trabka-Janik E, et al: Gap junctional currents in adult mammalian sinus nodal cell pairs. Circ Res 71:229, 1992.
102. Rook MB, Jongsma HJ, van Ginneken ACG: Properties of single gap junctional channels between isolated neonatal rat heart cells. Am J Physiol 255:H770, 1988.
103. Spray DC, Burt JM: Structure-activity relations of the cardiac gap junctional channel. Am J Physiol 258:C195, 1990.

104. Löffelholz K, Pappano AJ: The parasympathetic neuroeffector junction of the heart. Pharmacol Rev 37:1, 1985.
105. Randal WC, Ardell JL: Nervous control of the heart: Anatomy and pathophysiology. In DP Zipes, J Jalife (eds): Cardiac Electrophysiology: From Cell to Bedside. Philadelphia, PA, WB Saunders, 1990, pp. 291–299.
106. Levy MN: Cardiac sympathetic-parasympathetic interactions. Fed Proc 43:2598, 1984.
107. Lindemann JP, Watanabe AM: Sympathetic control of cardiac electrical activity. In DP Zipes, J Jalife (eds): Cardiac Electrophysiology: From Cell to Bedside. Philadelphia, PA, WB Saunders, 1990, pp. 277–283.
108. Jalife J, Hamilton AJ, Lamanna VR, et al: Effects of current flow on pacemaker activity of the isolated kitten sinoatrial node. Am J Physiol 238:H307, 1980.
109. Kodama I, Boyett MR: Regional differences in the electrical activity of the rabbit sinus node. Pflügers Arch 404:214, 1985.
110. Van der Pol B, Van der Mark J: The heartbeat considered as a relaxation oscillator and an electrical model of the heart. Phil Mag 6:763, 1928.
111. Fessard A: Auto-rythmicité et synchronisations interneuroniques a l'intérieur d'organes électriques isolés. CR Soc Bio 136:114, 1942.
112. Fessard A: Hypothése sur le mécanisme d'intervention du facteur électrique dans la synchronisation interneuronique. CR Soc Biol 136:268, 1942.
113. Segers M: Les phenomenes de synchronisation au niveau du coeur. Arch Int Physiol 54:87, 1946.
114. Weidmann S: Effect of current flow on the membrane potential of cardiac muscle. J Physiol (Lond) 115:227, 1950.
115. Perkel DH, Schulman JH, Bullock TH: Pacemaker neurons: Effects of regularly spaced synaptic input. Science 145:61, 1964.
116. Jalife J, Antzelevitch C: Phase resetting and annihilation of pacemaker activity in cardiac tissues. Science 206:695, 1979.
117. Clay JR, Guevara MR, Shrier A: Phase resetting of the rhythmic activity of embryonic heart cell aggregates: Experiment and theory. Biophys J 45:699, 1984.
118. Guevara MR, Glass L: Phase-locking, period doubling bifurcations and chaos in a mathematical model of a periodically driven oscillator: A theory for the entrainment of biological oscillators and the generation of cardiac dysrhythmias. J Math Biol 14:1, 1982.
119. Guevara MR, Shrier A: Phase resetting in a model of cardiac Purkinje fibre. Biophys J 52:265, 1987.
120. Michaels DC, Matyas EP, Jalife J: Experimental and mathematical observations on pacemaker interactions as a mechanism of synchronization in the sinoatrial node. In DP Zipes, J Jalife (eds): Cardiac Electrophysiology: From Cell to Bedside. Philadelphia, PA, WB Saunders, 1990, pp. 182–192.
121. Landau M, Lorente P, Michaels D, et al: Bistabilities and annihilation phenomena in electrophysiological cardiac models. Circ Res 66:1658, 1990.
122. Pittendrigh C: On the mechanism of the entrainment of a circadian rhythm by light cycles. In J Aschoff (ed): Circadian Clocks. Amsterdam, North Holland, 1965.
123. Buck J, Buck E: Synchronous fireflies. Sci Am 234:74, 1976.
124. Ypey DL, Clapham DE, DeHaan RL: Development of electrical coupling and action potential synchrony between paired aggregates of embryonic heart cells. Membrane Biol 51:75, 1970.
125. Clapham DE, Shrier A, DeHaan RL: Junctional resistance and action potential delay between embryonic heart cell aggregates. J Gen Physiol 75:633, 1980.
126. Veenstra RD, DeHaan RL: Electrotonic interactions between aggregates of chick embryo cardiac pacemaker cells. Am J Physiol 250:H453, 1986.
127. James TN: Cardiac innervation: Anatomic and pharmacologic relations. Bull NY Acad Med 43:1041, 1967.
128. Pappano A: Parasympathetic control of cardiac electrical activity. In DP Zipes, J

Jalife (eds): Cardiac Electrophysiology: From Cell to Bedside. Philadelphia, PA, WB Saunders, 1990, pp. 271–277.
129. Noma A, Trautwein W: Relaxation of the ACh-induced potassium current in the rabbit sinoatrial node cell. Pflügers Arch 377:193, 1978.
130. Osterrieder W, Noma A, Trautwein W: On the kinetics of the potassium channel activated by acetylcholine in the S-A node of the rabbit heart. Pflügers Arch 386:101, 1980.
131. Sakmann B, Noma A, Trautwein W: Acetylcholine activation of single muscarinic K+ channels in isolated pacemaker cells of the mammalian heart. Nature 303:250, 1983.
132. Reuter H: Calcium channel modulation by neurotransmitters, enzymes and drugs. Nature 301:569, 1983.
133. Jewett DL: Activity of single efferent fibres in the cervical vagus nerve of the dog, with special reference to possible cardioinhibitory fibres. J Physiol (Lond) 175:321, 1964.
134. Katona PG, Poitras JW, Barnett GO, et al: Cardiac vagal efferent activity and heart period in the carotid sinus reflex. Am J Physiol 218:1030, 1970.
135. Levy MN, Martin PJ, Iano T, et al: Effects of single vagal stimulus on heart rate and atrioventricular conduction. Am J Physiol 218:1256, 1970.
136. Jalife J, Moe GK: Phasic effects of vagal stimulation on pacemaker activity of the isolated sinus node of the young cat. Circ Res 45:595, 1979.
137. Jalife J, Slenter VAJ, Salata JJ: Dynamic vagal control of pacemaker activity in the mammalian sinoatrial node. Circ Res 52:642, 1983.
138. Michaels DC, Matyas EP, Jalife J: A mathematical model of the effects of acetylcholine pulses on sinoatrial pacemaker activity. Circ Res 55:89, 1984.
139. Yang T, Jacobstein MD, Levy MN: Sustained increases in heart rate induced by timed repetition of vagal stimulation in dogs. Am J Physiol 249:H703, 1985.
140. Kunze DL: Reflex discharge patterns of cardiac vagal efferent fibres. J Physiol (Lond) 222:1, 1972.
141. Levy MN, Iano T, Zieske H: Effects of repetitive bursts of vagal activity on heart rate. Circ Res 30:186, 1972.
142. Trautwein W, Kameyama M: Intracellular control of calcium and potassium currents in cardiac cells. Jpn Heart J 27:31, 1986.
143. Brown HF, DiFrancesco D, Noble SJ: How does adrenaline accelerate the heart? Nature 290:31, 1979.
144. Noma A, Kotake H, Irisawa H: Slow inward current and its role mediating the chronotropic effect of epinephrine in the rabbit sino-atrial node. Pflügers Arch 388:1, 1980.
145. DiFrancesco D, Ferroni A, Mazzanti M, et al: Properties of the hyperpolarizing-activated current (i_f) in cells isolated from the rabbit sino-atrial node. J Physiol (Lond) 377:61, 1986.
146. Kameyama M, Hoffman F, Trautwein W: On the mechanism of β-adrenergic regulation of the Ca channel in guinea pig heart. Pflügers Arch 405:285, 1985.
147. Tohse N, Kameyama M, Irisawa H: Intracellular Ca^{2+} and protein kinase C modulate K^+ current in guinea pig heart cells. Am J Physiol 253:H1321, 1987.
148. Walsh KB, Kass RS: Regulation of heart potassium channel by protein kinase A and C. Science 242:67, 1988.
149. DiFrancesco D: Current i_f and the neuronal modulation of heart rate. In DP Zipes, J Jalife (eds): Cardiac Electrophysiology: From Cell to Bedside. Philadelphia, PA, WB Saunders, 1990, pp. 28–35.
150. Rosen MR, Bilezikian JP, Cohen IS, et al: α-adrenergic modulation of cardiac rhythm. In DP Zipes, J Jalife (eds): Cardiac Electrophysiology: From Cell to Bedside. Philadelphia, PA, WB Saunders, 1990, pp. 300–304.
151. Boineau JP, Schuessler RB, Henkel DB, et al: Widespread distribution and rate differentiation of atrial pacemaker complex. Am J Physiol 239:H406, 1980.

152. Joyner RW, van Capelle FJL: Propagation through electrically coupled cells: How a small SA node drives a large atrium. Biophys J 50:1157, 1986.
153. Kamino K: Optical approaches to ontogeny of electrical activity and related functional organization during early heart development. Physiol Rev 71:53, 1991.
154. Reiffel JA: Clinical electrophysiology of the sinus node in man. In T Mazgalev, LS Dreifus, EL Michaelson (eds): Electrophysiology of the Sinoatrial and Atrioventricular Nodes. New York, NY, Allan R Liss, 1988, pp. 239–257.
155. Bonke FIM, Kirchhof CJHJ, Allessie MA: Sinus node reentry. In DP Zipes, J Jalife (eds): Cardiac Electrophysiology: From Cell to Bedside. Philadelphia, PA, WB Saunders, 1990, pp. 526–530.
156. Han J, Malozzi AM, Moe GK: Sino-atrial reciprocation in the isolated rabbit heart. Circ Res 22:355, 1968.
157. Allessie MA, Bonke FIM: Direct demonstration of sinus node reentry in the rabbit heart. Circ Res 44:557, 1979.
158. Jalife J, Davidenko JM, Michaels DC: A new perspective on the mechanisms of arrhythmias and sudden cardiac death: Spiral waves of excitation in heart muscle. J Cardiovasc Electrophysiol 2(suppl):S133, 1991.
159. Allessie MA, Kirchhof CJHJ, Bonke FIM: The role of the sinus node in supraventricular arrhythmias. In T Mazgalev, LS Dreifus, EL Michaelson (eds): Electrophysiology of the Sinoatrial and Atrioventricular Nodes. New York, NY, Allan R Liss, 1988, pp. 53–66.
160. Anumonwo JMB, Jalife J: Initiation and modulation of pacemaker activity in cardiac cells. In C Fisch, B Surawicz (eds): Cardiac Electrophysiology and Arrhythmias. New York, NY, Elsevier, 1991, pp. 35–47.

CHAPTER 13

Regulation of the Pacemaker Current by Acetylcholine

D. DiFrancesco

Historically, the vagal modulation of the heartbeat has been one of the first aspects of cardiac function investigated by electrophysiological means. In the early 1950s, several laboratories applied the newborn microelectrode technique to study the vagal control of cardiac pacing and opened the way to the electrophysiological approach to cardiac function and its modulation by neurotransmitters.[1–4] By using nerve-muscle preparations, it was possible to show in these early studies that stimulation of vagal efferents led to hyperpolarization of the membrane potential and the consequent slowing of pacing rate.

This first evidence that vagal stimulation hyperpolarized the membrane by increasing the K permeability was later confirmed by several studies in both amphibian and mammalian cardiac preparations.[5–11] Also, the properties of the acetylcholine- (ACh-) dependent K component were investigated in detail in pacemaker tissues [12–14] and analyzed at the single-channel level in the rabbit sinoatrial (SA) node.[15]

The bulk of evidence from these experiments established the view that the main process responsible for the negative chronotropic effect of ACh was the activation of a K conductance. Several observations, however, indicated that, in pacemaker cells, substantial slowing could be elicited by moderate vagal stimulation or low doses of ACh, in the absence of significant membrane hyperpolarization.[12,16] This finding led to the suggestion that inhibition of the Ca current could be involved,[16] a hypothesis that was not however, supported by evidence that showed that moderate ACh concentrations are effective on the basal Ca current in intact SA node preparations.

More recently, the "potassium" hypothesis has been challenged by new evidence involving a different current, the hyperpolarization-activated, "pacemaker" current i_f, which is also strongly affected by ACh.[17–19] In this chapter, the properties of the pacemaker current, its modulation by ACh, and the relevance of this mechanism to the vagal control of pacing are briefly reviewed.

The work reviewed here was supported by the Consiglio Nazionale delle Ricerche and partly by the National Institutes of Health.
From *Vagal Control of the Heart: Experimental Basis and Clinical Implications* edited by MN Levy, PJ Schwartz © 1994, Futura Publishing Co. Inc., Armonk, NY.

Differential Actions of Acetylcholine on Sinoatrial Node Spontaneous Activity

According to the early data on the action of ACh, slowing of spontaneous activity was directly correlated to the membrane hyperpolarization caused by ACh itself. As mentioned above, however, it was also observed in different studies[16] that slowing associated with moderate vagal stimulation or low ACh doses could occur in the absence of hyperpolarization of the maximum diastolic potential (MDP). The same experimental observation can be made in the mammalian SA node, as shown in Figure 1. In this figure, the action of different ACh concentrations is shown on spontaneous activity of an isolated SA node myocyte. It is apparent that during perfusion with the highest concentration used (1 μM, Fig. 1c), the MDP is hyperpolarized and slowing occurs. Indeed, even if not apparent in Figure 1, beating is arrested during the perfusion with this concentration of ACh. The lowest ACh dose used, however (0.01 μM, Fig. 1a), causes a substantial rate slowing without any hyperpolarization of the MDP, while at the concentration of 0.1 μM (Fig. 1b), intermediate effects are observed. At low doses of ACh, the action potential shape is not modified by the neurotransmitter, while at high doses, the increased K permeability results in a shortening of action potential duration. Thus, hyperpolarization of the membrane and, more generally, an increased K permeability do not appear to be necessary conditions for slowing to occur.

Comparison Between the Effects of Acetylcholine and Current Injection on Rhythm

Further insight into the mechanism by which low doses of ACh slow rhythm in SA node cells is to compare the actions of ACh and membrane hyperpolarization.[18] Indeed, if the major slowing action of ACh results from a membrane hyperpolarization due to opening of K channels, then hyperpolarizing a SA node myocyte by current injection should have a similar effect. The protocol of Figure 2, however, indicates that just the opposite occurs. Whereas perfusion of ACh (0.03 μM) slows markedly, as expected, the spontaneous activity of a single SA node myocyte (Fig. 2B), in the same cell the injection of a 60-pA hyperpolarizing current gives rise to only a minor slowing. In contrast with the noticeable hyperpolarization caused by current injection (about 5 mV), ACh slows the diastolic depolarization and rhythm in the absence of an obvious hyperpolarization of the MDP. This finding indicates that the major action of ACh is not performed via an increased K permeability but, as discussed below, via inhibition of the current i_f.

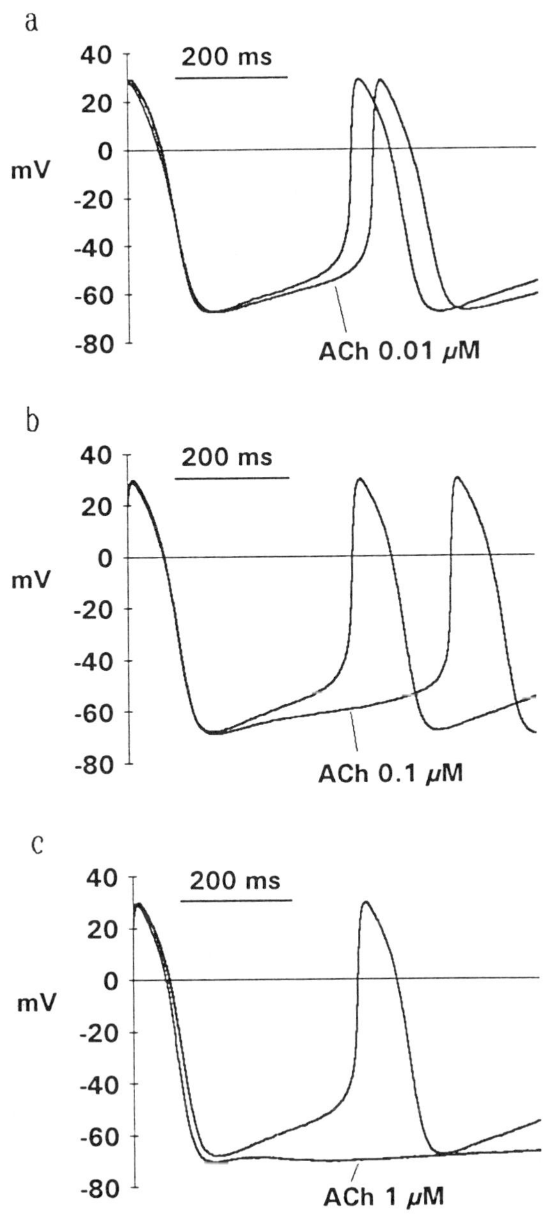

Figure 1. *Effects of ACh on spontaneous activity of a single SA node myocyte. Each panel shows two superimposed voltage traces, one recorded in control Tyrode's solution and one during perfusion with ACh 0.01 μM (a), 0.1 μM (b), and 1 μM (c), as indicated. Traces are triggered at the onset of action potential depolarization so as to allow comparison of the changes induced by ACh in the action potential configuration and in the diastolic depolarization. See further explanation in the text.*

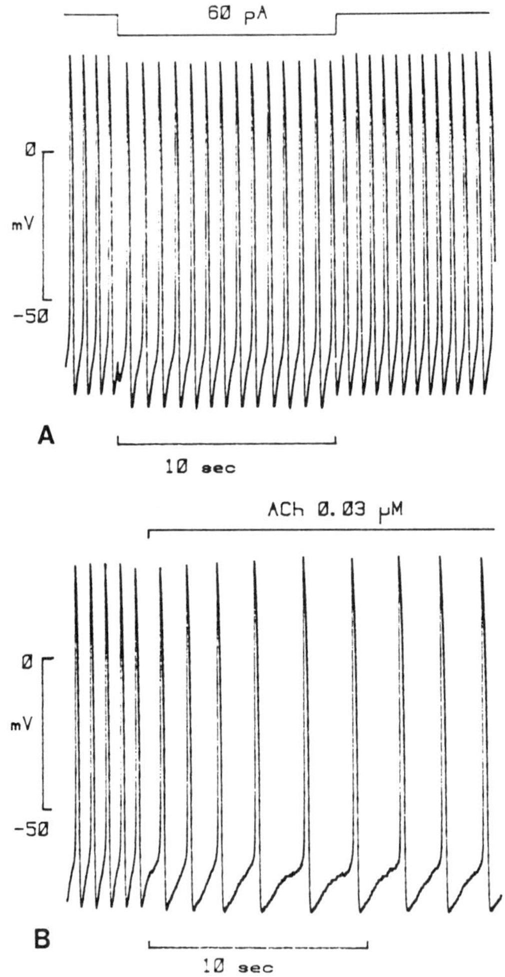

Figure 2. *Comparison between the effects of hyperpolarizing current injection and ACh on spontaneous activity. A: Current-clamp hyperpolarization of the MDP is induced in a beating SA node cell by passing 60 pA through the recording pipette. This action hyperpolarizes the MDP by about 5 mV, but does not substantially decrease the spontaneous frequency. B: Superfusion of the same cell with ACh 0.03 μM has a marked slowing action without causing membrane hyperpolarization.*

Current i_f and its Inhibition by Acetylcholine

When the hyperpolarization-activated current i_f was first described in the SA node in 1979,[20] its involvement in the catecholamine-induced acceleration of rhythm was apparent. The possibility that i_f also played a role in the slowing action of cholinergic stimulation, however, was investigated only several years later.[21] This occurrence was possibly due to the fact that a mechanism specifically involved in the ACh modulation of rhythm, the activation of a K conductance, had long been known and, therefore, the existence of other mechanisms for the same action was not actively pursued. It was thus by chance that, while studying the type of muscarinic receptor (mAChR) responsible for the K current activation in the SA node (Terry E. Egan, Susan J. Noble, and D. DiFrancesco, unpublished observation), a marked inhibition of i_f by ACh was found. This inhibitory action was then studied in detail.[17] The essential features of the action of ACh on currents in isolated SA node myocytes is shown in Figure 3. In Figure 3a, the action of ACh (1 μM) is shown on currents recorded in normal Tyrode's solution in a single SA node myocyte. Clearly, ACh induces a large outward displacement of the holding current at −38 mV, which reflects activation of the ACh-dependent K current $i_{K,ACh}$.[13] An increase in the instantaneous current in the outward direction due to the same

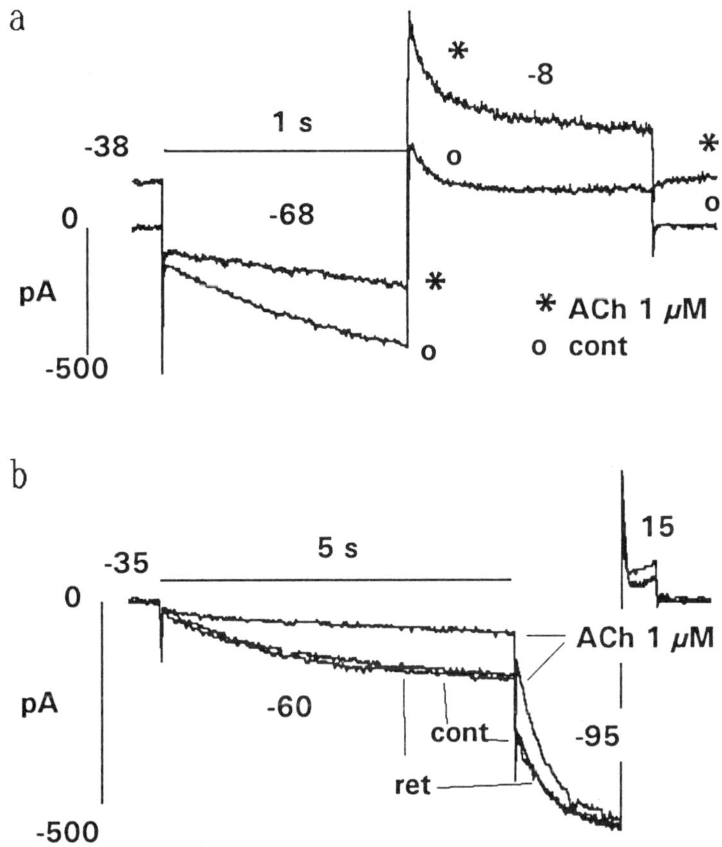

Figure 3. *Action of ACh on ionic currents in a single SA node myocyte. Currents are recorded during voltage-clamp steps to the voltages indicated. a: Perfusion with ACh 1 μM (*) on a cell perfused with normal Tyrode solution induces, with respect to control (o), an increase in K flux, as revealed by an outward displacement of the current trace at −38 and −8 mV, as well as a reduction of i_f at −68 mV. b: In the presence of barium 1 mM, the ACh-dependent K current ($i_{K,ACh}$) is blocked and the action of ACh 1 μM on i_f can be analyzed more properly. From the three-pulse protocol shown here, ACh acts by shifting the i_f activation curve without decreasing the current fully-activated amplitude at −95 mV.*

K conductance is also observed on depolarization to −8 mV (followed by relaxation) and, with a reduced amplitude, on hyperpolarization to −68 mV. Together with an increased K current, however, a reduced amplitude of i_f recorded at −68 mV is also apparent.

To investigate whether the i_f reduction is due to a genuine action of ACh on i_f rather than an indirect result of $i_{K,ACh}$ activation (for example, due to relaxation), ACh can be perfused in the presence of barium, which blocks the K current but leaves i_f essentially unaltered.[17,18] After block of $i_{K,ACh}$ by barium, the extent of i_f inhibition by ACh is then fully appreciated, as shown in Figure 2b. The three step protocol used here also allows for discrimination between different modes of action of ACh, and indicates that ACh does not reduce i_f to the same degree at every potential. Indeed, i_f is decreased at −60 mV, but is increased during the following step to −95 mV by ACh, so that the fully-activated current at the latter voltage is unaltered. This finding implies that, with ACh, the fraction of i_f activated at −60 mV is reduced, while the fraction at −95 is correspondingly increased. Thus, the i_f inhibition by ACh does not involve a reduction of the current fully-activated current/voltage (I/V) relation, and is due rather to a shift of the i_f activation curve to the negative direction.

Although the experimental observation of the ACh-induced i_f inhibition was made a few years later than that of the catecholamine-induced i_f activation, it soon became clear that the two actions had much to share. A first clue to the hypothesis of a common pathway came from evidence that the two neurotransmitters had exactly symmetrical actions on i_f. Indeed, both adrenaline and ACh shift the i_f activation curve along the voltage axis (to the left and to the right, respectively) without affecting the current fully-activated I/V relation. Further studies then showed that, like adrenaline, ACh exerted its action on i_f via interaction with adenylyl cyclase (AC). This finding was inferred by several observations, including the finding that the ACh action was muscarinic and mediated by pertussis toxin- (PTX-) sensitive guanine nucleotide-binding proteins (G-proteins), and by direct experimental evidence of the involvement of AC.[19]

Further, these results underlined the relevance of adenosine 3'5'-cyclic phosphate (cyclic AMP) as a second messenger in the neurotransmitter regulation of i_f. While it had been previously demonstrated that β-adrenergic stimulation of i_f depended upon an elevation of intracellular cyclic AMP,[22,23] it was then also shown that muscarinic stimulation inhibited i_f via a reduction of cyclic AMP. The cyclic AMP level is upregulated by β-adrenergic stimulation, and downregulated by muscarinic stimulation in cardiac cells. Thus, these data indicated that the sensitivity of i_f to neurotransmitters simply reflected a sensitivity to cyclic AMP.

This is by no means a property specific to i_f, and is shared by several ionic currents including calcium and potassium currents of SA node myocytes (for a review, see Hartzell[24]). Interestingly, i_f is inhibited by fairly low ACh concentrations in the absence of previous β-stimulation. This finding was interpreted to indicate that the basal activity of AC in the SA node cells could be sufficiently large to be depressed by muscarinic stimulation.[19] Evidence supporting this view was subsequently found in the Purkinje fiber, where it was shown that a given dose of ACh could not normally inhibit i_f, but did so after current activation by epinephrine.[25] This observation agrees with the view that, in the Purkinje fiber, AC activity and the basal cyclic AMP level is lower than in the SA node, as also predicted by the more negative position of the i_f activation curve in this preparation.[26]

Differential Actions of Acetylcholine on i_f and $i_{K,ACh}$

The finding of the ACh-induced i_f inhibition soon raised a few obvious questions: did this action contribute to the rate slowing caused by ACh and, if so, why were at least two different mechanisms involved in the vagal control of pacing and what were their relative roles? Answers to these questions came from the investigation of the relative efficiency of ACh in its action on the currents i_f and $i_{K,ACh}$. The basic experimental observation of this study[21] is illustrated in Figure 4. In this figure, ACh, at the concentration of 0.01 μM, is able to inhibit the current i_f recorded during a hyperpolarization to −90 mV (upper diagram), but is unable to activate $i_{K,ACh}$. This latter effect, revealed as an outward shift of the current trace at −40 and 0 mV and an inward shift at −90 mV, is only barely visible at the ACh concentration of 0.1 μM (middle diagram) and clearly apparent at 1 μM (lower diagram). Thus, when different concentrations of ACh are perfused on a single pacemaker cell, the effects on i_f and on the K conductance can be easily separated. These data indicate that the ACh doses effective on i_f are much lower than those required to activate $i_{K,ACh}$. A more complete quantitative analysis of this difference can be performed by plotting, as shown in Figure 5, the dose-response relationships for the i_f inhibition and $i_{K,ACh}$ activation by ACh.[21]

The i_f dose-response curve (measured in terms of the displacement of the activation curve in mV) is clearly centered around lower concentrations than the $i_{K,ACh}$ curve (measured as steady-state current normalized to cell capacity). Thus, the half-maximal ACh concentration required for $i_{K,ACh}$ activation (0.260 μM) is 20-fold higher than that required for i_f inhibition (0.013 μM). The result in Figure 5 illustrates an important property of the ACh action on the two currents: up to 0.01 to 0.03 μM, the threshold for activation of $i_{K,ACh}$, the only action of ACh is to inhibit i_f. If we now turn to the observation in Figure 1 above, the relevance of this result to the issue of the origin of the slowing action of ACh becomes clear. Indeed, in agreement with the fact that modifications of the repolarization process and the action potential duration only appear at ACh concentrations above 0.01 μM, these data indicate that in the low concentration range, ACh slows rhythm by inhibiting i_f, and not by activating a K conductance.

It may be interesting to note in this context that some authors[27] have suggested the existence of different sets of mAChRs to explain different responses to ionophoretically-applied ACh and vagal stimulation. This suggestion is partly based on evidence that ACh-induced slowing is accompanied by MDP hyperpolarization, whereas moderate vagal stimulation only acts on the

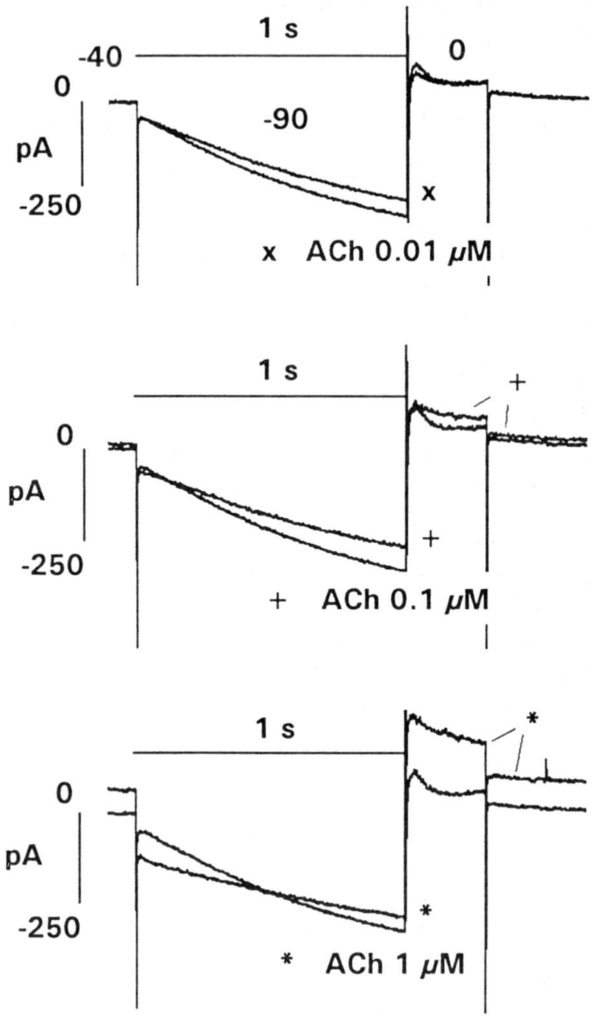

Figure 4. *Separation of the effects of ACh on i_f and $i_{K,ACh}$. A single SA node cell is perfused with three different ACh concentrations: 0.01 μM (upper diagram, x), 0.1 μM (middle diagram, +), and 1 μM (bottom diagram, *). Steps from −40 mV to −90 mV are used to activate i_f. Notice that with ACh 0.01 μM, i_f is depressed but no change is apparent in the steady-state current at any potential. An increased outward component at −40 and 0 mV (inward at −90 mV) is just apparent, on the other hand, with 0.1-μM ACh, and more marked with 1-μM ACh, suggesting that the concentration threshold for activation of the ACh-dependent K conductance is just below 0.1 μM.*

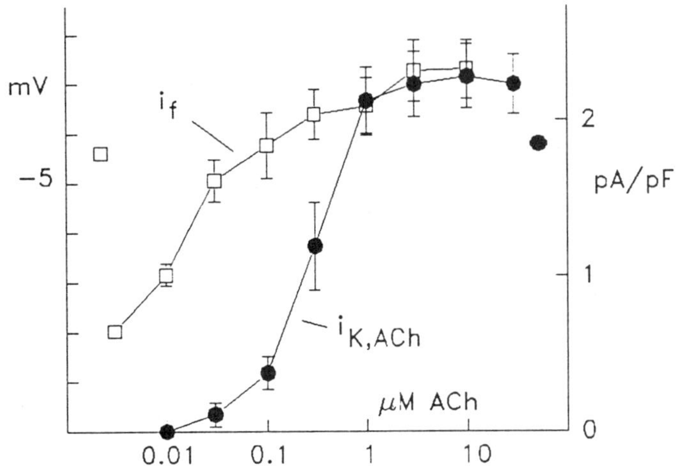

Figure 5. *Dose-response relationship for the activation of $i_{K,ACh}$ and the inhibition of i_f by ACh. Plotted are mean ± s.e.m. values of the steady-state amplitude of $i_{K,ACh}$ at −35 mV after normalization to cell capacity (filled circles), and of the negative shifts of the i_f activation curve (open squares). The half-maximal ACh concentrations are 0.013 μM for the i_f curve, and 0.260 μM for the $i_{K,ACh}$ curve.*[21]

diastolic depolarization, and that barium blocks ACh-induced, but not vagal-induced, hyperpolarization. This last finding also leads these authors to suggest that ACh reduces a voltage-independent Na conductance. Two relevant facts should also, however, be taken into account in this respect. One, low ACh concentrations do indeed slow diastolic depolarization without affecting the MDP[21] (see Figs. 1 and 2), which can be attributed to a specific ACh action on i_f. Two, direct evidence for an independent-resting Na component involved in pacemaking and modulated by ACh is lacking, and barium-resistant hyperpolarizations caused by moderate vagal stimulation can be explained by i_f inhibition if this current is sufficiently activated in the range of −35 to −40 mV (see Fig. 2B).[28] Furthermore, restricted access to nerve terminals could at least partly reduce the action of barium on the effects of vagal stimulation. Thus, although it is likely that mAChRs are concentrated in regions surrounding nerve terminals, the evidence that supports the existence of different sets of receptors available to vagal stimulation and externally applied ACh, and of a resting ACh-inhibited Na current, can possibly be explained by the differential action of ACh on i_f and $i_{K,ACh}$ based on concentration, as described in the SA node.[21]

Comparison Between Acetylcholine Action on i_f and the Ca Current

ACh is known to decrease the Ca current after β-adrenergic stimulation, although its inhibitory effect on basal Ca current is still controversial.[24]

Different results have been reported on the action of ACh on i_{Ca} in the SA node. For example, while some authors[13] report no significant effect on multicellular preparations at micromolar concentrations, in isolated nodal myocytes other authors[19,29] report partial inhibition at submillimolar concentrations. Clearly, single-cell data may be affected by some degree of variation intrinsic to single-cell preparations. Due to this variability, and in the light of the high sensitivity of i_f to ACh discussed above, it may be interesting to compare the response of i_{Ca} and i_f to low ACh concentrations in the same isolated nodal cell so as to establish the degree of specificity of the neurotransmitter action. An experiment in which this comparison was made is shown in Figure 6. The voltage-clamp protocol used here was such as to allow the simultaneous measurement of the neurotransmitter-sensitive Ca current component (L-component, i_L) and i_f, which were dissected using appropriate intracellular and extracellular solutions. This experiment indicates that, as expected, perfusion with ACh 0.03 μM inhibited i_f, and that this same concentration did not modify the Ca current. Thus, the action of ACh in the range of up to 0.01 to 0.03 μM can be considered as essentially specific on i_f in the SA node.

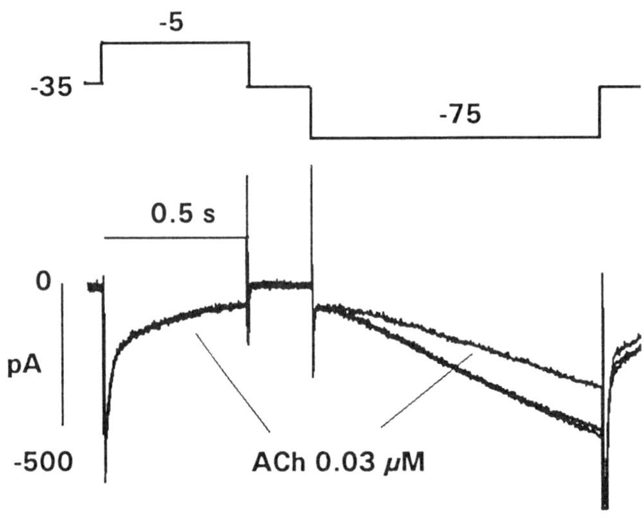

Figure 6. *Comparison of ACh actions on i_f and the L-component of the Ca current (i_L). To improve dissection of these two components, in the intracellular-like solution of the whole-cell pipette, KCl was replaced by CsCl (130 mM), and the standard Ca concentration of the extracellular solution (1.8 mM) was replaced by (mM): $CaCl_2$, 0.5; $BaCl_2$, 2. Upper diagram: Voltage protocol used to activate i_L and, subsequently, i_f. The protocol was repeated every 3 s. Lower diagram: Current traces recorded before, during, and after perfusion with ACh 0.03 μM as indicated. Control and return traces were almost perfectly superimposable. Notice that ACh reduced i_f, but had no effect on i_L.*

Modulation of i_f by Cyclic AMP

As discussed above, both adrenergic and cholinergic neurotransmitters, in opposite ways, modulate i_f by controlling the activity of AC and the intracellular level of cyclic AMP, which acts as a second messenger for i_f regulation. As it is well established that the cyclic AMP-mediated modulation of other cardiac channels (like the L-type Ca channel and the delayed K channel) occurs via phosphorylation by cyclic AMP-dependent protein kinase A (PKA),[24] it was natural to expect that i_f modulation by cyclic AMP was also mediated by a phosphorylation process. It has recently been found, however, that, surprisingly, cyclic AMP modulates i_f independently of phosphorylation, via a mechanism involving a direct interaction of cyclic AMP with the intracellular side of the channels.[30] Thus, ACh-induced downregulation of cyclic AMP represents a mechanism able to modulate rhythm not only with remarkable efficiency, but also at a speed that would not be possible through a metabolic-dependent pathway.

Conclusion

The term "pacemaker" refers to the involvement of the current i_f in the generation of the diastolic depolarization phase of the action potential, which is responsible for spontaneous activity in pacemaker cells. This involvement was apparent since the current was first described in the SA node,[20] and its identity with the pacemaker current in Purkinje fibers, previously incorrectly described in terms of a pure K current,[29] was clarified. The view that i_f activation is the leading process in the generation of diastolic depolarization in SA node myocytes has recently received substantial experimental support. For example, it has been shown that the threshold of current activation, although variable, is usually in the range of -35 to -40 mV,[31] far less negative than previously thought.[32] Further, the very existence in the pacemaker range of a net inward background current sufficiently large to contribute significantly to diastolic depolarization has been questioned.[33] The latter is a necessary condition for the hypothesis that the decay of the current i_{Kl} is a key process in the generation of the pacemaker depolarization.[34] A further important observation in the assessment of the role of i_f in pacemaking relates to its modulation by neurotransmitters. As originally found,[20] i_f is modified by adrenaline in a way compatible with its being responsible for the positive chronotropic action of catecholamines. It should be noted that the "i_K-decay" hypothesis would be unable to explain the acceleration caused by catecholamines. Indeed, it is known that adrenaline increases i_{Kl},[35,36] a process that would lead to a rate slowing if i_{Kl} decay was the process responsible for generation of the diastolic depolarization.

The ACh-dependence of i_f reviewed here adds further consistency to the hypothesis that i_f activation is the main process responsible for the generation and control of the diastolic depolarization. For example, if the current i_f had little role in contributing to the diastolic depolarization under normal conditions, it would not be possible to slow spontaneous rhythm by a specific inhibition of i_f. The evidence that low concentrations of ACh specifically inhibiting i_f are capable of reducing the pacemaker depolarization rate confirms the relevance of i_f activation as a key process in the generation of this phase. Thus, the i_f properties appear to be specifically designed for the generation and neurotransmitter-mediated control of the diastolic depolarization rate and, consequently, of spontaneous rhythm.

In conclusion, the classical concept that vagal modulation of rate is mediated by a K conductance needs to be reconsidered in the light of the finding that the pacemaker i_f current is modulated by ACh. The evidence that the same low doses of ACh that inhibit i_f, without activating $i_{K,ACh}$ or modifying the Ca current, have a marked slowing action on rate implies that the modulating action of ACh is specifically mediated by i_f in the low concentration range.

Under normal conditions, vagal tone prevails. In this case, the ACh concentrations involved are low and the only current system that is likely to be involved in underlying vagal control of rate is i_f. Like all biochemical reactions mediated by second messengers, modulation via cyclic AMP is highly efficient and, in the light of the recent findings that cyclic AMP regulates i_f channels directly,[30] fast. According to this assumption, activation of the K conductance at higher ACh concentrations would intervene only under conditions of a strong vagal discharge, possibly during an emergency, during which rate slowing would be accompanied by depressed excitability. In accordance with this point of view, it is interesting to note that the coupling between the mAChR and K channel is directly operated by G-proteins,[37,38] with a mechanism that ensures a very quick, albeit not highly efficient modulation.

References

1. Burgen ASV, Terroux KG: On the negative inotropic effect in cat's auricle. J Physiol (Lond) 120:449, 1953.
2. Hoffman BF, Suckling EE: Cardiac cellular potentials: Effect of vagal stimulation and acetylcholine. Am J Physiol 173:312, 1953.
3. del Castillo J, Katz B: Production of membrane potential changes in the frog's heart by inhibitory nerve impulses. Nature 175:1035, 1955.
4. Hutter O, Trautwein W: Vagal and sympathetic effects on the pacemaker fibres in the sinus venosus of the heart. J Gen Physiol 39:715, 1956.
5. Giles W, Noble SJ: Changes in membrane currents in bullfrog atrium produced by acetylcholine. J Physiol (Lond) 261:103, 1976.
6. Ten Eick R, Nawrath H, McDonald TF, et al: On the mechanism of the negative inotropic effect of acetylcholine. Pflügers Arch 361:207, 1976.
7. Ikemoto Y, Goto M: Nature of the negative inotropic effect of acetylcholine on the myocardium: An elucidation on the bullfrog atrium. Proc Japan Acad 51:501, 1975.
8. Garnier D, Nargeot J, Ojeda C, et al: The action of acetylcholine on background conductance in frog atrial trabeculae. J Physiol (Lond) 274:381, 1978.
9. Carmeliet E, Mubagwa K: Changes by acetylcholine of membrane currents in rabbit cardiac Purkinje fibres. J Physiol (Lond) 371:201, 1986.

10. Hartzell CH, Simmons MA: Comparison of effects of acetylcholine on calcium and potassium currents in frog atrium and ventricle. J Physiol (Lond) 389:411, 1987.
11. Boyett MR, Kirby MS, Orchard CH, et al: The negative inotropic effect of acetylcholine on ferret ventricular myocardium. J Physiol (Lond) 404:613, 1988.
12. Bouman LN, Gerlings ED, Biersteker A: Electrical activity of the sino-auricolar node during vagal stimulation. Acta Physiol Pharmacol (Netherlands) 12:282, 1963.
13. Noma A, Trautwein W: Relaxation of the ACh-induced potassium current in the rabbit sino-atrial node. Pflügers Arch 377:193, 1978.
14. Hartzell HC: Adenosine receptors in frog sinus venosus: Slow inhibitory potentials produced by adenine compounds and acetylcholine. J Physiol (Lond) 293:23, 1979.
15. Sakmann B, Noma A, Trautwein W: Acetylcholine activation of single muscarinic K channels in isolated pacemaker cells of the mammalian heart. Nature 303:250, 1983.
16. Shibata EF, Giles W, Pollack GH: Threshold effects of acetylcholine on primary pacemaker cells of the rabbit sino-atrial node. Proc R Soc Lond (Biol) 223:355, 1985.
17. DiFrancesco D, Tromba C: Acetylcholine inhibits activation of the cardiac pacemaker current, i_f. Pflügers Arch 410:139, 1987.
18. DiFrancesco D, Tromba C: Inhibition of the hyperpolarizing-activated current, i_f, induced by acetylcholine in rabbit sino-atrial node myocytes. J Physiol (Lond) 405:477, 1988.
19. DiFrancesco D, Tromba C: Muscarinic control of the hyperpolarizing-activated current i_f in rabbit sino-atrial node myocytes. J Physiol (Lond) 405:493, 1988.
20. Brown HF, DiFrancesco D, Noble SJ: How does adrenaline accelerate the heart? Nature 280:235, 1979.
21. DiFrancesco D, Ducouret P, Robinson RB: Muscarinic modulation of cardiac rate at low acetylcholine concentrations. Science 243:669, 1989.
22. Tsien RW: Effect of epinephrine on the pacemaker potassium current of cardiac Purkinje fibres. J Gen Physiol 64:293, 1974.
23. DiFrancesco D, Ferroni A, Mazzanti M, et al: Properties of the hyperpolarizing-activated current (i_f) in cells isolated from the rabbit sino-atrial node. J Physiol (Lond) 377:61, 1986.
24. Hartzell HC: Regulation of cardiac ion channels by catecholamines, acetylcholine and second messenger systems. Prog Biophys Mol Biol 52:165, 1988.
25. Chang F, Gao J, Tromba C, et al: Acetylcholine reverses effects of β-agonists on pacemaker current in canine Purkinje fibres but has no direct action. Circ Res 66:633, 1990.
26. DiFrancesco D: A study of the ionic nature of the pacemaker current in calf Purkinje fibres. J Physiol (Lond) 314:377, 1981.
27. Hirst GDS, Edwards FR, Bramich NJ, et al: Neural control of cardiac pacemaker potentials. News Physiol Sci 6:185, 1991.
28. DiFrancesco D: The hyperpolarization-activated current, i_f, and cardiac pacemaking. In MR Rosen, MJ Janse, AL Wit (eds): Cardiac Electrophysiology: A Textbook. Mount Kisco, NY, Futura Publishing Co, 1990, p. 117.
29. Brown HF, Denyer JC: Low-dose acetylcholine reduces calcium current in isolated sino-atrial node cells of rabbit. J Physiol (Lond) 410:65P, 1989.
30. DiFrancesco D, Tortora P: Direct activation of cardiac pacemaker channels by intracellular cyclic AMP. Nature 351:145, 1991.
31. DiFrancesco D, Noble D: The current i_f and its contribution to cardiac pacemaking. In JW Jacklet (ed): Neuronal and Cellular Oscillators. New York, Marcel Dekker, 1989, p. 31.
32. Yanagihara K, Irisawa H: Inward current activated during hyperpolarization in the rabbit sinoatrial node cell. Pflügers Arch 385:11, 1980.
33. DiFrancesco D: The contribution of the hyperpolarization-activated current (i_f) to the generation of spontaneous activity in rabbit sino-atrial node myocytes. J Physiol (Lond) 434:23, 1991.
34. Denyer JC, Brown HF: Pacemaking in rabbit isolated sino-atrial node cells during

Cs^+ block of the hyperpolarization-activated current i_f. J Physiol (Lond) 429:401, 1990.
35. Brown HF, DiFrancesco D: Voltage clamp investigations of membrane currents underlying pacemaker activity in rabbit sino-atrial node. J Physiol (Lond) 308:331, 1980.
36. Bennet P, Mckinney L, Begenisich T, et al: Adrenergic modulation of the delayed rectifier potassium channel in calf Purkinje fibres. Biophys J 49:839, 1986.
37. Pfaffinger PJ, Martin JM, Hunter DD, et al: GTP-binding proteins couple cardiac muscarinic receptors to a K channel. Nature 317:536, 1985.
38. Yatani A, Codina J, Brown AM, et al: Direct activation of mammalian atrial muscarinic potassium channels by GTP regulatory protein G_K. Science 235:207, 1987.

CHAPTER 14

Vagal Control of Atrioventricular Conduction

P. Martin

Both autonomic divisions richly innervate the atrioventricular (AV) nodal region of the heart.[1] Parasympathetic activity may profoundly alter AV conduction, especially on a beat-by-beat basis.[2] Although the AV node may also be quite sensitive to sympathetic regulation,[3,4] the vast majority of work, from the early part of this century through today, has focused on the vagal control of AV conduction time (AVCT).[5–7] The parasympathetic innervation of the AV nodal region is described in Ch. 2. This chapter begins by briefly discussing the electrophysiology of vagal activity and AV nodal function. It then describes the effects of continuous trains and brief bursts of vagal stimuli on AVCT, the complex interactions of AVCT responses with simultaneously changing heart periods, the phenomena of "fade" or desensitization of the AVCT responses to continuous vagal stimuli, vagal control of antegrade (A-V) versus retrograde (V-A) conduction times and, finally, vagal control of AVCT in man. This discussion is not an exhaustive review and, due to space limitations, many contributions to these topics are not cited as only key references have been supplied for each.

Electrophysiology of Vagal Effects

The electrophysiology of the autonomic effects on AV conduction is complex but is beginning to be understood. Vagal activity is expressed almost purely via muscarinic receptors (mAChRs). Atropine abolishes essentially all cardiac responses to acetylcholine (ACh).[8] ACh hyperpolarizes the cell membrane and flattens the phase 4 pacemaker potentials of both AV and sinoatrial (SA) nodal cells.[8] This action is the result of a large increase in an inwardly-rectifying K conductance, probably that responsible for the background current commonly designated I_{K1}, and a decrease in the inward pacemaker current, I_f.[8] ACh also reduces the action potential duration and amplitude in

From *Vagal Control of the Heart: Experimental Basis and Clinical Implications* edited by MN Levy, PJ Schwartz

cells of both nodes[9]; these effects are likely due to the muscarinic inhibition of the slow inward current, I_{Ca}.[8] These effects are not uniform throughout the AV node, however, but are much more pronounced in the central, N, region. This finding was recently shown using postganglionic vagal stimulation (PGVS) techniques by which the stimulation site could be localized to nodal areas of about 0.25 mm^2.[10]

Figure 1 illustrates a typical result. All panels of Figure 1 were obtained with identical PGVS parameters (including the onset time of the stimulus burst in the cardiac cycle, A-St), but at the three positions indicated by the stars. Panels 1e and 1f were recorded with the PGVS electrode in the atrio-nodal (AN) and nodal-His (NH) regions, respectively (open straight arrows), while panels 1a to 1d were recorded with the PGVS in the N region of the AV node. When the stimulating electrode was in the AN or the NH region, there was little effect on the overall AVCT or on the action potentials near to the electrode (panels 1e and 1f). The effects were pronounced, however, when the electrode was placed in the N region. Panels 1a to 1d were recorded from sites within the dotted area of Figure 1, a region about 1.5 to 2.5 mm long. When the PGVS (solid horizontal bar) was at the more posterior of the two N

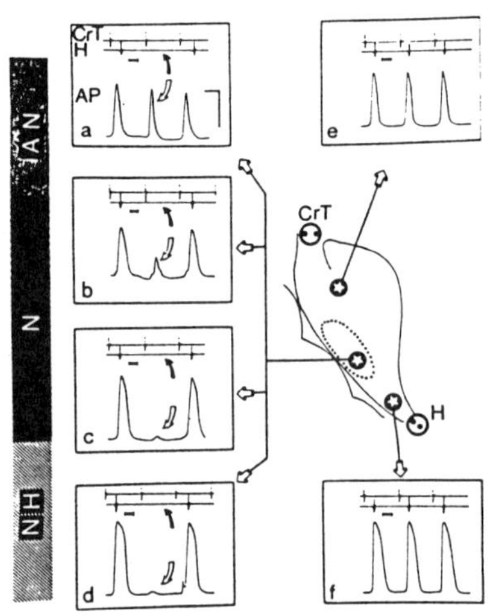

Figure 1. *Typical regional AV nodal electrophysiological responses to brief bursts of vagal stimuli. All panels were obtained with identical PGVS parameters (including the onset time of the stimulus burst in the cardiac cycle, A-St, indicated by the short horizontal bar below the H tracing in each panel), but with the stimulation electrode at the three positions indicated by the stars. The analog recordings in panels e and f were with the PGVS and recording electrodes in the AN and NH regions, respectively (open straight arrows), of the AV node. Panels a to d were with the PGVS in the N region, while panel a was recorded from the AN, panels b and c from the N, and panel d from the NH region. Calibration shown in panel a: horizontal, 200 msec; vertical, 50 mV (AP). Reproduced by permission of the American Heart Association, Inc. from Imaizumi S, Mazgalev T, Dreifus LS, et al: Morphological and electrophysiological correlates of atrioventricular nodal response to increased vagal activity. Circulation 82:955, 1990.*

recording sites (panel 1b), it markedly hyperpolarized phase 4, notched the action potential (open curved arrow), and blocked conduction (solid curved arrow). Stimulation at the more anterior N recording site (panel 1c) induced less hyperpolarization and only a local response (open curved arrow). This site was apparently just distal to the site of the AV nodal block (solid curved arrow). Stimulation at an AN recording site (panel 1a) had little effect. The small hyperpolarization was probably due to electrotonic influences of nearby depressed N cells (panels 1b and 1c). There was also only a little effect at the NH site (panel 1d) except for the predictable conduction block (curved arrows). Figure 1 illustrates the consistent finding that vagal stimuli[9] or ACh[11] have prepotent effects on action potentials and conduction times in the central N region of the AV node, and less or no effect in the more distal, transitional AN and NH regions.

The time in the cardiac cycle at which a vagal stimulus burst is given (A-St) is also an important determinant of the AV nodal cellular response. Figure 2 shows the effects of five different A-St intervals on the phase 4 potential of a cell in the N region.[12] The PGVS was given at the AV node only, and at A-St intervals of 0, 200, 300, 400, and 500 milliseconds (horizontal bars over the H tracing). The number 1 designates the control trace with no vagal stimulus, and the numbers 2 to 6 designate the corresponding traces from the order in which the His electrograms appeared. Note the great difference in the degree of hyperpolarization that occurred dependent upon the A-St interval. The dependency of the general AV nodal conduction time response on A-St is more fully developed below.

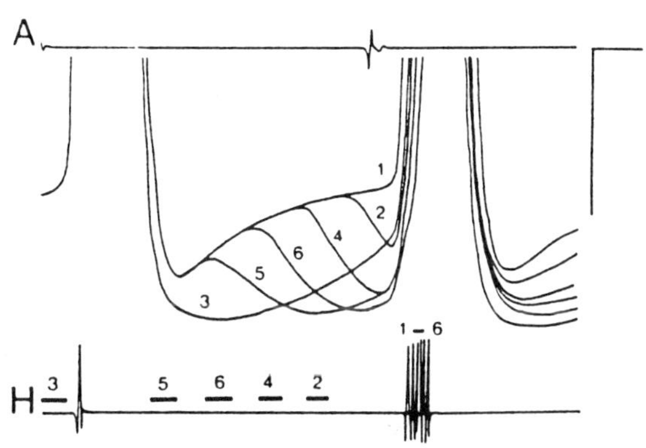

Figure 2. *The effect of five different A-St intervals on the phase 4 potential of a cell in the N region (same impalement, all superimposed recordings). The PGVS was given at the AV node only, and at A-St of 0, 200, 300, 400, and 500 msec (horizontal bars over the H tracing). The number 1 designates the control trace with no vagal stimulus, and the numbers 2 to 6 designate traces sequentially corresponding to the order in which the His electrograms appeared. Calibration marks are 100 msec horizontal, and 20 mV vertical (AP). Reproduced with permission from the American Physiological Society from Mazgalev T, Dreifus LS, Michelson EL, et al: Vagally induced hyperpolarization in atrioventricular node. Am J Physiol 251:H631–643, 1986.*

Effects of Vagal Nerve Stimulation on Atrioventricular Conduction Time

The right and left vagi have long been considered to innervate primarily the SA and AV nodes, respectively. The innervation, however, is more complex. It is useful to distinguish studies with continuous trains of vagal stimuli from those with only brief bursts of stimuli. In the unpaced heart, supramaximal trains of stimuli to various branches of the vagi induce bradydysrhythmias with fixed or changing degrees of heart block.[13] Although these responses are a monotonically increasing function of stimulus amplitude, AV conduction may be prolonged by 50% to 70% before block appears.[13–15] Continuous trains of supramaximal stimuli increase AVCT after a latency of less than one second.[14] Continuous trains of stimuli to the left vagus, but not the right, may induce second degree heart block in some dogs.[15]

From these findings, it was concluded that the AV node may comprise two physiologically separate areas. One area, innervated preferentially by the right vagus, determines the conduction velocity across the node. A second area, supplied preferentially by the left vagus, may completely block AV transmission.[15] This interpretation may be clouded, however, because the heart period (duration of the cardiac cycle) was not fixed while the AVCT was measured. As discussed below, heart period is a potent independent influence on AV conduction, so the pure effect of vagal stimulation alone must be studied without concomitant changes in heart period.

In recent years, most studies of the vagal control of AV conduction have employed brief bursts of stimuli, rather than continuous trains. A prime reason is that spontaneous efferent activity in vivo occurs as discrete bursts of nerve impulses (where the bursts are correlated with systolic pressure pulses).[16] Further, since the transient effects of vagal stimuli can appear and decay so rapidly (within about 200 milliseconds and about a second, respectively[17]), the dynamics of vagal nerve ending processes and their electrophysiological effects can only be studied well with the use of brief vagal bursts. The entire time-course of the AVCT response to a brief vagal burst may be less than just the latency period alone of the AVCT response to a brief burst of sympathetic activity.[18] If the pure AV nodal responses to brief vagal activity alone are sought, however, it is important to fix the heart period. When the heart was not paced, it was found that the AVCT responses to brief vagal bursts were very variable, i.e., the responses could increase or decrease, depending on the timing of the stimulus burst in the cardiac cycle.[18] This variability was ascribed to the interaction of vagal activity and the effects on AVCT of concomitant, rapid changes in heart period. When the heart period was fixed and brief vagal bursts reapplied, AVCT only increased.[19]

The "vagal effect curve" is a useful tool for the analysis of AVCT responses to brief vagal stimuli. These curves indicate the time-course of the composite of the responses to many stimulus bursts, i.e., the time history of the vagal effect on AVCT. Figure 3 is a typical example of three such curves recorded in our laboratory, where each curve was derived under identical circumstances, but

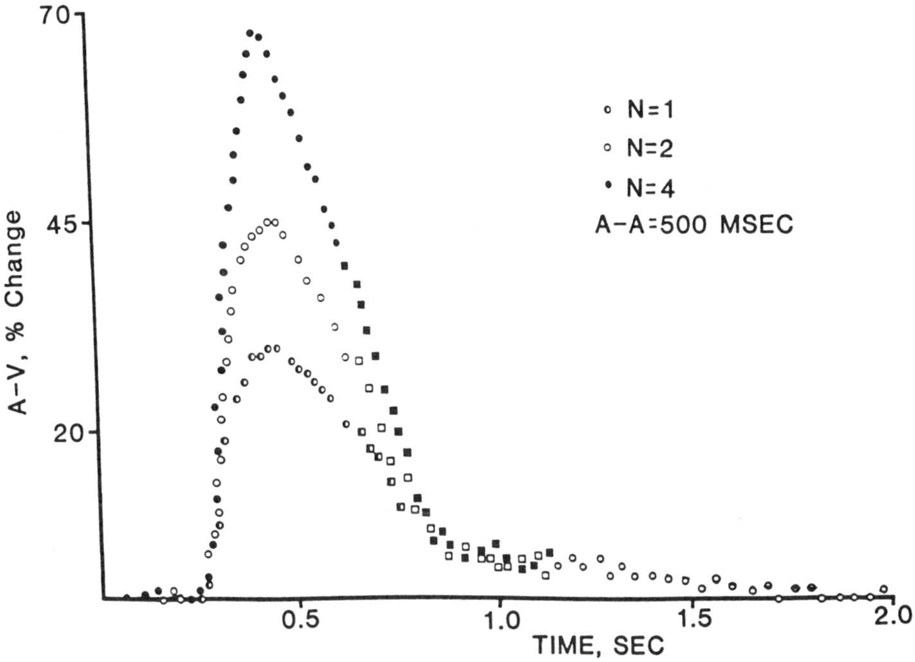

Figure 3. *Typical vagal effect curve for three levels of vagal stimuli (N = 1, 2, and 4 stimuli/burst) when the heart was paced at an A-A interval of 500 msec. Curve indicates the time-course of the composite of the responses to many stimulus bursts, i.e., the time history of the vagal effect on AVCT. The x-axis represents the time that has elapsed since a brief vagal stimulus has been given. The y-axis represents the beat-to-beat (percent) changes in AVCT following such a stimulus. (This figure represents original data of the author.)*

with a different stimulus intensity level (number of stimuli/burst). The x-axis represents the time that has elapsed since a brief vagal stimulus has been given. The y-axis represents the beat-to-beat changes in AVCT following such a stimulus. Each stimulus burst contributes three to five points to the complete curve, and the data points from a single stimulus burst are separated from each other by about one heart period along the time axis.

These curves clearly indicate that the AVCT response depends strongly on the phase of the stimulus, i.e., the time in the cardiac cycle at which the stimulus occurs. For example, note in Figure 3 that there is no detectable response for the first 200 to 250 milliseconds after the stimulus. The response rises rapidly thereafter, and reaches a peak at about 450 to 550 milliseconds after the stimulus. It is largely complete by about 1 second after the stimulus. Thus, if a stimulus burst occurs less than about 200 milliseconds before the AV node is excited, there is no effect on that very next AVCT. But the subsequent AVCT is prolonged maximally if the stimulus occurs about 500 milliseconds before the next AV nodal excitation in a paced heart. Thus, the time-course of the AVCT response to parasympathetic activity has a rapid onset and a slower decay, but the whole response is rapid enough to permit beat-to-beat control, e.g., via the baroreceptor reflex or central mechanisms.[19]

Interactions of Heart Period and Vagal Activity on Atrioventricular Conduction

Only in recent years have we gained a quantitative appreciation of the strength of the interaction between dynamically changing heart periods and vagal activity on AVCT. Continuous trains of vagal stimuli, in the unpaced cat heart, had the greatest effect on AVCT at low stimulus amplitude levels, where the chronotropic effect was weakest.[20] At high amplitude levels, where the chronotropic effect was greatest, AVCT was actually less (conduction was faster) than control. Thus, it was concluded that the degree of vagal inhibition of AVCT strongly depends on the concomitant chronotropic response.[20] The AVCT response to a step-wise change in atrial pacing rate can be described as a single exponential. The time constant of this exponential increased by a factor of four as the frequency of vagal stimulation increased from 0 to 10 Hz.[21] Further, this increase in time constant was independent of sympathetic activity, and changes in conduction through atrial and ventricular tissue played no role; i.e., the phenomenon represented purely a vagal-AV nodal interaction.[21]

Brief vagal stimuli was used to characterize the dynamic interaction between vagal activity and heart period.[22] We first obtained a vagal effect curve for AVCT when the heart was not paced (Fig. 4, curve U). This finding represents the combined effect of vagal activity and dynamically changing heart periods on AVCT. Note that the AVCT response to vagal stimulus bursts is considerably faster than control during certain times after the stimulus (the two large negative excursions of curve U of Fig. 4). We also stored in the computer the simultaneous changes in heart period (Fig. 4, curve AA) that occurred with this set of vagal stimuli. The heart was then paced at a fixed rate and identical vagal stimulus parameters were used to obtain a second vagal effect curve (Fig. 4, curve P). This curve represents the sole effect of vagal activity on AVCT, and it is purely an inhibitory response (curve P of Fig. 4 is positive). The changing A-A intervals were then used (Fig. 4, curve AA), previously stored as curve U of Figure 4, to pace the heart and measure the AVCT responses, but now in the absence of any vagal activity. This action yielded another curve, called the Playback curve (Fig. 4, curve PB), which represents the pure effect of rapid changes in heart period alone on AVCT.

Note particularly that the excursions of curve U are considerably more negative than those of curve PB. This finding was termed a paradoxical response, because under these conditions, AV conduction was actually faster with vagal activity than without! A new curve, called the Difference curve (Fig. 4, curve D), was next derived by subtracting the unpaced from the paced responses (curve U from curve P). The direct vagal effect was presumably the same for both curves. After such an algebraic subtraction, therefore, the only effect on AVCT remaining should be that of the rapidly changing heart periods. Thus, if the relation between vagal activity and heart period were linear, the Playback and Difference curves should be identical. Curves PB and D are clearly different over most of the time axis of Figure 4, and this finding was

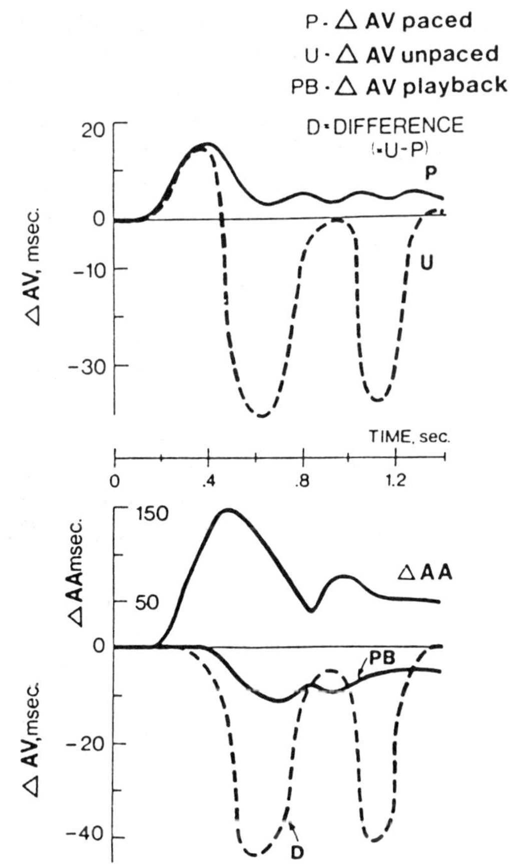

Figure 4. *Vagal effect curves with the same stimulus parameters and from the same dog, but under different pacing conditions. Upper panel: Vagal effect curves for the paced and unpaced hearts (curves P and U). Lower panel: Vagal effect curve for heart period (curve AA) measured at the same time as curve U in upper panel. Playback curve (curve PB) measures AVCT in response to dynamic changes in A-A intervals only, with no vagal stimuli. Difference curve (curve D) is derived by algebraically subtracting the curve of the paced heart from that of the unpaced heart preparation (see text). Reproduced by permission of the American Heart Association, Inc. from Martin P: Paradoxical dynamic interaction of heart period and vagal activity on atrioventricular conduction in the dog. Circ Res 40:84–85, 1977.*

true for the composite data as well. We thus concluded that there is a nonlinear dynamic interaction prevailing between vagal activity and heart period. Further work led us to postulate that shifting pacemaker sites, changing atrial activation patterns, and specific properties of AV nodal function could all contribute to the paradoxical response.[22]

More recent studies have shown that AVCT depends very clearly on the atrial pacing site. Shifting the pacing site by only one cm may result in a consistent heart block and AV nodal accommodation (slow continuous change in AVCT after a step change in pacing interval).[23] AVCT and, particularly, AV nodal accommodation may also depend on the level and direction of the change of heart period, on the pacing-induced release of neurotransmitters,[23] and on the direction and mode of entry of the atrial impulse to the AV node.[24] Any of these factors may interact with the pure vagal inhibition of AVCT.

The rate-dependent properties of AV nodal transmission can be ascribed to three physiological processes: AV nodal recovery, facilitation, and fatigue. Each of these is subject to vagal modulation.[25] AV nodal recovery is also referred to as the effective refractory period and is measured with the extrastimulus technique of inserting a premature S2 stimulus after a steady train of S1 stimuli. Pacing intervals are measured as A-A intervals, and AVCT is measured by the atrial-His (A-H) interval. The relationship that defines AV nodal recovery is derived by making S2 progressively more premature, i.e., by shortening the A_1-A_2 interval, and measuring the resultant A_2-H_2 interval. This functional dependence is usually characterized by plotting A_2-H_2 as a function of H_1-A_2, as indicated by the solid line in the lower panel of Figure 5.

Facilitation is a process by which a first premature beat, A_2, may actually decrease the AVCT for a subsequent premature beat, A_3. For example, an A_2 may result in a leftward shift of the AV Recovery Time curve (A_3-H_3 versus H_2-A_3, dot-dash curve of lower panel of Fig. 5). Fatigue is a slow increase in AVCT, over several minutes, induced by a sudden decrease in A_1-A_1 intervals at a constant His-atrial (H-A) interval (dashed curve, lower panel of Fig. 5). Because H-A is maintained constant, fatigue is independent of the AV nodal recovery process. The total vagal effect on AVCT can thus be broken down into four components:

1. an increase due to delayed recovery (increase in the effective refractory period);
2. an increase due to less facilitation (reduced leftward shift of the recovery characteristic);
3. increased fatigue; and
4. a tonic component that is independent of any of the above.[25]

The proportion that each of these components contributes to the total vagal effect is shown in the upper panel of Figure 5. Thus, in the results of the lower panel of Figure 5, vagal stimulation increased AVCT (A-H interval) by about 25 milliseconds for all A-H intervals greater than about 500 milliseconds. As H-A decreased, the vagal effect increased, until at an H-A interval of about 120 milliseconds, the vagal effect had been amplified by over fivefold.[25] This amplification of the vagal effect at shorter coupling intervals has some important implications for the vagal modulation of arrhythmias, as discussed below.

A related phenomenon involving extrastimuli is the so-called AV nodal "gap." This phenomenon refers to the paradoxical behavior whereby AV conduction of atrial impulses with a certain coupling interval are blocked (the gap), while those with a shorter interval are actually conducted. This gap behavior is markedly influenced by brief vagal stimuli.[26] Figure 6 illustrates the phenomenon. Panels a and b are analog tracings from a cell in the N region

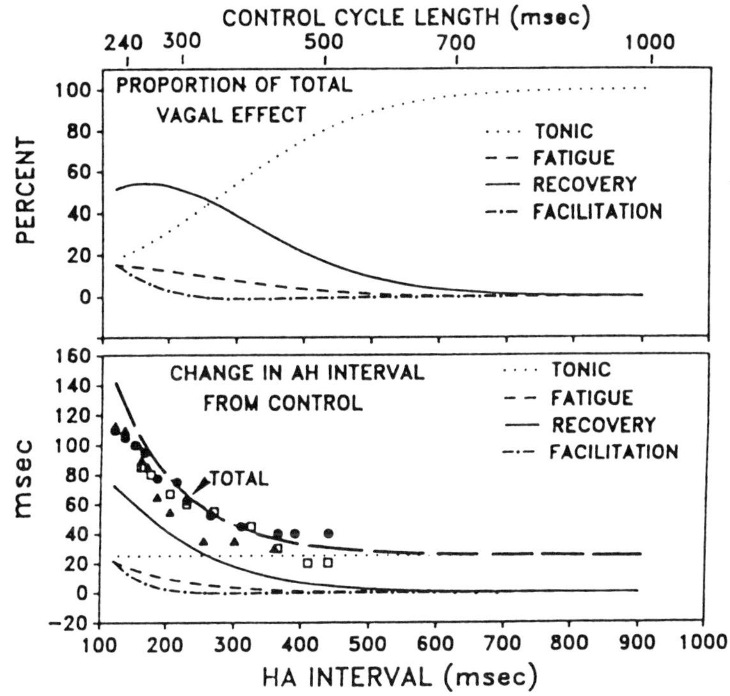

Figure 5. *Bottom panel: The effects of vagal activity on changes in the AH interval due to the nodal mechanisms of fatigue, recovery, and facilitation. The various lines are the contributions due to the three mechanisms postulated by the model, while each set of symbols is from an individual experiment. Top panel: The proportion of the total vagal effect due to each of the mechanisms, plus a tonic effect, varies with the steady-state HA intervals. Reproduced by permission of the American Heart Association, Inc. from Nayebpour M, Talajic M, Villemaire C, et al: Vagal modulation of the rate-dependent properties of the atrioventricular node. Circ Res 67:1152–1166, 1990.*

(AP) where the coupling interval has been increased from 200 to 500 milliseconds. The PGVS burst (horizontal bar above the His recordings) was delivered at a phase of 100 and 200 milliseconds, respectively, in panels a and b. Panel c shows the corresponding AV nodal conduction curves (A_2-H_2 versus A_1-A_2). The gaps in conduction are indicated by the lack of His potentials in panels a and b, and by the shaded portions of panel c. Note that the gap in panel a (for A_1-A_2 of 250 to 400 milliseconds) is much larger than in panel b (for A_1-A_2 of 380 to 420 milliseconds). Thus, not only the presence but also the specific characteristics of the vagal stimuli are important.

Figure 7 proposes a model to explain this phenomenon.[26] The curve with connected stars (Fig. 7) is the normal refractory characteristic relating an inverse measure of excitability (e.g., conduction time) to prematurity. The curve connecting the circles represents the bell-shaped time-course of the vagally-induced depression of excitability, and the solid curve is the summation of these two effects. AV nodal block occurs when the threshold of excitability exceeds some critical value (the dotted line). The left region of

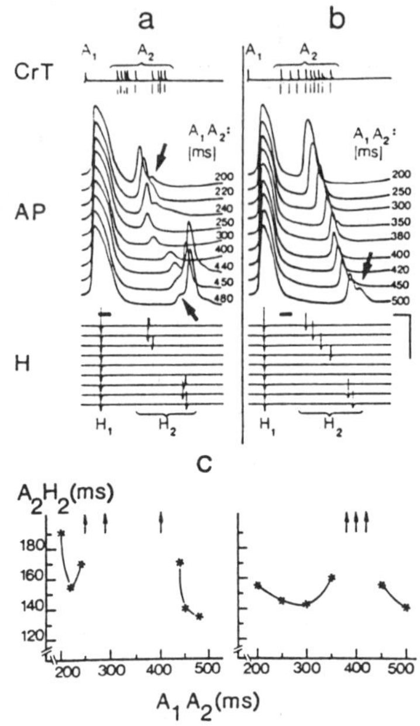

Figure 6. *The effect of brief vagal stimulus bursts (short horizontal bars above the His [H] tracings) on the AV nodal gap phenomenon at different A-St intervals (panel a, 100 msec; panel b, 200 msec). The crista terminalis (CrT) tracings are superimposed. Action potentials (AP) were recorded from the same N cell in all tracings. The number to the right of each AP tracing indicates the A_1-A_2 coupling interval. Panel c shows the corresponding AV nodal conduction curves, where the gap is indicated by the arrows. Reproduced by permission of the American Heart Association, Inc. from Mazgalev T, Dreifus LS, Michelson EL: A new mechanism for atrioventricular nodal gap—vagal modulation of conduction. Circulation 79:417–430, 1989.*

block is the expected block due to the absolute refractory properties of AV nodal conduction. The right region of block is due to the combined relative refractoriness and the vagal effect, where this combination is manifest over the shaded region of A_1-A_2 values, the gap.

In a recent study of the interaction of heart period and vagal activity on AV conduction, the nerve branches that separately innervate the SA and AV nodes were stimulated.[27] These discrete intrapericardial branches were then inactivated separately to demonstrate that the vagal control of SA and of AV nodes may be independent.[27] Building on this work, parasympathetic ganglia were stimulated in the right pulmonary vein fat pad (PVFP). These ganglia send fibers to the SA node and little or none to the AV node.[28] We also stimulated ganglia at the junction of the inferior vena cava-inferior left atrium (IVC-ILA). These ganglia innervate selectively the AV node with little or no crossover to the SA node. Separate vagal control of SA and AV nodal function could thus be elicited. Our results suggested that the direct depression of AVCT by vagal stimulation is attenuated by prolongation of the heart period when that prolongation is induced by independent vagal activity to the SA

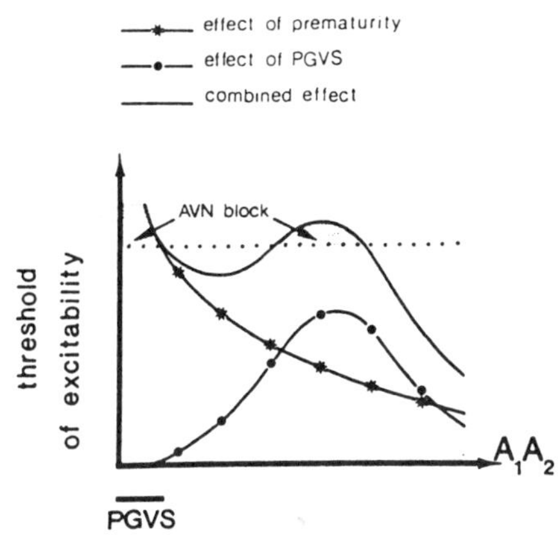

Figure 7. *A model proposed to explain the effects of vagal activity on the gap phenomenon. The curve connecting the stars is the normal AV nodal refractory characteristic. The curve connecting the circles represents the time-course of the depression of excitability due to the vagal effect, and the solid curve is the summation of these two effects. The vagal stimulus burst is assumed to have been given at the origin of the time axis. Reproduced by permission of the American Heart Association, Inc. from Mazgalev T, Dreifus LS, Michelson EL: A new mechanism for atrioventricular nodal gap—vagal modulation of conduction. Circulation 79:417–430, 1989.*

node.[29] Furthermore, this attenuation reflects some mechanisms that are independent of the phase of the vagal stimulus in the cardiac cycle, and also other mechanisms that are phase-dependent.

Progressive Depression of the Atrioventricular Nodal Responses to Vagal Stimuli

We found that the magnitude of the AVCT response to a brief vagal burst depended very strongly on the time that had elapsed since any prior vagal activity.[30] Figure 8 illustrates the beat-by-beat AVCT responses to a series of identical brief vagal stimulus bursts. The peak magnitudes of the AVCT responses to the first and second stimulus bursts are designated P_1 and P_2, respectively. The numbers to the left of each tracing indicate the time that had elapsed between the two stimulus bursts, and the numbers to the right of each tracing indicate the ratio P_2/P_1. The ratio is minimum when the time between stimuli was about five seconds. Note, however, that when the stimuli are very close, the ratio may actually exceed unity. This result is probably due to the nonlinear addition of the effects of the AVCT response to ACh with the effects of the local concentration of ACh that remains from a prior stimulus.[19] This nonlinear additive effect may thus mask a more severe depression than is actually reflected by the P_2/P_1 ratio that prevails at the shortest times between the two stimulus bursts. It may be presumed that about four to five seconds after a stimulus burst, virtually all local ACh has been inactivated.[19] Therefore, from 4 to 5 seconds to about 60 seconds, the effect of the first stimulus only

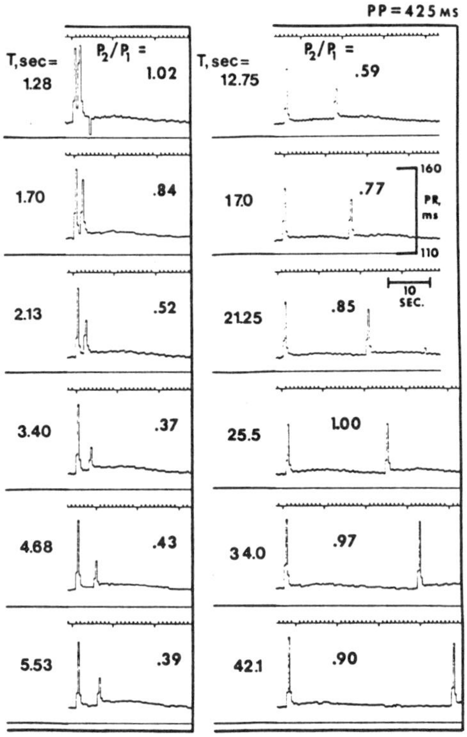

Figure 8. *The AV nodal response to a brief vagal stimulus burst depends upon the recent past history of vagal activity. The tracings in each panel show the beat-by-beat AVCT responses to successive, identical brief vagal stimulus bursts. The peak magnitudes of the AVCT responses to the first and second stimulus bursts are designated P_1 and P_2, respectively. The numbers to the left of each analog tracing indicate how much time in seconds have elapsed between the two identical stimulus bursts, and the numbers to the right of each tracing indicate the ratio P_2/P_1. Reproduced by permission of the American Heart Association, Inc. from Martin P: Depression of atrioventricular sensitivity in the dog by successive brief bursts of vagal stimulation. Circ Res 38:448–453, 1976.*

inhibits the effect of the second. This depression of the effects of a second stimulus by a first, for a given preparation, is independent of the absolute magnitude of P_1, no matter how that amplitude is changed (stimulus intensity or phase). The P_2/P_1 ratio is also invariant, after appropriate normalizations, when the vagus nerve from one side is used to evoke P_1 and the vagus from the other side is used to evoke P_2. From these data, it was concluded that the mechanism that gradually depresses AV sensitivity lies in changes of ACh inactivation, receptor sensitivity, or effector responsiveness, but not in mechanisms purely associated with the synthesis, storage, or release of ACh.[30] We subsequently determined that cardiac inotropic and chronotropic responses to a similar regimen of variably spaced stimulus bursts exhibited a nearly identical pattern of depression of the P_2/P_1 ratio.[31] Thus, this phenomenon is not unique for the vagal effects on conduction velocity, but is probably associated with the action of ACh on the cell membrane rather than on intracellular processes.

A related phenomenon may also be elicited by continuous vagal stimulation. When steady stimulus trains are applied to the vagi, the rapid initial increase in heart period is usually followed by a more gradual return of the response back toward control until some final steady-state elevation of heart period is attained.[32] Loeb et al[32] did not observe a "fading " of the AVCT responses to similar trains of vagal stimuli. They thus concluded that mAChR behavior may be different at the SA and AV nodes. We subsequently observed that, after the initial rapid depression, slow secondary changes in the inotropic[33] and dromotropic[34] responses could be elicited. Figure 9 illustrates this behavior for AVCT. Panels A, B, and C of Figure 9 indicate that, at least for the AV node, the phenomenon is more complex than a simple "fading" of the response back toward control, e.g., as might be produced by slow receptor desensitization. Although panel C does show such a fade, under some conditions the response may actually increase slowly (panel A), or only show a small secondary change (panel B).

We concluded that two opposing mechanisms may be responsible for the slow secondary changes in the dromotropic responses to a sudden sustained increase in vagal activity. The first mechanism may involve receptor desensitization and resembles the fade of other cardiac responses. The second, opposing mechanism involved in the slow secondary augmentation of the dromotropic responses may be related to the diffusion of ACh into the AV nodal region from surrounding atrial tissue, or to a slow cumulative change in AV nodal refractoriness.[34]

Loeb and deTarnowsky subsequently infused ACh into the AV nodal artery at concentrations sufficient to cause various degrees of heart block, and they found that these changes were maintained for the duration of the infusions.[35] They did not observe any fade of the near-maximal AV nodal responses to maintained ACh infusion. They again concluded that ACh affects chronotropic and dromotropic responses differently. Salata et al,[36] however, recorded action potentials from an isolated, rabbit AV node treated with verapamil. They found that the hyperpolarization induced by brief vagal

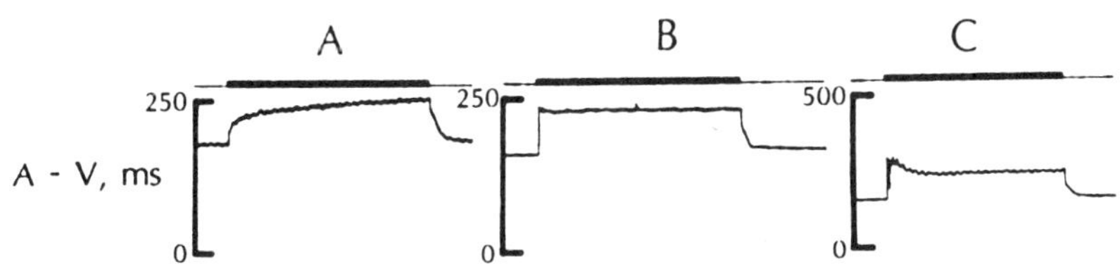

Figure 9. *Three different types of slow secondary AVCT responses to continuous trains of vagal stimuli. Stimulus trains were applied for 5 min in each panel. The response types in panels A, B, and C represent 62%, 20%, and 18%, respectively of the total. Note that the AVCT scale in C is half the sensitivity of A and B. Reproduced with permission from the American Physiological Society from Martin P: Secondary AV conduction responses during tonic vagal stimulation. Am J Physiol 245:H584-H591, 1983.*

stimuli faded with a time-course similar to that of the SA nodal responses. These workers thus suggested that fade was characteristic of AV dromotropic responses, at least at the stimulus levels they employed. Thus, although the fades of chronotropic and inotropic responses are similar and predictable, the slow secondary changes of dromotropic responses seem more complex and are not so predictable. The receptor dynamics may be different at the AV node, and the dromotropic responses may vary more with the experimental conditions.

Vagal Control of Antegrade and Retrograde Conduction

V-A conduction through the AV node is almost always slower than A-V conduction in all species studied.[37–41] Several mechanisms bear on this finding:

1. the functional refractory period is longer for V-A than for A-V conduction[37];
2. the effective path length is different in the two directions, i.e., the functional boundary between the AV node and atrium shifts with the direction of propagation[38];
3. A-V wavefronts may accelerate as they pass through certain regions of the AV node, whereas V-A wavefronts decelerate[37];
4. nodal conduction depends on the characteristics of the incident excitation,[10,11,17,19,24–26,37–40] and wavefronts that arrive from the His bundle differ from those that arrive from the atrium; and
5. the asymmetric structure of the AV node may cause the longitudinal resistance to conduction to be higher in the V-A than in the A-V direction.[39]

It is not so clear, however, how the vagally-induced cholinergic depression of AVCT differs with the direction of propagation through the AV node. Such cholinergic effects are not clearly different for A-V and V-A conduction in the dog,[42] rabbit,[9] and human hearts.[43] Also, such cholinergic effects on V-A conduction exceed those on A-V conduction in man.[44] Finally, the effects on V-A conduction exceed those on A-V conduction in the rabbit heart.[38,45] In most of these studies, however, the methods (pharmacological blockade or ACh infusions) used to compare the A-V and V-A effects were indirect, or the ACh processes could have become saturated by the continuous trains of vagal stimuli that were used.

A recent study in isolated rabbit hearts clearly showed that brief vagal stimuli had a considerably greater direct effect on A-V than on V-A conduction.[38] It was reasoned that the vagus would depress conduction more severely in the V-A direction, because conduction was inherently more depressed. We therefore used brief vagal stimuli in an intact dog preparation to study this problem.[41] We found that the V-A conduction was depressed twice as much as

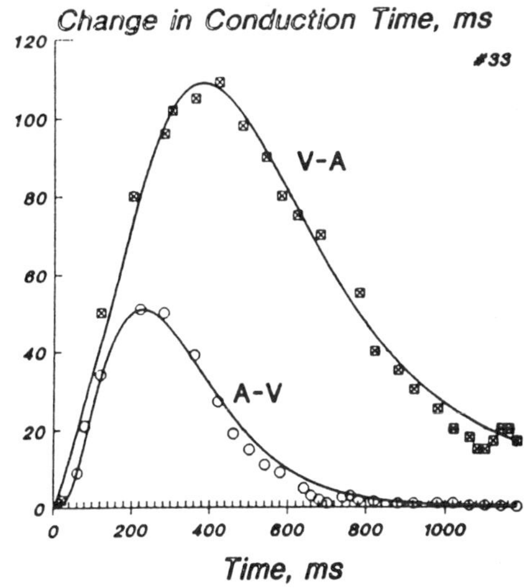

Figure 10. *Typical vagal effect curves for identical stimuli from one animal, but the heart was paced either in the A-V or V-A directions. Note that the latencies (pure time delays before any physiological effect is detectable, about 200 msec) have been subtracted out of these curves. This process makes fitting the curves with an analytic function (smooth lines) more practical. Reproduced with permission from the American Physiological Society from Martin PJ: Brief vagal stimuli and AV conduction in dogs: Effects on retrograde exceed antegrade. Am J Physiol 257:H812-H817, 1989.*

A-V conduction by vagal stimulation. This finding is illustrated by Figure 10, which is based on a typical animal, and it was verified by the composite data.[41] It was thus concluded that the cholinergic control of A-V and V-A conduction varies among species. The responses in the dog are perhaps closer to those of man. The general patterns of A-V and V-A responses in man are more similar to those in dogs than to those in rabbits.

Note also in Figure 10 that the time-courses of the descending portions of these curves appear to differ considerably. To check this finding, we normalized the composite V-A curve to the peak amplitude of the composite A-V curve, as shown in Figure 11, and analyzed it by fitting a single exponential function to the downslope of each curve. We found that the time constant for V-A conduction was 267 milliseconds, whereas that for A-V was 180 milliseconds ($p<.0001$). It was concluded from this study that factors other than diffusion and inactivation of ACh (which, presumably, should be the same for both A-V and V-A conduction) contribute importantly to the time-course of the effect of a given vagal stimulus burst on conduction through the AV node. Prior quantitative models of the vagal control of AVCT have assumed that the time-course of the vagal effect is very similar to the time-course of the local ACh concentration at the AV node.[19] These results indicate that additional factors, perhaps electrotonic effects on membrane processes, also affect the time-course of the vagal control of AVCT substantially.

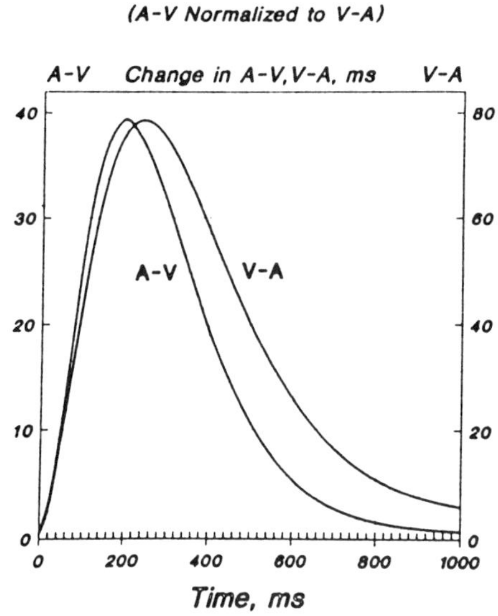

Figure 11. *Composite vagal effect curves for A-V and V-A conduction, but normalized for the same peak amplitude to show differences in curve widths and decay time-courses. Reproduced with permission from the American Physiological Society from Martin PJ: Brief vagal stimuli and AV conduction in dogs: Effects on retrograde exceed antegrade. Am J Physiol 257:H812-H817, 1989.*

Effects of Vagal Activity on Atrioventricular Conduction in Man

The vagal contribution to certain types of clinical arrhythmias is covered in other chapters of this book, but some aspects of the general topic will be discussed briefly here. Most studies of AV nodal responses to vagal activity in man have been indirect, i.e., by studying electrocardiographic P-R intervals during certain arrhythmias thought to be related to autonomic activity, or by drawing inferences from electrocardiograms after autonomic blockade. Paroxysmal block within the NH system has commonly been attributed to vagally-induced bradycardia.[46] Rardon and Bailey[47] noted that the vagus could influence the initiation or termination of certain arrhythmias, and that vagal tone or vagal stimulation could terminate certain ventricular tachycardias in man. Patients with abnormal AV nodal function may be more sensitive than others to vagal activity; i.e., the sensitivity of the AV node to a given vagal stimulus depends on the baseline state of AV nodal conduction.[48] The importance of a vagal contribution to certain arrhythmias was elegantly expounded by Moe et al,[49] who concluded that several types of conduction disturbances, particularly "supernormal conduction," could as well be directly ascribed to the effects of vagal activity. An analysis of clinical electrocardiograms recently led us to ascribe a potential role of brief bursts of vagal activity to the pathogenesis of several common types of conduction disturbances, including: ventriculophasic sinus arrhythmia with various degrees of AV block, various patterns of AV dissociation, prolongation of AV conduction after premature beats, supernormal AVCTs, Wenckebach periodicities, and alternation of AVCTs.[50] It was recently confirmed that an appropriately timed, brief vagal stimulus burst placed in each cardiac cycle in dogs could directly induce many patterns of Wenckebach periodicities.[51]

Two techniques developed in animals for the stimulation of efferent vagal nerve fibers may be used for studies in man. One of these is the use of a transvenous stimulating catheter in the right pulmonary artery. Efferent vagal fibers pass over this artery to the heart, and may be field-stimulated with the catheter.[52] The other technic involves placing a stimulus electrode over one of the two fat pads that contain the parasympathetic ganglia to the SA and AV nodes.[28] Preliminary data indicate that the latter technique, particularly, is effective in the operating room.[53] These technics may permit one to determine the applicability of much of the animal data to the vagal control of cardiac function in man.

References

1. Randall WC, Ardell JL: Differential innervation of the heart. In DP Zipes, J Jalife (eds): Cardiac Electrophysiology and Arrhythmias. New York, NY, Grune & Stratton, 1985, p. 137.
2. Warner MR, deTarnowsky JM, Whitson CC, et al: Beat-by-beat modulation of AV conduction. II. Autonomic neural mechanisms. Am J Physiol 251:H1134, 1986.
3. Randall WC, Ardell JL, O'Toole MJ, et al: Differential autonomic control of SAN and AVN regions of the canine heart: Structure and function. In T Mazgalev, LS Dreifus, EL Michelson (eds): Electrophysiology of the Sinoatrial and Atrioventricular Nodes. New York, NY, Alan R Liss Inc, 1988, p. 15.
4. Urthaler F, Neely BH, Hageman GR, et al: Differential sympathetic-parasympathetic interactions in sinus node and AV junction. Am J Physiol 250:H43, 1986.
5. Cohn AE, Lewis T: The predominant influence of the left vagus nerve upon conduction between the auricles and ventricles of the dog. J Exp Med 18:739, 1913.
6. Martin P: The influence of the parasympathetic nervous system on atrioventricular conduction. Circ Res 41:593, 1977.
7. Page RL, Tang ASL, Prystowsky EN: Effect of continuous enhanced vagal tone on atrioventricular nodal and sinoatrial nodal function in humans. Circ Res 68:1614, 1991.
8. Hewett KW: Membrane effects of muscarinic agonists. In MR Rosen, MJ Janse, AL Wit (eds): Cardiac Electrophysiology: A Textbook. Mount Kisco, NY, Futura Publishing Company Inc, 1990, p. 877.
9. West TC, Toda N: Response of the A-V node of the rabbit to stimulation of intracardiac cholinergic nerves. Circ Res 20:18, 1967.
10. Imaizumi S, Mazgalev T, Dreifus LS, et al: Morphological and electrophysiological correlates of atrioventricular nodal response to increased vagal activity. Circulation 82:951, 1990.
11. Tse WW: Suppressive effect of acetylcholine on action potentials of canine paranodal fibers. Am J Physiol 251:H710, 1986.
12. Mazgalev T, Dreifus LS, Michelson EL, et al: Vagally induced hyperpolarization in atrioventricular node. Am J Physiol 251:H631, 1986.
13. Hageman GR, Randall WC, Armour JA: Direct and reflex cardiac bradydysrhythmias from small vagal nerve stimulation. Am Heart J 89:338, 1975.

14. Irisawa H, Caldwell WM, Wilson MF: Neural regulation of atrioventricular conduction. Jpn J Physiol 21:15, 1971.
15. Hamlin RL, Smith CR: Effects of vagal stimulation on S-A and A-V nodes. Am J Physiol 215:560, 1968.
16. Jewett DL: Activity of single efferent fibers in the cervical vagus nerve of the dog, with reference to possible cardioinhibitory fibers. J Physiol (Lond) 175:321, 1964.
17. Spear JF, Moore EN: Influence of brief vagal and stellate nerve stimulation on pacemaker activity and conduction within the atrioventricular conduction system of the dog. Circ Res 32:27, 1973.
18. Levy MN, Martin PJ, Iano T, et al: The effects of single vagal stimuli on heart rate and atrioventricular conduction. Am J Physiol 218:1256, 1970.
19. Martin P: Dynamic vagal control of atrial-ventricular condition: Theoretical and experimental studies. Ann Biomed Eng 3:275, 1975.
20. Pavlov V: Dependence of the atrioventricular conduction on the cardiac rate upon increased vagal activity. Agressologie 16:9, 1975.
21. De Beer EL, Boom HBK, Naafs B: The combined influence of the stimulus frequency of the vagal nerves and the atrial stimulus interval on the atrioventricular conduction time. Cardiovasc Res 11:47, 1977.
22. Martin P: Paradoxical dynamic interaction of heart period and vagal activity on atrioventricular conduction in the dog. Circ Res 40:81, 1977.
23. Loeb JM, deTarnowsky JM: Modulation of atrioventricular conduction in vivo: Integration of heart rate and autonomic neural input. In T Mazgalev, LS Dreifus, EL Michelson (eds): Electrophysiology of the Sinoatrial and Atrioventricular Nodes. New York, NY, Alan R Liss Inc, 1988, p. 169.
24. Janse MJ: Influence of the direction of the atrial wave front on atrioventricular nodal transmission in isolated hearts of rabbits. Circ Res 25:439, 1969.
25. Nayebpour M, Talajic M, Villemaire C, et al: Vagal modulation of the rate-dependent properties of the atrioventricular node. Circ Res 67:1152, 1990.
26. Mazgalev T, Dreifus LS, Michelson EL: A new mechanism for atrioventricular nodal gap—vagal modulation of conduction. Circulation 79:417, 1989.
27. O'Toole MF, Ardell JL, Randall WC: Functional interdependence of discrete vagal projections to SA and AV nodes. Am J Physiol 251:H398, 1986.
28. Wallick DW, Martin PJ: Separate parasympathetic control of heart rate and atrioventricular conduction of dogs. Am J Physiol 259:H536, 1990.
29. Furukawa Y, Wallick DW, Carlson MD, et al: Prolongation of cardiac cycle length attenuates negative dromotropic response to selective vagal stimuli. J Auton Nerv Syst 28:43, 1989.
30. Martin P: Depression of atrioventricular sensitivity in the dog by successive brief bursts of vagal stimulation. Circ Res 38:448, 1976.
31. Martin P: Time-dependent heart period and contractility responses to successive brief vagal stimuli. Am J Physiol 239:H494, 1980.
32. Loeb JM, Dalton DP, Moran JM: Sensitivity differences of SA and AV node to vagal stimulation: Attenuation of vagal effects at SA node. Am J Physiol 241:H684, 1981.
33. Martin P, Levy MN, Matsuda Y: Fade of cardiac responses during tonic vagal stimulation. Am J Physiol 243:H219, 1982.
34. Martin P: Secondary AV conduction responses during tonic vagal stimulation. Am J Physiol 245:H584, 1983.
35. Loeb JM, deTarnowsky JM: Maintained prolongation of AV conduction time by acetylcholine. Eur J Pharmacol 100:351, 1984.
36. Salata J, Slenter VAJ, Jalife J: Biphasic decay of muscarinic response to acetylcholine in SA and AV nodes. Circulation 68(suppl III):III-154, 1983.
37. Akhtar MA, Damato AN, Batsford WP, et al: A comparative analysis of antegrade and retrograde conduction patterns in man. Circulation 52:766, 1975.
38. Mitsuoka T, Mazgalev T, Dreifus LS, et al: Differential vagal effects on antegrade vs. retrograde atrioventricular conduction. Am J Physiol 253:H1059, 1987.

39. Spach MS, Lieberman M, Scott JG, et al: Excitation sequences of the atrial septum and the AV node in isolated hearts of the dog and rabbit. Circ Res 29:156, 1971.
40. Zipes DP, Mendez C, Moe GK: Evidence for summation and voltage dependency in rabbit atrioventricular nodal fibers. Circ Res 32:170, 1973.
41. Martin PJ: Brief vagal stimuli and AV conduction in dogs: Effects on retrograde exceed antegrade. Am J Physiol 257:H812, 1989.
42. Urthaler FB, Neely BH, Hageman GR, et al: Differential sympathetic-parasympathetic interactions in sinus node and AV junction. Am J Physiol 250:H43, 1986.
43. Paparella NP, Albani B, Pirani R, et al: Effects of autonomic blockade on dual atrioventricular nodal pathways pattern. J Electrocardiol 19:269, 1986.
44. Mahmud RS, Denker ST, Lehmann MH, et al: Unidirectional retrograde atrioventricular nodal block in man: Determinants of reversibility by vagal antagonism. Am Heart J 110:568, 1985.
45. Hoffman BF, Paes de Carvalho A, DeMello WC, et al: Electrical activity of the atrio-ventricular node. Circ Res 7:11–18, 1959.
46. Zaman L, Moleiro F, Rozanski JJ, et al: Multiple electrophysiologic manifestations and clinical implications of vagally mediated AV block. Am Heart J 106:92, 1983.
47. Rardon DP, Bailey JC: Parasympathetic effects on electrophysiologic properties of cardiac ventricular tissue. J Am Coll Cardiol 2:1200, 1983.
48. Prystowsky EN, Page RL: Electrophysiology and autonomic influences of the human atrioventricular node. In T Mazgalev, LS Dreifus, EL Michelson (eds): Electrophysiology of the Sinoatrial and Atrioventricular Nodes. New York, NY, Alan R Liss, Inc, 1988, p. 259.
49. Moe GK, Childers RW, Merideth J: An appraisal of 'supernormal' A-V conduction. Circulation 38:5, 1968.
50. Jedlicka J, Martin P: Time course of vagal effects studied in clinical electrocardiograms. Eur Heart J 8:762, 1987.
51. Wallick DW, Martin PJ: Brief vagal bursts can induce Wenckebach arrhythmia. Am J Physiol 257:H935, 1989.
52. Cooper TB, Hageman GR, James TN, et al: Neural effects on sinus rate and atrioventricular conduction produced by electrical stimulation from a transvenous electrode catheter in the canine right pulmonary artery. Circ Res 46:48, 1980.
53. Carlson MD, Geha AS, Hsu J, et al: Selective stimulation of parasympathetic nerve fibers to the human sinoatrial node. Circulation 85:1311–1317, 1992.

CHAPTER 15

Vagal Control of Myocardial Contractility

M.N. Levy, A.J. Pappano

The predominant effect of the vagus nerves on myocardial contractility is inhibitory, although facilitatory effects may be observed. Furthermore, the vagus nerves exert disparate effects on the different chambers of the heart. The inhibitory effects on the atria are very potent in most vertebrate species, whereas the effects on the ventricles are usually less pronounced and they vary considerably among different classes of vertebrates. In most mammals, for example, the vagal influence on the ventricles is not very strong, whereas it is much more powerful in birds. In this chapter, the inhibitory effects of the vagus nerves on atrial and ventricular contractility are first considered, and then some of the facilitatory effects are discussed.

Vagal Inhibition of Atrial Contractility

Muscarinic Agonists

The powerful inhibitory effects of vagal activity and muscarinic agonists on atrial contractility have been recognized for over a century. The most detailed early studies were published by Gesell[1] in 1916 and by Wiggers[2] in 1917. Acetylcholine (ACh) and other muscarinic agonists hyperpolarize the resting cell membrane, markedly diminish the duration of the atrial action potential, and profoundly reduce the force of atrial contraction (Fig. 1).[3–7]

Muscarinic agonists decrease atrial contractile force partly because they diminish action potential duration and they reduce the Ca^{++} conductance of the atrial cell membranes.[4,8–10] The pronounced reduction in action potential duration allows less time for Ca^{++} influx into the cell during the abbreviated plateau, and the diminished Ca^{++} conductance permits less Ca^{++} influx per unit time. The decreased duration of the action potential is a consequence of

From *Vagal Control of the Heart: Experimental Basis and Clinical Implications* edited by MN Levy, PJ Schwartz

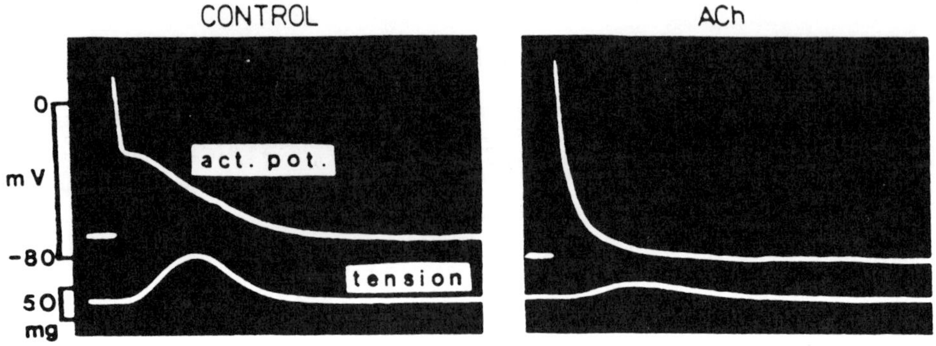

Figure 1. *The action potential (upper tracing) and contractile tension (lower tracing) recorded from a canine atrial fiber under control conditions (left panel) and in the presence of 2×10^{-6} M acetylcholine (ACh). Modified with permission from Ten Eick R, Nawrath H, McDonald TF, et al: On the mechanism of the negative inotropic effect of acetylcholine. Pflügers Arch 361:210, 1976.*

the activation of ACh regulated K^+ channels in the atrial cell membranes. The resulting outward K^+ current hastens repolarization. The impairment of Ca^{++} conductance probably operates mainly through the regulation of L-type Ca^{++} channels by the adenylyl cyclase (AC) system.

The effects of muscarinic agonists on Ca^{++} conductance are achieved by direct and indirect mechanisms.[5,6,8–10] The indirect mechanisms have been defined more completely. They involve a cholinergic antagonism of the concurrent facilitatory effects of any prevailing sympathoadrenal influences on the AC system. β-adrenergic agonists interact with β-adrenergic receptors (β-AR) to enhance AC activity via G_s proteins. This interaction elevates adenosine 3′5′-cyclic monophosphate (cyclic AMP) in the atrial myocytes, and thereby activates L-type Ca^{++} channels in the cell membranes. Muscarinic agonists, on the other hand, interact with muscarinic receptors (mAChRs) in the cell membranes to inhibit AC via G_i proteins, and thereby attenuate the rise in cyclic AMP evoked by the prevailing sympathoadrenal activity. Hence, muscarinic agonists would act indirectly by antagonizing the adrenergic effects on the membrane Ca^{++} channels. This mechanism is discussed in detail in Ch. 11.

The direct effects of muscarinic agonists on Ca^{++} conductance are those that might operate even if the intracellular cyclic AMP concentration was not elevated. The direct effects have not been elucidated as clearly or as convincingly as have the indirect effects. Evidence has been adduced that indicates that muscarinic agonists raise intracellular cyclic guanosine monophosphate (cGMP) concentrations, and that this nucleotide itself may diminish Ca^{++} influx into myocytes or it may act to reduce intracellular levels of cyclic AMP and, thereby, decrease Ca^{++} influx.[9,10] Contradictory results have also been obtained, however, and, therefore, the details of this mechanism remain controversial.[9–11]

Vagus Nerve Activity

The effects of vagus nerve activity on atrial contractility resemble those of exogenous ACh and other muscarinic agonists. Many investigators have documented the profound inhibitory effect of vagal stimulation on atrial contractile force or on atrial pressure generation.[12–19] Thus, augmented vagal activity diminishes the atrial contribution to ventricular filling.[18] Similarly, by weakening atrial contraction, increased vagal activity might impair the normal closure of the atrioventricular (AV) valves.[12,20,21]

The effect of vagal activity on atrial contraction is profound. Even a single electrical pulse to the vagus nerves can diminish vagal contraction by more than 50% and two or three pulses in rapid succession can reduce contraction by almost 100% (Fig. 2).[16] This negative inotropic effect of vagal activity is more pronounced the longer the cardiac cycle length (Fig. 2)[16]

The reason for the cycle length dependence of this negative inotropic influence has not been elucidated. The mechanism may be related, however, to an interaction between influences exerted by two types of K^+ channels: namely, the ACh-regulated K^+ channels and the K^+ channels that conduct the transient outward current, i_{to}. The ACh-regulated K^+ channels are abundant in atrial cell membranes.[7,8] Activation of these channels by neurally released ACh increases the outward K^+ current, $i_{K,ACh}$. Repolarization is thereby hastened and the action potential duration is abridged.[8]

The second K^+ channel that may contribute to this interaction is the channel that conducts i_{to}. This channel is also abundant in atrial myocytes, and it affects atrial action potential duration.[7,8] The outward K^+ current, i_{to}, that

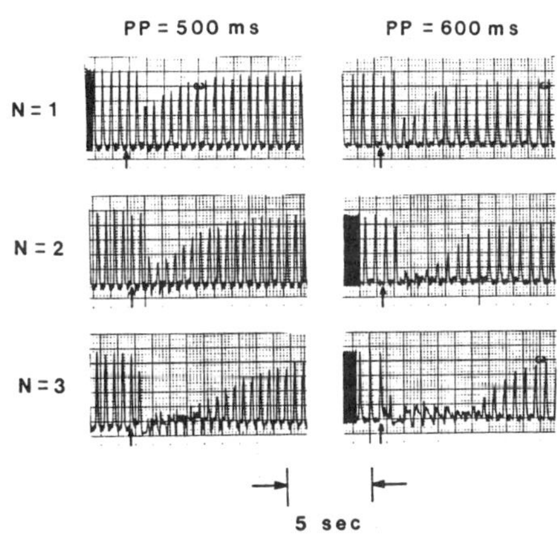

Figure 2. *Changes in pressure in an atrial balloon induced by vagal stimulus bursts that contain either 1, 2, or 3 pulses (N) per burst. The stimuli were delivered at the time marked by the arrow in each panel. The hearts were paced at cycle lengths (PP intervals) of 500 and 600 msec. Reproduced with permission from Martin P: Atrial inotropic responses to brief vagal stimuli: Frequency-force interactions. Am J Physiol 239:H333, 1980.*

passes through this channel is very sensitive to changes in cardiac cycle length.[7] As the cycle length is progressively increased, the K^+ current is augmented and the atrial action potential duration therefore diminishes (Fig. 3).[7] Thus, the vagal activation of the ACh-regulated K^+ channels and the augmentation of i_{to} by an increase in cycle length both act to diminish atrial action potential duration. This action, in turn, diminishes Ca^{++} influx into the atrial myocytes, and thereby diminishes atrial contractility.[4,8] This mechanism may then explain, at least partially, why an increase in cardiac cycle length intensifies the negative inotropic influence of vagal activity on the atrial myocytes.

Brown and Eccles[22] pointed out more than 50 years ago that the change in cardiac cycle length produced by a brief burst of vagal stimulation depended on the time (or phase) within the cardiac cycle that the stimulus was delivered. To define this "phase dependency," they delivered stimuli at different times in the cardiac cycle and allowed enough time after each stimulus to permit the heart to recover fully from the effects of the preceding stimulus. They could then construct a "vagal effect curve" from the responses to the entire series of such stimuli.[22]

Martin[16] used this technic to define the phase dependency of the atrial response to brief bursts of vagal stimuli in anesthetized dogs. He verified that

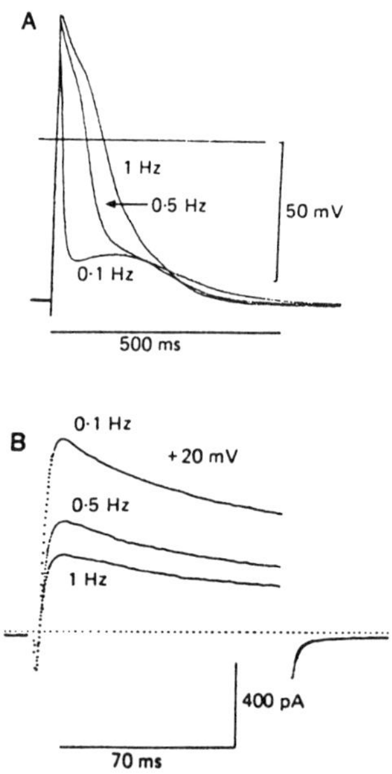

Figure 3. *Frequency dependence of atrial action potential durations (A) and transient outward current (B). Stimuli or voltage pulses (from a holding potential of −80 to +20 mV) were applied at the indicated frequencies. Note that decreasing the stimulus frequency (A) or voltage clamp frequency (B) diminishes the amplitude and duration of the action potential and increases the transient outward current. Modified with permission from Giles WR, Imaizumi Y: Comparison of potassium currents in rabbit atrial and ventricular cells. J Physiol (Lond) 405:123, 1988.*

when the heart was allowed to beat spontaneously, the phase dependency of the responses of the sinoatrial (SA) node pacemaker cells to vagal stimuli was characterized by a triphasic vagal effect curve (Fig. 4A) that closely resembled those obtained by Brown and Eccles[22] and many other investigators.

To derive the vagal effect curve for atrial contractility, Martin placed a small balloon in the right auricle and measured the pressure that the atrial contractions generated in the balloon.[16] He paced the heart at a constant frequency and scanned the cardiac cycle with a vagal stimulation regimen similar to that used to characterize the chronotropic responses. The vagal effect curve derived for the atrium is shown in Figure 4B. The maximum reduction in the atrial pressure (ΔAP) occurred about 2.5 seconds after the vagal stimulus (at t = 0 seconds). This finding corresponds to the fourth contraction after the stimulus, at the pacing frequency used in that experiment. The inhibitory effect of the vagal stimulus then decayed over the subsequent 15 seconds.

The time dependency is also illustrated by experiments in which vagal stimulus bursts were delivered once per cardiac cycle, and the time within the

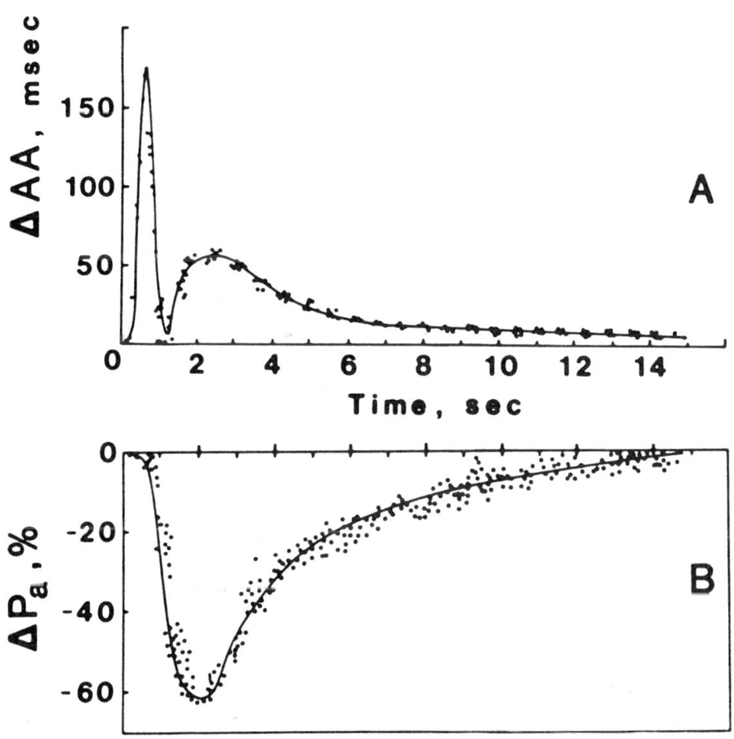

Figure 4. *Vagal effect curves for cardiac cycle length (ΔAA, top panel) in the spontaneously beating heart and for pressure generated in an atrial balloon (ΔPa, lower panel) in the artificially-paced heart of an anesthetized dog. The curves were derived from a sequence of stimulus bursts given at various times in the cardiac cycle. Reproduced with permission from Martin P: Atrial inotropic responses to brief vagal stimuli: Frequency-force interactions. Am J Physiol 239:H333, 1980.*

cardiac cycle was changed by a small constant amount each cycle. The results of such an experiment are shown in Figure 5.[18] In each panel, the lower tracing shows how the atrial contraction was affected by the A-St interval (upper tracing). A-St is the time from an atrial depolarization (A wave of the atrial electrogram) until the subsequent vagal stimulus (St). Figure 5 shows that, as the timing was gradually varied from cycle to cycle, the atrial contraction changed. The extent of the change varied depending on the number (N) of stimulus pulses in each burst (N = 2 or 6), on the time interval (I) between the pulses in a burst (I = 5 or 25 milliseconds), and on the atrial cycle length (A-A = 400 or 500 milliseconds).[18]

The relation between the atrial contraction amplitude and the A-St interval in Figure 5B has been replotted in Figure 6. In this portion of the experiment, the atria were paced at an A-A interval of 500 milliseconds. The atrial contraction amplitude was minimum when the A-St interval was about 150 milliseconds, and it was maximum when the A-St interval was about 450 milliseconds.[18] This phase dependency varied slightly, depending upon whether the A-St intervals were increasing or decreasing (as denoted by the arrows); that is, some hysteresis prevailed.

The minimum contraction amplitude elicited by vagal stimuli delivered at A-St intervals of about 150 milliseconds denotes that stimulation at this time in the cycle evokes the maximum inhibition (Fig. 6). Thus, the maximum

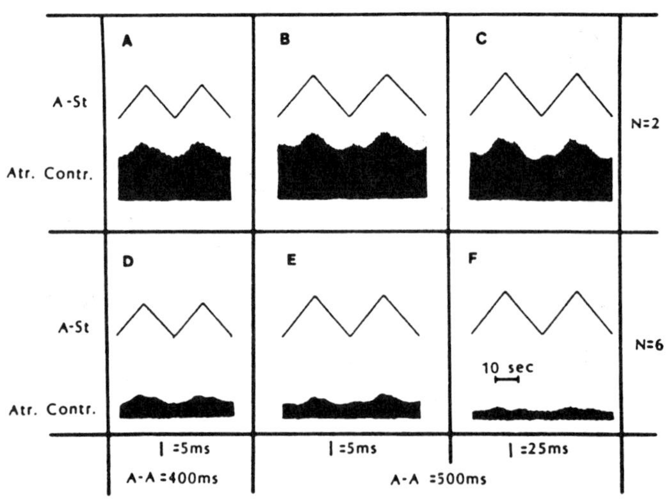

Figure 5. *The effects of one burst of vagal stimulation per cardiac cycle on atrial contraction in an anesthetized dog. The time interval (A-St interval) from the beginning of atrial depolarization (A wave) until the beginning of the vagal stimulus (St) was varied by a constant amount each cardiac cycle. The number (N) of pulses in each stimulus burst was either 2 or 6. The interval (I) between pulses in the bursts was either 5 or 25 msec, and the atria were paced at cycle lengths (A-A intervals) of either 400 or 500 msec. Reproduced by permission of the American Heart Association, Inc. from Martin PJ, Levy JR, Wexberg S, et al: Phasic effects of repetitive vagal stimulation on atrial contraction. Circ Res 52:657, 1983.*

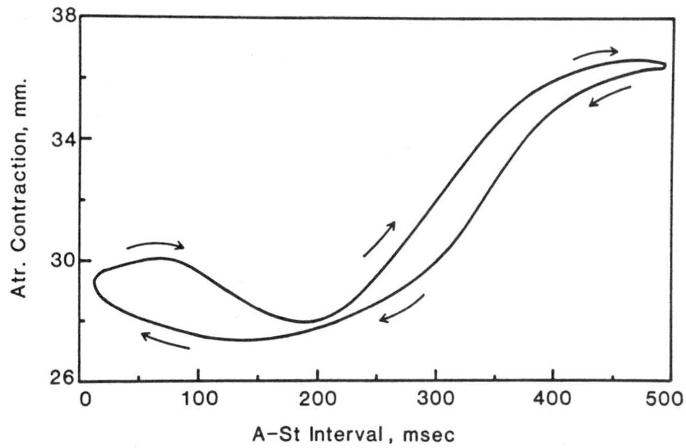

Figure 6. *The atrial contraction amplitude as a function of the A-St interval for the data shown in Figure 5. The atrial contraction amplitudes obtained during the ascending A-St interval ramps are denoted by the rightward arrows. Those obtained during the descending ramps are denoted by the leftward arrows. Reproduced by permission of the American Heart Association, Inc. from Martin PJ, Levy JR, Wexberg S, et al: Phasic effects of repetitive vagal stimulation on atrial contraction. Circ Res 52:657, 1983.*

inhibition was achieved when the stimulus was given about 350 milliseconds before the next atrial depolarization (A-A = 500 milliseconds). Conversely, the minimum inhibitory effect was achieved when the stimulus was delivered only about 50 milliseconds before the next atrial depolarization.

This phase dependency of the atrial response to such phase-coupled stimulation provides some valuable insight into the nature of vagal neurotransmission in the atria. Two important features of vagal neurotransmission must prevail for the atrial response to be phase-dependent: one, the neurally released ACh must be degraded quickly and, two, a rapid mechanism must initiate the change in contractility.

With regard to the first of these neurotransmission characteristics, rapid hydrolysis of the neurally released ACh is achieved by the acetylcholinesterase, (AChE) that is abundant in atrial tissue.[3,5,6,23,24] If a substantial fraction of the ACh was not degraded within the time of one cardiac cycle, the concentration of ACh at the surface of the atrial myocytes would not vary substantially during the cardiac cycle.[23,24] Hence, the time between atrial depolarization and vagal stimulation would not affect the contractile response to that vagal stimulus.

With regard to the second characteristic of vagal neurotransmission, the inhibition of atrial contractility by the vagal stimuli must be mediated at least partly by a rapid, direct mechanism. An indirect mechanism, notably one that operates via the AC system, would be too sluggish to display any detectable phase dependency.[3,5,6,9,10] The data shown in Figures 4 and 5 indicate that the vagal effects are exerted within one cardiac cycle. For example, vagal stimuli delivered within 50 milliseconds of an atrial depolarization (i.e., A-St = 450 to

500 milliseconds when the A-A interval is 500 milliseconds) cannot affect the very next atrial depolarization (Fig. 6) because the latent period for vagal stimulation to affect the ionic conductance of the atrial cell membrane exceeds 50 milliseconds.[5,6,23,24] Stimuli delivered more than 100 milliseconds before the next atrial depolarization, however, do decrease the amplitude of the very next atrial contraction (Fig. 6), and the maximum inhibition prevails when the stimuli occur about 350 milliseconds before the next atrial depolarization (A-St = 150 milliseconds). When the vagal stimuli are delivered at this time in the cycle, the peak ACh concentration in the neighborhood of the myocardial cell membranes is probably attained at the time of the next atrial depolarization.[23,24]

These rapid effects are probably mediated via the ACh-regulated K^+ channels.[7–10,23] The mAChRs in the sarcolemma of the atrial myocytes are coupled to these channels via guanine nucleotide-binding proteins (G-proteins).[8–10] A slow second messenger system is not interposed. Hence, the signalling system is rapid enough to permit beat-by-beat regulation of atrial contractility. Occupation of the mAChRs by vagally released ACh quickly activates the $i_{K(ACh)}$ current,[7–10] and thereby diminishes the action potential duration. This mechanism, in turn, curtails the influx of Ca^{++} into the atrial myocytes, and diminishes their contractility, as described above. This rapid process is certainly not the exclusive mechanism by which vagal activity regulates atrial contractility, but it is probably the principle mechanism for exerting beat-by-beat control.

Vagal Inhibition of Ventricular Contractility

Muscarinic Agonists

Muscarinic agonists have only a moderate influence on ventricular myocardial cells in most mammalian species[3,5,6]; the ferret is an exception.[25] The negative inotropic effects of ACh on the ventricles vary substantially with the background level of sympathetic neural activity.[3,5,6,11,26,27] For example, when Hollenberg et al[26] infused ACh directly into the left anterior descending coronary artery (LAD) of anesthetized dogs, left ventricular contractile force was only slightly reduced during the infusion (Fig. 7). A prominent "rebound" was evident, however, immediately after the infusion was terminated. The mechanism responsible for this rebound is described in the next section of this chapter. When an identical ACh infusion was given during tonic sympathetic nerve stimulation (Fig. 8) or during an intravenous infusion of norepinephrine (NE), however, the reduction of ventricular contractile force was much more pronounced. These results suggest that muscarinic agonists diminish ventricular contractility via an indirect mechanism, principally by antagonizing the facilitatory effect of concomitant sympathoadrenal activity on the AC system. This topic is discussed in detail in Ch. 11.

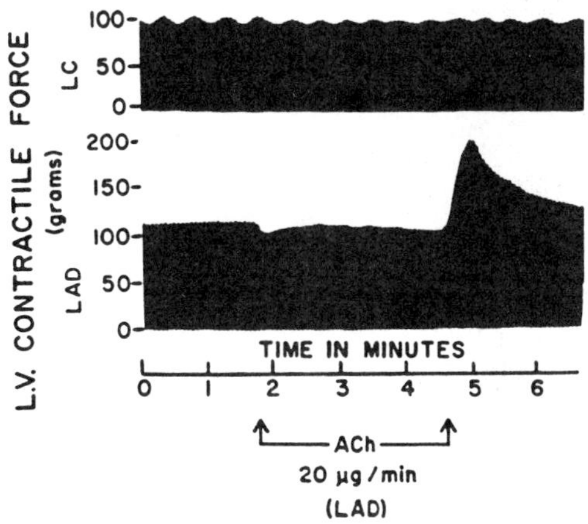

Figure 7. *Effects of an infusion of acetylcholine (ACh), 20 μg/min, into the left anterior descending (LAD) coronary artery on left ventricular contractile force during, and immediately after, intracoronary infusion. In the myocardial region supplied by the LAD coronary artery, ACh slightly reduced contractile force during the infusion, but elicited a pronounced rebound in force immediately after the infusion stopped. ACh had no effect on contractile force in the myocardial region supplied by the left circumflex (LC) coronary artery. Modified by permission of the American Heart Association, Inc. from Hollenberg M, Carriere S, Barger AC: Biphasic action of acetylcholine on ventricular myocardium. Circ Res 16:527, 1965.*

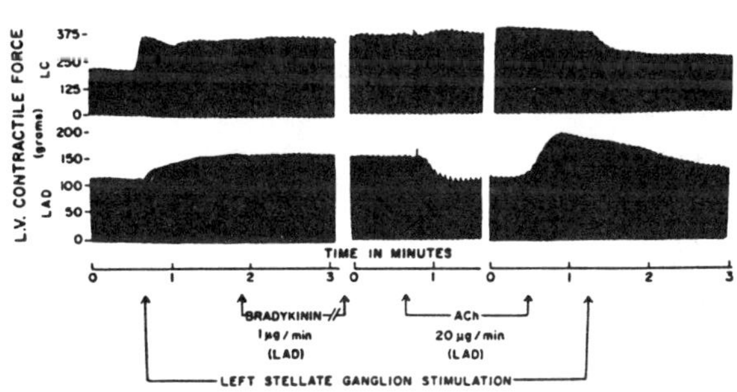

Figure 8. *Effects of intracoronary infusions of ACh (20 μg/min) and of bradykinin (1 μg/min) into the left anterior descending (LAD) coronary artery on left ventricular contractile force during left stellate ganglion stimulation in the same animal from which Figure 7 was recorded. ACh diminished contractile force in the myocardial region supplied by the LAD coronary artery, but not in the region supplied by the left circumflex (LC) coronary artery. Bradykinin is a potent coronary vasodilator, as is ACh. Bradykinin, however, had no detectable effect on myocardial contractile force, which suggests that the negative inotropic effect of ACh cannot be explained by its vasodilator effect. Modified by permission of the American Heart Association, Inc. from Hollenberg M, Carriere S, Barger AC: Biphasic action of acetylcholine on ventricular myocardium. Circ Res 16:527, 1965.*

Vagus Nerve Activity

Until about 30 years ago, anatomical and functional studies strongly favored the conclusion that the vagus nerves did not innervate the ventricles in mammals.[28,29] Studies conducted on anesthetized dogs in our laboratory[30] in 1965 challenged this prevailing view. Since the animals had been placed on total heart bypass, it was possible to rigorously control the heart rate, preload, afterload, atrial transport function, and coronary perfusion pressure. Our experimental results indicated that vagal stimulation did indeed diminish ventricular contractility (Fig. 9). The reductions in contractility varied directly with the frequency of vagal stimulation, and they paralleled the changes in heart rate induced in the spontaneously beating heart (Fig. 9).

Subsequent studies from our laboratory showed that the inhibitory effects of vagal activity were more pronounced the greater the prevailing level of sympathoadrenal activity.[31] The experiment shown in Figure 10 was conducted on the isovolumically contracting left ventricle of an anesthetized dog on total heart bypass.[31] After panels A and B had been recorded, additional fluid was added to a balloon in the left ventricle. Panels A to C show the responses to supramaximal vagal stimulation at a frequency of 20 Hz. In panel D, the fluid volume in the left ventricular balloon was restored to that which existed in panel A. The left stellate ganglion was stimulated between event marks 1 and 3. The vagus nerve was stimulated concomitantly (event mark D)

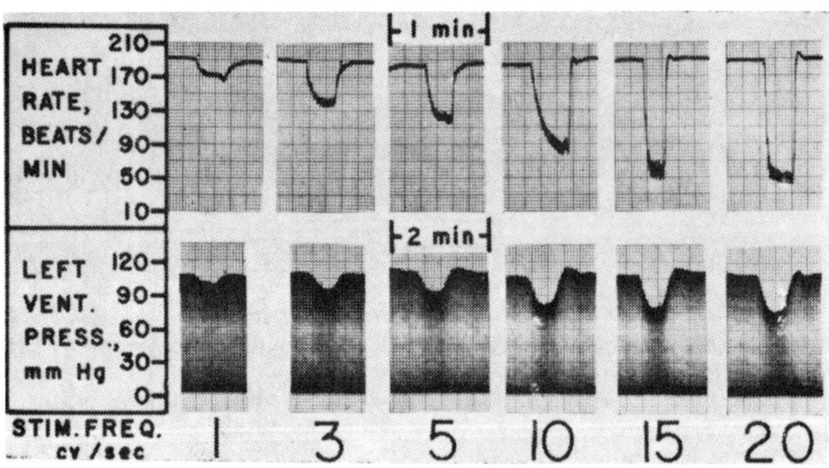

Figure 9. *Effects of right vagus nerve stimulation (10 V, 5 msec) on heart rate and left ventricular pressure in a canine isovolumetric left ventricle preparation. Left ventricular pressure was recorded while the atria and ventricles were paced simultaneously at 210 beats/min. The vagus nerve was stimulated at the frequencies (Hz) denoted by the numbers below each panel. The stimulation frequencies were delivered in a random sequence. Reproduced by permission of the American Heart Association, Inc. from DeGeest H, Levy MN, Zieske H, et al: Depression of ventricular contractility by stimulation of the vagus nerves. Circ Res 17:222, 1965.*

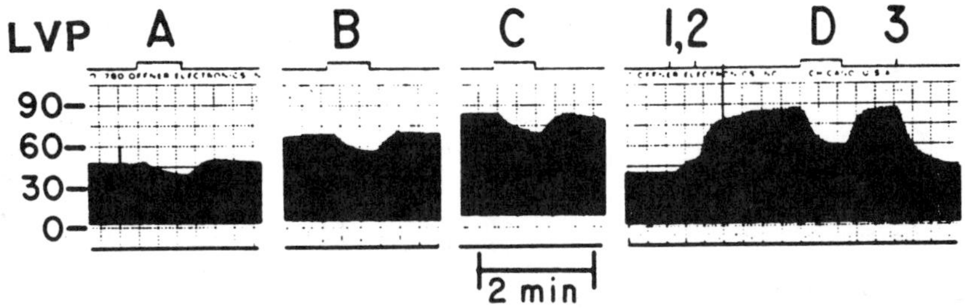

Figure 10. *Effects of vagal stimulation on left ventricular pressure (mm Hg) in the presence and absence of concurrent sympathetic stimulation in a canine isovolumetric left ventricle preparation. During event marks A, B, C, and D, the cardiac end of the transected right vagus nerve was stimulated electrically with pulses of 10 V, 5 msec, 20 Hz. Fluid volumes in a balloon in the left ventricle in each panel were, from left to right, 1.0, 2.0, 3.0, and 0.8 ml. Between marks 1 and 2 in the fourth panel, the left stellate ganglion was stimulated with pulses of 3.0 V, 5 msec, 2 Hz. Between marks 2 and 3, the stimulus intensity was increased to 3.5 V. Reproduced by permission of the American Heart Association, Inc. from Levy MN, Ng M, Martin P, et al: Sympathetic and parasympathetic interactions upon the left ventricle of the dog. Circ Res 19:5, 1966.*

at a frequency again of 20 Hz. Vagal stimulation alone (panels A, B, and C) decreased peak left ventricular pressure by 21%, regardless of the differences in contractile strength caused by the disparate fluid volumes in the ventricular balloon. During concomitant sympathetic stimulation (panel D), however, vagal stimulation diminished peak left ventricular pressure by 35%. Hence, the negative inotropic effect of vagal stimulation was substantially greater in the presence than in the absence of tonic sympathetic activity. These effects of vagal stimulation paralleled the responses to intracoronary ACh infusions reported by Hollenberg et al.[26]

In some of our experiments, the ventricular responses to vagal stimulation alone were virtually undetectable, and they only became manifest when the vagus was stimulated in the presence of a significant background level of sympathoadrenal activity. Such an experiment, illustrated in Figure 11, was also conducted on an isovolumically contracting left ventricle preparation.[32] At event marks A and C, the vagus nerves were stimulated supramaximally at a frequency of 20 Hz. Note that the left ventricular pressure changed very slightly or not at all during the stimulation. The only change of any consequence was a positive inotropic rebound immediately after cessation of vagal stimulation. When the same vagal stimulation (event mark B) was applied during concurrent stimulation of the cardiac sympathetic nerves (between marks 1 and 2), however, vagal stimulation diminished left ventricular pressure substantially.[32] The absence of any detectable change in ventricular performance during vagal stimulation alone strongly suggests that the vagal influence on ventricular myocardial contractility is mediated mainly by an indirect mechanism; that is, by opposing the inotropic influence of concomitant sympathoadrenal activity.[9,10]

The negative inotropic effect of vagal activity on the mammalian ventricles has been confirmed in various other canine preparations and in other

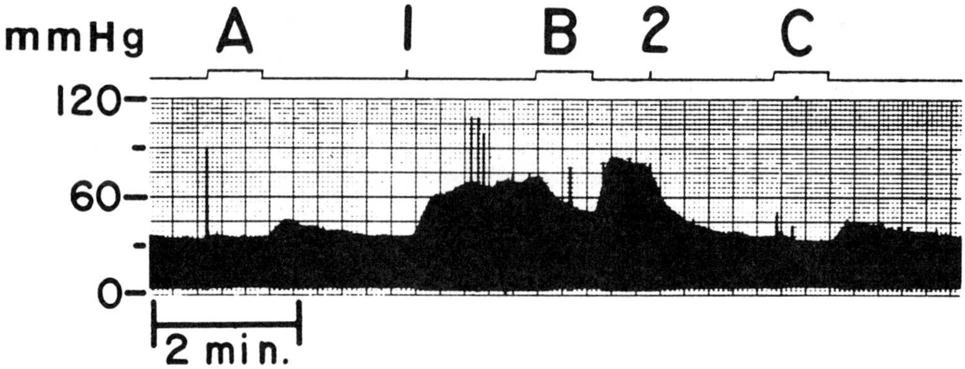

Figure 11. *Changes in left ventricular pressure induced by stimulation of the cardiac nerves in a canine isovolumetric left ventricle preparation that was paced at a constant frequency. During event marks A, B, and C, the cervical vagi were stimulated supramaximally at a frequency of 20 Hz. Between event marks 1 and 2, the left stellate ganglion was stimulated supramaximally at a frequency of 2 Hz. Reproduced with permission from Levy MN: Neural control of the heart: Sympathetic-vagal interactions. In J Baan, A Noordergraaf, J Raines (eds): Cardiovascular Systems Dynamics. Cambridge, MA, MIT Press, 1978, p. 365.*

mammals, including humans. Vagal stimulation causes the ventricular function curves to be shifted in the direction that denotes depressed contractility, it significantly reduces the maximum rate of rise of intraventricular pressure, and it diminishes ventricular contractile force.[5,6] One reason why the vagal effects on ventricular contractility had not been established sooner is probably related to its dependence on the prevailing background of cardiac sympathetic tone. The vagal effect is usually not very conspicuous in the absence of concurrent sympathetic activity.

Vagal Stimulation of Cardiac Contractions

Evidence for Stimulant Effects of the Vagus Nerve or Muscarinic Agonists

There are many examples of vagal or muscarinic stimulation of the heart-beat. In the SA node, vagal stimulation elicits a triphasic chronotropic response (early deceleration, acceleration, delayed deceleration). The phase of acceleration, which is muscarinic in nature, has been observed by many investigators.[22,33–37] When pertussis toxin (PTX) has inactivated the inhibitory G-proteins G_i/G_o, carbachol (CCh) accelerates the frequency of spontaneous impulse generation without any sign of inhibition in the chick SA node.[38] Feline atrial muscle displays a rebound positive inotropic effect to vagal stimulation.[39] Either ACh or CCh increases atrial contraction force in chicks treated with PTX.[40] Positive chronotropic[41] and inotropic[42,43] responses to ACh have been registered in mammalian Purkinje fibers. Sometimes, a rebound positive chronotropic effect of ACh occurs in rabbit Purkinje fibers,[44,45] as has also been reported for the SA node from the same animal.[46] A rebound positive inotropic effect of intracoronary ACh has been reported in the canine ventricle (see Fig. 7).[26] Stimulation of cervical vagus nerves also evokes a rebound positive inotropic effect in the absence or presence of stellate ganglion stimulation to the paced canine ventricle (see Fig. 11).[32] In the reserpine-treated guinea pig ventricle, ACh or CCh elicits concentration-dependent increases of contraction force.[47,48] Summarily, vagal stimulation or choline esters can elicit stimulant effects in pacemaker, conducting, and contractile cardiac tissues.[49]

Mechanism(s) for Cardiac Stimulation by the Vagus Nerve or Muscarinic Agonist

The stimulant effects (depolarization, positive inotropic or chronotropic actions) of either vagal stimulation or certain muscarinic agonists can occur in the absence of sympathetic influences.[9,10,27,50] These stimulant effects are also independent of G_i/G_o because they are more easily detected in the presence of PTX, which suppresses the transduction of inhibitory signals by G_i/G_o.[9–11,50] The ability of atropine to suppress the stimulant as well as inhibitory effects, however, indicates that a mAChR is involved.

Two mechanisms have been advanced to account for the stimulant effects of vagal stimulation or muscarinic agonists on the heartbeat.[49] The first of these is that vagal stimulation or muscarinic agonists increase the intracellular Na^+ concentration ($[Na^+]_i$) by raising membrane permeability to Na^+. Inferential evidence for this mechanism was adduced from experiments in the SA node of rabbits,[51] dogs,[52] cats,[33] and very young embryonic chicks.[53] Experiments in atrial tissues,[40] Purkinje fibers,[43] and in ventricular muscle[47,48] also provided evidence consistent with this hypothesis.

Direct evidence that ACh or CCh increases membrane permeability to Na^+ was obtained in single guinea pig ventricular myocytes with a voltage clamp technique.[54] In these cells, ACh or CCh induced an inward current, provided that the Na gradient was inwardly directed across the plasma membrane. An example of this effect is shown in Figure 12. At a concentration (3×10^{-4}M) that was maximal for its positive inotropic effect,[47] CCh depolarized the membrane (Fig. 12a) and induced an inward current (Fig. 12b) carried primarily by Na^+.[54] Moreover, the apparent reversal potential for the CCh-induced current was shifted by 61 mV toward more negative potentials by a 10-fold reduction of $[Na^+]_o$. An alternative explanation for the positive inotropic effect of ACh in sheep Purkinje fibers was that the muscarinic agonist inhibited the Na/K pump and thereby caused $[Na^+]_i$ accumulation by a digitalis glycoside-like action.[43] This mechanism has been excluded for ventricular muscle[47,54] and is at variance with the results obtained by Carmeliet and Ramon[55] in sheep Purkinje fibers. In all cardiac tissues examined, the increased membrane permeability to Na caused by muscarinic agonist is not sensitive to blockade by tetrodotoxin (TTX).[49]

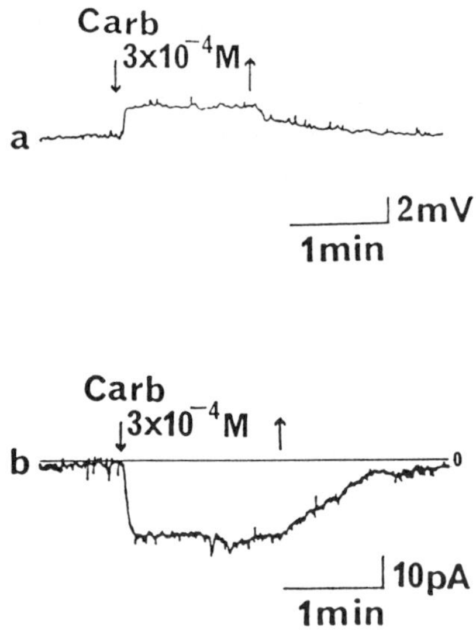

Figure 12. *Depolarization (a) and inward current (b) induced by carbachol (Carb) in isolated guinea pig ventricular myocytes. In the presence of Tyrode's solution with 20-mM Cs^+, addition of Carb for the period between the arrows depolarized the membrane by 3 mV (a) and induced an inward current of 22 pA (b). These effects were sustained during exposure to Carb. Reproduced with permission from Matsumoto K, Pappano AJ: Sodium-dependent membrane current induced by carbachol in single guinea-pig ventricular myocytes. J Physiol (Lond) 415:487, 1989.*

Activation of Na-Ca exchange by muscarinic agonist-induced elevation of $[Na^+]_i$ has been proposed to account for the positive inotropic effect.[47,48] This proposal was substantiated by the observation that an increase of $[Ca^{2+}]_i$ occurred subsequently to the increase of $[Na^+]_i$ produced by CCh.[56] Interestingly, the muscarinic agonist-induced increase of $[Ca^{2+}]_i$ required $[Na^+]_o$ and $[Ca^{2+}]_o$ and it was not sensitive to blockade by either caffeine or ryanodine, which deplete Ca^{2+} from the sarcoplasmic reticulum.[56]

Another mechanism by which muscarinic agonists might increase the force of contraction is through phospholipid signalling pathways. Muscarinic agonists, ACh and CCh, activate phospholipase C (PLC) to generate the second messengers, inositol 1,4,5-trisphosphate (IP_3) and diacylglycerol (DAG)[57] and also activate phospholipase D.[58] Moreover, CCh activates a phosphatidylcholine-specific PLC,[59] and by this pathway generates four times as much DAG as from activation of phosphatidylinositol-specific PLC.[60] Positive inotropic effects of muscarinic agonists can be traced to these phospholipid-signalling systems through several pathways. First, treatment of ventricular muscle with phospholipase D elicits a positive inotropic action[61] and it also stimulates Na-Ca exchange in sarcolemmal vesicles from the heart.[62] Whether the activation of phospholipase D and stimulation of Na-Ca exchange lead to the positive inotropic action in the presence of CCh is not known.

An alternative mechanism for the positive inotropic action of ACh and CCh is accumulation of the Ca-mobilizing intracellular messenger, IP_3.[40]

Accumulation of IP_3 precedes the positive inotropic effect of CCh in atria from guinea pigs treated with PTX to inactivate G_i/G_o and the negative inotropic effect.[63] In turn, IP_3 increases developed tension in cardiac cells with hyperpermeable plasma membranes or in mechanically-skinned cardiac myocytes.[49] In this instance, IP_3 mobilizes Ca^{2+} from the sarcoplasmic reticulum.

As shown in Figure 13, addition of a maximally effective concentration of IP_3 induced a tension transient (~40% of maximal tension of T_{max}) that was briefer and smaller than that subsequently induced by caffeine (Fig. 13A). When caffeine was added first, subsequent exposure to IP_3 was largely without effect (Fig. 13B). This binding indicates that IP_3 released calcium from a caffeine-sensitive store, the sarcoplasmic reticulum. This observation seems at odds with the finding that the CCh-induced rise in $[Ca^{2+}]_i$ does not depend on release of Ca^{2+} from caffeine- or ryanodine-sensitive intracellular stores.[56] If CCh mobilized Ca^{2+} by increasing IP_3, stimulation of Na-Ca exchange current would ensue, as has been reported.[64]

At present, one can only speculate as to whether stimulation of Na-Ca exchange current by IP_3 helps to reconcile the discrepancy concerning the origin of the Ca required for the positive inotropic effect of CCh. If the IP_3 pathway was involved, there is much evidence for a role of Na-Ca exchange in

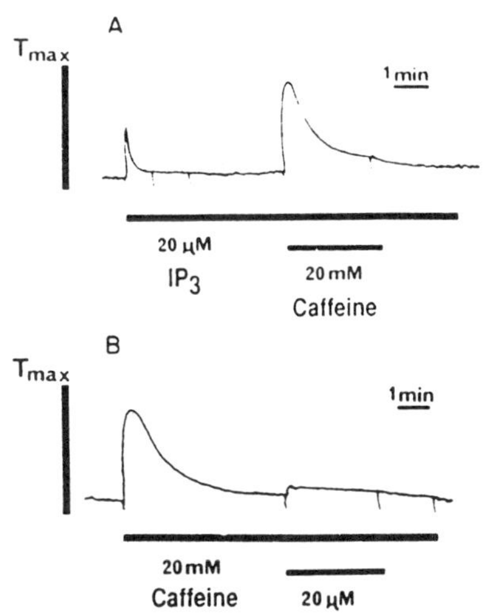

Figure 13. *Interactions between IP_3 and caffeine in a saponin-permeabilized chick atrial muscle bundle. T_{max} indicates maximum tension generated by a solution with pCa = 5.0 in the presence of 70 μM EGTA. Bathing solution set at pCa = 7.0 with EGTA = 70 μM. A: Sequential responses to IP_3 (20 μM) followed by caffeine (20 μM). IP_3 was present throughout the period shown by the bold horizontal line. B: Response to caffeine followed by exposure to IP_3. Caffeine present during the time indicated by bold horizontal line. The response to IP_3 was 43% of T_{max} (A); in B, the response to IP_3 was 8% of T_{max} because caffeine had depleted calcium from the IP_3-sensitive store. Reproduced with permission from Vites AM, Pappano A: Inositol 1,4,5-trisphosphate increases tension by releasing intracellular Ca^{2+} in permeabilized atrial muscle. Am J Physiol 258 (Heart Circ Physiol 27):H1745-H1752, 1990.*

regulating force development in heart muscle.[65,66] As speculated in a recent review,[49] the stimulation of IP_3 accumulation may amplify, rather than initiate, the positive inotropic of CCh, because agents that act primarily to increase Na^+ permeability and thereby Na-Ca exchange, eventually activate PLC through an increase of $[Ca^{2+}]_i$. It should be remembered that the effect of muscarinic agonists on Na^+ permeability and on phospholipid signalling are similar in:

1. agonist selectivity; ACh and CCh, but not oxotremorine;
2. concentration dependence; concentrations $>10^{-6}$M;
3. resistance to suppression by PTX; G_i/G_o not involved; and
4. sensitivity to blockade by atropine.

Physiological Significance

The reports that high concentrations of muscarinic agonist are needed to evoke stimulant effects on the contraction force of cardiac tissues seemingly belies the physiological importance of this phenomenon. There are two reasons to suggest that this phenomenon is physiologically significant. First, the stimulant effects can be elicited in response to vagal stimulation. Second, rapid application of ACh ($t_{1/2}<250$ milliseconds) at lower concentrations (10^{-7} to 10^{-6}M) was accompanied by rebound positive chronotropic effects in the rabbit SA node.[46] These observations may be taken as indices of a physiological role of the stimulant effects that limit the inhibition of the heartbeat by the vagus nerve.[49]

References

1. Gesell RA: Cardiodynamics in heart block as affected by auricular systole, auricular fibrillation and stimulation of the vagus nerve. Am J Physiol 40:267, 1916.
2. Wiggers CJ: The physiology of the mammalian auricle. II. The influence of the vagus nerves on the fractionate contraction of the right auricle. Am J Physiol 42:133, 1917.
3. Higgins CB, Vatner SF, Braunwald E: Parasympathetic control of the heart. Pharmacol Rev 25:120, 1973.
4. Ten Eick R, Nawrath H, McDonald TF, et al: On the mechanism of the negative inotropic effect of acetylcholine. Pflügers Arch 361:207, 1976.
5. Levy MN, Martin PJ: Neural control of the heart. In R Berne, N Sperelakis (eds): Handbook of Physiology. Section 2: Cardiovascular System. Vol. I: Heart. Bethesda, MD, American Physiological Society, 1979, p. 581.
6. Löffelholz K, Pappano AJ: The parasympathetic neuroeffector junction of the heart. Pharmacol Rev 37:1, 1985.
7. Giles WR, Imaizumi Y: Comparison of potassium currents in rabbit atrial and ventricular cells. J Physiol (Lond) 405:123, 1988.
8. Shumaker JM, Clark JW, Giles WR, et al: A model of the muscarinic receptor-induced changes in K^+-current and action potentials in the bullfrog atrial cell. Biophys J 57:567, 1990.

9. Sorota S, Pappano AJ: Muscarinic receptor-effector coupling in the heart. In MR Rosen, MJ Janse, AL Wit (eds): Cardiac Electrophysiology: A Textbook. Mount Kisco, NY, Futura Publishing Company Inc, 1990, p. 803.
10. Pappano A: Parasympathetic control of cardiac electrical activity. In DP Zipes, J Jalife (eds): Cardiac Electrophysiology: From Cell to Bedside. Philadelphia, PA, WB Saunders Co, 1990, p. 271.
11. Hartzell HC: Regulation of cardiac ion channels by catecholamines, acetylcholine and second messenger systems. Prog Biophys Mol Biol 52:165, 1988.
12. Sarnoff SJ, Gilmore JP, Mitchell JH: Influence of atrial contraction and relaxation on closure of mitral valve. Circ Res 11:26, 1962.
13. Randall WC, Priola DV, Ulmer RH: A functional study of the distribution of cardiac sympathetic nerves. Am J Physiol 205:1227, 1963.
14. Williams JF Jr, Sonnenblick EH, Braunwald E: Determinants of atrial contractile force in the intact heart. Am J Physiol 209:1061, 1965.
15. Armour JA, Randall WC, Sinha S: Localized myocardial responses to stimulation of small cardiac branches of the vagus. Am J Physiol 228:141, 1975.
16. Martin P: Atrial inotropic responses to brief vagal stimuli: Frequency-force interactions. Am J Physiol 239:H333, 1980.
17. Martin P, Levy MN, Matsuda Y: Fade of cardiac responses during tonic vagal stimulation. Am J Physiol 243:H219, 1982.
18. Martin PJ, Levy JR, Wexberg S, et al: Phasic effects of repetitive vagal stimulation on atrial contraction. Circ Res 52:657, 1983.
19. Mitchell JH, Gilmore JP, Sarnoff SJ: The transport function of the atrium. Am J Cardiol 9:237, 1962.
20. Williams JCP, Vandenberg RA, Sturm RI, et al: Presystolic atriogenic mitral reflux developed at abnormally long PR intervals. Cardiovasc Res 3:271, 1968.
21. Zaky A, Steinmetz E, Feigenbaum H: Role of atrium in closure of mitral valve in man. Am J Physiol 217:1652, 1969.
22. Brown GL, Eccles JE: The action of a single vagal volley on the rhythm of the heart beat. J Physiol (Lond) 82:211, 1934.
23. Dexter F, Levy MN, Rudy Y: Mathematical model of the changes in heart rate elicited by vagal stimulation. Circ Res 65:1330, 1989.
24. Dexter F, Saidel GM, Levy MN: Mathematical model of dependence of heart rate on tissue concentration of acetylcholine. Am J Physiol 256:H520, 1989.
25. Boyett MR, Kirby MS, Orchard CH, et al: The negative inotropic effect of acetylcholine on ferret ventricular myocardium. J Physiol (Lond) 404:613, 1988.
26. Hollenberg M, Carriere S, Barger AC: Biphasic action of acetylcholine on ventricular myocardium. Circ Res 16:527, 1965.
27. Levy MN, Zieske H: Comparison of the cardiac effects of vagus nerve stimulation and of acetylcholine infusions. Am J Physiol 216:890, 1969.
28. Wiggers CJ: Physiology in Health and Disease. 5th ed. Philadelphia, PA, Lea & Febiger, 1949, p. 530.
29. Sarnoff SJ, Mitchell JH: The control of the function of the heart. In WF Hamilton (ed): Handbook of Physiology. Section 2. Volume I. Circulation. Washington, DC, American Physiological Society, 1962, p. 489.
30. DeGeest H, Levy MN, Zieske H, et al: Depression of ventricular contractility by stimulation of the vagus nerves. Circ Res 17:222, 1965.
31. Levy MN, Ng M, Martin P, et al: Sympathetic and parasympathetic interactions upon the left ventricle of the dog. Circ Res 19:5, 1966.
32. Levy MN: Neural control of the heart: Sympathetic-vagal interactions. In J Baan, A Noordergraaf, J Raines (eds): Cardiovascular System Dynamics. Cambridge, MA, MIT Press, 1978, p. 365.
33. Burke GH, Calaresu FR: An experimental analysis of the tachycardia that follows vagal stimulation. J Physiol (Lond) 226:491, 1972.
34. Iano TL, Levy MN, Lee MH: An acceleratory component of the parasympathetic control of heart rate. Am J Physiol 224:997, 1973.

35. Moore EN, Spear JF, Kronhaus KD: The effects of brief vagal and sympathetic stimulation on rate and rhythm changes in the sinus node. In LN Bouman, HJ Jongsma (eds): Cardiac Rate and Rhythm. Boston, MA, Martinus Nijhoff, 1982, p. 543.
36. Michaels DC, Matyas EP, Jalife J: A mathematical model of the effects of acetylcholine pulses on sinoatrial pacemaker activity. Circ Res 55:89, 1984.
37. Prystowsky EN, Zipes DP: Observations on postvagal tachycardia in humans. In DP Zipes, J Jalife (eds): Cardiac Electrophysiology and Arrhythmias. New York, NY, Grune & Stratton Inc, 1985, p. 177.
38. Agnarsson U, Tajima T, Pappano AJ: Carbachol depolarizes and accelerates pacemaker activity in the sinoatrial node of chicks treated with pertussis toxin. J Pharmacol Exp Ther 247:150, 1988.
39. Endoh M, Blinks JR: Effects of endogenous neurotransmitters on calcium transients in mammalian atrial muscle. In WW Fleming, KH Graefe, SZ Langer, et al (eds): Neuronal and Extraneuronal Events in Autonomic Pharmacology. New York, NY, Raven Press, 1984, p. 221.
40. Tajima T, Tsuji Y, Brown JH, et al: Pertussis toxin-insensitive phosphoinositide hydrolysis, membrane depolarization, and positive inotropic effect of carbachol in chick atria. Circ Res 61:436, 1987.
41. Carmeliet E, Ramon J: Electrophysiological effects of acetylcholine in sheep cardiac Purkinje fibers. Pflügers Arch 387:197, 1980.
42. Gilmour RF Jr, Zipes DP: Positive inotropic effect of acetylcholine in canine cardiac Purkinje fibers. Am J Physiol 249 (Heart Circ Physiol 18): H735, 1985.
43. Iacono G, Vassalle M: Acetylcholine increases intracellular sodium activity in sheep cardiac Purkinje fibers. Am J Physiol 256 (Heart Circ Physiol 25): H1407, 1989.
44. Mubagwa K, Carmeliet E: Effects of acetylcholine on electrophysiological properties of rabbit cardiac Purkinje fibers. Circ Res 53:740, 1983.
45. Carmeliet E, Mubagwa K: Desensitization of the acetylcholine-induced increase of potassium conductance in rabbit cardiac Purkinje fibres. J Physiol (Lond) 371:239, 1986.
46. Boyett MR, Roberts A: The fade of the response to acetylcholine at the rabbit isolated sino-atrial node. J Physiol (Lond) 393:171, 1987.
47. Korth M, Kühlkamp V: Muscarinic receptor-mediated increase of intracellular Na^+ -ion activity and force of contraction. Pflügers Arch 403:266, 1985.
48. Korth M, Kühlkamp V: Muscarinic receptors mediate negative and positive inotropic effects in mammalian ventricular myocardium: Differentiation by agonists. Br J Pharmacol 90:81, 1987.
49. Pappano AJ: Vagal stimulation of the heartbeat: Muscarinic receptor hypothesis. J Cardiovasc Electrophysiol 2:262, 1991.
50. Pappano AJ, Mubagwa K: Actions of muscarinic agents and adenosine on the heart. In H Fozzard, E Haber, R Jennings, et al (eds): The Heart and Cardiovascular System. 2nd ed. New York, NY, Raven Press, 1992, p. 1765.
51. Toda N, West TC: Interactions of K, Na and vagal stimulation in the S-A node of the rabbit. Am J Physiol 212:416, 1967.
52. Chiba S, Levy MN, Zieske H: Chronotropic response to acetylcholine injected into the sinus node artery of the isolated atrium of the dog. Cardiovasc Res 9:127, 1975.
53. Pappano AJ: Sodium-dependent depolarization of non-innervated embryonic chick heart by acetylcholine. J Pharmacol Exp Ther 180:340, 1972.
54. Matsumoto K, Pappano AJ: Sodium-dependent membrane current induced by carbachol in single guinea-pig ventricular myocytes. J Physiol (Lond) 415:487, 1989.
55. Carmeliet E, Ramon J: Effect of acetylcholine on time-independent currents in sheep cardiac Purkinje fibers. Pflügers Arch 387:207, 1980.
56. Korth M, Sharma VK, Sheu SS: Stimulation of muscarinic receptors raises free

intracellular Ca^{2+} concentration in rat ventricular myocytes. Circ Res 62:1080, 1988.
57. Brown JH, McDonough PM: Muscarinic cholinergic receptor regulation of inositol phospholipid metabolism and calcium mobilization. In JH Brown (ed): The Muscarinic Receptors. Clifton, NJ, Humana Press, 1989, p. 259.
58. Corradetti R, Lindmar R, Löffelholz K: Mobilization of cellular choline by stimulation of muscarine receptors in isolated chicken heart and rat cortex in vivo. J Pharmacol Exp Ther 226:826, 1983.
59. Löffelholz K: Receptor-regulation of choline phospholipid hydrolysis: A novel source of diacylglycerol and phosphatidic acid. Biochem Pharmacol 38:1543, 1989.
60. Martinson EA, Goldstein D, Brown JH: Muscarinic receptor activation of phosphatidylcholine hydrolysis. J Biol Chem 264:14748, 1989.
61. Langer GA, Rich TL: Phospholipase D produces increased contractile force in rabbit ventricular muscle. Circ Res 56:146, 1985.
62. Philipson KD, Nishimoto AY: Stimulation of Na^{+}-Ca^{2+} exchange in cardiac sarcolemmal vesicles by phospholipase D. J Biol Chem 259:16, 1984.
63. Kohl C, Schmitz W, Scholz H: Positive inotropic effect of carbachol and inositol phosphate levels in mammalian atria after pretreatment with pertussis toxin. J Pharmacol Exp Ther 254:894, 1990.
64. Gilbert JC, Shirayama T, Pappano AJ: Inositol trisphosphate promotes Na-Ca exchange current by releasing calcium from sarcoplasmic reticulum in cardiac myocytes. Circ Res 69:1632–1639, 1991.
65. LeBlanc N, Hume JR: Sodium current-induced release of calcium from cardiac sarcoplasmic reticulum. Science 248:372, 1990.
66. Earm YE, Noble D: A model of the single atrial cell: Relation between calcium current and calcium release. Proc R Soc Lond (Biol) 240:83, 1990.

CHAPTER 16

Vagal Control of Myocardial Refractoriness

M.R. Warner, D.P. Zipes

This chapter provides an overview of parasympathetic influences on cardiac refractoriness. Parasympathetic effects on refractoriness vary both quantitatively and qualitatively depending on the cardiac structure. Indeed, vagal stimulation markedly shortens the atrial effective refractory period (ERP), but only slightly lengthens ventricular refractoriness. Vagal effects on refractoriness of the sinoatrial (SA) and atrioventricular (AV) nodes, atrial and ventricular muscle, Purkinje fibers, and AV accessory pathways are discussed. Where possible, clinical implications about these vagally-induced changes in refractoriness are presented.

Sinus and Atrioventricular Nodal Refractoriness

The SA and AV nodes are richly innervated by the parasympathetic nervous system, and vagal activation depresses automaticity and conduction in these tissues.[1–5] In addition, neurally-released and exogenous acetylcholine (ACh) prolong SA and AV nodal ERPs.[6–13] In isolated rabbit right atrial preparations,[6] ACh (5×10^{-7}M) increased the mean ERP of the SA node from 183 ± 16 to 210 ± 24 milliseconds ($n = 8$) and prolonged SA node action potential duration. Many investigators have shown similar vagal effects on AV nodal refractoriness and AV nodal action potential duration.[8–12] ACh evokes these changes in refractoriness by directly altering the electrophysiological properties of the SA and AV nodal slow response action potentials.[1,9,13] ACh hyperpolarizes the cell membrane and decreases the slope of phase 4 depolarization.

Phasic changes in vagal activity associated with the respiratory cycle and arterial baroreflexes also modulate AV nodal refractoriness.[8,9,11,14–16] The beat-to-beat changes in vagal tone can evoke various manifestations of first-

From *Vagal Control of the Heart: Experimental Basis and Clinical Implications* edited by MN Levy, PJ Schwartz © 1994, Futura Publishing Co. Inc., Armonk, NY.

and second-degree heart block, including Wenckebach periodicity, that have been observed both experimentally and clinically.[8,9,11,14–16]

Atrial Refractoriness

Parasympathetic activation and exogenous ACh markedly abbreviate the action potential duration of atrial myocardial cells[17–19] and shorten the atrial ERP.[20–23] By measuring atrial action potentials with intracellular microelectrode techniques, Hoffman and Suckling[17] (Fig. 1) demonstrated that ACh shortened the action potential duration in canine atrial tissue both in vitro and in vivo. Alessi and coworkers[21] found, however, that the effects of vagal stimulation or reflex vagal activation on atrial refractoriness were not distributed uniformly over the atria. Thus, vagal activation evoked pronounced decreases in the atrial ERP at some points on the atria, but produced little change in refractoriness at others (Fig. 2). The authors concluded that vagal stimulation enhanced the likelihood for the atria to fibrillate due to the

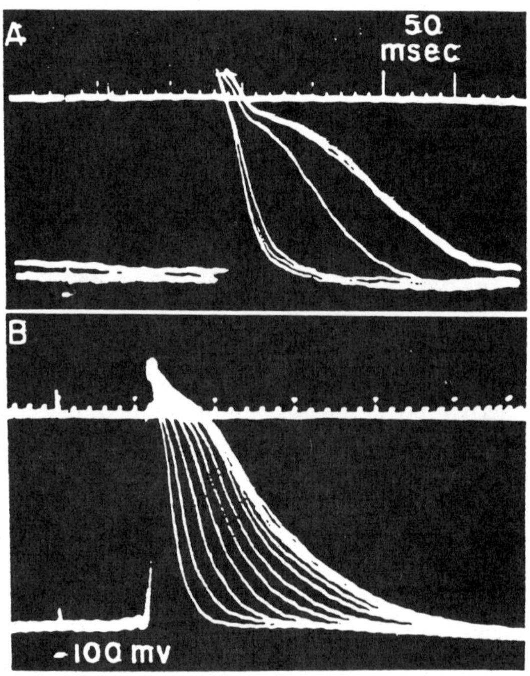

Figure 1. *Superimposed intracellular recordings of action potentials measured from a single atrial fiber in the anesthetized dog. A: Two control records (curves to the right) and records showing the sequential changes evoked by vagal stimulation. B: Superimposed atrial action potential recordings showing recovery after the termination of vagal stimulation. The hatched time line represents zero potential. Reproduced with permission from Hoffman BF, Suckling EE: Cardiac cellular potentials: Effect of vagal stimulation and acetylcholine. Am J Physiol 173:313, 1953.*

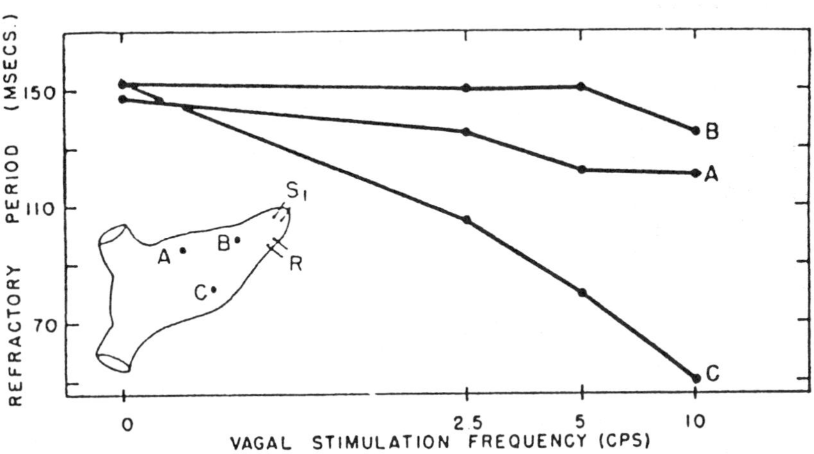

Figure 2. *Representative example of vagal effects on atrial effective refractory period measured at three different atrial sites in an anesthetized dog. Vagal stimulation had appreciably greater effects on atrial refractoriness at site C than at sites A and B. Reproduced with permission from Alessi R, Nusynowitz M, Abildskov JA, et al: Nonuniform distribution of vagal effects on the atrial refractory period. Am J Physiol 194:407, 1958.*

vagally-induced abbreviation of atrial ERP and to the inhomogeneity of vagal effects on atrial refractoriness.[21]

Zipes et al[22] explored further the regional variation of vagal influences on atrial refractoriness by measuring ERPs at several atrial sites while individually stimulating the right or left vagus in anesthetized dogs. Rather than being totally heterogeneous as implied by Alessi et al,[21] they found functional evidence for distinct patterns of vagal innervation of the atria. Right or left vagal stimulation evoked the greatest shortening of atrial ERP in the region of the SA node (Fig. 3). At most right atrial sites, the ERP shortened significantly more during right than during left vagal stimulation. At all left atrial sites, however, the ERP shortened to a similar extent during right or left vagal stimulation. As hypothesized by Alessi et al,[21] it is probable that atrial tissue adjacent to vagal nerve endings is exposed to higher concentrations of ACh and thereby exhibits greater shortening of ERP than does tissue remote from sites of ACh release. The data from our laboratory[22] support this hypothesis, in that vagal stimulation evoked the greatest shortening of refractory period in the SA node region, which is more densely innervated by parasympathetic fibers than other atrial sites.[4] Imaizumi et al[5] also showed that the magnitude of vagal effects at the AV node was correlated with the density of vagal innervation.

In conscious humans, increases in vagal activity also shorten the atrial ERP. Neck suction applied through a lead collar stimulates the carotid sinus baroreceptors and evokes an increase in cardiac vagal tone.[23] In 12 patients, increasing vagal tone with neck suction shortened the atrial ERP from a control of 241 ± 24 to 230 ± 20 milliseconds and decreased the atrial functional refractory period from 272 ± 32 to 262 ± 29 milliseconds. In two patients,

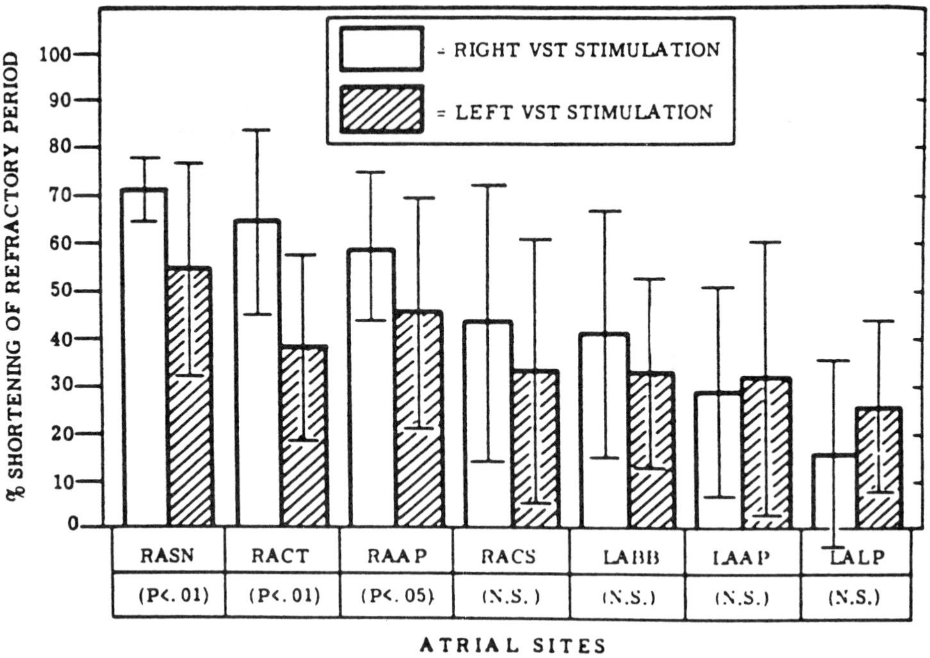

Figure 3. *Effects of right and left vago-sympathetic trunk (VST) stimulation on atrial ERP in anesthetized dogs. Values are the percent shortening from the control atrial ERP (means ± SD; n = 9 to 17). RASN: right atrium sinus node; RACT: right atrium sulcus terminalis; RAAP: right atrial appendage; RACS: right atrium coronary sinus; LABB: left atrium interatrial band of Bachman's bundle; LAAP: left atrial appendage; and LALP: low posterior left atrium. Reproduced with permission from Zipes DP, Mihalick MJ, Robbins GT: Effects of selective vagal and stellate ganglion stimulation on atrial refractoriness. Cardiovasc Res 8:652, 1974.*

atropine abolished the effects of neck suction on atrial refractoriness. This finding indicates that the vagal effects were mediated by activation of muscarinic receptors (mAChRs).

In contrast to these results, other data[24] suggest that vagal tone prolongs rather than shortens atrial refractoriness in humans. In these studies, the investigators showed that atropine shortened atrial refractoriness, and they concluded that vagal stimulation would have opposite effects. It is important to stress that vagal effects on atrial refractoriness were assessed indirectly by measuring refractory periods before and after atropine. In addition to blocking postsynaptic mAChRs, atropine blocks presynaptic mAChRs on sympathetic nerve endings. Such a blockade leads to an increase in norepinephrine (NE) release.[1–3] Moreover, postsynaptic effects of sympathetic activity, ordinarily modulated by vagal actions, are unopposed after atropine. It is likely that the shortening of refractoriness after atropine reflected, in part, unopposed sympathetic effects on the atria, because direct vagal activation shortens atrial action potential duration[17,18] and refractoriness.[20–23]

Ventricular Refractoriness

Although it is clear that vagal stimulation prolongs ventricular refractoriness, whether it does so directly or by opposing sympathetic activity is still not completely resolved.[25–32] Initial studies of vagal effects on ventricular refractoriness were done in anesthetized dogs with cardiac sympathetic nerves intact.[27,28] Figure 4 shows that bilateral vagal stimulation significantly prolonged left ventricular epicardial and endocardial ERPs in anesthetized dogs. The influence of vagal stimulation on ventricular refractoriness, however, was abolished after β-adrenergic receptor (β-AR) blockade.[27,28] These data suggest that vagal stimulation did not directly affect ventricular refractoriness, but that it did prolong the ventricular ERP by antagonizing the effects of tonic sympathetic activity.

To characterize the autonomic interactions in the control of ventricular refractoriness, Nattel et al[29] measured the effects of various frequencies of sympathetic and vagal stimulation on the ventricular ERP in anesthetized dogs. As found in previous studies,[25,27,28] vagal stimulation did not appreciably lengthen the ventricular ERP in the absence of concomitant sympathetic

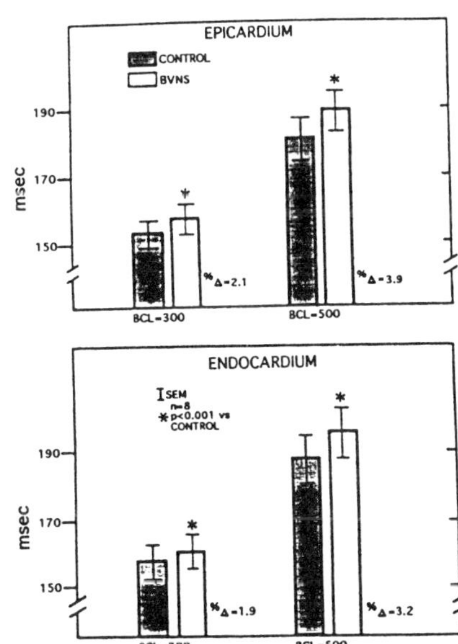

Figure 4. *Effects of bilateral vagal nerve stimulation (BVNS) on ventricular epicardial and endocardial ERPs measured at pacing cycle lengths (BCL) of 300 and 500 msec. The y-axis represents ERP in msec. Vagal stimulation significantly prolonged the ERP measured in the epicardium and endocardium at both pacing cycle lengths. The percent vagally-induced changes in refractory period were similar in the epicardium and endocardium. Reproduced by permission of the American Heart Association, Inc., from Martins JB, Zipes DP: Effects of sympathetic and vagal nerves on recovery properties of the endocardium and epicardium of the canine left ventricle. Circ Res 46:106, 1980.*

activity. Vagal stimulation, however, evoked a frequency-dependent attenuation of sympathetic effects on ventricular refractoriness. Thus, vagal stimulation, by antagonizing the effects of sympathetic activity, prolonged the ventricular ERP. Both presynaptic and postsynaptic mechanisms may contribute to the vagal antagonism of sympathetic effects on ventricular refractoriness.[1–3,33] Presynaptically, for example, ACh inhibits the release of NE from sympathetic nerve endings and, postsynaptically, ACh attenuates sympathetically-evoked adenosine 3′5′-cyclic phosphate (cyclic AMP) accumulation.[1–3]

In contrast to findings in anesthetized animals, data from conscious human subjects suggest that vagal activity modulates ventricular refractoriness independent of concomitant sympathetic activity.[26,30,31] The influence of vagal tone on right ventricular refractoriness in humans was assessed by administering atropine and propranolol to block MAChRs and β-ARs, respectively.[30,31] Because atropine given either alone or after propranolol shortened the ventricular ERP (Fig. 5), it was inferred that resting vagal tone had a direct effect on right ventricular refractory periods in humans.[30,31] Moreover, Morady et al[30] demonstrated that decreases in the ventricular ERP after atropine were more pronounced during a continuous infusion of isoproterenol, a β-AR agonist. Thus, in humans, the data suggest that resting vagal tone directly modulates ventricular refractoriness as well as antagonizes the effects of β-AR activation.

Measurement of ventricular refractory periods before and after atropine provides only indirect evidence of how vagal activity may potentially modulate ventricular refractoriness. Thus, to assess directly the vagal effects on ventricular refractoriness, Ellenbogen et al[26] increased cardiac vagal tone in humans by stimulating either carotid sinus baroreceptors with neck suction or carotid and aortic baroreceptors with phenylephrine-induced increases in systolic pressure. Figure 6 shows that before neck suction, the right ventricular ERP

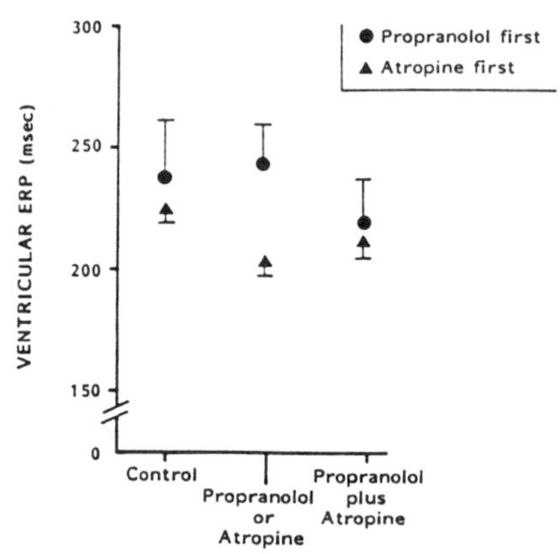

Figure 5. *Right ventricular ERPs before and after autonomic blockade in humans. The ventricular ERP was significantly shorter than control after atropine plus propranolol. Values are means ±SD (n = 3 to 8). Reproduced by permission of the American Heart Association, Inc. from Prystowsky EN, Jackman WM, Rinkenberger RL, et al: Effect of autonomic blockade on ventricular refractoriness and atrioventricular nodal conduction in humans. Evidence supporting a direct cholinergic action on ventricular muscle refractoriness. Circ Res 49:514, 1981.*

was 235 milliseconds, and during neck suction, when vagal tone was enhanced, the ERP increased to 240 milliseconds. The mean increase in the ventricular ERP during neck suction was 4 ± 1 milliseconds (n = 26). In 18 of 26 patients, however, the refractory period increased by 5 to 25 milliseconds, whereas in the remaining 8 patients, refractoriness was not altered during neck suction. When baroreceptors were activated by acutely elevating arterial pressure with phenylephrine, the ventricular ERP was prolonged an average of 5 ± 2 milliseconds (n = 6). In 2 patients, neck suction prolonged the ventricular ERP after β-AR blockade with propranolol. These data indicate that reflex increases in vagal tone prolonged the ventricular ERP in humans and confirm the results obtained after atropine alone.[30,31] In anesthetized dogs, Martins[12] also demonstrated that baroreceptor-induced increases in vagal tone prolonged the ventricular ERP. Both withdrawal of sympathetic tone and an increase in vagal tone, however, contributed to the baroreceptor-evoked prolongation of ventricular refractoriness.

In addition to efferent vagal activity, afferent vagal activity also appears to influence ventricular refractoriness.[34,35] Stimulation of cardiac vagal afferent fibers increases cardiac efferent vagal activity and decreases cardiac efferent sympathetic activity.[1] Schwartz et al,[34] in studies in anesthetized dogs treated with atropine, demonstrated that bilateral vagotomy decreased the ventricular ERP by three milliseconds. The authors concluded that afferent vagal activity inhibited efferent sympathetic outflow. Thus, when the vagi were sectioned bilaterally, the inhibitory effect of vagal afferent activity on sympathetic efferents was abolished, and this outcome led to a sympatheti-

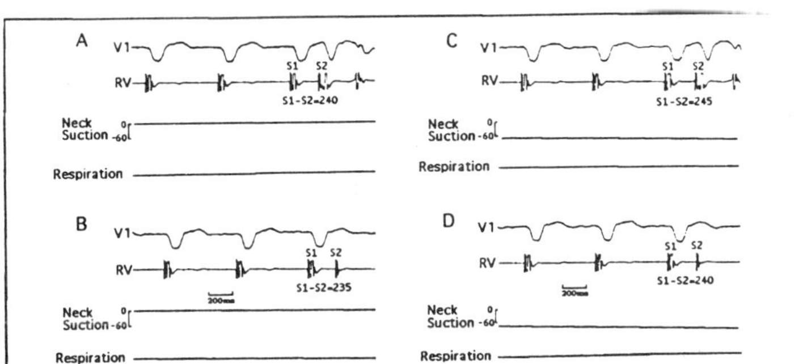

Figure 6. *Representative example in a resting human of the effect of reflexly increasing vagal tone with neck suction on ventricular refractoriness. From top to bottom in each panel are lead V_1 of the electrocardiogram, a right ventricular electrogram (RV), intracollar pressure (neck suction), and respiration. Panels A and B show that, without neck suction, the right ventricular ERP was 235 msec. Panels C and D show that, during neck suction at -60 mm Hg, the right ventricular ERP increased to 240 msec. Ventricular pacing at 600 msec (S_1-S_1) was used to determine the ERP and the coupling interval of the extrastimulus (S_2) was reduced by 5 msec. Measurements were obtained during held expiration to minimize catheter movement and respiratory-related changes in vagal tone. Reproduced with permission from Ellenbogen KA, Smith ML, Eckberg DL: Increased vagal cardiac nerve traffic prolongs ventricular refractoriness in patients undergoing electrophysiology testing. Am J Cardiol 65:1356, 1990.*

cally-evoked reduction in the ventricular ERP. In anesthetized cats with cardiac sympathetic and parasympathetic neurons intact, stimulation of vagal efferents in the caudovagal nerve prolonged the ventricular refractory period.[35] Prolongation of the ventricular ERP during afferent vagal stimulation was the result of both an increase in efferent vagal activity and a decrease in efferent sympathetic activity. Thus, vagal afferents modulate ventricular refractoriness by altering sympathetic and parasympathetic efferent outflow.

To delineate the location of the vagal fibers that modulate ventricular refractoriness, Zipes and his associates[36–40] measured vagal effects on ventricular ERP before and after surgically or chemically ablating nerve fibers in the ventricular epicardium or endocardium. In anesthetized dogs, they measured the effects of vagal and sympathetic stimulation on ventricular ERP before and after encircling (1- to 2-cm diameter) an area of the anterior left ventricular epicardium with phenol.[36] Phenol is a caustic agent that produces necrosis to a depth of 0.25 to 0.5 mm. The phenol was applied to only the perimeter of the circle, and a multipolar electrode for measuring ERPs was placed in the center of the epicardium encircled by phenol. Since vagal stimulation evokes greater increases in the ventricular ERP in the presence than in the absence of β-AR stimulation,[29,30,36] Zipes measured vagally-induced changes in refractoriness during a continuous infusion of NE.[40] Before and after phenol application, vagal stimulation prolonged the ventricular ERP by three to five milliseconds. In the same animals, however, sympathetically-induced shortening of the ventricular ERP was abolished after phenol application. These data support the hypothesis that sympathetic fibers travel in the ventricular epicardium, and nerve transmission in these fibers can be interrupted by epicardial phenol application (Fig. 7). Since the functional effects of vagal stimulation remained after phenol, these data also indicated that the vagal efferent fibers innervating the anterior left ventricle reside not in the epicardium, but either intramurally or in the endocardium.

To determine the pathway of efferent vagal innervation in the left ventricle, Chilson et al[38] showed in a subsequent study that a circumferential endocardial incision made to a depth of 2 mm eliminated vagally-induced prolongation of ERPs at endocardial and epicardial sites apical to the incision. The endocardial incision did not alter the vagal effects on ventricular refractoriness at sites basal to the incision. These data suggest that efferent vagal fibers affecting ventricular refractoriness reside in the endocardium of the left ventricle.

Although most vagal efferent fibers that affect ventricular refractoriness travel in the ventricular endocardium (Fig. 7),[36,38] the pathway of efferent vagal innervation from atria to ventricles remained unclear. To delineate the route that efferent vagal fibers travel to reach the left ventricle, Takahashi et al[37] measured vagally-induced ventricular ERP changes before and after applying phenol to selected sites on the epicardial surface of the heart. During a continuous NE infusion, they measured vagal effects on refractoriness at three left ventricular sites aligned vertically from apex to base (Fig. 8; sites 1,

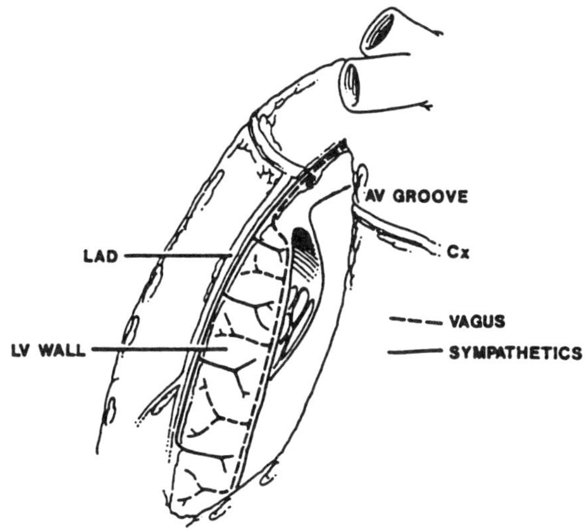

Figure 7. *Schematic of a saggital section through the left ventricle (LV) showing pathways of parasympathetic (vagus) and sympathetic nerves. Most postganglionic sympathetic axons are located superficially in the periadventitia of coronary arteries. Postganglionic parasympathetic axons cross the atrioventricular (AV) groove in the subepicardium, but are then located in the ventricular subendocardium. LAD: left anterior descending coronary artery; Cx: circumflex coronary artery. Reproduced by permission of the American Heart Association, Inc. from Zipes DP: Influence of myocardial ischemia and infarction on autonomic innervation of heart. Circulation 82:1096, 1990.*

2, and 3). After they obtained control measurements of vagal effects on ventricular refractoriness at the three electrode sites, they applied four lines of phenol (Fig. 8; lines A, B, C, D) sequentially from apex to base. The final line of phenol (Fig. 8, line D) was applied to the area of the AV groove. The vagally-induced prolongation of ventricular refractoriness at the three test sites was significantly attenuated only after application of phenol to the AV groove (line D). They concluded, therefore, that most efferent vagal fibers reach the ventricle by traversing the AV groove within 0.25 to 0.5 mm of the epicardial surface. Within 1 to 2 cm of the AV groove, however, the vagal efferent fibers in the ventricular epicardium penetrate the left ventricle and travel an intramural or subendocardial course (Fig. 7).

In agreement with these data, Blomquist and coworkers[41] demonstrated that efferent vagal axons present in the ventricles originate in supraventricular ganglia and reach the ventricles by traveling within the superficial layer of the AV groove. The vagal fibers that are located superficially in the AV groove may be prone to damage during certain surgical procedures. For example, in anesthetized dogs, surgical dissection or cryolesion in the AV groove (e.g., surgery for Wolff-Parkinson-White syndrome) attenuated the vagal effects on ventricular refractoriness.[39]

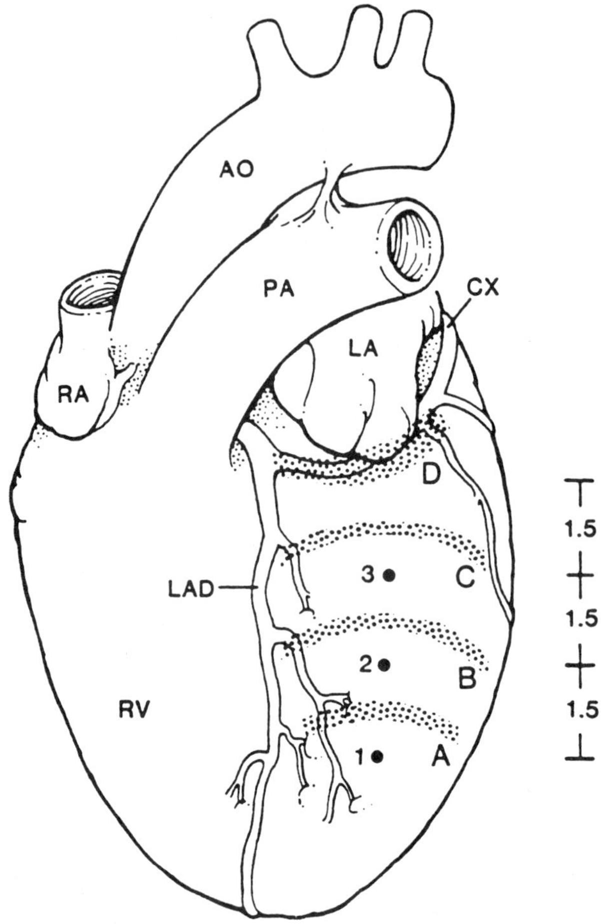

Figure 8. *Schematic representation of the sites of phenol application (stippled lines A, B, C, and D) to the surface of the heart. Distance between phenol stripes was 1.5 cm. Sites labelled 1, 2, and 3 denote location of electrodes for ERP measurements. AO: aorta; PA: pulmonary artery; RA: right atrium; LA: left atrium; RV: right ventricle; LAD: left anterior descending coronary artery; and CX: circumflex coronary artery. Reproduced with permission from Takahashi N, Barber MJ, Zipes DP: Efferent vagal innervation of the ventricle. Am J Physiol 248:H91, 1985.*

Purkinje Fiber Refractoriness

Parasympathetic effects on Purkinje fiber repolarization and refractoriness have been studied extensively by recording Purkinje fiber action potentials in vitro with intracellular microelectrode techniques.[32,42–45] The effects of ACh on Purkinje fiber repolarization appear to be species-dependent. In isolated canine cardiac Purkinje fibers, ACh had either no effect[43,45] or shortened the action potential duration.[42] In contrast, in isolated sheep Purkinje fibers, ACh prolonged the action potential duration in a dose-dependent manner.[44] Although ACh alone has various effects on Purkinje fiber repolarization, in canine cardiac Purkinje fibers, ACh consistently attenuated isoproterenol-induced shortening of action potential duration.[43,45] ACh antagonized adrenergic effects on Purkinje fiber action potential duration by presynaptic and postsynaptic mechanisms.[33]

Wendt and Martins[46] examined sympathetic and parasympathetic influences on the relative refractory period of Purkinje fibers in anesthetized dogs. Vagal stimulation alone did not appreciably affect the Purkinje relative refractory period, but it did increase the ERP of the adjacent ventricular muscle (Fig. 9). Vagal activation did, however, prolong the Purkinje relative refractory period in the presence of physostigmine, an acetylcholinesterase (AChE) inhibitor. Since the cardiac sympathetic nerves were intact during the physostigmine administration, it is unclear whether the enhanced vagal tone prolonged the Purkinje relative refractory period directly or indirectly by antagonizing tonic sympathetic effects. Indeed, vagal activation attenuated sympathetically-induced shortening of Purkinje relative refractory period in this preparation (Fig. 9). These data correlate with in vitro results that showed

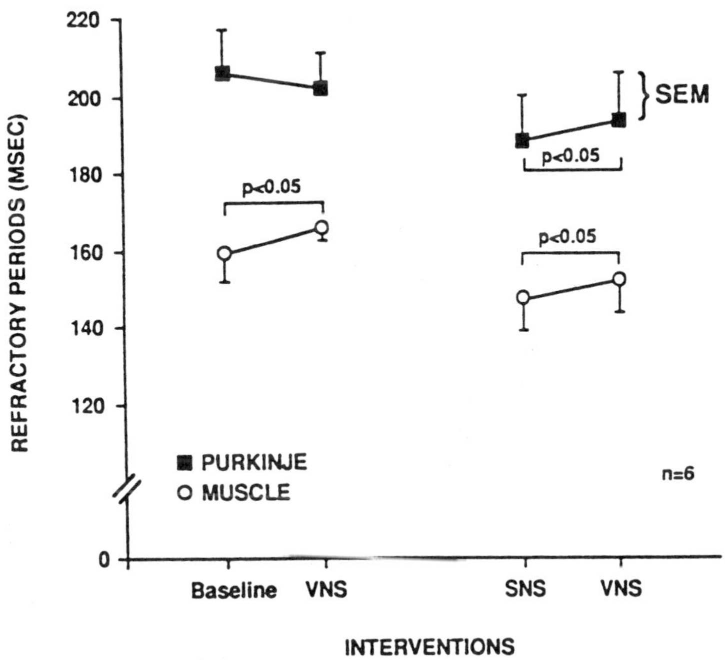

Figure 9. *Effects of vagal nerve stimulation (VNS) alone (left panel) and in combination with sympathetic nerve stimulation (SNS, right panel) on Purkinje relative refractory period (Purkinje) and ventricular endocardial ERP (Muscle) in anesthetized dogs. VNS alone significantly prolonged endocardial muscle ERP, but not Purkinje relative refractory period. During SNS, VNS significantly prolonged refractoriness of ventricular muscle and Purkinje. Reproduced with permission from Wendt DJ, Martins JB: Autonomic neural regulation of intact Purkinje system of dogs. Am J Physiol 258:H1424, 1990.*

that ACh antagonized β receptor-induced shortening of Purkinje fiber action potential duration.[43,45] Interestingly, Wendt and Martins[46] also showed that α-adrenergic receptor activation slightly prolonged the Purkinje relative refractory period, an effect that was enhanced by concomitant vagal stimulation.

Accessory Pathway Refractoriness

Morady et al[47] examined the effects of vagal tone on the ERP of accessory AV connections in patients with the Wolff-Parkinson-White syndrome. Patients included in the study had only a single accessory AV pathway. Atropine, either alone or in combination with propranolol, significantly shortened the anterograde and retrograde ERPs of the accessory AV connection. Thus, the authors inferred that resting vagal tone exerted an inhibitory effect on refractoriness of the accessory AV connection and that this effect was independent of the underlying sympathetic activity. Although the effects of changes in vagal activity were not measured directly, these data suggest that vagal tone lengthens the refractory periods of accessory AV pathways. Because vagal activation shortens atrial ERPs[20–23] and lengthens ventricular ERPs,[26,30,31] the results of this study suggest that at least a portion of the accessory AV connection in this group of patients had properties of ventricular rather than of atrial muscle.

Clinical Implications of Vagal Modulation of Cardiac Refractoriness

The experimental and clinical evidence discussed in this chapter indicates that vagal activation modulates refractoriness of all cardiac tissue, including the SA and AV nodes, Purkinje fibers, accessory AV pathways, and atrial and ventricular muscle. By altering cardiac refractoriness, changes in vagal tone can initiate, maintain, or terminate cardiac arrhythmias.[48,49] For example, maneuvers that increase vagal tone (e.g., carotid sinus massage, Valsalva, etc.) have been associated with the emergence of paroxysmal atrial fibrillation in humans.[49] The marked shortening of atrial refractoriness and the nonuniform distribution of vagal effects contribute to the vagally-induced initiation and maintenance of atrial fibrillation. In contrast to its effects on the atria, vagal activation, by lengthening the AV nodal ERP, terminates some tachyarrhythmias, including AV nodal and AV reentrant supraventricular tachycardia. In the ventricles, vagal activation increases the ventricular fibrillation threshold,[50,51] protects against reperfusion arrhythmias,[51] and, in some patients, consistently terminates ventricular tachycardia.[49,52,53] Vagal activation may mediate these responses, in part, by prolonging ventricular refractoriness both directly and indirectly by antagonizing sympathetic effects on refractoriness. Indeed, if the ventricular arrhythmia depends on a reentrant circuit, small vagally-induced changes in refractoriness at a critical point in the circuit could terminate the reentrant arrhythmia.

Although vagal activity only slightly prolongs refractoriness in normal ventricular muscle, in abnormal myocardium, the vagal effects may become more pronounced. Myocardial ischemia or infarction can partially or totally denervate myocardial tissue and thereby induce a denervation supersensitivity in the damaged ventricular muscle and at noninfarcted sites apical to that zone.[54–57] Responses to vagal stimulation in the partially denervated myocardium may be greater than in the neighboring, normally innervated myocardium.

References

1. Corr PB, Yamada KA, Witkowski FX: Mechanisms controlling cardiac autonomic function and their relation to arrhythmogenesis. In HA Fozzard et al (eds): The Heart and Cardiovascular System. New York, NY, Raven Press, 1986, p. 1343.
2. Levy MN, Martin PJ: Neural control of the heart. In RM Berne, N Sperelakis (eds): Handbook of Physiology. Section 2: The Cardiovascular System-the Heart, Vol. I. Bethesada, MD, American Physiological Society, 1979, p. 581.
3. Löffelholz K, Pappano AJ: The parasympathetic neuroeffector junction of the heart. Pharmacol Rev 37:1, 1985.
4. Brown OM: Cat heart acetylcholine: Structural proof and distribution. Am J Physiol 231:781, 1976.
5. Imaizumi S, Mazgalev T, Dreifus LS, et al: Morphological and electrophysiological correlates of atrioventricular nodal response to increased vagal activity. Circulation 82:951, 1990.
6. Prystowsky EN, Grant AO, Wallace AG, et al: An analysis of the effects of acetylcholine on conduction and refractoriness in the rabbit sinus node. Circ Res 44:112, 1979.
7. Kerr CR: Effects of acetylcholine, propranolol, and verapamil on sinus node refractoriness of the rabbit. Can J Physiol Pharmacol 67:1232, 1989.
8. Moe GK, Childers RW, Meredith J: An appraisal of "supernormal" A-V conduction. Circulation 38:5, 1968.
9. Childers R: The AV node: Normal and abnormal physiology. Prog Cardiovasc Dis 19:361, 1977.
10. Linhart JW, Braunwald E, Ross J: Determinants of the duration of the refractory period of the atrioventricular nodal system in man. J Clin Invest 44:883, 1965.
11. Gambetta M, Denes P, Childers RW: Vagally induced second degree A-V block Mobitz type I, and the hyporeactive SA node. Chest 62:152, 1972.
12. Martins JB: Carotid sinus baroreflex influence on electrophysiologic properties of the canine atrioventricular node and ventricle. Am J Cardiol 54:431, 1984.
13. Toda N, West TC: Changes in sino-atrial node transmembrane potentials on vagal stimulation of the isolated rabbit right atrium. Nature 205:808, 1965.
14. Jalife J, Moe GK: Phasic responses of the SA and AV nodes to vagal stimulation. In MB Rosenbaum, MV Elizari (eds): Frontiers of Cardiac Electrophysiology. Boston, MA, Martinus Nijhoff Publishers, 1983, p. 501.
15. Warner MR, Loeb JM: Beat-by-beat modulation of AV conduction. I. Heart rate and respiratory influences. Am J Physiol 251:H1126, 1986.
16. Zipes DP, Mendez C, Moe G: Some examples of Wenckebach periodicity in cardiac tissues, with an appraisal of mechanisms. In MB Rosenbaum, MV Elizari (eds): Frontiers of Cardiac Electrophysiology. Boston, MA, Martinus Nijhoff Publishers, 1983, p. 357.
17. Hoffman BF, Suckling EE: Cardiac cellular potentials: Effect of vagal stimulation and acetylcholine. Am J Physiol 173:312, 1953.

18. Ninomiya I: Direct evidence of nonuniform distribution of vagal effects on dog atria. Circ Res 19:576, 1966.
19. Hordof AJ, Spotnitz A, Mary-Rabine L, et al: The cellular electrophysiologic effects of digitalis on human atrial fibers. Circulation 57:223, 1978.
20. Hoffman BF, Siebens AA, Brooks C: Effect of vagal stimulation on cardiac excitability. Am J Physiol 169:377, 1952.
21. Alessi R, Nusynowitz M, Abildskov JA, et al: Nonuniform distribution of vagal effects on the atrial refractory period. Am J Physiol 194:406, 1958.
22. Zipes DP, Mihalick MJ, Robbins GT: Effects of selective vagal and stellate ganglion stimulation on atrial refractoriness. Cardiovasc Res 8:647, 1974.
23. Prystowsky EN, Naccarelli GV, Jackman WM, et al: Enhanced parasympathetic tone shortens atrial refractoriness in man. Am J Cardiol 51:96, 1983.
24. Dhingra RC, Amat-Y-Leon F, Wyndham C, et al: Electrophysiologic effects of atropine on human sinus node and atrium. Am J Cardiol 38:429, 1976.
25. Amlie JP, Refsum H: Vagus-induced changes in ventricular electrophysiology of the dog heart with and without beta-blockade. J Cardiovasc Pharmacol 3:1203, 1981.
26. Ellenbogan KA, Smith ML, Eckberg DL: Increased vagal cardiac nerve traffic prolongs ventricular refractoriness in patients undergoing electrophysiology testing. Am J Cardiol 65:1345, 1990.
27. Kolman BS, Verrier RL, Lown B: Effect of vagus nerve stimulation upon the excitability of the canine ventricle. Role of sympathetic-parasympathetic interactions. Am J Cardiol 37:1041, 1976.
28. Martins JB, Zipes DP: Effects of sympathetic and vagal nerves on recovery properties of the endocardium and epicardium of the canine left ventricle. Circ Res 46:100, 1980.
29. Nattel S, Euler DE, Spear JF, et al: Autonomic control of ventricular refractoriness. Am J Physiol 241:H878, 1981.
30. Morady F, Kou WH, Nelson SD, et al: Accentuated antagonism between beta-adrenergic and vagal effects on ventricular refractoriness in humans. Circulation 77:289, 1988.
31. Prystowsky EN, Jackman WM, Rinkenberger RL, et al: Effect of autonomic blockade on ventricular refractoriness and atrioventricular nodal conduction in humans. Evidence supporting a direct cholinergic action on ventricular muscle refractoriness. Circ Res 49:511, 1981.
32. Rardon DP, Bailey JC: Parasympathetic effects on electrophysiologic properties of cardiac ventricular tissue. J Am Coll Cardiol 2:1200, 1983.
33. Gilmour RF, Zipes DP: Evidence for prejunctional and postjunctional antagonism of the sympathetic neuroeffector junction by acetylcholine in canine cardiac Purkinje fibers. J Am Coll Cardiol 3:760, 1984.
34. Schwartz PJ, Verrier RL, Lown B: Effect of stellectomy and vagotomy on ventricular refractoriness in dogs. Circ Res 40:536, 1977.
35. Blair RW, Shimizu T, Bishop VS: The role of vagal afferents in the reflex control of the left ventricular refractory period in the cat. Circ Res 46:378, 1980.
36. Martins JB, Zipes DP: Epicardial phenol interrupts refractory period responses to sympathetic but not vagal stimulation in canine left ventricular epicardium and endocardium. Circ Res 47:33, 1980.
37. Takahashi N, Barber MJ, Zipes DP: Efferent vagal innervation of the ventricle. Am J Physiol 248:H89, 1985.
38. Chilson DA, Peigh P, Mahomed Y, et al: Encircling endocardial incision interrupts efferent vagal-induced prolongation of endocardial and epicardial refractoriness in the dog. J Am Coll Cardiol 5:290, 1985.
39. Inoue H, Mahomed Y, Kovacs RJ, et al: Surgery for Wolff-Parkinson-White syndrome interrupts efferent vagal innervation to the left ventricle and to the atrioventricular node in the canine heart. Cardiovasc Res 22:163, 1988.

40. Zipes DP: Influence of myocardial ischemia and infarction on autonomic innervation of heart. Circulation 82:1095, 1990.
41. Blomquist TM, Priola DV, Romero AM: Source of intrinsic innervation of canine ventricles: A functional study. Am J Physiol 252:H638, 1987.
42. Gadsby DC, Wit AL, Cranefield PF: The effects of acetylcholine on the electrical activity of canine cardiac Purkinje fibers. Circ Res 43:29, 1978.
43. Bailey JC, Watanabe AM, Besch HR, et al: Acetylcholine antagonism of the electrophysiological effects of isoproterenol on canine cardiac Purkinje fibers. Circ Res 44:378, 1979.
44. Lipsius SL, Gibbons WR: Acetylcholine lengthens action potentials of sheep cardiac Purkinje fibers. Am J Physiol 238:H237, 1980.
45. Hamra M, Viamonte VM, Rosen MR: Transmembrane potential characteristics and muscarinic and beta-adrenergic responsiveness in Purkinje fibers from a canine model of lethal ventricular arrhythmias. J Cardiovasc Electrophysiol 2:108, 1991.
46. Wendt DJ, Martins JB: Autonomic neural regulation of intact Purkinje system of dogs. Am J Physiol 258:H1420, 1990.
47. Morady F, Kadish AH, Schmaltz S: Effects of resting vagal tone on accessory atrioventricular connections. Circulation 81:86, 1990.
48. Moe GK, Abildskov JA: Atrial fibrillation as a self-sustaining arrhythmia independent of focal discharge. Am Heart J 58:59, 1959.
49. Waxman MB, Wald RW, Cameron D: Interactions between the autonomic nervous system and tachycardias in man. Cardiol Clin 1:143, 1983.
50. Kent KM, Smith ER, Redwood DR, et al: Electrical stability of ischemic myocardium: Influences of heart rate and vagal stimulation. Circulation 47:291, 1973.
51. Corr PB, Gillis RA: Autonomic neural influences on the dysrhythmias resulting from myocardial infarction. Circ Res 43:1, 1978.
52. Waxman MB, Wald RW: Termination of ventricular tachycardia by an increase in cardiac vagal drive. Circulation 56:385, 1977.
53. Hess DS, Hanlon T, Scheinman M, et al: Termination of ventricular tachycardia by carotid sinus massage. Circulation 65:627, 1982.
54. Inoue H, Zipes DP: Time course of denervation of efferent sympathetic and vagal nerves after occlusion of the coronary artery in the canine heart. Circ Res 62:1111, 1988.
55. Kaseda S, Zipes DP: Supersensitivity to acetylcholine of canine sinus and atrioventricular nodes after parasympathetic denervation. Am J Physiol 24:H534, 1988.
56. Barber MJ, Mueller TM, Davies BG, et al: Interruption of sympathetic and vagal-mediated afferent responses by transmural myocardial infarction. Circulation 72:623, 1985.
57. Barber MJ, Mueller TM, Henry DP, et al: Transmural myocardial infarction in the dog produces sympathectomy in noninfarcted myocardium. Circulation 67:787, 1983.

CHAPTER 17

Vagal Control of Coronary Blood Flow

E.O. Feigl

Activation of parasympathetic fibers to the heart produces a slowing of the heart rate, decreased contractility, and a fall in blood pressure that results in decreased myocardial metabolism. The diminished myocardial oxygen consumption results in a decrease in coronary blood flow by a local metabolic mechanism.

In dogs, when the heart is electrically paced at a constant rate, vagal stimulation results in an increase in coronary flow independent of the negative chronotropic and inotropic effects of parasympathetic activation (Fig. 1).[1,2] Bolus injections of acetylcholine (ACh) in dogs produces dilation of epicardial coronary vessels that is longer lasting than the augmented flow.[3,4] In species other than dogs, the effects of ACh on the coronary circulation are complicated.[5]

In baboons, continuous intracoronary infusions of low doses of ACh resulted in increases in coronary blood flow and coronary venous oxygen tension without changes in myocardial oxygen consumption, a clear indication of vasodilation (Fig. 2).[6] At high doses, the negative inotropic effect of ACh dominated and a net decrease in coronary blood flow was observed, although coronary venous oxygen tension still increased. Vagal stimulation in baboons produced a modest increase in coronary blood flow. Intracoronary bolus injections of high doses of ACh produced coronary vasoconstriction potent enough to cause a diminution of cardiac contraction.[7]

In goats, a weak coronary vasodilation was observed at low doses of ACh, and a marked decrease in coronary flow and myocardial oxygen consumption was found with high doses.[8] In calves, intracoronary bolus doses of ACh resulted in prompt transient decreases in coronary flow; however, myocardial oxygen consumption was not determined, so it is difficult to interpret the relative importance of coronary vascular and myocardial effects.[9] In pigs, intracoronary bolus doses of ACh also produced transient decreases in coronary flow, but myocardial oxygen consumption was not measured.[10] Porcine epicardial coronary arteries constrict in response to intracoronary injections

From *Vagal Control of the Heart: Experimental Basis and Clinical Implications* edited by MN Levy, PJ Schwartz © 1994, Futura Publishing Co. Inc., Armonk, NY.

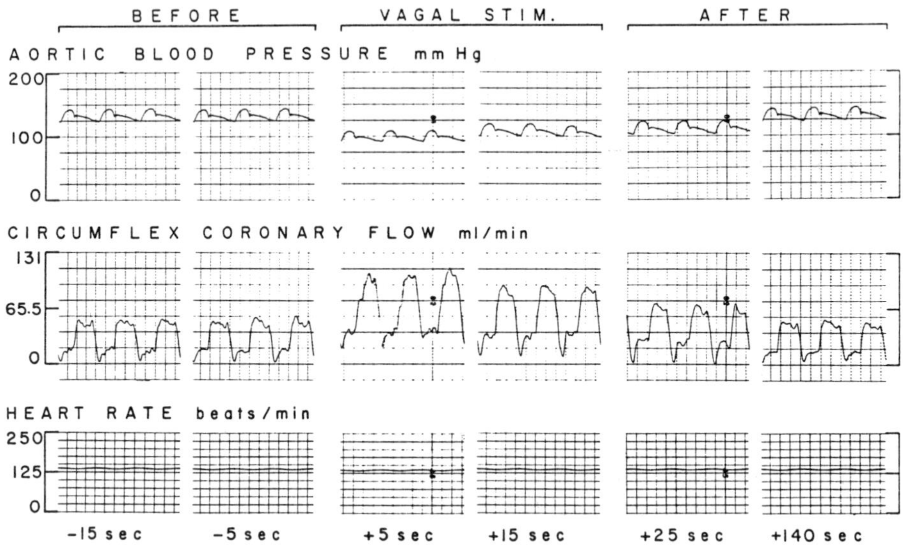

Figure 1. *Effects of a 20-s vagal stimulation (30 Hz, 8 V, 2 msec) in a chloralose-anesthetized dog. Blood pressure fell and circumflex coronary artery blood flow increased in both systole and diastole. Heart rate was constantly paced. Reproduced by permission of the American Heart Association, Inc. from Feigl EO: Parasympathetic control of coronary blood flow in dogs. Circ Res 25:512, 1969.*

of ACh.[11] Human responses to ACh are discussed in the section on atherosclerosis.

Endothelium-Derived Relaxing Factor

The effect of ACh on the coronary circulation depends on a muscarinic action on both endothelium and vascular smooth muscle.[12,13] ACh stimulates endothelial cells to release endothelium-derived relaxing factor (EDRF), which causes relaxation by stimulating soluble guanylate cyclase in the adjacent smooth muscle. At the present time, EDRF is thought to be the nitric oxide free radical (·NO) or a precursor that releases ·NO. In the absence of endothelium, ACh causes contraction in many vessels,[5] although cholinergic relaxation is observed in the ear artery of the cat.[14] Thus, whether ACh causes a net dilation or constriction depends on the balance between the muscarinic effects on endothelium and vascular smooth muscle. The balance between endothelial-mediated dilation and smooth muscle vasoconstriction depends on the dose of ACh, as described above in the baboon. At low infusion rates, dilation is dominant, while at very high doses, vasoconstriction is the net effect. The net balance between EDRF dilation and smooth muscle constriction also varies

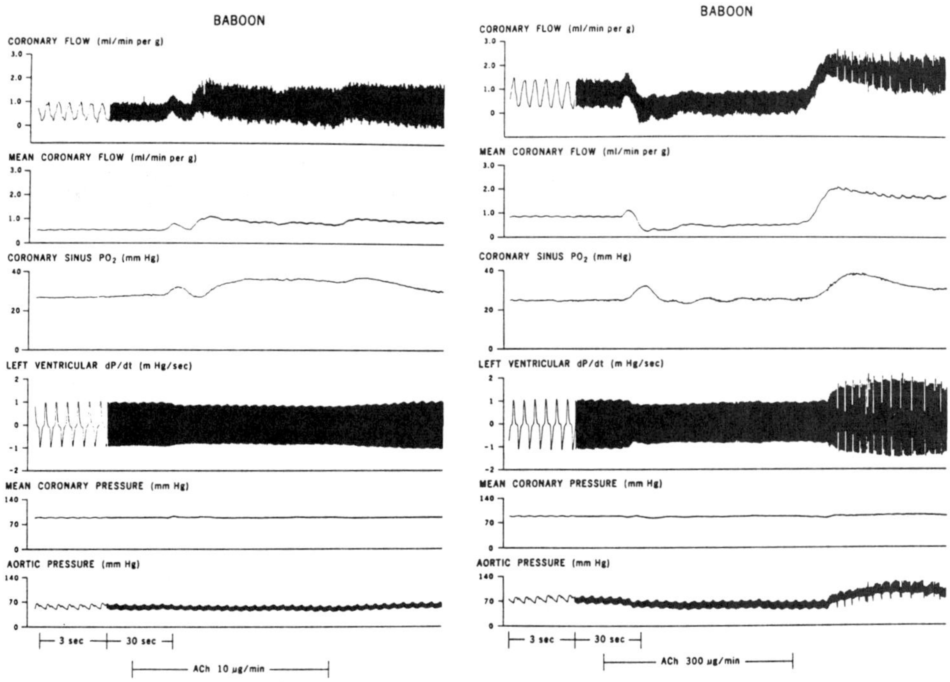

Figure 2. *Effects of two doses of intracoronary ACh in one baboon. During infusion of 10 μg/min ACh (at steady portion of response, left panel), coronary blood flow was increased by 50% over control values. Coronary sinus oxygen tension (PO_2) was also increased for the period of infusion. With 300 μg/min ACh (right panel), coronary blood flow increased transiently. This effect was followed by a 43% decrease in flow that was sustained for the duration of the infusion. Coronary sinus PO_2 increased at start of infusion, then returned toward baseline. Reproduced by permission of the American Heart Association, Inc. from Van Winkle DM, Feigl EO: Acetylcholine causes coronary vasodilation in dogs and baboons. Circ Res 65:1580, 1989.*

among different species,[5] with increases in flow the only effect observed in dogs[2] and decreases in flow the only effect reported in calves[9] and pigs.[10]

EDRF is synthesized from the guanidino nitrogen atoms of L-arginine by a ·NO synthase,[15] and the synthesis of EDRF can be blocked by L-arginine analogs that are false substrates for the synthase.

Figure 3 illustrates that the arginine analog L-nitro-arginine methyl ester (L-NAME) blunted both the coronary vasodilation due to intracoronary injection of ACh and parasympathetic coronary vasodilation due to electrical stimulation of the vagus nerves, but did not diminish the response to nitroglycerin, which is an EDRF-independent vasodilator. These results indicate that parasympathetic coronary vasodilation is mediated via EDRF. Since parasympathetic innervation ends at the adventitial-medial border, presumably the ACh from vagal fibers diffuses across the media to reach the endothelium where EDRF is released.

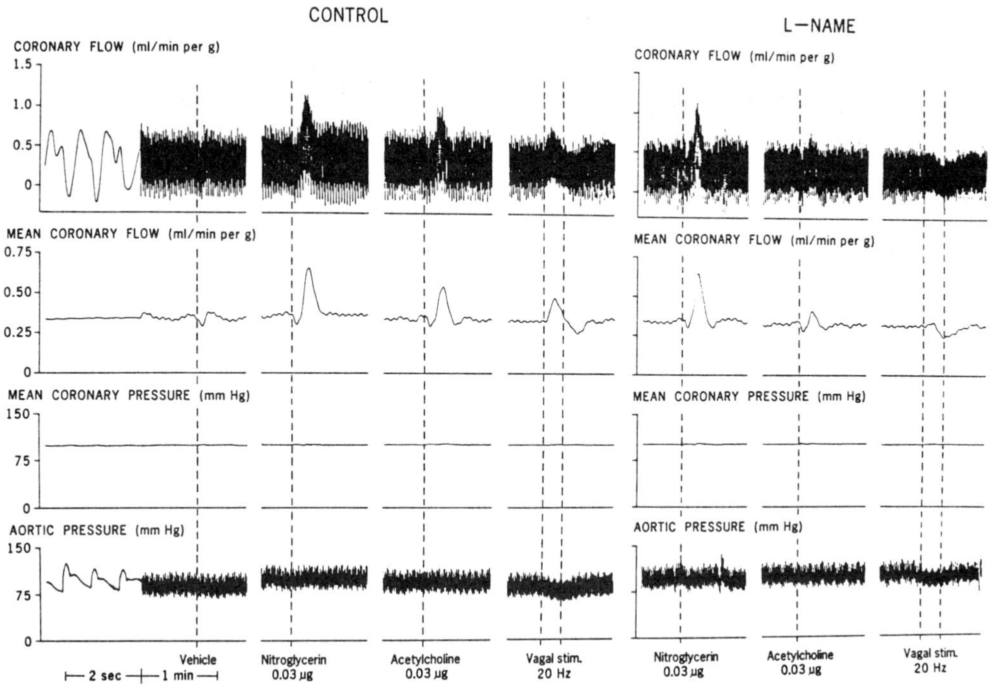

Figure 3. *An example, from one dog, of the hemodynamic responses to vagal stimulation and intracoronary administration of vehicle, nitroglycerin, and ACh before (CONTROL) and during intracoronary infusion of L-NAME. The small decrease in flow immediately following injections is an artifact generated by the pump that maintained coronary perfusion pressure. Nitroglycerin and ACh increased coronary flow, without affecting arterial pressure. Bilateral stimulation of the vagus nerves (20 Hz, 0.6 msec, 7 V) produced a transient increase in coronary flow and a concomitant decrease in arterial pressure. L-NAME infusion (intracoronary blood concentration 300 μM) significantly reduced the coronary responses to ACh and vagal stimulation, but not to nitroglycerin. Note that the decrease in contractility associated with vagal stimulation was not affected by L-NAME.*

Receptor Subtype

The coronary effects of vagal activation or ACh are blocked by atropine, indicating that muscarinic receptors (mAChRs) are involved. mAChRs are members of the superfamily of seven-helix receptors that includes α_{-2}, β_{-1}, β_2-adrenergic receptors (β-Ar), and some types of serotonin receptors. These receptors have seven membrane-spanning regions and transduce their signals via one or more guanosine nucleotide-binding proteins (G-proteins). The mAChRs have been pharmacologically classified into three groups—M_1, M_2, M_3—by selective antagonists pirenzepine (PZ) (M_1), AF-DX 116 (M_2), and *p*-fluorohexahydrosiladifenidol (M_3). mAChRs have also been characterized into five groups (m_1 through m_5) according to their molecular sequence, where m_1, m_2, and m_3 are thought to correspond respectively to M_1, M_2, and M_3.[16,17]

Gross and coworkers[18,19] suggest that cholinergic endothelium-dependent coronary vasodilation in dogs is predominantly mediated by M_1 (PZ-sensitive) receptors. Although methacholine constriction of bovine coronary artery rings (where the endothelium is stripped away) is blunted by either PZ (M_1) or AF-DX 116 (M_2),[20] bovine coronary smooth muscle probably has *p*-fluorohexahydrosiladifenidol (M_3) receptors.[21]

Transmural Flow

The inner layer of the left ventricle normally receives 10% to 20% more blood flow than the outer layer in unstressed hearts.[2] However, the inner layer of the left ventricle is much more susceptible to underperfusion than the outer layer, and a fall in the inner/outer flow ratio to values below approximately 0.9 usually indicates subendocardial ischemia. Therefore, agents that selectively dilate the coronary circulation in the inner layer of the left ventricle might have therapeutic potential. The intracoronary infusion of ACh increases the inner/outer flow ratio.[19,22,23] However, the vasodilation produced by vagal activation increases coronary blood flow uniformly across the left ventricular wall (Fig. 4).[23–25]

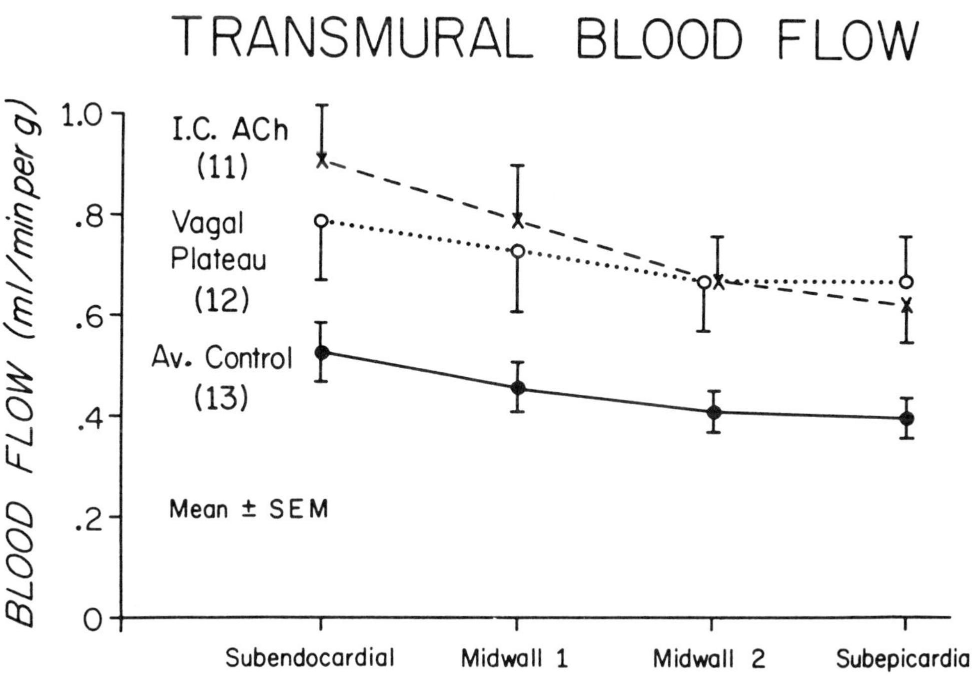

Figure 4. *Steady-state vagal stimulation increased coronary blood flow equally in all transmural layers of the left ventricle. In contrast, intracoronary ACh (I.C. ACh) infusion preferentially vasodilated subendocardium. Mean values ± SEM. Reproduced with permission from Reid JVO, Ito BR, Huang AH, et al: Parasympathetic control of transmural coronary blood flow in dogs. Am J Physiol 249:H341, 1985.*

Parasympathetic Reflex Coronary Control

Parasympathetic reflex coronary vasodilation has been observed in a number of conditions where vagal bradycardia occurs. Thus far, reflex parasympathetic coronary control has only been studied in dogs.

Carotid Sinus Baroreceptor Reflex

Elevation of carotid sinus blood pressure results in a reflex inhibition of sympathetic fiber discharge to the heart and peripheral vasculature and a reflex activation of parasympathetic fibers to the heart, producing bradycardia. If the coronary artery is perfused at constant pressure and the heart is paced at a constant rate while pressure in the vascularly isolated carotid sinuses is elevated, then a parasympathetic coronary vasodilation may be observed (Fig. 5).[26] A reflex inhibition of sympathetic coronary vasoconstriction is also present.

Carotid Body Chemoreceptor Reflex

Physiologically, the carotid body chemoreceptors respond to arterial hypoxemia and, to a lesser extent, hypercarbia. The receptors also respond to injections of nicotine. The cardiac effect of activating carotid body receptors is reflex parasympathetic bradycardia. A reflex parasympathetic coronary vasodilation in response to intracarotid bolus injections of nicotine has been observed in several laboratories.[27–29] However, it is difficult to know how a nicotine injection corresponds to the physiological stimulus of hypoxia. When the carotid bodies are perfused with hypoxic-hypercarbic blood, there is only a transient reflex parasympathetic coronary vasodilation (Fig. 6).[30]

Ventricular Receptors

Mechano- and chemoreceptors in the wall of the left ventricle can be stimulated nonspecifically by intracoronary injections of *Veratrum* alkaloids. This finding is the basis of the Bezold-Jarisch reflex, in which intracoronary injection of veratridine results in vagal bradycardia and peripheral vasodilation by inhibition of sympathetic discharge. If the heart is paced at a constant rate, injection of veratridine into one coronary branch produces a reflex parasympathetic coronary vasodilation in other branches that did not receive any veratridine (Fig. 7).[24,31,32] A similar parasympathetic reflex coronary vasodilation can be elicited by intracoronary injection of ouabain.[33] The physiological function of parasympathetic coronary vasodilation as part of the Bezold-Jarisch reflex has not been clearly demonstrated. Ventricular chemore-

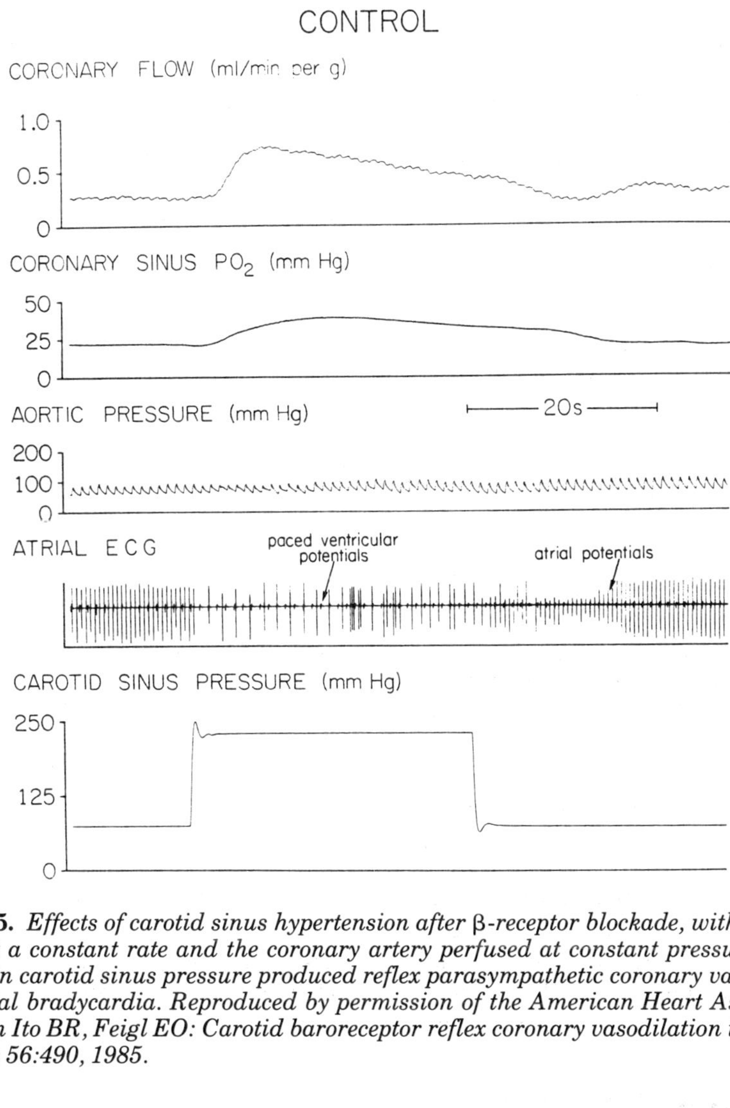

Figure 5. *Effects of carotid sinus hypertension after β-receptor blockade, with the heart paced at a constant rate and the coronary artery perfused at constant pressure. A step change in carotid sinus pressure produced reflex parasympathetic coronary vasodilation and atrial bradycardia. Reproduced by permission of the American Heart Association, Inc. from Ito BR, Feigl EO: Carotid baroreceptor reflex coronary vasodilation in the dog. Circ Res 56:490, 1985.*

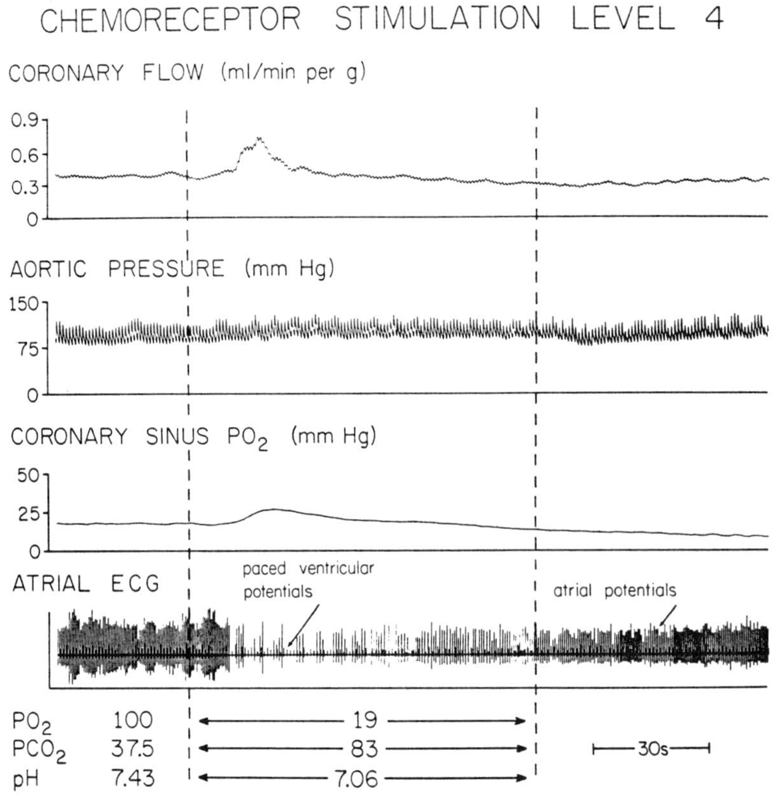

Figure 6. *Effects of a step 90-s hypoxic-hypercarbic perfusion of carotid bodies with ventricle paced at a constant rate in a β-receptor blocked dog. There was a parasympathetic reflex increase in coronary blood flow and coronary sinus PO_2 and atrial bradycardia. Values for PO_2, PCO_2, and pH of carotid perfusion blood before and during chemoreceptor stimulation are given. Reproduced with permission from Ito BR, Feigl EO: Carotid chemoreceptor reflex parasympathetic coronary vasodilation in the dog. Am J Physiol 249:H1170, 1985.*

ceptors are activated during myocardial ischemia, and mechanoreceptors may be activated by ventricular bulging in an ischemic area. Since the coronary vasculature is not maximally dilated at low perfusion pressures that cause functional impairment,[34] it is possible that reflex parasympathetic coronary vasodilation protects underperfused myocardium.

Pulmonary Chemoreflex

Right atrial, but not left atrial, injections of capsaicin produce reflex bradycardia, systemic hypotension, and apnea by stimulating pulmonary receptors with vagal C-fiber afferent connections. If the reflex bradycardia is prevented by cardiac pacing, then a parasympathetic coronary vasodilation may be demonstrated during the pulmonary chemoreflex.[25,35] Pulmonary C-fibers are stimulated during embolization or inhalation of irritant gases, but

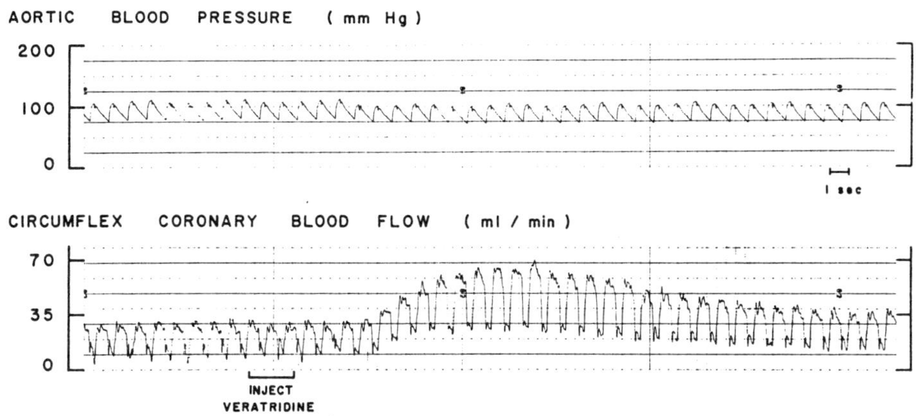

Figure 7. *Effect of 5 μg of veratridine injected into the anterior descending and septal coronary arteries after α- and β-receptor blockade with the heart electrically paced at a constant rate. Veratridine injected in the anterior descending coronary artery produced reflex parasympathetic vasodilation in the circumflex coronary artery, which received no veratridine. Reproduced by permission of the American Heart Association, Inc. from Feigl EO: Reflex parasympathetic coronary vasodilation elicited from cardiac receptors in the dog. Circ Res 37:177, 1975.*

the physiological importance of a reflex coronary vasodilation during such conditions is unclear.

Atherosclerosis

In 1986, Ludmer et al[36] reported that the intracoronary infusion of ACh produced epicardial coronary artery dilation in normal subjects, but produced paradoxical constriction in patients with early or advanced coronary atherosclerosis. This observation has been confirmed in other laboratories.[37,38] Paradoxical constriction of epicardial coronary arteries may be observed even in vessels with angiographically smooth lumens and it is postulated that this occurrence may be an early marker of endothelial dysfunction in atherosclerosis, since the constriction correlates well with age[38] and risk factors for coronary artery disease.[39] The coronary arteries of transplanted hearts undergo an accelerated form of atherosclerosis, and paradoxical cholinergic constriction is also observed in these patients.[40,41]

An intriguing question is whether the endothelial dysfunction, as demonstrated by an absence of a cholinergic EDRF response, is part of the atherosclerotic process or just a nonspecific correlation. The ·NO radical may act as a protective factor against oxygen free radicals found in arterial blood, and the loss of function might be part of the atherosclerosis process.[42]

Most of coronary vascular resistance is in the microcirculation, which does not develop atherosclerosis, and intracoronary infusion of ACh produces coronary vasodilation in normal subjects and patients with coronary atherosclerosis.[41,43]

Coronary spasm (otherwise known as variant angina or Prinzmetal's angina) represents a special syndrome that is probably separate from the epicardial coronary artery constriction that is observed in ordinary atherosclerotic patients.[44] The characteristic lesion in variant angina is a segmental spasm that occludes, or nearly occludes, the coronary artery lumen. Ergonovine is usually used to provoke spasm in patients with variant angina, but histamine, epinephrine, hyperventilation, and other interventions can also induce spasm in these patients.[45] Yasue and coworkers[46,47] have demonstrated that intracoronary injections of ACh can precipitate spasm in patients with variant angina, and they suggest that parasympathetic discharge to an arterial segment with impaired endothelial function may be the cause of variant angina. This finding is a tempting hypothesis for the genesis of coronary spasm and variant angina but, as Cannon[48] points out, there is probably another unknown factor involved, otherwise coronary spasm would be more common.

Conclusions

ACh has four main effects on the heart: bradycardia, decreased contractility, EDRF-dependent vasodilation, and EDRF-independent vascular smooth muscle constriction. The net effect of ACh or parasympathetic activation on coronary blood flow depends on the balance among these four factors. This balance depends upon the dose of ACh, the species, and the presence or absence of coronary atherosclerosis. If cholinergic bradycardia is prevented by cardiac pacing, then with low doses of ACh, coronary vasodilation can be observed in dogs, baboons, and humans. In baboons, the negative inotropic effects become dominant at high doses and coronary blood flow decreases secondary to the decrease in myocardial oxygen consumption, whereas with very high bolus doses of ACh, the EDRF-independent vasoconstriction predominates. Normal human epicardial coronary arteries dilate in response to ACh, but there is a paradoxical constriction in atherosclerotic vessels. Even vessels with angiographically smooth lumens may manifest paradoxical constriction, and it is thought that paradoxical constriction is an early marker of endothelial dysfunction in the atherosclerotic process. Coronary flow is primarily controlled by microvessels that do not develop atherosclerosis, and intracoronary ACh increases coronary blood flow in both normal subjects and patients with atherosclerosis.

Variant angina with segmental occlusive spasm of an epicardial coronary artery can be precipitated with intracoronary infusions of ACh and it is postulated that spasm is triggered by parasympathetic discharge to a vessel segment with damaged endothelium. However, there is likely to be some additional factor in variant angina, since most patients develop paradoxical constriction, but not occlusive spasm, during ACh infusion.

Although there has been good progress in understanding the actions of ACh on the coronary circulation, the role of the parasympathetic nervous system in coronary vascular disease remains unclear.

References

1. Feigl EO: Parasympathetic control of coronary blood flow in dogs. Circ Res 25:509, 1969.
2. Feigl EO: Coronary physiology. Physiol Rev 63:1, 1983.
3. Cox DA, Hintze TH, Vatner SF: Effects of acetylcholine on large and small coronary arteries in conscious dogs. J Pharmacol Exp Ther 225:764, 1983.
4. Chu A, Murray JJ, Lin C-C, et al: Preferential proximal coronary dilation by activators of guanylate cyclase in awake dogs. Am J Physiol 259:H340, 1990.
5. Kalsner S: Cholinergic constriction in the general circulation and its role in coronary artery spasm. Circ Res 65:237, 1989.
6. Van Winkle DM, Feigl EO: Acetylcholine causes coronary vasodilation in dogs and baboons. Circ Res 65:1580, 1989.
7. Knight DR, Shen K-Z, Young MA, et al: Acetylcholine-induced coronary vasoconstriction and vasodilation in tranquilized baboons. Circ Res 69:706–713, 1991.
8. Feigl EO, Van Winkle DM, Miyashiro JK: Cholinergic vasodilatation of coronary resistance vessels in dogs, baboons and goats. Blood Vessels 27:94, 1990.
9. Young MA, Knight DR, Vatner SF: Parasympathetic coronary vasoconstriction induced by nicotine in conscious calves. Circ Res 62:891, 1988.
10. Cowan CL, McKenzie JE: Cholinergic regulation of resting coronary blood flow in domestic swine. Am J Physiol 259:H109, 1990.
11. Kawamura A, Fujiwara H, Onodera T, et al: Response of large and small coronary arteries of pigs to intracoronary injection of acetylcholine: Angiographic and histologic analysis. Int J Cardiol 25:289, 1989.
12. Furchgott RF: Role of endothelium in responses of vascular smooth muscle. Circ Res 53:557, 1983.
13. Bassenge E, Busse R: Endothelial modulation of coronary tone. Prog Cardiovasc Dis 30:349, 1988.
14. Brayden JE, Bevan JA: Neurogenic muscarinic vasodilation in the cat. An example of endothelial cell-independent cholinergic relaxation. Circ Res 56:205, 1985.
15. Moncada S, Higgs EA: Nitric Oxide from L-Arginine: A Bioregulatory System. Amsterdam, Elsevier, 1990.
16. Birdsall N, Buckley N, Doods H, et al: Nomenclature for muscarinic receptor subtypes recommended by symposium. TIPS 10(suppl IV), 1989.
17. Goyal RK: Muscarinic receptor subtypes: Physiology and clinical implications. N Engl J Med 321:1022, 1989.
18. Pelc LR, Gross GJ, Warltier DC: Changes in regional myocardial perfusion by muscarinic receptor subtypes in dogs. Cardiovasc Res 20:482, 1986.
19. Pelc LR, Daemmgen JW, Gross GJ, et al: Muscarinic receptor subtypes mediating myocardial blood flow redistribution. J Cardiovasc Pharmacol 11:424, 1988.
20. Duckles SP: Vascular muscarinic receptors - pharmacological characterization in the bovine coronary artery. J Pharmacol Exp Ther 246:929, 1988.
21. Duckles SP, Garcia-Villalon AL: Characterization of vascular muscarinic receptors—Rabbit ear artery and bovine coronary artery coronary smooth muscle cells. J Pharmacol Exp Ther 253:608, 1990.
22. Gross GJ, Buck JD, Warltier DC: Transmural distribution of blood flow during activation of coronary muscarinic receptors. Am J Physiol 240:H941, 1981.
23. Reid JVO, Ito BR, Huang AH, et al: Parasympathetic control of transmural coronary blood flow in dogs. Am J Physiol 249:H337, 1985.
24. Clozel JP, Pisarri TE, Coleridge HM, et al: Reflex coronary vasodilatation evoked by chemical stimulation of cardiac afferent vagal C fibres in dogs. J Physiol (Lond) 428:215, 1990.
25. Clozel JP, Roberts AM, Hoffman JIE, et al: Vagal chemoreflex coronary vasodilation evoked by stimulating pulmonary C-fibers in dogs. Circ Res 57:450, 1985.

26. Ito BR, Feigl EO: Carotid baroreceptor reflex coronary vasodilation in the dog. Circ Res 56:486, 1985.
27. Hashimoto K, Igarashi S, Uei I, et al: Carotid chemoreceptor reflex effects on coronary flow and heart rate. Am J Physiol 206:536, 1964.
28. Hackett JG, Abboud FM, Mark AL, et al: Coronary vascular responses to stimulation of chemoreceptors and baroreceptors. Evidence for reflex activation of vagal cholinergic innervation. Circ Res 31:8, 1972.
29. Vatner SF, McRitchie RJ: Interaction of the chemoreflex and the pulmonary inflation reflex in the regulation of coronary circulation in conscious dogs. Circ Res 37:664, 1975.
30. Ito BR, Feigl EO: Carotid chemoreceptor reflex parasympathetic coronary vasodilation in the dog. Am J Physiol 249:H1167, 1985.
31. Feigl EO: Reflex parasympathetic coronary vasodilation elicited from cardiac receptors in the dog. Circ Res 37:175, 1975.
32. Zucker IH, Cornish KG, Hackley J, et al: Effects of left ventricular receptor stimulation on coronary blood flow in conscious dogs. Circ Res 61(suppl II):II–54, 1987.
33. Trimarco B, Chierchia S, Ricciardelli B, et al: Ouabain-induced reflex coronary vasodilatation mediated by cardiac receptors. Am J Physiol 246:H664, 1984.
34. Aversano T, Becker LC: Persistence of coronary vasodilator reserve despite functionally significant flow reduction. Am J Physiol 248:H403, 1985.
35. Ordway GA, Pitetti KH: Stimulation of pulmonary C fibres decreases coronary arterial resistance in dogs. J Physiol (Lond) 371:277, 1986.
36. Ludmer PL, Selwyn AP, Shook TL, et al: Paradoxical vasoconstriction induced by acetylcholine in atherosclerotic coronary arteries. N Engl J Med 315:1046, 1986.
37. Werns SW, Walton JA, Hsia HH, et al: Evidence of endothelial dysfunction in angiographically normal coronary arteries of patients with coronary artery disease. Circulation 79:287, 1989.
38. Yasue H, Matsuyama K, Okumura K, et al: Responses of angiographically normal human coronary arteries to intracoronary injection of acetylcholine by age and segment. Possible role of early coronary atherosclerosis. Circulation 81:482, 1990.
39. Vita JA, Treasure CB, Nabel EG, et al: Coronary vasomotor response to acetylcholine relates to risk factors for coronary artery disease. Circulation 81:491, 1990.
40. Fish RD, Nabel EG, Selwyn AP, et al: Responses of coronary arteries of cardiac transplant patients to acetylcholine. J Clin Invest 81:21, 1988.
41. Hodgson JMcB, Marshall JJ: Direct vasoconstriction and endothelium-dependent vasodilation. Mechanisms of acetylcholine effects on coronary flow and arterial diameter in patients with nonstenotic coronary arteries. Circulation 79:1043, 1989.
42. Feigl EO: EDRF—a protective factor? Nature 331:490, 1988.
43. Horio Y, Yasue H, Okumura K, et al: Effects of intracoronary injection of acetylcholine on coronary arterial hemodynamics and diameter. Am J Cardiol 62:887, 1988.
44. Maseri A, Davies G, Hackett D, et al: Coronary artery spasm and vasoconstriction. The case for a distinction. Circulation 81:1983, 1990.
45. Kaski JC, Crea F, Meran D, et al: Local coronary supersensitivity to diverse vasoconstrictive stimuli in patients with variant angina. Circulation 74:1255, 1986.
46. Yasue H, Horio Y, Nakamura N, et al: Induction of coronary artery spasm by acetylcholine in patients with variant angina: Possible role of the parasympathetic nervous system in the pathogenesis of coronary artery spasm. Circulation 74:955, 1986.
47. Okumura K, Yasue H, Matsuyama K, et al: Sensitivity and specificity of intracoronary injection of acetylcholine for the induction of coronary artery spasm. J Am Coll Cardiol 12:883, 1988.
48. Cannon RO III: Acetylcholine and coronary artery spasm: Important insight or squeeze play? J Am Coll Cardiol 12:889, 1988.

CHAPTER 18

Effects of Neuropeptides on the Vagal Neuroeffector Junction

E.K. Potter

It is now over 20 years since Levy reported his classical work on interactions between the sympathetic and the parasympathetic nerves of the heart, and accounted for his findings in terms of the interactions between norepinephrine (NE) and acetylcholine (ACh) released from the nerves.[1,2] Since that time, several neuropeptides have been identified in these nerves, co-localized with the classical neurotransmitters, and interactions at the heart following activation of these nerves can no longer be interpreted simply as interactions between NE and ACh. The observed physiological response now seems more likely to result from interactions between the classical transmitters and neuropeptides released together with them.

Although a precise functional or physiological role has not yet been fully delineated for the neuropeptides, many have been identified in the autonomic nerves to the heart and several have been shown to modify effector function. This chapter discusses the effect of these peptides on vagal effector action. Unfortunately, the physiology of neuropeptides is a step behind the immunohistochemical identification of their location. Therefore, much more is known about their location, co-localization, and structure than is known about their function. Actions of some peptides, however, particularly those found in the cardiovascular system, are being studied. This review starts with the neuropeptide that has attracted the most attention recently in this context: neuropeptide Y (NPY), a 36 amino acid peptide, identified initially in porcine brain in 1982 and then in sympathetic nerves co-localized with NE.[3,4] NPY has many actions in the nervous system, both centrally and peripherally.[5,6] Although much work has therefore concentrated on NPY, a second sympathetic co-transmitter, galanin (GAL),[7] has also been identified in cardiovascular autonomic nerves in some species. Other peptides that have been shown to have an action on vagal effector action and that are reviewed here include enkephalin, also localized in sympathetic nerves,[8] and the circulating

From *Vagal Control of the Heart: Experimental Basis and Clinical Implications* edited by MN Levy, PJ Schwartz © 1994, Futura Publishing Co. Inc., Armonk, NY.

hormones angiotensin and vasopressin. It is also possible that peptides released from the vagus itself have some modifying action on the heart. These peptides include vasoactive intestinal polypeptide (VIP),[9–11] peptide histidine isoleucine (PHI),[12] often co-localized with VIP, and somatostatin.[13] The cardiac action of peptides which are localized in sensory nerves in some species,[11] such as substance P (SP) and calcitonin gene-related peptide (CGRP), and neurotensin (NT), which is found in perivascular nerves in the heart in some species,[11] are also briefly reviewed here.

Neuropeptide Y

NPY was first identified from porcine brain in 1982 by Tatemoto,[14] and has since been identified in many, possibly all, sympathetic neurons supplying the heart and cardiovascular system in many species including cat, rat, mouse, guinea pig, cow, dog, and man.[14–24] Its amino acid sequence is remarkably well conserved. Rat, rabbit, guinea pig, and human forms are identical, and only one amino acid is different from the porcine form.[25] NPY has potent prejunctional and postjunctional effects on vascular reactivity.[26] In addition, exogenous NPY has been demonstrated to have a potent and prolonged inhibitory effect on vagal control of heart rate.[27–29] This inhibition of cardiac vagal action follows periods of cardiac sympathetic nerve stimulation in anesthetized dogs, and it has been proposed to be mediated by endogenous NPY, acting as a sympathetic co-transmitter. The vagal inhibitory action of sympathetic stimulation is blocked by guanethidine, an agent known to block release of both NE and NPY from sympathetic nerves.[30,31] However, the inhibitory action survives α- and β-adrenoceptor (β-AR) blockade, and is not mimicked by exogenous NE, so it cannot be attributed to NE. It is mimicked by exogenous NPY. Furthermore, NPY and fragments of the NPY molecule can be collected in coronary sinus blood during sympathetic stimulation.[32] Figure 1 shows records from an anesthetized dog in which cardiac vagal action was inhibited for over an hour after a period of cardiac sympathetic nerve stimulation. Although the frequency of sympathetic stimulation used in the experiment illustrated in Figure 1 is high (16 Hz), similar inhibitory effects can be seen after stimulation at lower, more physiological frequencies.[29,33]

Attenuation of cardiac vagal action following sympathetic stimulation has been shown to be dependent upon the peak frequency of stimulation. High-frequency, intermittent stimulation of the sympathetic nerve produced greater and more prolonged vagal inhibition than low-frequency (5 Hz), continuous stimulation with the same total number of impulses.[33] Previous studies have demonstrated that bursts of high-frequency stimuli more effectively release neuropeptide transmitters than continuous stimuli with the same mean frequency.[34,35] It has also been demonstrated that repeated stimulation of the cut, cardiac sympathetic nerve reduces the ability of such stimulation to attenuate vagal action at the heart.[36] This marked decline in the effect of sympathetic nerve stimulation in attenuating cardiac vagal action cannot be ascribed to a failure of the electrical stimulus to be reliably transmitted to the nerve

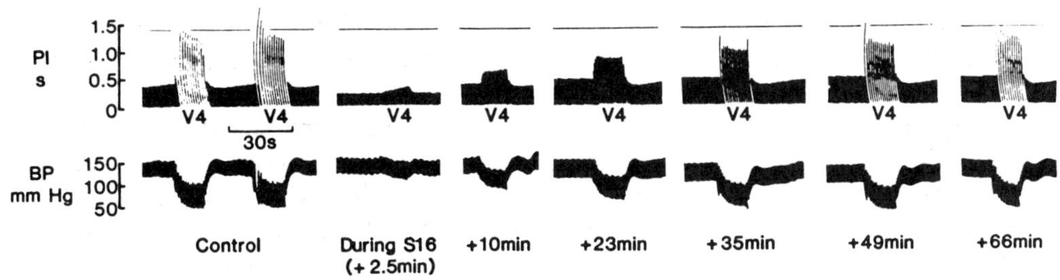

Figure 1. *Records from an anesthetized, vagotomized dog show pulse interval (PI) in the top trace and arterial blood pressure (BP) in the bottom trace. PI is increased intermittently by stimulation of the vagus nerve at 4 Hz (V4) for 15 s. The first panel shows the control increase in PI evoked by two episodes of vagal stimulation. The second panel shows the increase in PI evoked by the same vagal stimulation during a period of stimulation of the right cardiac sympathetic nerve at 16 Hz for 3 min (S16). Note the decrease in resting PI, and attenuation of vagal action. Subsequent panels are taken at various time intervals (indicated) following cessation of sympathetic stimulation. Note it takes over 1 h before the standard vagal stimulus can increase PI as effectively as it did before sympathetic stimulation. Reprinted from Pharmacol Ther, 37, Potter EK, Neuropeptide Y as an autonomic neurotransmitter, 251–273, Copyright 1988, with kind permission from Pergamon Press Ltd, Headington Hill Hall, Oxford OX3 OBW, UK.*

terminals, because the effect of sympathetic nerve stimulation in increasing heart rate (presumably, the immediate action of released NE) did not change significantly during the course of the experiments demonstrating the effect. Nor can the findings be attributed to a general desensitization of tissues to released NPY, because the effect of exogenous NPY on cardiac vagal action was similar whether injected at the beginning or end of the decline. Thus, the observed decline in the effect of sympathetic nerve stimulation in attenuating vagal action, while leaving the effect on increasing heart rate unchanged, suggests that the inhibition of the vagus nerve is mediated, at least in part, by a depletable transmitter, conforming in this respect to the properties of a peptide transmitter. Such a peptide is likely to be NPY.[36]

Release of NPY is modulated in the presence of α-adrenoceptor agonists and antagonists. In the pithed guinea pig, clonidine reduced the increase in plasma NPY induced by preganglionic nerve stimulation (8 Hz) by almost 50%. This effect was reversed by the α_2-adrenoceptor antagonist yohimbine, which causes a threefold increase in plasma NPY.[37] In the pig, overflow of NPY from the heart induced by sympathetic stimulation at 10 Hz was enhanced about threefold by α-adrenoceptor blockade with phenoxybenzamine.[21,35] Recent experiments sought to demonstrate the effect of the α-adrenoceptor antagonist phentolamine on the sympathetically-induced vagal attenuation, and in these the sympathetic nerves were stimulated for 1 minute at a high frequency of 20 Hz. The increased enhancing effect of α-blocking drugs is more easily demonstrable at high frequencies of stimulation,[38] and prolonged attenuation of cardiac vagal action has been demonstrated at this frequency.[27–29] Therefore, there is a parallel modulation by adrenoceptor agonists of the release of NPY and of its inhibitory effect on cardiac vagal action.[29,39]

The site at which cardiac vagal action is inhibited by sympathetic stimulation and by exogenous NPY is not postsynaptic at the cardiac pacemaker cells.[40] In both the anesthetized dog and the isolated atrial preparation, the direct slowing of the pacemaker after addition of a cholinomimetic agent was not altered in the presence of NPY nor, in the dog, by stimulation of the cardiac sympathetic nerve. In the isolated atrial preparation, NPY was shown to exert its inhibitory action at the postganglionic nerve terminal, because vagal transmission was blocked at the ganglion with hexamethonium. A presynaptic inhibitory action on vagal transmission had earlier been suggested by Lundberg et al,[41] but their experiments could not distinguish between preganglionic and postganglionic presynaptic actions, nor between these and a postsynaptic action at the vagal ganglion near the heart. These experiments show that NPY exerts its effect prejunctionally at the postganglionic nerve terminals. It is possible that NPY has an additional action at the ganglion, as this would not have been revealed in these experiments (Fig. 2). This peptidergic interaction of vagus and sympathetic nerves at the sinoatrial (SA) node has recently been confirmed and extended to include documentation of a similar interaction at the atrioventricular (AV) node and on atrial contractile strength (Fig. 3).[42,43] These studies therefore show a powerful and prolonged presynaptic inhibitory effect on vagal control of the heart by NPY. It seems likely that this finding may prove to be just one manifestation of a general phenomenon, as NPY also modulates cholinergic activity at other sympathetic/parasympathetic sites.[44,45]

NPY is released from sympathetic nerves when they are activated in many forms of stress; for example, during cardiothoracic surgery or exercise.[46,47] High circulating levels of NPY are also found in some forms of hypertension and in patients with congestive heart failure.[48–50] Therefore, it is probable that NPY becomes a factor in vagal control of the heart, especially at times when sympathetic outflow is increased. This finding has important implications for reflexes that modify or control heart rate through the vagus nerve.

Galanin

GAL is a 29 amino acid peptide first isolated from porcine intestine in 1983[51] and since found throughout the central and peripheral nervous systems.[52] GAL has been identified in sympathetic postganglionic neurons in the cat, where it is co-localized with NE and NPY.[7,53] In the cat, as in the dog, stimulation of the cardiac sympathetic nerve is followed by a prolonged attenuation of cardiac vagal action that survives α-adrenoceptor and β-AR blockade and is not mimicked by NE, but is also blocked by guanethidine. In the cat, however, it is GAL, and not NPY, that mimics the prolonged attenuation of cardiac vagal action.[54] NPY has no inhibitory effect on cardiac vagal action in the cat. These effects are shown in Figure 4. In the Australian possum (*Trichosurus vulpecula*), GAL, but *not* NPY, is co-localized with NE in thoracic sympathetic ganglia.[55] Interestingly, prolonged vagal inhibition is also evoked by sympathetic stimulation in this species, but NPY has little or no vagal

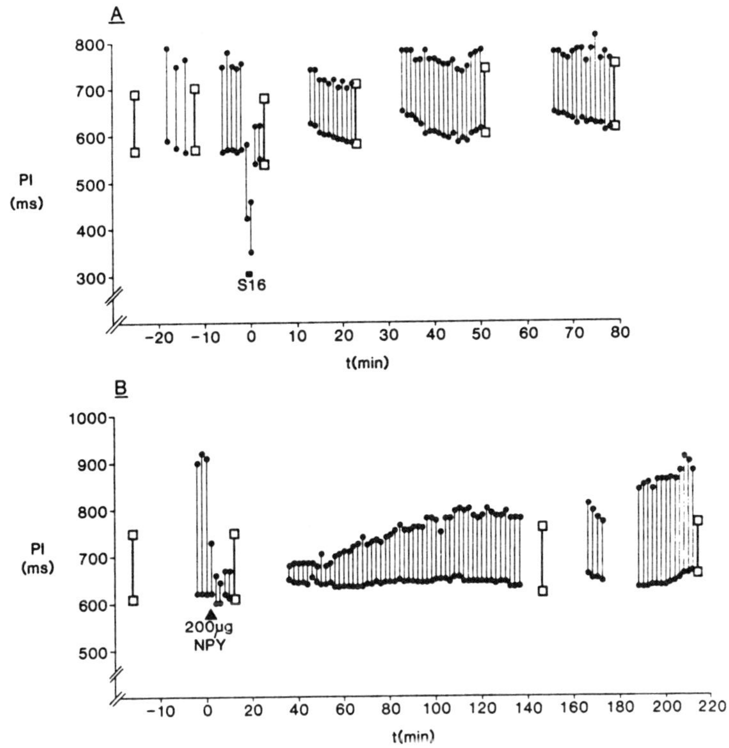

Figure 2. *Data from an anesthetized dog with both vagus nerves cut, and without adrenoceptor blockade, are shown. A: The change in pulse interval (PI) evoked by stimulating the right vagus nerve at 4 Hz for 15 s every 2 min (closed circles) or by a bolus injection of the parasympathomimetic agent bethanechol (open squares). Each pair of points joined by a line shows the PI immediately before vagal stimulation or administration of bethanechol (lower point), and at the peak attained during such intervention (upper point). The peripheral stump of the cut right cardiac sympathetic nerve was stimulated at 16 Hz for 1 min (at marker, S16) in A. Note resting PI (lower symbol of each joined pair) is decreased by sympathetic stimulation as is the peak PI attained in response to vagal stimulation (upper symbol of each joined pair). The PI in the absence of vagal stimulation however, returns very soon to control levels, but the prolongation of PI caused by vagal stimulation remains attenuated for over 30 min afterwards. The change in PI evoked by a bolus intravenous injection of bethanechol (250 µg) is similar whether given before or after sympathetic stimulation. B: Data show the change in PI evoked by stimulating the right vagus nerve at 4 Hz for 15 s every 2 min (closed circles) or by injection of bethanechol (open squares). A bolus, intravenous dose of NPY (200 µg) was given at the marker, and there was marked and prolonged inhibition of vagal effectiveness (lasting 180 min). The change in PI evoked by injection of bethanechol was similar before or after injection of NPY. Note the different scale on time axes in A and B. Reproduced with permission from Potter EK: Presynaptic inhibition of cardiac vagal postganglionic nerves by neuropeptide Y. Neurosci Lett 83:101–106, 1987.*

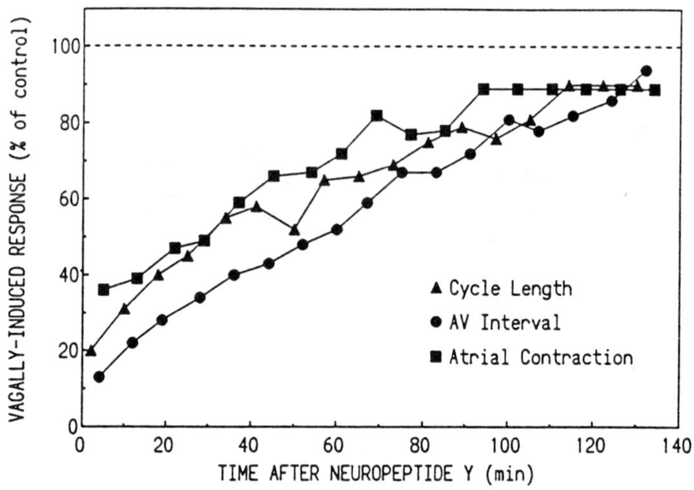

Figure 3. *Graph showing the recovery of vagally-induced atrial contraction (■) cardiac cycle length (▲), and AV interval responses (●), after exogenous NPY in a representative animal. The vagally-induced responses, expressed as percent of control, are plotted as a function of the time, after neuropeptide Y administration, in minutes. The dashed horizontal line represents 100% of the control vagally-induced cardiac responses. Reproduced by permission of the American Heart Association, Inc. from Warner MR, Levy MN: Inhibition of cardiac vagal effects by neurally released and exogenous neuropeptide Y. Circ Res 65:1536–1546, 1989.*

inhibitory action in this species.[56] GAL, however, mimics the effect of sympathetic stimulation in the possum as in the cat. In the dog, GAL has little effect on cardiac vagal action, although here also it is co-localized with NPY and NE.[57]

Thus, it seems that either NPY or GAL, two quite different peptides that are known to be co-localized with NE in sympathetic neurons, can modulate cardiac vagal action in different species. Why one peptide acts in one species, in a role apparently filled by the other in other species, remains obscure. Nor is it clear why both peptides should exist together in the sympathetic nerves of some species in which only one of the pair has the demonstrable vagal inhibitory role. Other roles, yet to be delineated, seem likely.

Enkephalin

Enkephalin-like immunoreactivity has been identified in human sympathetic ganglia[58] in a separate population of neurons from those containing NPY,[8] and in sympathetic nerves in the heart of the guinea pig.[59] Significant increases in the levels of plasma pro-enkephalin have been measured after cardiac sympathetic nerve stimulation in the guinea pig.[60] Recently, an interaction between sympathetic and parasympathetic nerves attributed to

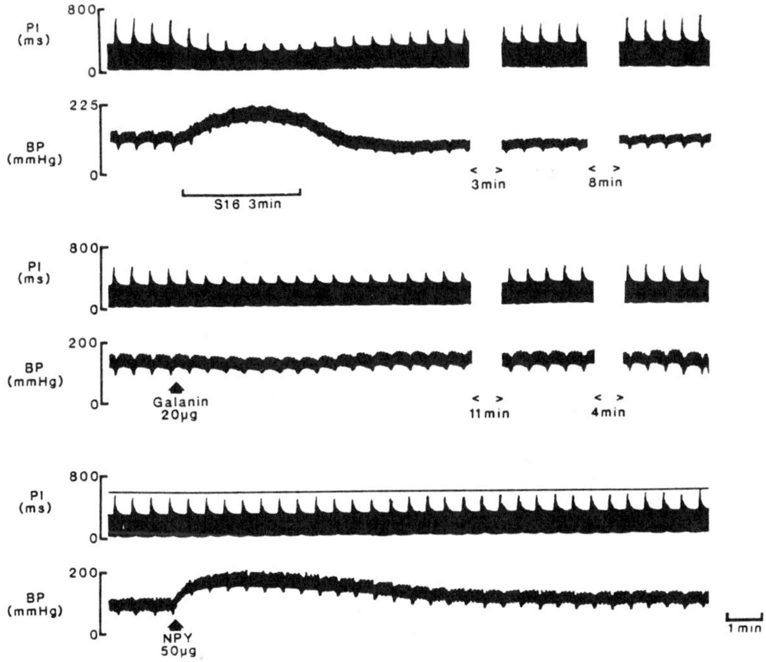

Figure 4. *Records of pulse interval (PI) and blood pressure (BP) from an anesthetized cat, showing the effects of stimulation of the cardiac sympathetic nerve, intravenous GAL, and intravenous NPY. All experiments were carried out in the presence of effective β-AR blockade. An increase in PI was evoked every 30 s by stimulating the peripheral, cut end of the right vagus. Sympathetic stimulation caused a prolonged inhibition of cardiac vagal action. GAL caused a similar prolonged attenuation of vagal effects on PI. GAL also had a slight depressor action. NPY caused only a marginal inhibition of vagally-induced changes in PI. NPY was a powerful pressor agent. Reproduced with permission from Revington ML, Potter EK, McCloskey DI: Prolonged inhibition of cardiac vagal action following sympathetic stimulation and galanin in anaesthetized cats. J Physiol (Lond) 431:495–503, 1990.*

release of opioid peptides has been described.[61] In the anesthetized dog, Koyanagawa et al[61] reported that inhibition of cardiac vagal action during sympathetic stimulation was significantly reversed by large doses of naloxone. On the basis of this finding, they attributed the inhibitory effect to opioid peptides released during stimulation of the cardiac sympathetic nerves. Exogenous opioids have been shown to inhibit cholinergic action by decreasing ACh release,[62–64] and an early study has shown a presynaptic inhibition of vagal action by morphine.[65] These studies point to a role for modulation of cardiac vagal action by opioids released during sympathetic nerve stimulation. Any opioid inhibitory effect must only be transient, however, because the *prolonged* attenuation of cardiac vagal action attributed to NPY, also released during sympathetic nerve stimulation, is *not* reversed in the presence of naloxone (Potter, unpublished results).

Angiotensin

Angiotensin II raises blood pressure by acting within the central nervous system (CNS) as well as by acting directly on peripheral arterioles.[66] In addition, there is an inhibitory action by systemic angiotensin on the central neural pathways leading to cardiac vagal motoneuronal excitation.[67] Angiotensin II also has an inhibitory action at the vagal neuroeffector junction. In isolated guinea pig atria, with one vagus attached, angiotensin inhibits the slowing of the heart evoked by stimulation of the vagus nerve, but not the slowing evoked directly by addition of a cholinomimetic.[68] This inhibitory effect on cardiac vagal action of angiotensin II is illustrated in Figure 5. The site of this inhibitory action has since been localized to nerve terminals at the intracardiac ganglion.[69] Binding sites for angiotensin have been identified in the heart at the intracardiac ganglia, on vagal nerve terminals in the heart, and in the SA node.[70] This finding supports a role for angiotensin in regulation of vagal control of the heart.

Vasopressin

Vasopressin is another circulating peptide with potent actions in the cardiovascular system. Its peripheral pressor action is, however, offset by potent stimulation of central vagal pathways. Its peripheral actions on vagal control of heart rate are variable and possibly related to its coronary vasoconstrictor effects. In the isolated, innervated guinea pig atria, vasopressin has no effect on cardiac vagal action.[71]

Vasoactive Intestinal Polypeptide

VIP has been identified in nerves in the heart in several species. VIP immunoreactive neurons occur in the SA and AV nodes, at intracardiac ganglia, and around coronary arteries.[11,16,72] It is found in cholinergic cells and in adrenergic neurons that also contain NPY. It has potent vasodilator effects and increases heart rate in anesthetized dogs by up to 80 beats/minute. These effects are direct,[73,74] however, and VIP has no effects on vagally-evoked decreases in heart rate.[75]

Peptide Histidine Isoleucine

PHI was originally isolated from porcine gut.[12] It has a distribution similar to VIP and also has a direct chronotropic effect on the heart in some species.[73,76]

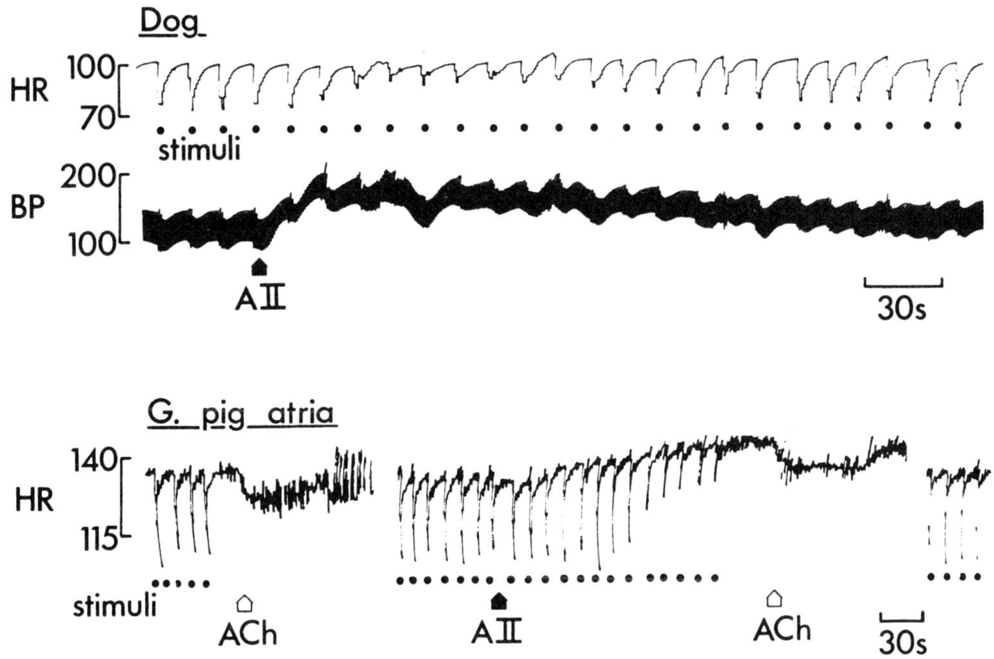

Figure 5. *Top panels are records of heart rate (HR) and blood pressure (BP) from an anesthetized dog after bilateral vagotomy and sympathetic blockade with propranolol (1 mg/kg). Markers indicate the times at which supramaximal stimuli were applied to the peripheral end of the right vagus (4 shocks 300 msec apart at 30 V, 1 msec). In the control conditions the stimuli elicited prompt and marked bradycardia. When angiotensin (5 μg I.V.) was given (at solid arrow), this response of heart rate was inhibited as BP rose, and returned to control levels as the BP response declined. Lower panels are records of heart rate (HR) from isolated, spontaneously-beating atria of guinea pig with the right vagus attached. Markers below the HR trace indicate the times at which supramaximal stimuli were delivered to the vagus (4 shocks, 300 msec apart at 3 V, 1 msec). In control conditions the stimuli elicited prompt and marked bradycardia. When angiotensin (5 μg) was given (at solid arrow), inhibition of this response became marked after 2 min. The full control response returned within 2 to 3 min of washing out the angiotensin (far right of record). ACh, whether given before the addition of angiotensin to the bath (at first unfilled arrow) or when angiotensin had its maximal inhibitory effect on the vagus (at second unfilled arrow), was equally effective in slowing the rate of beating of the atria (ACh concentration in bath 20 ng/ml). Reproduced with permission from Potter EK: Angiotensin inhibits action of vagus nerve at the heart. Br J Pharmacol 75:9–11, 1982.*

Substance P - Calcitonin Gene-Related Peptide

SP innervation of the mammalian heart has been identified in the areas of the SA and AV nodes as well as around arteries.[11,16,77–79] In guinea pig hearts, it is co-localized with CGRP,[80] but this finding is likely to be the case in many peripheral sensory nerves,[81] because coding for both peptides is on the same gene.[82] Both SP and CGRP decrease blood pressure and increase heart rate.[80] In isolated guinea pig hearts, CGRP causes a direct increase in heart rate. In guinea pigs, CGRP is thought to be responsible for the excess tachycardia of vagal origin.[83] Neither SP[75] nor CGRP (Potter, unpublished observations) modulate cardiac vagal action in anesthetized dogs.

Somatostatin

Somatostatin has been identified in cholinergic nerves in toads and in nerves presumed to be cholinergic in the heart in humans and guinea pigs, but there is wide species variation.[13,84–86] Somatostatin causes a direct bradycardia, and in toads it potentiates cardiac vagal action.[87] In the dorsal motor nucleus (DMN) of the vagus in rat brain stem slices, somatostatin inhibits vagal output by membrane hyperpolarization,[88] and in rat hippocampal slices, somatostatin increases ACh release.[89] In anesthetized dogs, however, somatostatin has no effect on cardiac vagal action[75]; therefore, its effects as well as its distribution are likely to be species-specific.

Neurotensin

NT is present in nerves to the mammalian heart and blood vessels.[11] In anesthetized dogs, NT has a direct positive chronotropic effect,[70] but has no effect on the slowing of the heart evoked by vagal stimulation.[75]

Conclusion

Many peptides have now been identified in the nerves to the heart. There is a wide species variation in the distribution of peptides, in co-localization with other neurotransmitters, and in actions of these peptides on the heart and on vagal control of the heart. The most studied peptide, NPY, has potent and prolonged inhibitory effects on vagal control of heart rate. In some species, however, it is GAL, a peptide often co-localized with NPY, that has inhibitory and prolonged effects on cardiac vagal action of this kind. It is clear that the description of actions of a particular peptide should be confined to the species in which it is studied, as it is clear that one function, such as inhibition of vagal action, can be carried out by different neuropeptides in different species.

References

1. Levy MN, Zieske H: Autonomic control of cardiac pacemaker activity and atrioventricular activity. J Appl Physiol 27:465, 1969.
2. Levy MN: Sympathetic-parasympathetic interactions in the heart. Circ Res 29:437, 1971.
3. Tatemoto K: Neuropeptide Y: Complete amino acid sequence of the brain peptide. Proc Natl Acad Sci USA 79:5485, 1982.
4. Tatemoto K, Carlquist M, Mutt V: Neuropeptide Y—a novel brain peptide with structural similarities to peptide YY and pancreatic polypeptide. Nature 296:659, 1982.
5. Potter EK: Neuropeptide Y as an autonomic neurotransmitter. Pharmacol Ther 37:251, 1988.
6. Potter EK: Neuropeptide Y as an automatic neurotransmitter. In C Bell (ed): Novel Peripheral Neurotransmitters. New York, NY, Pergamon Press, 1991, p. 81.
7. Kummer W: Galanin- and neuropeptide Y-like immunoreactivities coexist in paravertebral sympathetic neurones in the cat. Neurosci Lett 78:127, 1987.
8. Järvi R, Pelto-Huikko M: Localization of neuropeptide Y in human sympathetic ganglia: Correlation with met-enkephalin, tyrosine hydroxylase and acetylcholinestaerase. Histochem J 22:87, 1990.
9. Mutt V, Said SI: Structure of the porcine vasoctive intestinal octacosa peptide. The amino acid sequence. Use of Kallikrein in its determination. Eur J Biochem 42:581, 1974.
10. Lundberg JM, Hökfelt T, Schultzberg M, et al: Occurrence of vasoactive intestinal polypeptide (VIP)-like immunoreactivity in certain cholinergic neurons of the cat. Evidence from combined immunohistochemistry and acetylcholinesterase staining. Neuroscience 4:1539, 1979.
11. Weihe E, Reinecke N: Peptidergic innervation of the mammalian sinus nodes: Vasoactive intestinal polypeptide, neurotensin, substance P. Neurosci Lett 26:283, 1981.
12. Tatemoto K, Mutt V: Isolation and characterization of the intestinal peptide porcine PHI (PHI-27), a new member of the glucagon-secretin family. Proc Natl Acad Sci USA 78:6603, 1981.
13. Campbell G, Gibbins IL, Morris JL, et al: Somatostatin is contained in and released from cholinergic nerves in the heart of the toad *Bufo marinus*. Neuroscience 1:2013, 1982.
14. Lundberg JM, Tatemoto K: Pancreatic polypeptide family (APP, BPP, NPY and PYY) in relation to sympathetic vasoconstriction resistant to α-adrenoceptor blockade. Acta Physiol Scand 116:392, 1982.
15. Lundberg JM, Terenius L, Hökfelt T, et al: Neuropeptide Y (NPY)-like immunoreactivity in peripheral noradrenergic neurons and effects of NPY on sympathetic function. Acta Physiol Scand 116:477, 1982.
16. Furness JB, Costa M, Papka RE, et al: Neuropeptides contained in peripheral cardiovascular nerves. Clin Exp Hypertens A6(1–2):91, 1984.
17. Gu J, Adrian TE, Tatemoto K, et al: Neuropeptide tyrosine (NPY)—A major cardiac neuropeptide. Lancet 1:1008, 1983.
18. Sternini C, Brecha N: Distribution and colocalisation of neuropeptide Y and tyrosine hydroxylase-like immunoreactivity in the guinea pig heart. Cell Tissue Res 241:93, 1985.
19. Allen JM, Gjörstrup P, Björkman JA, et al: Studies on cardiac distribution and function of neuropeptide Y. Acta Physiol Scand 126:405, 1986.
20. Dalsgard C-J, Franco-Cereceda A, Saria A, et al: Distribution and origin of substance P and neuropeptide Y immunoreactive nerves in the guinea pig heart. Cell Tissue Res 243:477, 1986.

21. Rudehill A, Sollevi A, Franco-Cereceda A, et al: Neuropeptide Y (NPY) and the pig heart: Release and coronary vasoconstrictor effects. Peptides 1:821, 1986.
22. Purjeranta M, Rechardt L, Pelto-Huikko M, et al: Light and electron microscope demonstration of neuropeptide Y-like immunoreactive nerves in human cardiac muscle. Virchows Arch (A) 410:147, 1986.
23. Forsgren A: Neuropeptide Y-like immunoreactivity in relation to the distribution of sympathetic nerve fibres in the heart conduction system. J Mol Cell Cardiol 21:279, 1989.
24. Warner MR, Levy MN: Sinus and atrioventricular nodal distribution of sympathetic fibres that contain neuropeptide Y. Circ Res 67:713, 1990.
25. O'Hare MNT, Tenmoku S, Aakerlund L, et al: Neuropeptide Y in guinea pig, rabbit, rat and man. Identical amino acid sequence and oxidation of methienine - 17. Regul Pept 20:293, 1988.
26. Edvinsson L: The effects of neuropeptide Y on the circulation. ISI Atlas of Science. Pharmacology 2:357, 1988.
27. Potter EK: Prolonged non-adrenergic inhibition of cardiac vagal action by sympathetic stimulation: A role for neuropeptide Y? Proc Aust Physiol Pharmacol Soc 15:200, 1984.
28. Potter EK: Prolonged non-adrenergic inhibition of cardiac vagal action following sympathetic stimulation: Neuromodulation by neuropeptide Y? Neurosci Lett 54:117, 1985.
29. Warner MR, Levy MN: Neuropeptide Y as a putative modulator of the vagal effects on heart rate. Circ Res 64:882, 1989.
30. Lundberg JM, Änggård A, Theodorsson-Norheim E, et al: Guanethidine-sensitive release of neuropeptide Y-like immunoreactivity in the cat spleen by sympathetic nerve stimulation. Neurosci Lett 52:175, 1984.
31. Potter EK: Guanethidine blocks neuropeptide Y-like inhibitory action of sympathetic nerves on cardiac vagus. J Auton Nerv Syst 21:87, 1987.
32. Senanayake P, Warner NR, Levy MN, et al: Characterization of neuropeptide Y immunoreactivity in dog plasma by high performance liquid chromatography and radioimmunoassay. Ann NY Acad Sci 611:340, 1990.
33. Gardner TD, Potter EK: Dependence of non-adrenergic inhibition of cardiac vagal action on peak frequency of sympathetic stimulation in the dog. J Physiol (Lond) 405:115, 1988.
34. Allen JM, Bircham PM, Bloom SR, et al: Release of neuropeptide Y in response to splanchnic nerve stimulation in the conscious calf. J Physiol (Lond) 357:401, 1984.
35. Lundberg JM, Saria A, Franco-Cereceda A, et al: Frequency and reserpine dependent chemical coding of sympathetic transmission: Differential release of noradrenaline and neuropeptide Y from the pig spleen. Neurosci Lett 63:96, 1986.
36. Hall GT, Gardner TD, Potter EK: Attenuation of long-lasting effects of sympathetic stimulation after repeated stimulation. Circ Res 67:193, 1990.
37. Dahlof C, Dahlof P, Lundberg JM: Alpha$_2$ adrenoceptor-mediated inhibition of nerve stimulation-evoked release of neuropeptide Y (NPY)-like immunoreactivity in the pithed guinea pig. Eur J Pharmacol 131:279, 1986.
38. Langer SZ: Presynaptic regulation of release of catecholamines. Pharmacol Rev 32:337, 1981.
39. Hall GT, Potter EK: Attenuation of vagal action following sympathetic stimulation is modulated by prejunctional α_2-adrenoceptors in the dog. J Auton Nerve Syst 30:129, 1990.
40. Potter EK: Presynaptic inhibition of cardiac vagal postganglionic nerves by neuropeptide Y. Neurosci Lett 83:101, 1987.
41. Lundberg JM, Hua X-Y, Franco-Cereceda A: Effects of neuropeptide Y (NPY) on mechanical activity and neurotransmission in the heart, vas deferens and urinary bladder of the guinea pig. Acta Physiol Scand 121:325, 1984.

42. Pirola FT, Potter EK: Vagal action on atrioventricular conduction and its inhibition by sympathetic stimulation and neuropeptide-Y in anaesthetised dogs. J Auton Nerve Syst 31:1, 1990.
43. Warner MR, Levy MN: Inhibition of cardiac vagal effects by neurally released and exogenous neuropeptide Y. Circ Res 65:1536–1546, 1989.
44. Stjernquist M, Emson P, Owman CH, et al: Neuropeptide Y in the female reproductive tract of the rat. Distribution of nerve fibres and motor effects. Neurosci Lett 39:279, 1983.
45. Stretton CD, Barnes PJ: Modulation of cholinergic neurotransmission in guinea pig trachea by neuropeptide Y. Br J Pharmacol 93:672, 1988.
46. Morris MJ, Russell AE, Kapoor V, et al: Increases in plasma neuropeptide Y concentrations during sympathetic activation in man. J Auton Nerv Syst 17:143, 1986.
47. Lundberg JM, Torssel L, Sollevi A, et al: Neuropeptide Y and sympathetic vascular control on man. Regul Pept 13:41, 1985.
48. Maisel A, Scott NA, Moltusky HJ, et al: Elevation of plasma neuropeptide Y levels in congestive heart failure. Am J Med 86:43, 1989.
49. Hulting J, Sollevi A, Ullman B, et al: Plasma neuropeptide Y on admission to a coronary care unit: Raised levels in patients with left heart failure. Cardiovasc Res 24:102, 1990.
50. Edvinsson L, Ekman R, Hedner P, et al: Congestive heart failure: Involvement of perivascular peptides reflecting activity in sympathetic parasympathetic and afferent fibres. Eur J Clin Invest 20:85, 1990.
51. Tatemoto K, Rökaeus Å, Jörnvall H, et al: Galanin—a novel biologically active peptide from porcine intestine. FEBS Lett 164:124, 1983.
52. Rökaeus Å: Galanin— a newly isolated biologically active peptide. Trends Neurosci 10:158, 1987.
53. Lindh B, Lundberg JM, Hökfelt T: NPY-like galanin-, VIP/PHI-, CGRP- and substance P-immunoreactive neuronal subpopulation in cat autonomic and sensory ganglia and their projects. Cell Tissue Res 256:259, 1989.
54. Revington ML, Potter EK, McCloskey DI: Prolonged inhibition of cardiac vagal action following sympathetic stimulation and galanin in anaesthetized cats. J Physiol (Lond) 431:495, 1990.
55. Morris JL, Gibbins IL, Holmgren J: Galanin is more common than NPY in vascular sympathetic neurons of Australian marsupials. Regul Pept 37:101, 1992.
56. Courtice GP, Potter EK, McCloskey DI: Inhibition of cardiac vagal action by galanin but not neuropeptide Y in the brush-tailed possum, *Trichosurus Vulpecula.* Proc Aust Physiol Pharmacol Soc 21:50p, 1991.
57. Moriarty M, Potter EK, Gibbins I: Comparison of the inhibitory roles of neuropeptide Y and galanin on cardiac vagal action in the dog. Neurosci Lett 139:275–279, 1992.
58. Hervonen A, Linnoila I, Pickel VM, et al: Localization of [Met^5]- and [Leu^5]-enkephalin-like immunoreactivity in nerve terminals in human paravertebral sympathetic ganglia. Neuroscience 6:323, 1990.
59. Lang RE, Herman K, Dietz R, et al: Evidence for the presence of enkephalins in the heart. Life Sci 32:399, 1983.
60. Xiang JZ, Archelos J, Lang RE: Enkephalins in the heart. Clin Exp Hypertens (A)(10–11):1883, 1984.
61. Koyanagawa H, Musha T, Kanda A, et al: Inhibition of vagal transmission by cardiac sympathetic nerve stimulation in the dog: Possible involvement of opioid receptor. J Pharmacol Exp Ther 250:1092, 1989.
62. Weitzell R, Iles P, Starke K: Inhibition via opioid μ- and Δ-receptors of vagal transmission in rabbit isolated hearts. Naunyn Schmiedebergs Arch Pharmacol 328:186, 1984.

63. Wong-Dusting HK, Rand NJ: Effect of [D-Ala^2, Met^5] enkephalinamide and [-D Ala^2, D-Leu^5] enkephalin on cholinergic and noradrenergic neurotransmission in isolated atria. Eur J Pharmacol 111:65, 1985.
64. Musha T, Satoh E, Hiroshi K, et al: Effects of opioid agonists on sympathetic and parasympathetic transmission to the dog heart. J Pharmacol Exp Ther 250:1087, 1989.
65. Kennedy BL, West TC: Effect of morphine on electrically-induced release of autonomic mediators in the rabbit sino-atrial node. J Pharmacol Exp Ther 157:149, 1967.
66. Bickerton RJ, Buckley JP: Evidence for a central mechanism in angiotensin induced hypertension. Proc Soc Exp Biol Med 106:834, 1961.
67. Lumbers ER, McCloskey DI, Potter EK: Inhibition by angiotensin II of baroreceptor-evoked activity in cardiac vagal efferent nerves in the dog. J Physiol (Lond) 294:69, 1979.
68. Potter EK: Angiotensin inhibits action of vagus nerve at the heart. Br J Pharmacol 75:9, 1982.
69. Korner PI, Head GA, Badoer E, et al: Role of brain amine transmitters and some neuromodulators in blood pressure heart rate and baroreflex control. J Cardiovasc Pharmacol 10 (suppl 12):S26, 1987.
70. Allen AM, Yanada H, Mendelsohn FAO: In vitro autoradiographic localization of binding to angiotensin receptors. Int J Cardiol 228:25, 1990.
71. Courtice GP, Kwong TE, Lumbers ER, et al: Excitation of the cardiac vagus by vasopressin in mammals. J Physiol (Lond) 354:547–556, 1984.
72. Forsgren A: Vasoactive intestinal polypeptide-like immunoreactivity in the bovine heart: High degree of coexistence with neuropeptide Y-like immunoreactivity. Cell Tissue Res 256:125, 1989.
73. Rigel DF: Effects of neuropeptides on heart rate in dogs: Comparison of VIP, PHI, NPY, CGRP and NT. Am J Physiol 255:H311, 1988.
74. Rigel DF, Lathrop DA: Vasoactive intestinal polypeptide facilitates atrioventricular nodal conduction and shortens atrial and ventricular refractory periods in conscious and anaesthetized dogs. Circ Res 67:1323, 1990.
75. Kilborn MJ, Potter EK, McCloskey DI: Neuromodulation of the cardiac vagus: Comparison of neuropeptide Y and related peptides. Regul Pept 12:155, 1985.
76. Lyn WA, Dixon CNS, Yiangou Y, et al: Heart rate response to peptide histidine valine in human subjects is not mediated through β receptors. Regul Pept 29:251, 1990.
77. Weihe E, Reinecke N, Opherk D, et al: Peptidergic innervation (substance P) in the human heart. J Mol Cell Cardiol 13:331, 1981.
78. Papka RE, Furness JB, Della NG, et al: Time course of effect of capsaicin on ultrastructure and histochemistry of substance P—immunoreactive nerves associated with cardiovascular system of the guinea-pig. Neuroscience 12:1277, 1984.
79. Forsgren A: The distribution of nerve fibres showing substance P-like immunoreactivity in the conduction system of the bovine heart: Dense innervation in atrioventricular bundle. Anat Embryol (Berl) 179:485, 1989.
80. Lundberg JM, Franco-Cereceda A, Hökfelt T, et al: Co-existence of substance P and calcitonin gene-related peptide-like immunoreactivities in sensory nerves in relation to cardiovascular and bronchoconstrictor effects of capsaicin. Eur J Pharmacol 108:315, 1985.
81. Lee Y, Takami K, Kawai Y, et al: Distribution of calcitonin gene-related peptide in the rat peripheral nervous system with reference to its co-existence with substance P. Neuroscience 15:1227, 1985.
82. Nawa H, Hirose T, Takashima H, et al: Nucleotide sequences of cloned CDNAs for two types of bovine brain substance P precursor. Nature 306:32, 1983.
83. Saito A, Kimura S, Goto K: Calcitonin gene-related peptide as potential neurotransmitter in guinea pig right atrium. Am J Physiol 250:H693, 1986.

84. Hallemans R, Naeije R, Melot C, et al: Systemic and pulmonary haemodynamic effects of somatostatin. Lancet 1:1270, 1981.
85. Day SM, Gu J, Polak JM, et al: Somatostatin in the human heart and comparison with guinea pig and rat heart. Br Heart J 53:153, 1985.
86. Franco-Cereceda A, Lundberg JM, Hökfelt T: Somatostatin: An inhibitory parasympathetic transmitter in the human heart. Eur J Pharmacol 132:101, 1986.
87. Preston E, Courtice GP: Potentiation of cardiac vagal action by somatostatin in the toad *Bufo marinus*. Proc Aust Physiol Pharmacol Soc 21:174p, 1990.
88. Nabekura J, Mizuno Y, Oomura Y: Inhibitory effect of somatostatin on vagal motoneurons in the rat brain stem in vitro. Am J Phys 256:C155, 1989.
89. Araujo DN, Lapchak PA, Collier B, et al: Evidence that somatostatin enhances endogenous acetylcholine release in the rat hippocampus. J Neurochem 55:1546, 1990.

CHAPTER 19

Vagal Tachycardias

M.N. Levy

Although vagal activity usually decreases the heart rate, investigators have long recognized that vagal activity may actually increase the heart rate under certain conditions. One type of vagal tachycardia (hyperpolarization-induced tachycardia) only appears under restricted experimental conditions; that is, when the vagal stimuli are delivered each cardiac cycle near the beginning of the period of slow diastolic depolarization of the sinoatrial (SA) node pacemaker cells.[1,2] The released acetylcholine (ACh) hyperpolarizes the cell membranes and activates the hyperpolarization-activated (i_f) channels. The resulting influx of cations, mainly Na^+, increases the slope of diastolic depolarization and thereby increases the heart rate. This type of vagal tachycardia will not be discussed further in this chapter, but additional information about this topic is provided in Ch. 12.

When vagal activity is more sustained and is not confined to any specific portion of the cardiac cycle, vagal tachycardia may become manifest either immediately after vagal activation (postvagal tachycardia), or during vagal activation (vagally-induced tachycardia and excess tachycardia [ET]) if appropriate doses of muscarinic blocking agents, such as atropine, have been administered. These three forms of vagal tachycardia have been evoked experimentally by different maneuvers. More than one factor may mediate any of these tachycardias. One important factor, however, in the above tachycardias is the release of the neuropeptide, vasoactive intestinal polypeptide (VIP), which may be common to all three tachycardias. Each tachycardia is described in this chapter and compared with the others.

Postvagal Tachycardia

Ordinarily, the heart rate decreases during vagal stimulation. After stimulation has ceased, however, the bradycardia is often followed by a postvagal tachycardia; that is, an increase in heart rate above the control level

From *Vagal Control of the Heart: Experimental Basis and Clinical Implications* edited by MN Levy, PJ Schwartz © 1994, Futura Publishing Co. Inc., Armonk, NY.

(Fig. 1).[3] Such a response has been recognized for a century or more.[4] The bradycardia that occurs during vagal stimulation is usually associated with a reduction in arterial blood pressure.[3] The consequent unloading of the arterial baroreceptors reflexly increases cardiac sympathetic activity and reduces parasympathetic activity, both of which accelerate the heart.[5]

Substantial evidence indicates, however, that the baroreceptor reflex is not the only mechanism responsible for postvagal tachycardia, and it is probably not even the main mechanism. When the ventricles are paced during a period of vagal stimulation in anesthetized dogs to prevent the arterial blood pressure from falling, postvagal tachycardia is no less pronounced (Fig. 2).[6]

Both adrenergic and nonadrenergic mechanisms may mediate postvagal tachycardia. In the dog and many other mammals, vagal and sympathetic fibers in the neck and thorax constitute a common bundle, identified as the vago-sympathetic trunk. Electrical stimulation of this nerve trunk activates sympathetic as well as vagal fibers to the heart.[7] After vago-sympathetic trunk stimulation has ceased, the vagally-induced bradycardia quickly disappears, because the ACh that had been released during stimulation is rapidly hydrolyzed by the cholinesterase (ChE) that is so abundant in the SA node.[8] The norepinephrine (NE) that is also released during stimulation is removed largely by reuptake by the sympathetic nerve endings and by diffusion into the neighboring capillaries.[9] These NE removal processes are considerably slower than those that degrade ACh. Therefore, after cessation of vago-sympathetic nerve stimulation, some NE lingers in the cardiac interstitium after the ACh has disappeared. This residual NE is partly responsible for the postvagal tachycardia that appears after vago-sympathetic trunk stimulation.

Postvagal tachycardia can be substantial, however, even when efferent sympathetic nerves have not been activated. Adrenergic mechanisms may contribute to postvagal tachycardia even in animals that have been sympathectomized surgically. The postvagal tachycardia induced in atria removed from chronically sympathectomized cats was not significantly different from that elicited in atria from nonsympathectomized cats.[10] The ACh released from

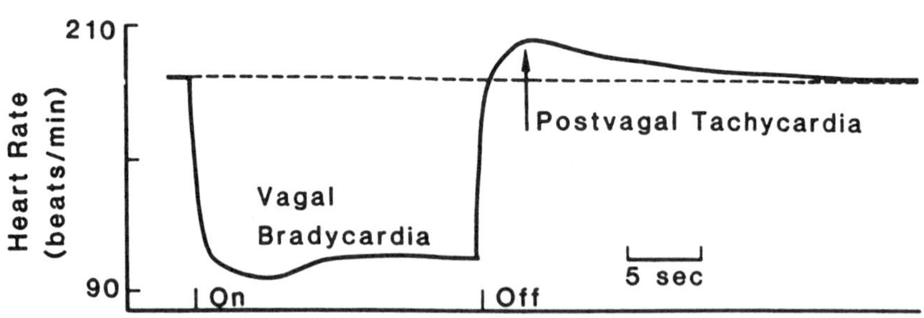

Figure 1. *Time-course of the changes in heart rate (beats/min) during and after stimulation of the right cervical vagus nerve (40 Hz, 0.1-msec pulses) for 60 s in an anesthetized cat. Modified with permission from Burke GH, Calaresu FR: An experimental analysis of the tachycardia that follows vagal stimulation. J Physiol (Lond) 226:491, 1972.*

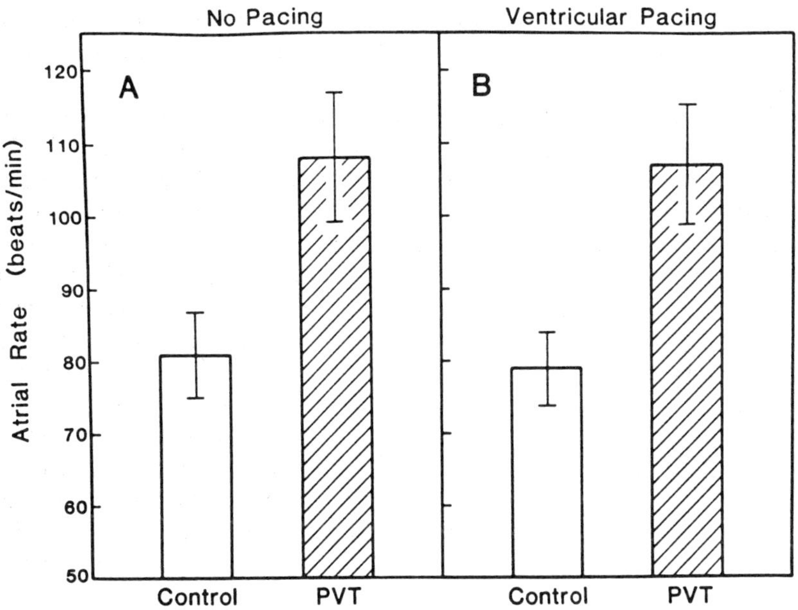

Figure 2. *The mean atrial rates (±SEM) before (control) and after (PVT) stimulation of the right vago-sympathetic nerve (7 to 15 V, 5 msec, 20 Hz) in a group of 10 anesthetized dogs. During one period of vagal stimulation (A), the ventricles were allowed to contract spontaneously. During a second period (B), the ventricles were paced artificially to prevent the arterial blood pressure from diminishing during vagal stimulation. Derived from Copen DL, Cirillo DP, Vassalle M: Tachycardia following vagal stimulation. Am J Physiol 215:696, 1968.*

vagal terminals may induce postvagal tachycardia partly by liberating catecholamines from chromaffin cells in the SA node region.[6,11,12] In experiments on anesthetized dogs, postvagal tachycardia was not significantly attenuated by doses of reserpine that almost abolished the chronotropic responses to stellate ganglion stimulation.[11] In such doses, reserpine depletes catecholamines in sympathetic nerves, but does not deplete them in the adrenal medulla, and presumably not in chromaffin cells elsewhere in the body.

Nonadrenergic mechanisms may also mediate postvagal tachycardia. Blockade of the β-adrenoceptors (β-ARs) does not abolish postvagal tachycardia in either human subjects[13] or in experimental animals.[3,14] The baroreceptor reflex has been induced by a neck suction device in human subjects.[13] The application of suction enhanced vagal tone reflexly, and when the neck suction was relieved, postvagal tachycardia supervened. Propranolol did not affect the postvagal response.

In anesthetized cats, an appreciable postvagal tachycardia could still be evoked after β-AR blockade.[3,14] Action potentials recorded from SA node pacemaker cells during the period of postvagal tachycardia did not resemble the alterations produced by catecholamines. While postvagal tachycardia prevailed, the maximum diastolic potential (MDP), the threshold potential, the overshoot of the action potential, and the slope of slow diastolic depolarization of the automatic cells were all augmented.[3] Catecholamines, by contrast, only increase the slope of diastolic depolarization.

The bradycardia evoked during vagal stimulation and the tachycardia that ensues after vagal stimulation vary with the stimulation frequency.[3,15] In the experiments[3] on anesthetized cats described above, the frequency dependence of the heart rate responses during vagal stimulation differed from that observed after cessation of vagal stimulation (Fig. 3). The heart rate was reduced maximally during vagal stimulation at frequencies of 20 to 40 Hz, whereas the maximal effects on the postvagal tachycardia were achieved with stimulation frequencies of 40 to 60 Hz. This frequency dependence suggests that the postvagal tachycardia may have been mediated by a neuropeptide. The neural stimulation frequencies that release neuropeptides maximally are typically higher than those that evoke the maximal release of the classical transmitters (NE and ACh).[16–18] The bradycardia evoked during vagal stimulation is undoubtedly mediated principally by ACh. The higher frequency maximum for inducing the postvagal tachycardia, compared to that needed for inducing the vagal bradycardia, suggests that the postvagal tachycardia may

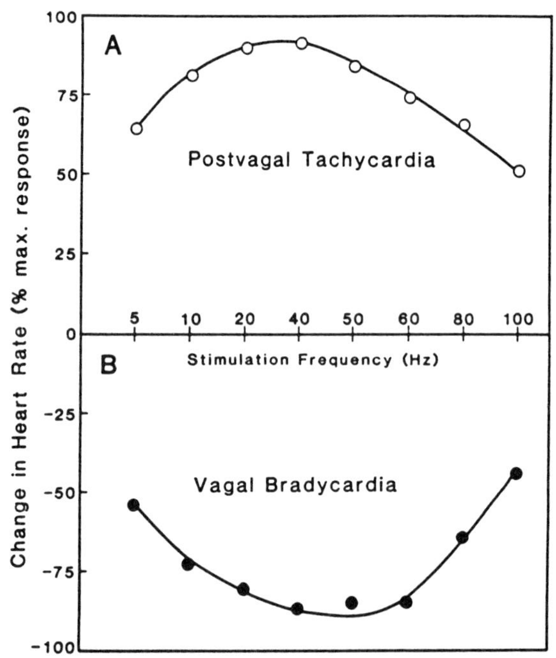

Figure 3. *The mean effects of changing the frequency of stimulation of the right cervical vagus nerve (30 s, 0.1-msec pulses) on the bradycardia induced during stimulation (B) and on the tachycardia observed after cessation of stimulation (A) in a group of eight anesthetized cats. In each animal, the changes in heart rate were expressed as the percentage of the maximum change observed during (B) and after (A) vagal stimulation. Modified with permission from Burke GH, Calaresu FR: An experimental analysis of the tachycardia that follows vagal stimulation. J Physiol (Lond) 226:491, 1972.*

have been mediated mainly by a neuropeptide (possibly VIP) that was released from the vagal nerve terminals together with ACh during neural stimulation.

Vagally-Induced Tachycardia

The increase in heart rate elicited by vagal stimulation after the administration of atropine has been recognized for several decades.[19–21] An example of this response,[22] now known as vagally-induced tachycardia, is shown in Figure 4. Stimulation of the right vago-sympathetic trunk in an anesthetized dog elicited a pronounced tachycardia. The heart rate initially rose in two steps, and the maximum increase in heart rate amounted to about 100 beats/minute.

Many factors, including some of those involved in postvagal tachycardia, probably contribute to this phenomenon. Intracranial stimulation of the vagal rootlets may increase the heart rate, either in the absence[19] or presence[20] of atropine. The cell bodies for the preganglionic vagal neurons that mediate this cardioacceleration are located mainly in the nucleus ambiguus (NA) in the dog.[23,24] Cardiac inhibition is also evoked from that same nucleus in the absence of atropine, but the pathways that conduct the inhibitory and facilitatory effects may differ.[23]

Adrenergic and nonadrenergic mechanisms probably both operate to generate vagally-induced tachycardia. In those species that possess vago-sympathetic trunks, stimulation of those trunks after atropine induces a tachycardia partly because the atropine leaves the effects of the sympathetic fibers unopposed in these combined nerves.[7,25,26] Furthermore, just as in postvagal tachycardia, the ACh released from vagal nerve endings may release NE from chromaffin cells in the SA node region.[6,11,12,26–28]

Vagally-induced tachycardia does not depend exclusively on adrenergic mechanisms, however. In the experiment shown in Figure 4, a fast and a slow component of the response was identified.[22] The fast component disappeared after β-receptor blockade (Fig. 5), after administration of bretylium (which inhibits the release of NE from sympathetic nerve fibers), and after "chemical sympathectomy" with 6-hydroxydopamine.[22,26] The slow component, however,

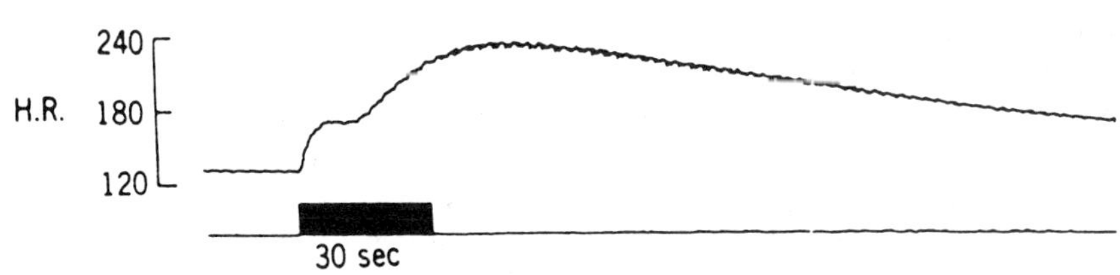

Figure 4. *The changes in heart rate (beats/min) induced by a 30-sec period of supramaximal right vago-sympathetic trunk stimulation (30 Hz, 5-msec pulses) in an anesthetized dog that had received atropine, but did not receive a β-AR antagonist. Modified with permission from Alter WA, Weiss GK, Priola DV: Vagally-induced tachycardia in atropinized dogs: Effect of beta-adrenergic blockade. Eur J Pharmacol 24:329, 1973.*

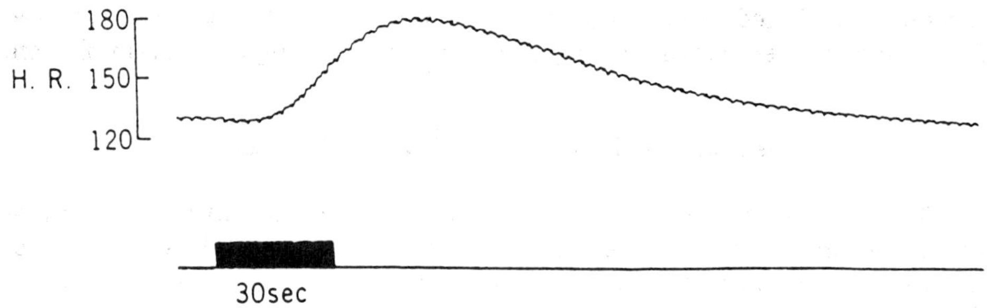

Figure 5. *The changes in heart rate (beats/min) induced by a 30-sec period of supramaximal right vago-sympathetic trunk stimulation (30 Hz, 5-msec pulses) in an anesthetized dog that had received atropine, practolol, and propranolol. Modified with permission from Alter WA, Weiss GK, Priola DV: Vagally-induced tachycardia in atropinized dogs: Effect of beta-adrenergic blockade. Eur J Pharmacol 24:329, 1973.*

persisted after all these interventions. Hence, the slow component does not depend on activation of β-ARs. The mean latent period for the overall response was two seconds, but after the fast component had been eliminated pharmacologically, the mean latent period became 23 seconds. The latent period for the fast component (two seconds) equalled that for the response to sympathetic stimulation in the same animals. Also, the time required for the recovery of the slow component was almost three times as long as the time required for the recovery of the chronotropic response to sympathetic stimulation.[22] These characteristics of the slow component of vagally-induced tachycardia resemble those elicited by neuropeptides, as discussed in the next section.

Excess Tachycardia

In experiments on chronically instrumented, unanesthetized dogs, Rigel et al[29] observed that the tachycardia induced by blocking the cardiac muscarinic receptors (mAChRs) was substantially greater than that induced by blocking conduction in the vago-sympathetic trunks. They called this disparity in the evoked changes in heart rate excess tachycardia (ET).

The phenomenon of ET is illustrated in Figure 6. In the depicted experiment, the animal had already received propranolol (1 mg/kg) to block the β-ARs, and its control heart rate was about 50 beats/minute (1, upper panel). Coolant at −5°C was then circulated through coils that were implanted around both vago-sympathetic trunks to block neural conduction. The heart rate increased to about 125 beats/minute when conduction was fully blocked (2, upper panel). Rewarming the vagi (3, upper panel) soon restored heart rate to its control value. Thus, blocking vagal conduction increased heart rate by about 75 beats/minute.

In the lower panel of Figure 6, vagal cooling was repeated (4, lower panel) with similar results.[29] Atropine methylbromide (0.11 mg/kg) was then given to block the cardiac mAChRs (5, lower panel); heart rate increased by about 10

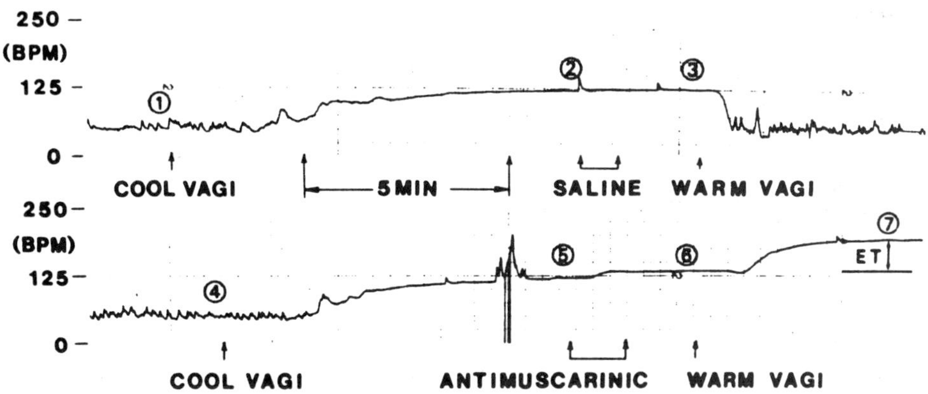

Figure 6. *Cold-blocking the vagus nerves (1) in a conscious, chronically instrumented dog that had received propranolol (1 mg/kg) evoked a substantial increase (2) in heart rate (BPM, beats/min). Rewarming the vagi (3) restored heart rate to its control value. Vagal cooling (4) again increased the heart rate (5), and subsequent administration of atropine methylbromide (0.11 mg/kg) caused a slight additional increase in heart rate (6). Subsequent rewarming of the vagi evoked the excess tachycardia (ET) of about 55 beats/min (7). Reproduced with permission from Rigel DF, Lipson D, Katona PG: Excess tachycardia: Heart rate after antimuscarinic agents in conscious dogs. Am J Physiol 246:H168, 1984.*

beats/minute. Vagal conduction was then restored by rewarming the vagi (6, lower panel). Heart rate then increased by about 55 beats/minute after conduction was fully restored (7, lower panel). This increment in heart rate elicited by restoring vagal conduction after muscarinic blockade is the ET. Three different antimuscarinic agents were used in these experiments. The extent of the ET was not significantly affected by the different abilities of these muscarinic blocking drugs to cross the blood-brain barrier.[29]

Rigel et al[29] concluded that ET depended entirely upon efferent vagal activity. ET was abolished by blocking vagal conduction and was reinstituted by restoring vagal conduction (Fig. 6). Furthermore, the ET could be altered by changing vagal tone reflexly (Fig. 7). When these investigators increased arterial blood pressure by injecting phenylephrine (P), the ET was augmented, whereas when they reduced blood pressure by injecting nitroprusside (N), the ET waned. The bolus injections of P and N changed blood pressure abruptly, but the heart rate responses were delayed and gradual (Fig. 7). The long latency and the sluggish rise and decay times of the responses, plus the failure of the responses to be attenuated by propranolol, resembled the characteristics of the slow component of vagally-induced tachcardia (Fig. 5). Catecholamines released by ACh could not have mediated the ET, because this response was not attenuated by adrenergic antagonists.[29]

The temporal characteristics of ET and of the slow component of vagally-induced tachycardia suggested to Rigel[30] that these responses may be mediated by the release of a neuropeptide from the vagal nerve endings in the heart. Therefore, he evaluated the direct effects of several neuropeptides, namely VIP, peptide histidine isoleucine (PHI), neuropeptide Y (NPY), calcitonin

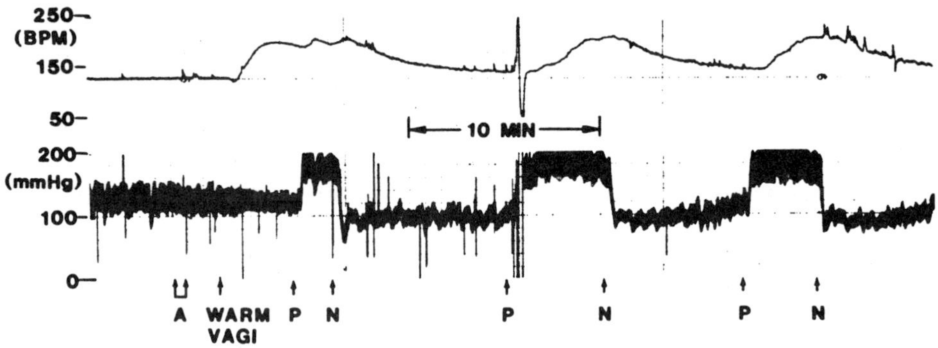

Figure 7. *The effects on heart rate (beats/min) of changing the arterial blood pressure (mm Hg) by injecting phenylephrine (P) or nitroprusside (N) in a conscious, chronically instrumented dog. At the beginning of this experiment (left margin), vagal conduction had been cold-blocked. Atropine sulfate, 0.1 mg/kg, was injected at A, and then vagal conduction was restored by warming the vagi. Reproduced with permission from Rigel DF, Lipson D, Katona PG: Excess tachycardia: Heart rate after antimuscarinic agents in conscious dogs. Am J Physiol 246:H168, 1984.*

gene-related peptide (CGRP), and neurotensin (NT), on the SA node automatic cells in anesthetized dogs. All of these neuropeptides have been identified in neurons in the SA node region.[31–34] The most likely peptide candidates to mediate these tachycardias, however, are VIP and PHI, because they are co-localized in parasympathetic nerves together with ACh, and they are all released together in response to parasympathetic stimulation.[35,36] VIP and PHI receptors have been identified in the heart, and VIP and PHI stimulate adenylyl cyclase (AC) in heart cell membranes.[37]

The changes in heart rate produced by the injection of VIP and PHI directly into the SA node artery in Rigel's experiments[30] are shown in Figure 8, and these responses may be compared with those elicited by injections of glucagon (GLN) and NE. The heart rate increased much more gradually in response to each of the peptides than in response to NE, and the tachycardias induced by the peptides persisted much longer than did the one evoked by NE. The mean values of the 80% recovery times for VIP and PHI were about 5 and 10 minutes, respectively. The 80% recovery time is the time required for the response to return to a level that exceeds the control value by 20% of the peak response. The mean 80% recovery time for NE was much shorter (about 0.5 minutes), and that for GLN was much longer (about 35 minutes) than those for VIP and PHI. The time-courses of ETs and vagally-induced tachycardias more closely resembled those in response to VIP than to those in response to the other peptides.

Dose-response curves were generated for these various peptides and compared with that for NE.[30] VIP, PHI, and glucagon were all found to be as effective as NE in increasing heart rate when they were injected into the SA node artery; that is, they all achieved the same maximum increase in heart rate when administered in sufficiently high dosages. Only VIP, however, was more potent than NE, since VIP achieved half the maximum response at a dose

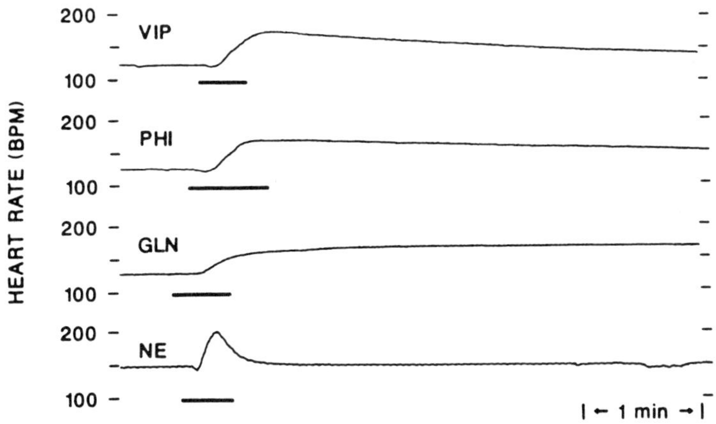

Figure 8. *The changes in heart rate (beats/min) induced by injecting (horizontal bars) vasoactive intestinal polypeptide (VIP, 63 pmol), peptide histidine isoleucine (PHI, 1 nmol), glucagon (GLN, 250 pmol), and norepinephrine (NE, 63 pmol) into the SA node artery in an anesthetized dog. Reproduced with permission from Rigel DF: Effects of neuropeptides on heart rate in dogs: Comparison of VIP, PHI, NPY, CGRP, and NT. Am J Physiol 255:H311, 1988.*

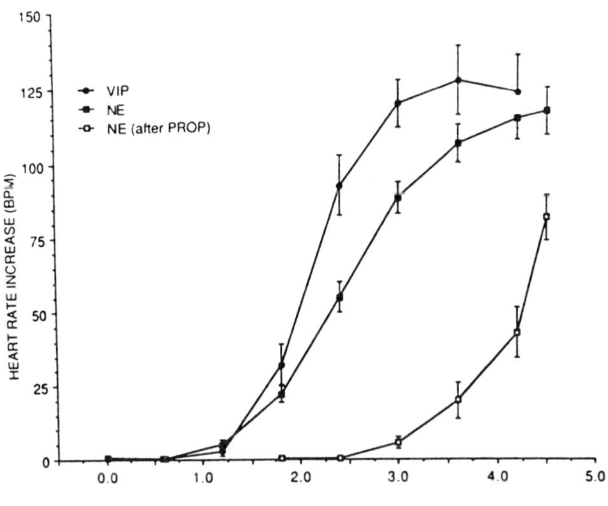

Figure 9. *The mean increases (±SEM) in heart rate (beats/min) induced by various doses of vasoactive intestinal polypeptide (VIP) and of norepinephrine (NE) before and after propranolol (PROP) in a group of seven anesthetized dogs. The VIP and NE were injected directly into the SA node artery. Reproduced with permission from Rigel DF: Effects of neuropeptides on heart rate in dogs: Comparison of VIP, PHI, NPY, CGRP, and NT. Am J Physiol 255:H311, 1988.*

(the ED_{50}) half as great (in pmol) as that required by NE (Fig. 9).[30] PHI was only about 5% as potent as NE.

Thus, VIP is most likely to be the neurotransmitter that mediates the postvagal tachycardias, vagally-induced tachycardias, and ETs. VIP is stored together with ACh in postganglionic parasympathetic neurons, and VIP receptors have been identified in cardiac tissues. Exogenous VIP, administered intravenously[38] or selectively to the SA node region,[30] evokes dose-dependent increases in heart rate. The tachycardia elicited by exogenous VIP reaches a maximum in about 40 seconds and returns slowly to control over about 5 minutes. The time-course of the VIP-induced tachycardia closely resembles the time-courses of the vagal tachycardias evoked in experimental animals. Therefore, VIP almost certainly may not be the sole or even the principal mediator. The elucidation of the precise mechanism must await future research, including the development of effective, specific antagonists for VIP and other neuropeptides.

References

1. Jalife J, Slenter VAJ, Salata JJ, et al: Dynamic vagal control of pacemaker activity in the mammalian sinoatrial node. Circ Res 52:642, 1983.
2. Yang T, Jacobstein MD, Levy MN: Sustained increases in heart rate induced by timed repetition of vagal stimulation in dogs. Am J Physiol 249:H703, 1985.
3. Burke GH, Calaresu FR: An experimental analysis of the tachycardia that follows vagal stimulation. J Physiol (Lond) 226:491, 1972.
4. Hunt R, Harrington DW: Notes on the physiology of the cardiac nerves of the opossum (dildelphys virginiana). J Exp Med 2:711, 1897.
5. Spyer KM: Neural mechanisms involved in cardiovascular control during affective behaviour. Trends Neurosci 12:506, 1989.
6. Copen DL, Cirillo DP, Vassalle M: Tachycardia following vagal stimulation. Am J Physiol 215:696, 1968.
7. Priola DV, Fulton RL: Positive and negative inotropic responses of the atria and ventricles to vagosympathetic stimulation in the isovolumic canine heart. Circ Res 25:265, 1969.
8. Dexter F, Saidel GM, Levy MN, et al: Mathematical model of dependence of heart rate on tissue concentration of acetylcholine. Am J Physiol 256:H520, 1989.
9. Levy MN, Masuda Y: The disposition of adrenergic neurotransmitter from cardiac tissues. In S Sideman, R Beyar (eds): Simulation and Control of the Cardiac System, Vol. III. Boca Raton, FL, CRC Press Inc, 1987, pp. 154–161.
10. Chiang TS, Leaders FE: Cardiostimulatory responses to vagal stimulation, nicotine, and tyramine. Am J Physiol 211:1443, 1966.
11. Vassalle M, Mandel WJ, Holder MS: Catecholamine stores under vagal control. Am J Physiol 218:115, 1970.
12. Loeb JM, Vassalle M: Adrenergic mechanisms in postvagal tachycardia. J Pharmacol Exp Ther 210:56, 1979.
13. Prystowsky EN, Zipes DP: Postvagal tachycardia. Am J Cardiol 55:995, 1985.
14. Raper C, Wale J: Sympathetic involvement in vagal escape and the effects of β-receptor blocking drugs. Eur J Pharmacol 8:47, 1969.
15. Celler BG: Characteristics of cardiac period responses to prolonged vagal stimulation in dogs. Med Biol Eng Comput 27:595, 1989.
16. Lundberg JM, Rudehill A, Sollevi A, et al: Frequency-and reserpine-dependent

chemical coding of sympathetic transmission: Differential release of noradrenaline and neuropeptide Y from pig spleen. Neurosci Lett 63:96, 1986.
17. Lundberg JM, Rudehill A, Sollevi A, et al: Co-release of neuropeptide Y and noradrenaline from pig spleen in vivo: Importance of subcellular storage, nerve impulse frequency and pattern, feedback regulation and resupply by axonal transport. Neuroscience 28:475, 1989.
18. Warner MR, Levy MN: Role of neuropeptide Y in neural control of the heart. J Cardiovasc Electrophysiol 1:80, 1990.
19. Jourdan F, Nowak SJG: Étude expérimentale chez le chien des fibres cardio-accélératrices du vague. Arch Int Pharmacodyn Ther 53:121, 1936.
20. Kabat H: The cardio-accelerator fibers in the vagus nerve of the dog. Am J Physiol 128:246, 1940.
21. Donald DE, Samueloff SL, Ferguson D: Mechanisms of tachycardia caused by atropine in conscious dogs. Am J Physiol 212:901, 1967.
22. Alter WA, Weiss GK, Priola DV: Vagally-induced tachycardia in atropinized dogs: Effect of beta-adrenergic blockade. Eur J Pharmacol 24:329, 1973.
23. Weiss GK, Priola DV: Brainstem sites for activation of vagal cardioaccelerator fibers in the dog. Am J Physiol 223:300, 1972.
24. Spyer KM: Neural organisation and control of the baroreceptor reflex. Rev Physiol Biochem Pharmacol 88:23, 1981.
25. Randall WC, Priola DV, Pace JB, et al: Ventricular augmentor fibers in the cervical vagosympathetic trunk. Proc Soc Exp Biol Med 124:1254, 1967.
26. Alter WA III, Weiss GK, Priola DV, et al: The effects of 6-hydroxydopamine on vagal cardioaccelerator systems. J Pharmacol Exp Ther 187:99, 1973.
27. Middleton S, Middleton HH, Toha J: Adrenergic mechanism of vagal cardiostimulation. Am J Physiol 158:31, 1949.
28. Antonaccio MJ, Robson RD: Pharmacological alterations of vagally induced tachycardia in anesthetized dogs. Eur J Pharmacol 25:19, 1974.
29. Rigel DF, Lipson D, Katona PG: Excess tachycardia: Heart rate after antimuscarinic agents in conscious dogs. Am J Physiol 246:H168, 1984.
30. Rigel DF: Effects of neuropeptides on heart rate in dogs: Comparison of VIP, PHI, NPY, CGRP, and NT. Am J Physiol 255:H311, 1988.
31. Lundberg J, Terenius L, Hokfelt T, et al: High levels of neuropeptide Y in peripheral noradrenergic neurons in various mammals including man. Neurosci Lett 42:167, 1983.
32. Reinecke M, Forssmann WG: Regulatory peptides (SP, NT, VIP, PHI, ENK) of autonomic nerves in the guinea pig heart. Clin Exp Hypertens: Part A—Theory Pract 6:1867, 1984.
33. Weihe E, Reinecke M, Forssmann WG: Distribution of vasoactive intestinal polypeptide-like immunoreactivity in the mammalian heart. Cell Tissue Res 236:527, 1984.
34. Saito A, Kimura S, Goto K: Calcitonin gene-related peptide as potential neurotransmitter in guinea pig right atrium. Am J Physiol 250:H693, 1986.
35. Lundberg JM: Evidence for coexistence of vasoactive intestinal peptide (VIP) and acetylcholine in neurons of cat exocrine glands: Morphological, biochemical, and functional studies. Acta Physiol Scand 496(suppl):1, 1981.
36. Yasui A, Naruse S, Yanaihara C, et al: Corelease of PHI and VIP by vagal stimulation in the dog. Am J Physiol 253:G13, 1987.
37. Christophe J, Waelbroeck M, Chatelain P, et al: Heart receptors for VIP, PHI and secretin are able to activate adenylate cyclase and to mediate inotropic and chronotropic effects. Species variations and physiopathology. Peptides 5:341, 1984.
38. Rigel DF, Lathrop DA: Vasoactive intestinal polypeptide facilitates atrioventricular nodal conduction and shortens atrial and ventricular refractory periods in conscious and anesthetized dogs. Circ Res 67:1323, 1990.

CHAPTER 20

Vagal Effects of Digitalis

M.R. Rosen

Withering[1] noted that the rapid irregular pulses of certain of his patients slowed and became more regular with the administration of foxglove. Clearly, in the dropsical patients treated by Withering, an improvement in the rhythm of the heart could be attributed to a variety of factors. Assuming many of his patients were in atrial fibrillation, with dilated hearts and with fluid overload, any reduction in the load, any decrease in heart size, and/or specific actions of digitalis on the heart might be held responsible for the improvement in rhythm. The actions of digitalis in modifying cardiac contraction, the relationship of this effect to the suppression of Na/K pumping, and questions related to cardiac size and fluid overload are detailed elsewhere.[2,3] The purpose of this chapter is to consider one specific effect of digitalis—that is, its interaction with the parasympathetic nervous system—and the impact of this interaction on the normal rhythm of the heart and on cardiac arrhythmias.

Of concern in reviewing the vagal effects of digitalis is that recent literature on the subject is scant. Indeed, most of the work referred to in this chapter was published before 1980. While this fact indicates that a great deal was known about the digitalis-parasympathetic neural interaction over a decade ago, it also raises concern that some of the questions inspired by earlier research have gone unanswered as investigators have shifted their attention to other frontiers. This development is unfortunate since digitalis remains an effective vagomimetic antiarrhythmic agent, and a great deal of benefit probably would accrue from its further study.

The Vagally-Mediated Effects of Digitalis on Normal Cardiac Rhythm

In the absence of cardiac disease, digitalis can be expected to have consistent effects on the rhythm of the heart, whether in humans or in experimental animals. Typically, sinoatrial (SA) rate slows, the PR interval

Certain of the studies referred to here were supported by USPHS-NHLBI grants HL-12738 and HL-28958.
From *Vagal Control of the Heart: Experimental Basis and Clinical Implications* edited by MN Levy, PJ Schwartz © 1994, Futura Publishing Co. Inc., Armonk, NY.

increases, and changes occur in the ST segment and T wave.[4] Those actions attributable to vagal effects of digitalis include both the slowing of SA rate and the prolongation of the PR interval.

Mechanism of Slowing of Sinus Rate

Spontaneous impulse initiation by the SA node is the result of a pacemaker current carried by Na^+ through the I_f channel.[5] This current is activated by hyperpolarization of the membrane, and, by bringing positive charge into the cell, it raises the cell to more positive membrane potentials, until threshold is reached and an action potential is initiated. Although there is intrinsic rhythmicity to the SA node pacemaker, its rate of impulse initiation is modulated by a variety of influences. Among the most important are sympathetic and parasympathetic stimulation. Sympathetic (β-adrenergic) stimulation augments the pacemaker current, such that SA rate increases. Parasympathetic (muscarinic) stimulation, both in its own right and as an antagonist to sympathetic stimulation, slows SA rate. Two mechanisms are involved here: over the higher range of acetylcholine (ACh) concentrations ($\geq 10^{-7}$ M), potassium conductance (gK) increases, generating a net outward current[6] that accelerates repolarization, hyperpolarizes the membrane, and decreases the slope of phase 4 depolarization, thereby decreasing automaticity (Fig. 1).[7] At a lower concentration range (10^{-9} M), ACh directly affects the I_f pacemaker current itself,[8] thereby reducing the slope of phase 4 and slowing the rate of impulse initiation. It has been hypothesized that the effect of ACh on the I_f pacemaker current is responsible for routine parasympathetic regulation of SA node automaticity, whereas the effect on gK potentiates this action at times of high vagal tone.[8]

The role of digitalis, here, is as follows: cardiac glycosides increase vagal release of ACh by augmenting efferent vagal activity.[9] As a result, in concentrations that do not exert a direct cardiac effect (i.e., do not significantly inhibit Na/K pumping by cardiac myocytes and induce resultant increases in free $[Ca^{2+}]_i$ and contractile force), digitalis acts via the enhancement of the actions

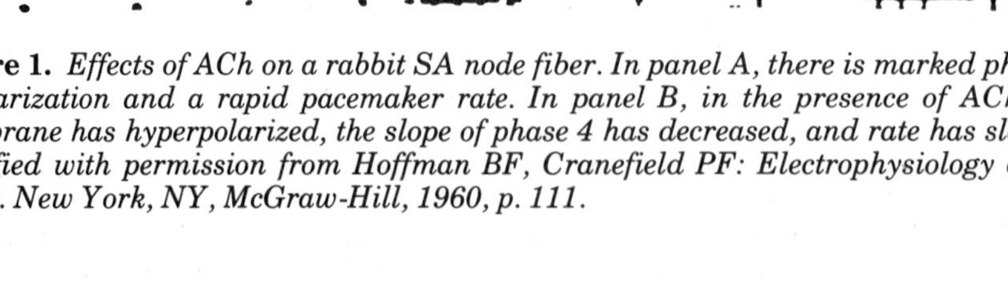

Figure 1. *Effects of ACh on a rabbit SA node fiber. In panel A, there is marked phase 4 depolarization and a rapid pacemaker rate. In panel B, in the presence of ACh, the membrane has hyperpolarized, the slope of phase 4 has decreased, and rate has slowed. Modified with permission from Hoffman BF, Cranefield PF: Electrophysiology of the Heart. New York, NY, McGraw-Hill, 1960, p. 111.*

of ACh and the slowing of the SA node pacemaker rate (although to what extent this mechanism is attributable to suppression of I_f versus enhancement of gK remains uncertain).

Mechanism of Prolongation of the PR Interval

In atrioventricular (AV) nodal tissues, ACh decreases I_{Ca}.[10] Since the AV nodal action potential is largely Ca^{2+}-dependent, any suppression of I_{iCa} would depress action potential amplitude and upstroke velocity, and with this action, slow conduction (Fig. 2). By increasing ACh release at the level of the AV node, digitalis would tend to slow conduction and increase the PR interval.

Mechanisms Whereby Digitalis Increases Acetylcholine Effect

There is general agreement that the combination of increased efferent vagal activity and decreased sympathetic tone are responsible for the increased ACh effect in the presence of digitalis.[11] There remains some uncertainty, however, about underlying mechanisms. It has been suggested that digitalis may increase active cation (Na and K) transport in efferent nerve terminals,

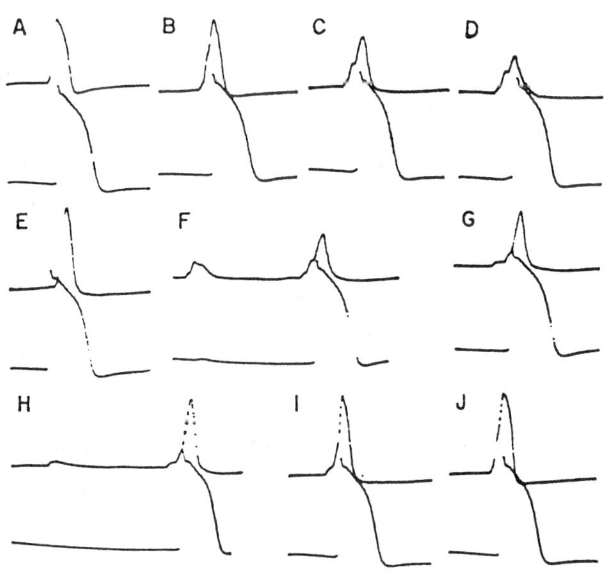

Figure 2. *Effects of ACh in a rabbit AV nodal fiber (upper trace) and His bundle fiber (lower trace). A: Control. Traces B through I show the effects of ACh. J: Recovery. Note the decrease in upstroke velocity of the action potential, its ultimate fragmentation, and decrease in amplitude. Note as well that after a critical loss in amplitude, there is failure to propagate to the His bundle. Modified with permission from Hoffman BF, Cranefield PF: Electrophysiology of the Heart. New York, NY, McGraw-Hill, 1960, p. 150.*

thereby sensitizing arterial baroreceptors.[12] Awareness of the effects of digitalis on central vagal nuclei and on the nodose ganglion[13] led Ten Eick and Hoffman to study its action on efferent vagal fibers, in which they found excitability to be increased.[14] An increase in the actual sensitivity of cardiac tissues to ACh in the presence of digitalis has been cited as well,[15] although the mechanism for this occurrence is uncertain.

Vagally-Mediated Effects of Digitalis on the Ventricles

Twenty years ago, it was generally believed that ACh had little or no effect on impulse initiation and propagation in specialized fibers of the ventricle.[16] It now is understood that muscarinic receptors (mAChRs) do exist in these ventricular tissues and that ACh reduces the slope of phase 4 depolarization and automatic activity in ventricular specialized fibers,[17,18] much as it does in the atrium. Similarly, ACh reduces the amplitude of delayed afterdepolarizations and triggered activity.[19] Nonetheless, the vagal innervation of the ventricle is far less dense than that of the atrium and is most prominent in the proximal septal regions.[20] Hence, the ability of digitalis to induce vagomimetic effects is limited by the distribution of nerve terminals. As a result, the actions of digitalis to suppress or prevent ventricular arrhythmias based on a vagal action are not seen as very significant.

An exception might be the induction of accentuated antagonism of sympathetic actions by digitalis, although this suggestion is highly speculative. ACh is known to induce "accentuated antagonism" of β-adrenergic catecholamine effects on the heart.[21] β-adrenergic amines tend to accelerate repolarization based on their ability to induce adenylyl cyclase (AC) activation and ATP metabolism via the guanosine triphosphate (GTP) regulatory protein G_s. This action of β-adrenergic amines is attenuated by mAChR stimulation, acting through the inhibitory protein G_i.[22] The result is lesser shortening of action potential duration and refractoriness by β-adrenergic amines in the presence of ACh than in its absence.[22] It is tempting to hypothesize that digitalis might potentiate accentuated antagonism of catecholamine effects on repolarization via its own vagomimetic action, but this idea has not yet been tested.

Antiarrhythmic Actions of Digitalis Mediated Via Vagal Effects

Digitalis finds use as an antiarrhythmic in instances of atrial tachycardias (especially those involving the AV node), and is most frequently used to increase AV block in settings of atrial flutter or fibrillation.[9] In experimental studies on animal and human tissues, the actions of digitalis on atrial fibers have been shown to hyperpolarize the membrane, an effect attributable to the actions of ACh on gK.[6] The increase in gK would also increase outward current during phase 4 and, thereby, suppress ectopic pacemaker activity (Fig. 3).[23]

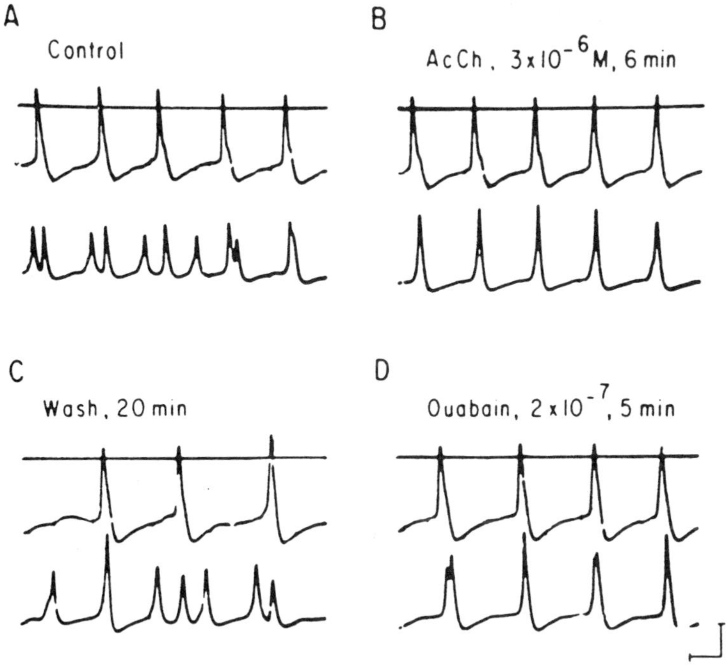

Figure 3. *Effects of ouabain and ACh on spontaneously-firing diseased human atrial fibers. Two impalements were made in the atrium. Panel A: Although both fibers are depressed, the one depicted on the lower trace is more depressed than the one on the upper trace. Ectopic activity occurring at the site on the lower trace is not propagated to that on the upper trace. Cycle length (upper trace) = 1050 msec. Panel B: ACh has induced hyperpolarization, resulting in improved conduction and cessation of the arrhythmia. Cycle length (upper trace) = 1300 msec. Panel C: Following washout of the ACh for 20 min, the control conditions have returned. Panel D: Ouabain has resulted in cessation of the arrhythmia. Vertical calibration = 20 mV; horizontal calibration = 500 msec. Reprinted by permission of the American Heart Association, Inc. from Hordof AJ, Spotnitz A, Mary-Rabine L, et al: The cellular electrophysiologic effects of digitalis on human atrial fibers. Circulation 57:228, 1978.*

The effects of digitalis on the normal AV node, described above, are of special importance in the management of atrial fibrillation and flutter. As conduction through the node is depressed and nodal refractoriness is prolonged, fewer impulses bombarding the node from its atrial margin can propagate to the ventricle and induce ventricular complexes.[4] The result is the prominent slowing of ventricular rate in patients who have atrial flutter or fibrillation and who are treated with digitalis.[4]

References

1. Withering W: An account of the foxglove and some of its medicinal uses. Classics of Medicine Library. Birmingham, AL, Gryphon, 1979, p. 1789.
2. Lee KS, Klaus W: The subcellular basis for the mechanism of action of cardiac glycosides. Pharmacol Rev 23:193, 1971.

3. Vassalle M: Cardiac glycosides: Regulation of force and rhythm. In RD Nathan (ed): Cardiac Muscle: The Regulation of Excitation and Contraction. New York, NY, Academic Press Inc, 1986, pp. 237–267.
4. Hoffman BF: The pharmacology of cardiac glycosides. In MR Rosen, BF Hoffman (eds): Cardiac Therapy. Boston, MA, Martinus Nijhoff Publishers, 1983, pp. 387–412.
5. DiFrancesco D, Ferroni A, Mazzanti M, et al: Properties of the hyperpolarizing-activated current (I_f) in cells isolated from the rabbit sinoatrial node. J Physiol (Lond) 377:61–88, 1986.
6. Noma A, Trautwein W: Relaxation of the ACh-induced potassium current in the rabbit sinoatrial node cell. Pflügers Arch 377:193–200, 1978.
7. Hoffman BF, Cranefield PF: Electrophysiology of the Heart. New York, NY, McGraw-Hill, 1960.
8. DiFrancesco D, Ducouret P, Robinson RB: Muscarinic modulation of cardiac rate at low acetylcholine concentrations. Science 243:669–671, 1989.
9. Hoffman BF, Bigger JT Jr: Digitalis and allied cardiac glycosides. In AG Gilman, LS Goodman, A Gilman (eds): The Pharmacological Basis of Therapeutics. 6th edition. New York, NY, Macmillan Publishing Co Inc, 1980, pp. 729–760.
10. Lindemann JP, Watanabe AM: Mechanisms of adrenergic and cholinergic regulation of myocardial contractility. In N Sperelakis (ed): Physiology and Pathophysiology of the Heart. 2nd edition. Boston, MA, Kluwer Academic Publishers, 1989, pp. 423–452.
11. McLain PL: Effects of cardiac glycosides on spontaneous efferent activity in vagus and sympathetic nerves of cats. Int J Neuropharmac 8:379–397, 1969.
12. Saum WR, Brown AM, Tuley FH: An electrogenic sodium pump and baroreceptor function in normotensive and spontaneously hypertensive rats. Circ Res 39:497–505, 1976.
13. Chai CY, Wang HH, Hoffman BF, et al: Mechanisms of bradycardia induced by digitalis substances. Am J Physiol 212:26–34, 1967.
14. Ten Eick RE, Hoffman BF: The effect of digitalis on the excitability of autonomic nerves. J Pharmacol Exp Ther 169:95–108, 1969.
15. Toda N, West TC: The influence of ouabain on cholinergic responses in the sinoatrial node. J Pharmacol Exp Ther 153:104–113, 1966.
16. Rosen MR, Hoffman BF: The vagus and the ventricles. Circ Res 42:1, 1978. Editorial.
17. Bailey JC, Greenspan K, Elizari MV, et al: Effects of acetylcholine on automaticity and conduction in the proximal portion of the His-Purkinje specialized conduction system of the dog. Circ Res 30:210–216, 1972.
18. Danilo P Jr, Rosen MR, Hordof AJ: Effects of acetylcholine on the ventricular specialized conducting system of neonatal and adult dogs. Circ Res 43:777–784, 1978.
19. Hashimoto K, Moe GK: Transient depolarizations induced by acetylstrophanthidin in specialized tissue of dog atrium and ventricle. Circ Res 32:618, 1973.
20. Kent KM, Epstein SE, Cooper T, et al: Cholinergic innervation of the canine and human ventricular conducting system. Circulation 50:948–955, 1974.
21. Levy MN: Sympathetic-parasympathetic interactions in the heart. Circ Res 29:437–445, 1971.
22. Bailey JC, Watanabe AM, Besch HR Jr, et al: Acetylcholine antagonism of the electrophysiological effects of isoproterenol on canine cardiac Purkinje fibers. Circ Res 44:378–383, 1979.
23. Hordof AJ, Spotnitz A, Mary-Rabine L, et al: The cellular electrophysiologic effects of digitalis on human atrial fibers. Circulation 57:223–229, 1978.

PART IV

Role in Cardiac Reflexes

CHAPTER 21

Role of Vagal Afferents in Cardiovascular Control

V.S. Bishop, S.E. DiCarlo

In the past several decades, there have been significant changes in our understanding of the neural mechanisms involved in the reflex control of the cardiovascular system. This understanding includes the recognition that sensory inputs, other than those from the arterial baroreceptors and chemoreceptors, contribute to the neurohumoral regulation of the cardiovascular system. In this regard, it is now apparent that cardiac receptors subserved by myelinated and unmyelinated vagal afferents are involved in the reflex regulation of the cardiovascular system in both physiological and pathophysiological states. Atrial receptors, connected to myelinated vagal afferents, are sensitive to small changes in atrial volume and are known to play a role in signalling changes in atrial filling and, consequently, in volume homeostasis. Although still not well defined, the reflex response to activation of these receptors includes an increase in sympathetic nerve activity (SNA) to the heart, but a decrease in SNA to the kidney.[1–3] Receptors connected to unmyelinated vagal afferents are widely distributed in the atria and ventricles.[3–5] The unmyelinated atrial receptors may be silent or may discharge at an irregular frequency. The spontaneous discharge is normally irregular, but some have a rhythm in phase with the V wave. The pressure threshold for these receptors is higher than that for the atrial receptors connected to myelinated afferents, but many have a threshold in the physiological range.[3,5] In the rat, Thorén[5] observed variations in the activity of the unmyelinated atrial receptors. Some receptors had a low threshold for activation and a relatively high level of activity that increased with atrial distension. In the rat, all of the vagal afferents were unmyelinated and no receptors were localized in the ventricles. Activation of these receptors resulted in a marked bradycardia and inhibition of activity in the renal and splanchnic sympathetic nerves.[5]

In most species, unmyelinated vagal afferents are also distributed in the walls of the left ventricle.[3–5] The discharge rate of single afferents is sparse and

From *Vagal Control of the Heart: Experimental Basis and Clinical Implications* edited by MN Levy, PJ Schwartz © 1994, Futura Publishing Co. Inc., Armonk, NY.

irregular. When these afferents are activated by probing the tissue or applying veratridine or capsaicin, the activity increases markedly.[3,4] In terms of their responses to mechanical and chemical stimuli,[6–8] at least two populations of cardiac receptors with unmyelinated vagal afferents have been identified. One group responds to mechanical stimuli and to the application of veratridine and nicotine. The other group is insensitive to mechanical stimuli, but is activated by veratridine, phenyl diguanide (5HT-3 receptors), bradykinin, and prostaglandins. In general, the reflex responses to activation of either the mechanosensitive or chemosensitive receptors are similar (bradycardia and peripheral vasodilation). The mechanosensitive receptors increase their discharge rate in response to increases in left ventricular end diastolic pressure (LVEDP). As LVEDP increases, the discharge rate also increases.[4] The activity of the receptors, however, occurs in early systole, and for a given increase in LVEDP, the discharge rate is greater if systolic pressure is also increased. This finding suggests that an increase in contractile force, resulting from the elevation in LVEDP, is the stimulus. In this regard, the tonic influence of these afferents can be modulated by changes in contractility.[3,9,10] Thus, alterations in contractility induced by SNA may act as a feedback mechanism to modulate the afferent activity of vagal afferents, providing a mechanism for the regulation of sympathetic outflow to the heart.

The natural stimuli for the chemosensitive vagal afferents may include bradykinin, prostaglandins, and serotonin.[6–8] It has been postulated that increases in myocardial oxygen demands or a reduction in myocardial perfusion may lead to an increased synthesis of bradykinin which, in turn, stimulates the production of prostaglandins. The resulting activation of the chemosensitive vagal afferents would modulate sympathetic outflow and vascular resistance.[11–13]

Tonic Influence

One of the important characteristics of the unmyelinated vagal afferents is that they exert a tonic inhibitory influence on SNA and arginine vasopressin (AVP) release.[3,14,15] Interruption of vagal afferent input to the central nervous system (CNS), either by sectioning the vagi in anesthetized aortic baroreceptor denervated animals,[16] by cold-blocking the vagi in conscious animals with prior aortic baroreceptor denervation,[15,17] or by injecting a local anesthetic agent into the pericardial sac to block cardiac afferents,[18,19] is characterized by increases in mean arterial pressure (MAP), peripheral vascular resistance (PVR), SNA, and plasma AVP concentration. The magnitude of the response varies inversely with the input from the arterial baroreceptors. For example, in aortic baroreceptor denervated animals in which the carotid sinuses are isolated, the MAP response to interruption of vagal afferents is greater at low carotid sinus pressures and has no effect at high carotid sinus pressures.[20,21] As would be expected from these studies, the response to interruption of vagal afferents is augmented in animals with sinoaortic denervation (SAD).[3,17]

Evidence that unmyelinated vagal afferents are responsible for this tonic influence is derived from studies in which MAP responses were determined during selective interruption of myelinated and unmyelinated fibers. The fiber type responsible for the tonic effects was determined by using anodal blockade to selectively interrupt transmission in myelinated fibers and, subsequently, blocking the remaining C-fibers with cold.[22] At least 80% of the total increase in MAP that results from blockade of all fibers was derived from blocking the C-fibers. This observation supports the view that the collective activity from the C-fibers constitutes a major modulatory input to the nucleus tractus solitarius (NTS).

Reflexes

More than three decades ago, Henry and Gauer[23,24] proposed that reflexes initiated from receptors located in the low pressure side of the circulation were important in volume homeostasis. These investigators found that distention of the atrium increased urine flow. The early investigations also focused on the excretion of water and the potential involvement of AVP in the reflex. Although the identification of the reflex mechanism responsible for the increase in renal excretory function has been controversial, increases in urinary volume and sodium excretion by mechanical distention of the atria and during volume expansion have been reported by numerous investigators.[1,2,5,25] Linden and colleagues[1,2] were the first to elucidate the reflex mechanism responsible for the natriuresis induced by atrial distention. Selective distention of the atria with small balloons was shown to decrease renal sympathetic nerve activity (RSNA) and the effect was blocked by vagotomy. Subsequent studies in conscious animals showed that reflexes initiated from cardiac receptors subserved by vagal afferents were responsible for the enhanced renal function in response to atrial distention.[25–27] There is still debate, however, as to whether cardiac denervation in conscious animals always eliminates the diuretic and natriuretic responses to volume expansion. Several investigators have reported that the natriuresis and diuresis due to atrial distention, but not due to volume expansion, is abolished by cardiac denervation in conscious animals.[26–28] One explanation for the differences is that volume expansion has a direct effect on renal hemodynamics, which influences renal function independent of the cardiac reflexes.

Other studies in conscious animals, however, have provided convincing evidence that reflexes initiated from cardiac vagal afferents contribute to the diuretic and natriuretic responses to volume expansion.[28–30] In dogs (both intact and SAD)[28,29] and in subhuman primates,[30] vagotomy markedly attenuated the increase in Na^+ excretion and urine volume in response to volume expansion. Note that the volume expansion had no effect on renal vascular resistance in either intact dogs or dogs with SAD, either before or after vagotomy, even though RSNA decreased in response to volume prior to vagotomy. These investigators also showed that renal denervation attenuated volume-induced diuresis and natriuresis in response to volume expansion. These results support earlier findings in the rat and dog, which showed that renal denervation altered the excretion of Na^+ in response to volume expansion.[31,32] In summary, the controversy concerning the role of cardiac vagal afferents in the regulation of sodium and water excretion during an acute volume expansion may be related to the initial sodium balance and hydration.[26]

Arginine Vasopressin

Abundant evidence indicates that cardiac vagal afferents and arterial baroreceptors contribute to the regulation of plasma AVP concentration.[15,25,33–40] Studies in anesthetized animals[33,36–38] and conscious animals[15,25,35,39–41] have shown that cardiac vagal afferents contribute to the regulation of plasma AVP concentrations. Unloading vagal afferents, either by vena caval occlusion or hemorrhage, leads to an increase in AVP.[34,37–42] In the absence of arterial baroreflexes, the increase in AVP is prevented by prior vagotomy. Also, activation of cardiac vagal afferents by atrial distension reduces plasma AVP concentrations.[25,42,43] In conscious dogs with aortic baroreceptors denervated, interruption of vagal afferents by cold-blocking the vagi elevates plasma AVP. This tonic inhibitory influence of the vagal afferents is enhanced if the carotid sinus baroreceptors are also denervated. Results from these and other studies suggest an interaction between the cardiac vagal afferents and the arterial baroreflex in the regulation of plasma AVP,[37,38] such that the removal or unloading of the receptors of either system enhances the response to the removal or unloading of the other system.[21]

A recent study in conscious dogs challenges the role of cardiac vagal afferents in mediating the reflex increase in plasma AVP in response to hemorrhage.[44] When increases in AVP were related to MAP, the response of AVP to hemorrhage was not altered by cardiac denervation, but was attenuated by SAD. When the data are evaluated, however, on the basis of the volume of hemorrhage (range 10 to 20 ml/kg), the release of AVP was generally greater after either cardiac or arterial baroreceptor denervation. This finding suggests that both reflexes contribute to the increase in AVP during blood loss. The apparent greater release of AVP in the absence of either input may be due to an interaction between the two reflexes.[14]

An important finding in the above-mentioned study[44] is that cardiac denervation attenuated the AVP response to hemorrhage in dogs with SAD, which indicates the potential role of cardiac afferents in modulating the AVP level in response to hemorrhage.

The separate and combined role of cardiac vagal afferents and arterial baroreflexes in the regulation of plasma AVP during blood loss has also been investigated in the conscious rabbit.[40] In the rabbit, the effects of hemorrhage (2% of the blood volume per minute, up to 35% of the blood volume) were studied in the intact animal and after cardiac denervation, SAD, or combined cardiac denervation and SAD. During the nonhypotensive phase, there was little effect of hemorrhage on plasma AVP levels. During the hypotensive phase (25% of the blood volume removed), however, there was a dramatic increase in AVP. This increase in AVP was almost entirely blocked by denervation of the cardiac receptors. Removal of the arterial baroreceptors with or without an intact cardiac innervation had no effect on the release of AVP. The increase in plasma AVP, however, did not contribute to the blood pressure response during hemorrhage. The arterial pressure response was dependent upon the arterial baroreflex. The plasma renin activity (PRA), which increased during the hemorrhage, appeared to be independent of the cardiac and arterial baroreflexes. This finding suggests that, under these conditions, renal perfusion pressure was the principal determinant of PRA.

Two important conclusions can be drawn from these two studies. One, the mechanisms regulating the release of AVP during hemorrhage are relatively insensitive and two, the blood pressure response depends largely on the arterial baroreflex regulation of vascular resistance. The interactions between the cardiac and arterial baroreflexes, however, may also influence the results of these studies which makes it difficult to judge the relative importance of the respective reflexes. Finally, it is still debatable as to the proper choice of the dependent variable when analyzing the relative roles of cardiac and arterial baroreflexes during hemorrhage. For example, when analyzing the contribution of cardiac afferents, is arterial pressure the appropriate dependent variable? In defining the role of arterial baroreflexes, should arterial pressure be the dependent variable after SAD?

The reflex release of AVP during decreases in afferent input from cardiopulmonary and arterial baroreflexes modulates the cardiopulmonary and arterial baroreflex regulation of the circulation.[45–47] For example, elevations in plasma AVP during bilateral vagal cold block exerted both vasoconstrictor affects and a central action that simultaneously inhibited the contribution of the sympathetic nervous system to the pressor response to vagal block.[45,46] In addition, osmotically-stimulated AVP augmented the inhibitory effects of the cardiopulmonary reflex, and this effect was mediated through the area postrema via the V_1 receptor.[48] For example, intracoronary infusion of veratridine significantly decreased arterial pressure (-10 mm Hg). After hypertonic saline infusion, the depressor response to veratridine was significantly enhanced (-18 mm Hg). Administration of the AVP V_1 antagonist prevented the enhanced depressor response to veratridine (-8 mm Hg) (Fig. 1). Lesions of the area postrema also eliminated the enhanced response to veratridine during hypertonic saline infusion. These data demonstrated that osmotically-released AVP acts at the area postrema to augment the cardiopulmonary baroreflex.

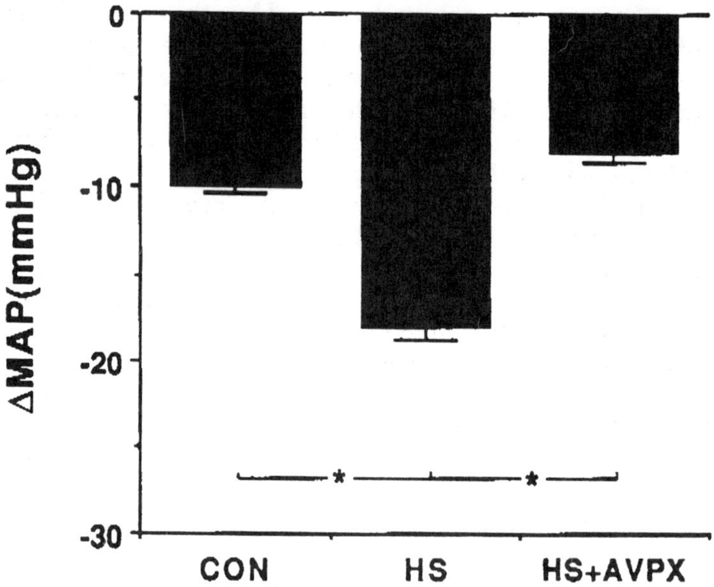

Figure 1. *Average depressor response to intracoronary infusion of veratridine in intact dogs under control conditions (CON), after infusion of hypertonic saline (HS), and after HS in the presence of AVP antagonist (HS + AVPX). ΔMAP: change in mean arterial pressure *$p<0.05$. Reproduced with permission from Hasser EM, DiCarlo SE, Applegate RJ, et al: Osmotically released vasopressin augments cardiopulmonary reflex inhibition of the circulation. Am J Physiol 254:R817, 1988.*

Renin

The elegant studies of Kirchheim and coworkers in 1985[49] and Persson et al in 1987[50] have provided a good understanding of the potential role of the cardiopulmonary afferents and the arterial baroreflexes in the modulation of renin release. In conscious dogs, increases in renin release occurred only when both the arterial and cardiopulmonary reflexes were eliminated. When either reflex was intact, the remaining reflex was able to oppose the effects of removing the other.

There are several factors to consider in the reflex regulation of renin release. First, renin release is pressure-dependent. Thus, the effects of interruption of the inhibitory influence of the cardiopulmonary vagal afferents may not augment renin release if MAP also increases. The neurogenic component of renin release may be offset by the increase in MAP, and thus renin release might be negligible. Second, after removal of both the cardiopulmonary vagal afferents and the arterial baroreceptors, renin release may increase even though the average MAP is elevated. Even if the average MAP is unaltered, however, the lability of MAP is increased, which results in frequent periods of hypotension. The increase in lability of MAP results in more frequent occurrences of MAP that are below the threshold for renin release. This action, together with a greater sympathetic component, may lead to an increased release of renin.

Hemorrhage

In contrast to the dominant role of cardiac afferents in mediating the sympathoinhibitory response during volume expansion, recent studies in conscious dogs and rabbits suggest that cardiac afferents contribute little to the hemodynamic and sympathoexcitatory responses to blood loss.[40,41,44,51,52] In conscious dogs and rabbits (intact or with SAD), the hemodynamic responses to hemorrhage were essentially unaltered by cardiac denervation.[40,44,51] The ability to maintain MAP during hemorrhage, however, was severely compromised in animals with SAD. These findings indicate that the arterial baroreflexes provide most of the reflex compensation to hemorrhage.

In conscious rabbits, the reflex increase in RSNA during moderate hemorrhage was essentially unaltered when the cardiac afferents were blocked by intrapericardial administration of procaine.[52] With severe hemorrhage (30% to 40% blood loss), however, blockade of cardiac receptors prevented the precipitous decrease in RSNA that occurs when the blood loss exceeds 20% to 25%. A similar inhibition of RSNA has been observed in anesthetized and conscious rats in response to severe hemorrhage.[53–55] In the rat, interruption of vagal afferents or interference with serotonergic mechanisms (interruption of serotonin synthesis or blockade of serotonin receptors) prevents the inhibition of RSNA.[54,55] These observations support the earlier work by Chen and coworkers[56] that showed that vagal afferents exert a tonic inhibitory effect on MAP during hemorrhage. In the anesthetized rabbit, interruption of vagal afferents resulted in an increase in MAP at different levels of hemorrhage. It has been postulated that the increased sympathoadrenal drive to the heart and the contraction of the heart around a small blood volume increase the activation of vagal afferent fibers.[53,57] In addition, studies in conscious dogs[9] and anesthetized cats[10] have provided evidence for a feedback relationship between cardiac vagal afferents and cardiac sympathetic efferent nerves. In these studies, increases in sympathetic drive to the heart augment the tonic inhibitory influence of vagal afferents. These findings suggest that the increased contractility resulting from activation of cardiac sympathetic nerves increases the activity of mechanosensitive vagal afferents. This effect would, in turn, result in a feedback inhibition of sympathetic activity.

In the conscious animal, the lack of an apparent role of vagal afferents in the response to moderate hemorrhage may be related to this feedback relationship between the cardiac vagal afferents and the cardiac sympathetic nerves. During hemorrhage, the expected decrease in vagal afferent activity, due to a reduction in central venous pressure, is counterbalanced by the effects of the augmented sympathoadrenal drive to the heart, which would increase vagal afferent activity. The net effect is little change in vagal afferent activity during moderate hemorrhage. Accordingly, removal of vagal afferents has little effect on the response to compensatory responses to moderate hemorrhage. During severe hemorrhage, however, the activation of the vagal afferents is likely to be more intense and, under these circumstances, it may contribute to the decrease in RSNA and MAP.

Exercise

Two mechanisms involved in the neural control of the circulation during exercise have been described: central command and the exercise pressor reflex. Although not well defined, central command refers to the central mechanisms responsible for the immediate autonomic adjustments at the onset of exercise. The concept of a parallel activation of cardiovascular and motor systems originated from the observation that heart rate (HR) and ventilation increased immediately at the onset of exercise. This central neural mechanism functions as a feed-forward control system.[58–60] The importance of central command in the sympathoexcitatory response to exercise, however, depends upon the type of exercise (dynamic versus static) and the muscle mass involved.

The mechanism(s) whereby central command may influence sympathetic outflow during exercise is unknown. One possibility is that central command may alter the response of barosensitive neurons in the NTS and result in an upward resetting of the operating point of the arterial baroreflex function. Data from animals with SAD support the concept that central command involves an interaction with the arterial baroreflex.[61–65] If central command operates independently of the baroreflex, one would expect to observe exaggerated increases in MAP, HR, and RSNA in animals with SAD during the onset of locomotion. This occurrence, however, is not the case. In the absence of functional arterial baroreflexes, spontaneous motor activity (such as postural changes, exploration, grooming, and eating) results in a decrease in arterial pressure.[64,65] A recent study in rabbits showed that, following SAD, the sympathoexcitatory response at the onset of exercise was changed to an inhibitory response (hypotension, bradycardia, and decreases in RSNA).[65] The results of these studies clearly show that functional baroreflexes are a major determinant of the sympathoexcitatory and hemodynamic responses to exercise or locomotion. The results are also consistent with the hypothesis that, during exercise, the operating point of the baroreflex is shifted toward higher pressures.[66]

Two additional studies support more directly an upward resetting of the arterial baroreflex during exercise. Walgenbach and Donald[67] studied the exercise response in aortic denervated dogs in which the carotid sinus could be isolated from the circulation and the pressure fixed at a given level. With the carotid sinus pressure fixed at systemic pressure, exercise resulted in an initial hypotension. This result was followed by an increase in arterial pressure that was substantially greater than that observed when the carotid sinuses were allowed to sense the systemic pressure. More recently, DiCarlo and Bishop[65] determined the role of the arterial baroreflex in the regulation of RSNA in exercising rabbits. Attenuation of the pressor response at the onset of exercise resulted in an exaggerated increase in RSNA. In rabbits with SAD, the onset of exercise was characterized by a decrease in MAP, HR, and RSNA. These two studies further supported the role of the arterial baroreflex during exercise. Furthermore, the sympathoexcitatory response appears to involve an upward shift of the operating point of the baroreflex function.[66]

The influence of cardiac vagal afferents on the sympathetic response during exercise is not well understood.[68–74] Since cardiac preload, afterload, and contractility are elevated during exercise,[75] one would expect the afferent activity of cardiac vagal afferents to be increased.[3,76] Accordingly, during exercise, cardiac vagal afferents may be important in suppressing sympathetic activity. Investigators have examined the influence of the cardiopulmonary receptors on forearm vascular resistance,[72,74] arterial pressure,[68,71] regional vascular resistance,[77] and efferent sympathetic nerve activity responses[69,70] during exercise. DiCarlo and Bishop,[77] examined the role of cardiac afferents in the regulation of mesenteric and renal vascular resistances during treadmill running in rabbits. Intrapericardial procainamide was used to selectively and reversibly denervate cardiac afferents. Figure 2 shows the percent change in renal (Panel A) and mesenteric (Panel B) vascular resistance during exercise under three experimental conditions: control, cardiac efferent blockade, and combined cardiac efferent and afferent blockade. As expected, during exercise, renal and mesenteric vascular resistance significantly increased (+37 ± 4% and +88 ± 9%, respectively). Cardiac efferent blockade did not significantly alter the renal or mesenteric vascular resistance (+43 ± 4% and +94 ± 9%, respectively) responses to exercise. Combined cardiac efferent and afferent blockade, however, significantly enhanced the renal (+62 ± 6%) and mesenteric (+134 ± 13%) resistance responses to exercise. These data demonstrate that cardiac afferents regulate renal and mesenteric vascular resistance during treadmill running in rabbits. Additional studies in humans[72,74,78] and animals[73] showed that cardiopulmonary receptors attenuate the exercise-induced reflex vasoconstriction during exercise. Other studies[69,70] indicated, however, that nonhypotensive lower body negative pressure (LBNP) did not augment muscle sympathetic nerve activity during static handgrip exercise in humans and vagal sectioning did not alter the arterial pressure response to treadmill exercise in dogs.[68,71]

The reasons for the discrepancies between the various studies investigating the role of arterial and cardiopulmonary reflexes in the exercise response could be due to a number of factors. First, the method using intrapericardial procainamide to assess the involvement of cardiac vagal afferents may be more selective than vagotomy. There is also concern that LBNP in humans unloads not only the cardiopulmonary but also the arterial baroreceptors.[79] Second, the type of exercise (static versus dynamic) may determine the extent of involvement of the reflex. The cardiovascular responses to exercise are determined by the intensity, duration, and mode of exercise. Exercise with relatively small muscle groups may elicit responses different from those evoked by whole body exercise. For example, when the mass of vasodilated muscle is too small to increase total vascular conductance substantially, it is not likely that the arterial and cardiopulmonary baroreflexes will have an important role in the regulation of peripheral resistance.[66,80] Static exercise, unlike dynamic exercise, does not increase cardiac filling pressures in young subjects without cardiopulmonary disease.[72,81]

Species differences may also account for the lack of agreement between studies. For example, the dog,[82] unlike humans[75] and rabbits,[80] has a large

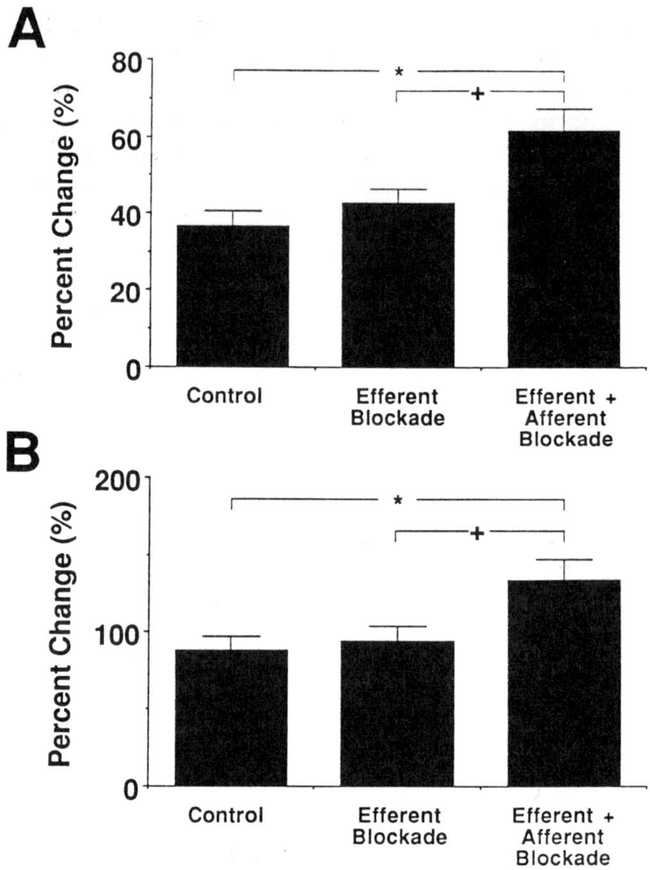

Figure 2. *Percent change in renal (Panel A) and mesenteric (Panel B) vascular resistance during exercise under the three experimental conditions of control, efferent blockade, and combined efferent and afferent blockade.* *$p<0.05$ *(control versus combined efferent and afferent blockade);* $+p<0.05$ *(efferent blockade versus combined efferent and afferent blockade). Reproduced with permission from DiCarlo SE, Bishop VS: Regional vascular resistance during exercise: Role of cardiac afferents and exercise training. Am J Physiol 258:H845, 1990.*

ratio of heart weight to body weight and a large cardiac reserve. With the large cardiac reserve, arterial and cardiopulmonary baroreceptors may be less important in regulating regional blood flow distribution during exercise.[80,83–86] Even during intense exercise, the normal dog can increase cardiac output to meet the demands of the exercising muscles without substantial redistribution of blood flow from visceral regions.[86,87] In dogs with heart failure (limited cardiac reserve), however, increases in metabolic demand during exercise require a redistribution of blood flow from the visceral regions,[85] a response observed in normal humans and rabbits.[58,73,77,88] Thus, it appears that, in species with limited cardiac output reserves, cardiopulmonary reflexes contribute to the regulation of blood flow distribution.

Exercise Training

A close evaluation of the literature examining the effects of endurance exercise training on the cardiopulmonary baroreflex regulation of the circulation reveals several major concerns. First, all investigations examining this question, except two,[80,83] have unloaded the baroreceptors with hypotensive[89–91] or nonhypotensive[74,92–95] levels of LBNP in the human model. Since even low levels (nonhypotensive) of LBNP may unload both arterial and cardiopulmonary baroreflexes,[79] only those studies that employed nonhypotensive levels of LBNP are discussed. Second, the studies using a human model and LBNP examined the effect of exercise training on the cardiopulmonary baroreflex regulation of the circulation at rest. To date, only one laboratory has examined the effects of endurance exercise training on the cardiopulmonary baroreflex regulation of the circulation during exercise.[77] Thus, with these points in mind, the influence of exercise training on the cardiopulmonary baroreflex regulation of the circulation at rest and during exercise are discussed below.

Although the effect of exercise training on the cardiac afferent regulation of the circulation is not well defined, it is known that exercise training results in significant increases in blood volume, cardiac mass, and contractility.[75,76,83,96] Since these factors influence cardiac vagal afferent activity,[97] it is logical to suspect that the tonic inhibitory influence of the cardiac receptors would be enhanced following training. DiCarlo and Bishop[80] recently reported that exercise training significantly enhanced the tonic inhibitory influence of cardiac afferents on arterial baroreflex function in conscious resting rabbits. This study was unique because the influence of the cardiopulmonary baroreflex on the entire arterial baroreflex function curve was examined. The investigators reported that, after training, the arterial baroreflex regulation of RSNA was reduced. This occurrence was characterized by a reduction in the maximum RSNA and the gain of the arterial baroreflex function curve (Fig. 3). This effect of training on the arterial baroreflex function appeared to result from an enhanced inhibitory influence of cardiac afferents on the arterial baroreflex regulation of RSNA, because blockade of cardiac afferents restored the arterial baroreflex function to a level similar to that observed in the untrained state (Fig. 3).

Although several studies demonstrated that the arterial baroreflex is attenuated in exercise-trained individuals and animals,[80,83,98–101] it now appears that the attenuated arterial baroreflex function associated with endurance exercise training is the result of an enhanced role of the cardiac afferents, and is not the result of an altered arterial baroreflex per se. Support for these findings are provided by Jingu and colleagues[92] in a longitudinal experimental design and by Takeshita and colleagues[102] in a cross-sectional experimental design. Jingu et al[92] reported a 2.5-fold augmentation in the forearm vascular resistance (FVR) response to LBNP at -10 mm Hg after endurance training in a group of middle-aged men and women. In addition, Takeshita et al[102] reported that the reflex control of FVR during LBNP (-10 mm Hg) was augmented in trained subjects. Mack and coworkers, however,[96] observed a

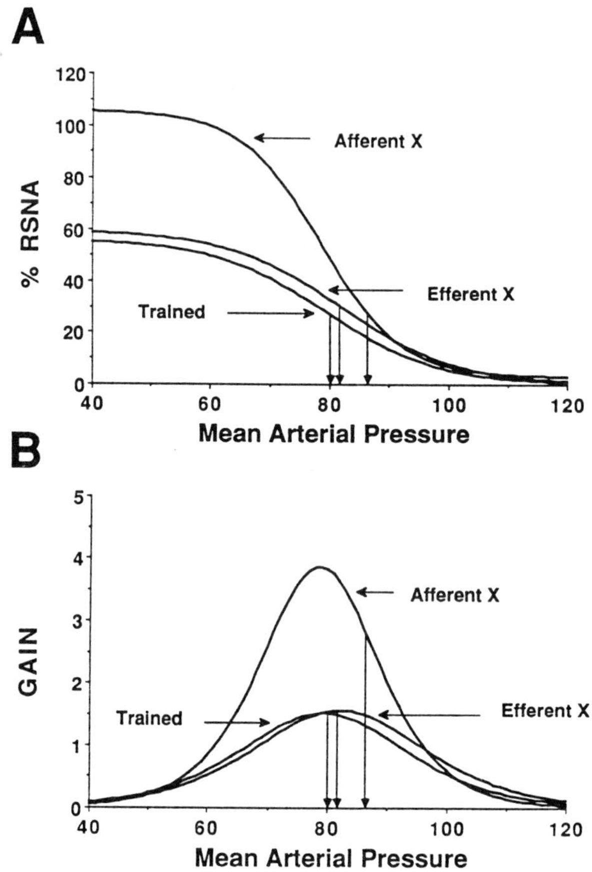

Figure 3. *Relationship between mean arterial pressure and RSNA fitted to a sigmoid logistic function in the trained condition (Trained), after efferent blockade (Efferent X), and after combined efferent and afferent blockade (Afferent X). Reproduced with permission from DiCarlo SE, Bishop VS: Exercise training enhances cardiac afferent inhibition of baroreflex function. Am J Physiol 258:H217, 1990.*

reduction in the FVR responses to LBNP (0 to 20 mm Hg) in trained subjects (cross sectional). These investigators reported a small reduction in pulse pressure during lower body suction of 20 mm Hg, which should have unloaded the arterial baroreflex. Finally, in a longitudinal experimental design, Vroman and colleagues[94] reported that training did not alter the FVR response to a nonhypotensive level (−10 mm Hg) of LBNP in a group of young subjects. The reflex forearm vasoconstriction in response to LBNP at −10 mm Hg may be largely determined by the cardiopulmonary receptors, because at this level of LBNP, blood pressure and heart rate do not change.[103] This concept, however, is not universally accepted.[79]

In summary, investigators using nonhypotensive levels of LBNP have reported unchanged,[94] augmented,[92,102] and attenuated[93,95] cardiopulmonary baroreflex responses at rest after training. Studies examining this question in chronically instrumented, conscious animals have demonstrated, however, an enhanced cardiopulmonary baroreflex regulation of the circulation at rest and during exercise after endurance exercise training.[77,83]

A recent study in chronically instrumented conscious rabbits[77] examined the effect of endurance exercise training on the cardiac afferent regulation of regional vascular resistance. This study was accomplished by measuring renal and mesenteric vascular resistance during dynamic treadmill running before and after reversible denervation of cardiac afferents (intrapericardial procainamide, 2%). These procedures were repeated, after an eight-week endurance exercise training program. The investigators reported that renal and mesenteric vascular resistance significantly increased during exercise (Fig. 2). Cardiac afferent blockade enhanced the vasoconstrictor responses in the renal and mesenteric vascular beds. Such findings demonstrate that cardiac afferents contribute to the regulation of renal and mesenteric vascular resistance during exercise (Fig. 2). In addition, this response to cardiac afferent blockade was enhanced after exercise training (Table 1). That is, training significantly altered the regulation of renal (22 ± 2 versus 37 ± 4%Δ) and mesenteric (46 ± 4 versus 88 ± 9%Δ) vascular resistance during exercise, such that the percent increase during exercise was significantly reduced after training. More importantly, cardiac afferents appeared to be responsible for the attenuation in renal and mesenteric vascular resistance after exercise training, because blockade of cardiac afferents with intrapericardial procainamide restored the vascular resistance to levels obtained in the untrained condition (Table 1). Thus, cardiac afferents contribute to the regulation of renal and mesenteric vascular resistance during exercise, and this effect is significantly enhanced after exercise training.

Table 1.

Percent Changes in Renal and Mesenteric Vascular Resistances During Exercise Before (Untrained) and After (Trained) Exercise Training.

	Control	*Efferent Blockade*	*Efferent and Afferent Blockade*
Renal Resistance, % Change			
Untrained	37±4	43±4	62±6+
Trained	22±2*	24±2*	68±6+
Mesenteric Resistance, % Change			
Untrained	88±9	94±9	134±13+
Trained	46±4*	49±4*	135±13+

Percent change from control in renal and mesenteric vascular resistance during exercise under the three experimental conditions of control, efferent blockade, and combined efferent and afferent blockade before (untrained) and after (trained) exercise training. *$p<0.05$ (untrained vs. trained); $^{+}p<0.05$ (efferent blockade versus combined efferent and afferent blockade). Reproduced with permission from DiCarlo SE, Bishop VS: Regional vascular resistance during exercise: Role of cardiac afferents and exercise training. Am J Physiol 258:H845, 1990.

Hypertension

In 1976, Kezdi[104] examined the reflex vasodilation of skeletal muscles to abrupt increases in left ventricular pressures in normotensive and hypertensive dogs. In hypertensive dogs, the reflex vasodilation was substantially impaired. Subsequent studies in a number of laboratories showed abnormalities in the cardiopulmonary baroreflexes.[105–107] When Dahl salt-sensitive rats are fed a low salt diet during the prehypertensive state, the arterial and cardiopulmonary baroreflexes are diminished.[105] This reduced function of the baroreflexes was postulated to be due to a decrease in afferent discharge. In contrast, the cardiopulmonary baroreflex in spontaneously-hypertensive rats was shown to be reset to a higher pressure, but the sensitivity of the reflex was unaltered. In rabbits with renal hypertension, the reflex inhibition of renal SNA to activation of either the mechanosensitive or chemosensitive cardiac receptors was substantially impaired in the absence of detectable cardiac abnormalities. These results suggest that the impairment of reflexes is not restricted to changes in cardiac function.[107]

In humans with borderline hypertension, there is evidence that the reflex response to unloading the cardiopulmonary receptors during LBNP is augmented.[108] Thus, the cardiopulmonary baroreflexes may oppose the increase in blood pressure initially and with the development of hypertension, the receptors may be reset to higher pressures.[109]

Myocardial Ischemia and Infarction

As mentioned previously, there are two types of vagal sensory endings in the left ventricle.[6–8] One type is mechanosensitive and the other type is chemosensitive. Until recently, most studies focused on the reflexes initiated from mechanosensitive endings. During myocardial ischemia and infarction, however, both types of nerve endings may be activated. Thus, the reflex bradycardia hypotension and sympathoinhibition during myocardial ischemia and infarction probably involves both types of vagal endings. In 1976, Thorén[110] provided direct evidence that vagal endings sensitive to mechanical events were activated during myocardial ischemia. The response of the endings during coronary artery occlusion was characterized by a rapid increase in discharge rate, followed by a return of activity toward control levels while the occlusion was maintained. This transient response of the mechanosensitive endings did not correlate with the reflex response to the acute ischemia, which suggests that other sensory receptors were involved.

Experimental studies show that the administration of prostaglandins elicits a reflex similar to the Bezold-Jarisch reflex.[111] Interruption of vagal afferents prevents this sympathoinhibitory action of prostaglandins. In anesthetized dogs, blockade of the synthesis of prostaglandins with indomethacin or meclofenamate attenuates the reflex inhibition of RSNA during coronary occlusion[12,13] and reperfusion.[13] These findings suggest that increased synthesis of prostaglandins during ischemia activates vagal endings in the left ventricle and initiates the reflex sympathoinhibitory response.

A recent study in conscious dogs showed that captopril alters the reflex control of sympathetic outflow as a result of the associated increase in synthesis of prostaglandins.[112] Administration of captopril decreased the MAP and RSNA. After treatment with a cyclo-oxygenase inhibitor, the decrease in MAP evoked by captopril was accompanied by an increase in RSNA. The above studies suggest that prostaglandins may play a role in cardiovascular regulation via an action involving the vagal chemosensitive endings.

References

1. Linden RJ: The function of atrial receptors. In R Hainsworth, PN McWilliam, DASG Mary (eds): Cardiogenic Reflexes. Oxford, Oxford University Press, 1987, p. 18.
2. Linden RJ, Kappagoda CT: Atrial Receptors. Cambridge, Cambridge University Press, 1982, p. 156.
3. Bishop VS, Malliani A, Thorén P: Cardiac mechanoreceptors. In JT Shepherd, FM Abboud (eds): Handbook of Physiology. Section 2: The Cardiovascular System, Vol. III, Part 2, Ch. 15. Bethesda, MD, American Physiological Society, 1983, p. 497.
4. Thorén PN: Characteristics of left ventricular receptors with nonmedullated vagal afferents in cats. Circ Res 40:415, 1977.
5. Thorén P: Role of cardiac vagal C-fibers in cardiovascular control. Rev Physiol Biochem Pharmacol 86:1, 1979.
6. Coleridge JCG, Coleridge HM: Chemoreflex regulation of the heart. In RM Berne, N Sperelakis, SR Geiger (eds): Handbook of Physiology. Section 2: The Cardiovascular System, Vol. I, Ch. 18. Bethesda, MD, American Physiological Society, 1979, p. 653.
7. Baker DG, Coleridge HM, Coleridge JCG: Vagal afferent C-fibers from the ventricle. In R Hainsworth, Kidd C, Linden RJ (eds): Cardiac Receptors. New York, NY, Cambridge University Press, 1979, p. 117.
8. Kaufman MP, Baker DG, Coleridge HM, et al: Stimulation by bradykinin of afferent vagal C-fibers with chemosensitive endings in the heart and aorta of the dog. Circ Res 46:476, 1980.
9. Barron KW, Bishop VS: The influence of vagal afferents on the left ventricular contractile response to intracoronary administration of catecholamines in the conscious dog. Circ Res 49:159, 1981.
10. Shimizu T, Peterson DF, Bishop VS: Role of cardiac sympathetics in the tonic circulatory restraint by vagal afferents. Am J Physiol 237:H528, 1979.
11. Staszewska-Barcsak J: Prostanoids and cardiac reflexes of sympathetic and vagal origin. Am J Cardiol 52:36A, 1983.
12. Zucker IH, Panzenbeck MJ, Barker S, et al: PGI_2 attenuates baroreflex control of renal nerve activity by a vagal mechanism. Am J Physiol 254:R424, 1988.
13. Thames MD, Minisi AJ: Reflex responses to myocardial ischemia and reperfusion: Role of prostaglandins. Circulation 80:1878, 1989.
14. Bishop VS, Hasser EM: Arterial and cardiopulmonary reflexes in the regulation of the neurohumoral drive to the circulation. Fed Proc 44:2377, 1985.
15. Bishop VS, Thames MD, Schmid PG: Effects of bilateral vagal cold block on vasopressin in conscious dogs. Am J Physiol 246:R566, 1984.
16. Mancia G, Donald DE, Shepherd JT: Inhibition of adrenergic outflow to peripheral blood vessels by vagal afferents from cardiopulmonary region in the dog. Circ Res 33:713, 1973.

17. Bishop VS, Peterson DF: The circulatory influences of vagal afferents at rest and during coronary occlusion in conscious dogs. Circ Res 43:840, 1978.
18. Arndt JO, Pasch U, Samodelov LF, et al: Reversible blockade of myelinated and non-myelinated cardiac afferents in cats by instillation of procaine into the pericardium. Cardiovasc Res 15:61, 1981.
19. Dorward PK, Riedel W, Burke SL, et al: The renal sympathetic baroreflex in the rabbit: Arterial and cardiac baroreceptor influences, resetting, and effect of anesthesia. Circ Res 57:618, 1985.
20. Mancia G, Shepherd JT, Donald DE: Interplay among carotid sinus, cardiopulmonary and carotid body reflexes in dogs. Am J Physiol 230:19, 1976.
21. Heesch CM, Bishop VS: Cardiovascular reflex modulation of plasma catecholamine concentrations in the anesthetized cat. Circ Res 51:391, 1982.
22. Thorén P, Shepherd JT, Donald DE: Anodal block of medullated cardiopulmonary vagal afferents in cats. J Appl Physiol 42:461, 1977.
23. Henry JP, Gauer OH, Reeves JL: Evidence of the atrial location of receptors influencing urine flow. Circ Res 41:85, 1956.
24. Gauer OH, Henry JP: Circulatory basis of fluid volume control. Physiol Rev 43:423, 1963.
25. Fater DC, Schultz HD, Sundet WD, et al: Effects of left atrial stretch in cardiac-denervated and intact conscious dogs. Am J Physiol 242:H1056, 1982.
26. Kaczmarczyk G, Drake A, Eisle R, et al: The role of the cardiac nerves in the regulation of sodium excretion in conscious dogs. Pflügers Arch 390:125, 1981.
27. Schultz HD, Fater DC, Sundet WD, et al: Reflexes elicited by acute stretch of atrial vs pulmonary receptors in conscious dog. Am J Physiol 242:H1065, 1982.
28. Sit SP, Morita H, Vatner SF: Responses of renal hemodynamics and function to acute volume expansion in the conscious dog. Circ Res 54:185, 1984.
29. Morita H, Manders WT, Skelton MM, et al: Vagal regulation of arginine vasopressin in conscious dogs. Am J Physiol 251:H19, 1986.
30. Vatner SF, Manders WT, Knight DR: Vagally mediated regulation of renal function in conscious primates. Am J Physiol 250:H546, 1986.
31. DiBona GF, Sawin LL: Renal nerve activity in conscious rats during volume expansion and depletion. Am J Physiol 248:F15, 1985.
32. Sadowski J, Kurkus J, Gellert R: Denervated and intact kidney responses to saline load in awake and anesthetized dogs. Am J Physiol 237:F262, 1979.
33. Brennan LA, Malvin RL, Jochim KE, et al: Influence of right and left atrial receptors on plasma concentrations of ADH and renin. Am J Physiol 221:273, 1971.
34. Claybough JR, Share L: Vasopressin, renin, and cardiovascular responses to continuous slow hemorrhage. Am J Physiol 224:519, 1973.
35. Kaczmarczyk G, Christe W, Mohnhaupt R, et al: An attempt to quantitate the contribution of antidiuretic hormone to the diuresis of left atrial distension in conscious dogs. Pflügers Arch 396:101, 1983.
36. Share L: Control of plasma ADH titer in hemorrhage: Role of atrial and arterial receptors. Am J Physiol 215:1384, 1968.
37. Thames MD, Schmid PG: Cardiopulmonary receptors with vagal afferents tonically inhibit ADH release in the dog. Am J Physiol 237:H299, 1979.
38. Thames MD, Schmid PG: Interaction between carotid and cardiopulmonary baroreflexes in control of plasma ADH. Am J Physiol 241:H431, 1981.
39. Wang BC, Sundet WD, Hakumäki MOK, et al: Vasopressin and renin responses to hemorrhage in conscious, cardiac-denervated dogs. Am J Physiol 245:H399, 1983.
40. Quail AW, Woods RL, Korner PI: Cardiac and arterial baroreceptor influences in release of vasopressin and renin during hemorrhage. Am J Physiol 252:H1120, 1987.
41. Quillen EW, Reid IA, Keil LC: Cardiac and arterial baroreceptor influences on plasma vasopressin and drinking. In AW Cowley Jr, J-F Liard, DA Ausiello (eds): Vasopressin: Cellular and Integrative Functions. New York, NY, Raven Press, 1988, p. 405.

42. Ramsay DJ, Thrasher TN, Metzler C, et al: Cardiovascular reflexes in the control of vasopressin secretion. In S Yoshida, L Share (eds): Recent Progress in Posterior Pituitary Hormones. New York, NY, Elsevier Science Publishing Co Inc, 1988, p. 57.
43. Shade RE, Share L: Volume control of plasma antidiuretic hormone concentration following acute blood volume expansion in the anesthetized dog. Endocrinology 97:1048, 1975.
44. Shen Y-T, Cowley AW Jr, Vatner SF: Relative roles of cardiac and arterial baroreceptors in vasopressin regulation during hemorrhage in conscious dogs. Circ Res 68:1422, 1991.
45. Applegate RJ, Hasser EM, Bishop VS: Vagal cold block in area postrema lesioned dogs: Interaction of vasopressin and the sympathetic nervous system. Am J Physiol 252:H135, 1987.
46. Hasser EM, Haywood JR, Johnson AK, et al: The role of vasopressin and the sympathetic nervous system in the cardiovascular response to vagal cold block in the conscious dog. Circ Res 55:454, 1984.
47. DiCarlo SE, Stahl LK, Hasser EM, et al: The role of vasopressin in the pressor response to bilateral carotid occlusion. J Auton Nerv Syst 27:1, 1989.
48. Hasser EM, DiCarlo SE, Applegate RJ, et al: Osmotically released vasopressin augments cardiopulmonary reflex inhibition of the circulation. Am J Physiol 254:R815, 1988.
49. Kirchheim HR, Finke R, Hackenthal E, et al: Baroreflex sympathetic activation increases threshold pressure for the pressure-dependent renin release in conscious dogs. Pflügers Arch 405:127, 1985.
50. Persson P, Ehmke H, Kirchheim H, et al: The influence of cardiopulmonary receptors on long-term blood pressure control and plasma renin activity in conscious dogs. Acta Physiol Scand 130:553, 1987.
51. Shen Y-T, Knight DR, Thomas JX Jr, et al: Relative roles of cardiac receptors and arterial baroreceptors during hemorrhage in conscious dogs. Circ Res 66:397, 1990.
52. Burke SL, Dorward PK: Influence of endogenous opiates and cardiac afferents on renal nerve activity during haemorrhage in conscious rabbits. J Physiol (Lond) 402:9, 1988.
53. Skoog P, Månsson J, Thorén P: Changes in renal sympathetic outflow during hypotensive hemorrhage in rats. Acta Physiol Scand 125:655, 1985.
54. Morgan DA, Thorén P, Wilczynski EA, et al: Serotonergic mechanisms mediate renal sympathoinhibition during severe hemorrhage in rats. Am J Physiol 255:H496, 1988.
55. Victor RG, Thorén P, Morgan DA, et al: Differential control of adrenal and renal sympathetic nerve activity during hemorrhagic hypotension in rats. Circ Res 64:686, 1989.
56. Chen HI, Stinnett HO, Peterson DF, et al: Enhancement of vagal restraint on systemic blood pressure during hemorrhage. Am J Physiol 234:H192, 1978.
57. Öberg B, Thorén P: Increased activity of left ventricular receptors with hemorrhage or occlusion of caval veins in the cat. A possible cause of the vaso-vagal reaction. Acta Physiol Scand 85:164, 1972.
58. Rowell LB: Circulatory adjustments to dynamic exericse. In LB Rowell (ed): Human Circulation Regulation During Physical Stress. New York, NY, Oxford University Press, 1986, p. 213.
59. Mitchell JH: Neural control of the circulation during exercise. Med Sci Sports Exerc 22:141, 1990.
60. Hobbs SF: Central command during exercise: Parallel activation of the cardiovascular and motor systems by descending command signals. In OA Smith, RA Galosy, SM Weiss (eds): Circulation, Neurobiology, and Behavior. New York, NY, Elsevier Science Publishing Co Inc, 1982, p. 217.
61. Alexander N, DeCuir M: Low arterial pressure in awake rabbits without carotid sinus and aortic nerves. Proc Soc Exp Biol Med 121:766, 1966.

62. Cowley AW Jr, Liard J-F, Guyton AC: Role of the baroreceptor reflex in daily control of arterial blood pressure and other variables in dogs. Circ Res 32:564, 1973.
63. Baccelli G, Albertini R, Del Bo A, et al: Role of sinoaortic reflexes in hemodynamic patterns of natural defense behaviors in the cat. Am J Physiol 240:H421, 1981.
64. Ludbrook J, Potocnik SJ: Circulatory changes during spontaneous motor activity: Role of arterial baroreflexes. Am J Physiol 250:H426, 1986.
65. DiCarlo SE, Bishop VS: Onset of exercise shifts the operating point of the arterial baroreflex to higher pressures. Am J Physiol 262:H303–307, 1992.
66. Rowell LB, O'Leary DS: Reflex control of the circulation during exercise: Chemoreflexes and mechanoreflexes. J Appl Physiol 69:407, 1990.
67. Walgenbach SC, Donald DE: Inhibition by carotid baroreflex of exercise-induced increases in arterial pressure. Circ Res 52:253, 1983.
68. Daskalopoulos DA, Shepherd JT, Walgenbach SC: Cardiopulmonary reflexes and blood pressure in exercising sinoaortic-denervated dogs. J Appl Physiol 57:1417, 1984.
69. Scherrer U, Vissing SF, Victor RG: Effects of lower-body negative pressure on sympathetic nerve responses to static exercise in humans. Microneurographic evidence against cardiac baroreflex modulation of the exercise pressor reflex. Circulation 78:49, 1988.
70. Seals DR: Cardiopulmonary baroreflexes do not modulate exercise-induced sympatho-excitation. J Appl Physiol 64:2197, 1988.
71. Walgenbach SC, Donald DE: Cardiopulmonary reflexes and arterial pressure during rest and exercise in dogs. Am J Physiol 244:H362, 1983.
72. Walker JL, Abboud FM, Mark AL, et al: Interaction of cardiopulmonary and somatic reflexes in humans. J Clin Invest 65:1491, 1980.
73. Ludbrook J, Graham WF: Circulatory responses to onset of exercise: Role of arterial and cardiac baroreflexes. Am J Physiol 248:H457, 1985.
74. Mack G, Nose H, Nadel ER: Role of cardiopulmonary baroreflexes during dynamic exercise. J Appl Physiol 65:1827, 1988.
75. Bloomqvist CG, Saltin B: Cardiovascular adaptations to physical training. Ann Rev Physiol 45:169, 1983.
76. Saltin B, Blomqvist G, Mitchell JH, et al: Response to exercise after bed rest and after training. Circulation 38(suppl VII):VII–1, 1968.
77. DiCarlo SE, Bishop VS: Regional vascular resistance during exercise: Role of cardiac afferents and exercise training. Am J Physiol 258:H842, 1990.
78. Thames MD, Abboud FM: Interaction of somatic and cardiopulmonary receptors in control of renal circulation. Am J Physiol 237:H560, 1979.
79. Cornish KG, Gilmore JP, McCulloch T: Central blood volume and blood pressure in conscious primates. Am J Physiol 254:H693, 1988.
80. DiCarlo SE, Bishop VS: Exercise training enhances cardiac afferent inhibition of baroreflex function. Am J Physiol 258:H212, 1990.
81. Stefadouros MA, Grossman W, Schahawy ME, et al: The effect of isometric exercise on the left ventricular volume in normal man. Circulation 49:1185, 1974.
82. Schaper W: Influence of physical exercise on coronary collateral blood flow in chronic experimental two vessel occlusion. Circulation 65:905, 1982.
83. DiCarlo SE, Bishop VS: Exercise training attenuates baroreflex regulation of nerve activity in conscious rabbits. Am J Physiol 255:H974, 1988.
84. Laughlin MH: Skeletal muscle blood flow capacity: Role of muscle pump in exercise hyperemia. Am J Physiol 253:H993, 1987.
85. Higgins CB, Vatner SF, Franklin D, et al: Effects of experimentally produced heart failure on the peripheral vascular response to severe exercise in conscious dogs. Circ Res 31:186, 1972.
86. Vatner SF: Effects of exercise on distribution of regional blood flows and resistances. In R Zebs (ed): The Peripheral Circulations. New York, NY, Grune & Stratton, 1975, p. 211.

87. Musch TI, Haidet GC, Ordway GA, et al: Training effects on regional blood flow response to maximal exercise in foxhounds. J Appl Physiol 62:1724, 1987.
88. Hales JRS, Ludbrook J: Baroreflex participation in redistribution of cardiac output at onset of exercise. J Appl Physiol 64:627, 1988.
89. Hudson DL, Smith ML, Raven PB: Physical fitness and hemodynamic response of women to lower body negative pressure. Med Sci Sports Exer 19:375, 1987.
90. Smith ML, Graitzer HM, Hudson DL, et al: Baroreflex function in endurance- and static exercise-trained men. J Appl Physiol 64:585, 1988.
91. Smith ML, Raven PB: Cardiovascular responses to lower body negative pressure in endurance- and static exercise-trained men. Med Sci Sports Exer 18:545, 1986.
92. Jingu S, Takeshita A, Imaizumi T, et al: Exercise training augments cardiopulmonary baroreflex control of forearm vascular resistance in middle-aged subjects. Jpn Circ J 52:162, 1988.
93. Seals DR, Chase PB: Influence of physical training on heart rate variability and baroreflex circulatory control. J Appl Physiol 66:1886, 1989.
94. Vroman NB, Healy JA, Kertzer R: Cardiovascular response to lower body negative pressure (LBNP) following endurance training. Aviat Space Environ Med 59:330, 1988.
95. Mack GW, Shi X, Nose H, et al: Diminished baroreflex control of forearm vascular resistance in physically fit humans. J Appl Physiol 63:105, 1987.
96. Scheuer J, Tipton CM: Cardiovascular adaptations to physical training. Ann Rev Physiol 39:221, 1977.
97. Mark AL, Mancia G: Cardiopulmonary baroreflexes in humans. In JT Shepherd, FM Abboud (eds): Handbook of Physiology. Section 2: The Cardiovascular System: Peripheral Circulation and Organ Blood Flow, Vol. III, Part 2, Ch. 21. Bethesda, MD, American Physiological Society, 1983, p. 795.
98. Barney JA, Ebert TJ, Groban L, et al: Vagal-cardiac activity and carotid-to-cardiac baroreflex responses in trained and untrained men. Fed Proc 44:818, 1985. Abstract.
99. Bedford TG, Tipton CM: Exercise training and the arterial baroreflex in the rat. J Appl Physiol 63:1926, 1987.
100. Klein KE, Bruner H, Jovy D, et al: Influence of stature and physical fitness on tilt-table and acceleration tolerance. Aerosp Med 40:293, 1969.
101. Stegemann J, Meier U, Skipka W, et al: Effects of a multi-hour immersion with intermittent exercise on urinary excretion and tilt table tolerance in athletes and nonathletes. Aviat Space Environ Med 46:26, 1975.
102. Takeshita A, Jingu S, Imaizumi T, et al: Augmented cardiopulmonary baroreflex control of forearm vascular resistance in young athletes. Circ Res 59:43, 1986.
103. Zoller RP, Mark AL, Abboud FM, et al: The role of low pressure baroreceptors in reflex vasoconstrictor responses in man. J Clin Invest 51:2967, 1972.
104. Kezdi P: Cardiac reflexes conducted by vagal afferents in normotensive and renal hypertensive dogs. Clin Sci 51:353, 1976.
105. Ferrari A, Gordon FJ, Mark AL: Impairment of cardiopulmonary baroreflexes in Dahl salt-sensitive rats fed low salt. Am J Physiol 247:H119, 1984.
106. Thorén P, Noresson E, Ricksten S-E: Resetting of cardiac C-fiber endings in the spontaneously hypertensive rat. Acta Physiol Scand 107:13, 1979.
107. Thames MD: Imparied responses of sympathetic nerves to cardiac receptor stimulation in hypertension. Hypertension 9:478, 1987.
108. Mark AL, Kerber RE: Augmentation of cardiopulmonary baroreflex control of forearm vascular resistance in borderline hypertension. Hypertension 4:39, 1982.
109. Mohanty PK, Thames MD, Sowers JR: Cardiopulmonary baroreflex is preserved in humans with established hypertension. Circulation 74(suppl III, Part III):III–18, 1985.
110. Thorén P: Activation of left ventricular receptors with nonmedullated vagal

afferent fibers during occlusion of the coronary artery in the cat. Am J Cardiol 37:1046, 1976.
111. Hintze TH, Kaley G: Ventricular receptors activated following myocardial prostaglandin synthesis initiate reflex hypotension, reduction in heart rate, and redistribution of cardiac output in the dog. Circ Res 54:239, 1984.
112. Zucker IH, Chen J-S, Wang W: Renal sympathetic nerve and hemodynamic responses to captopril in conscious dogs: Role of prostaglandins. Am J Physiol 260:H260, 1991.

CHAPTER 22

Vagal Afferent Modulation of Cardiac Pain

R.D. Foreman, M.J. Chandler

The role of vagal afferent fibers in cardiopulmonary function has been studied extensively. Activation of vagal afferent fibers can suppress sympathetic efferent activity and decrease hemodynamic responses.[1–5] Several groups of investigators have suggested that activation of vagal afferent fibers may modulate pain.[6–10] Vagal afferent stimulation suppresses responses of conscious animals to noxious somatic stimuli.[11] Experimental evidence shows that pain sensitivity is reduced in hypertensive rats.[12] Vagotomy increases pain sensitivity in these animals. Right cervical vagotomy reverses opioid-mediated analgesia in hot-plate assays of pain sensitivity in spontaneously hypertensive rats, and reduces stress-induced analgesia that results from intermittently shocking the foot of the rat.[8,13] Humans with borderline or essential hypertension have increased sensory and pain thresholds to tooth pulp stimulation,[14–17] which may result from activation of vagal afferent fibers.

Results of electrophysiological studies suggest that vagal afferent fibers may suppress potentially noxious information transmitted in a pain pathway. Studies in rats, cats, and monkeys showed that vagal stimulation reduces responses to noxious stimuli in spinothalamic tract (STT) and spinoreticular tract (SRT) neurons[6,18–21] and in dorsal horn neurons.[22,23] The first observation that the vagus could modulate cardiac afferent input was found serendipitously in our laboratory. An observation that transection of the vagus nerve changed activity of these neurons led to a series of studies that described vagal suppression of cardiopulmonary input (see the section below entitled "Vagal Afferents and the Spinothalamic Tract").[6,7,22]

Vagal suppression of pain sensitivity has gained interest in light of the number of reports about silent ischemia. Although several mechanisms have been proposed,[24] the ability of increased vagal activity to decrease pain sensitivity, increase pain thresholds, and suppress STT cell activity has led to

This work was supported in part by National Heart, Lung and Blood Institute Grant HL-22732 and the Presbyterian Health Foundation.
From *Vagal Control of the Heart: Experimental Basis and Clinical Implications* edited by MN Levy, PJ Schwartz © 1994, Futura Publishing Co. Inc., Armonk, NY.

the suggestion that the vagus may play a role in both asymptomatic myocardial ischemia and in unrecognized myocardial infarction.[7,10,25,26]

The purpose of this chapter is to discuss the role of the vagus in suppressing cardiac pain. The first section of the chapter discusses how the vagus modulates cardiac spinal afferent input to STT cells. The next section describes the central integration of vagal afferent input that modulates STT cell activity. The last section discusses neural mechanisms that may be involved in silent ischemia.

Vagal Modulation of Cardiac Spinal Afferent Input to Spinothalamic Tract Cells

Vagal Afferent Fibers

Myelinated and unmyelinated vagal afferent fibers transmit impulses from the heart to the brain stem. Myelinated fibers arise primarily from receptors located in the atria and venoatrial junction.[27–29] Fewer myelinated fibers originate from receptors located in the ventricles and coronary arteries.[30,31] In contrast, sensory endings of unmyelinated fibers are located in all chambers of the heart.[29,30,32–35] Although these kinds of studies provide information regarding the distribution of afferent fibers, they do not give an accurate picture about the density of afferents originating from receptors in different regions of the heart.

Unmyelinated fibers are a heterogeneous group that are separated primarily into fibers with chemosensitive or mechanosensitive endings. Chemosensitive endings do not appear to discharge with a cardiac rhythm[36] and are unresponsive to all but extreme vascular distensions.[36] These vagal receptors increase their discharge rate when the endogenous, potentially algesic chemical, bradykinin, is injected into the left atrium (Fig. 1A) or is applied to the surface of the heart (Fig. 1B).[36] Prostaglandin PGE_2 markedly increases activity of vagal afferents that fire irregularly and are relatively insensitive to increased ventricular pressure. Exogenous chemicals, such as capsaicin, phenylbiguanide, nicotine, and veratrum alkaloids, also excite these afferents.[32]

Mechanosensitive endings commonly display a more regular discharge pattern in control conditions, with one or two impulses occurring with each cardiac cycle.[32,35] Increased ventricular volume produced during venous infusion or aortic occlusion generates increased activity with a rhythmic discharge pattern in these endings.[35] Nicotine and veratrum alkaloids activate many of these afferents.[34,37] In contrast to chemosensitive endings, however, capsaicin, phenylbiguanide, bradykinin, and prostaglandins do not stimulate mechanosensitive endings.[32,36]

Myocardial ischemia excites unmyelinated vagal afferent fibers.[38] Recordings from single functional filaments of vagal afferent fibers have been made during occlusion of the coronary vessel supplying the myocardial region where sensory endings of the fiber are located. Generally, the latency of onset of

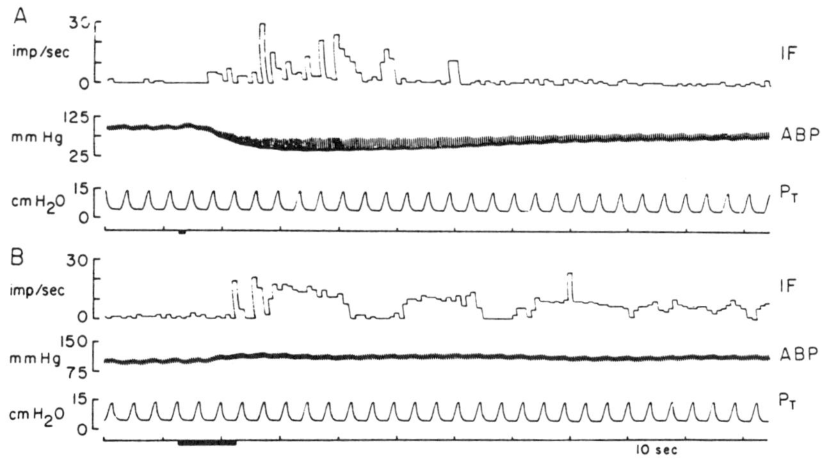

Figure 1. *Bradykinin activation of a chemosensitive C-fiber. The fiber ending is in the ventrolateral wall of the left ventricle near the epicardial surface. In panel A, bradykinin (0.5 μg/kg) is injected into the left atrium at the mark on the time trace. After an interval of 30 min between panels A and B, 1 ml of bradykinin (1 μg/ml) is dripped on the epicardium of the left ventricle during the signal on the time marker. IF: impulse frequency (impulses/s); ABP: arterial blood pressure recorded in the aortic arch; P_T: tracheal pressure with upstroke representing inflation. Reproduced by permission of the American Heart Association, Inc. from Kaufman MP, Baker DG, Coleridge HM, et al: Stimulation by bradykinin of afferent vagal C-fibers with chemosensitive endings in the heart and aorta of the dog. Circ Res 46:481, 1980.*

myocardial bulging and changes in the ST segment occur before activity increases in afferent fibers. The initial increase in receptor activity usually is correlated with cardiac rhythm, but becomes continuous as the occlusion is maintained. These afferents appear to have been selected for their mechanosensitivity. Therefore, responses of afferents with chemosensitive endings have not been studied. In summary, both chemosensitive and mechanosensitive afferents most likely increase their discharge rate during coronary artery occlusion. The assumption that chemosensitive afferents are excited by ischemia, however, is based on the observation that chemicals released during this occurrence excite them. Actual experiments to test this theory have not been done.

The Spinothalamic Tract

Before the role of vagal afferents in antinociception is discussed in detail, a summary of studies of the role of the STT in angina pectoris is presented. The STT is the classical pain pathway that transmits information about noxious somatic and visceral episodes to the thalamus and then to areas of the cortex that are involved with pain perception.[39] Therefore, the study of STT cells is essential in determining if noxious information arising from the heart is transmitted to areas involved with nociception. Most of these studies have been carried out in primates because they have a well-developed STT system and a heart that is large enough to perform cardiac experiments. Although electrical recordings are made from STT neurons in anesthetized animals, responses do not differ substantially from cell recordings made in conscious monkeys.[40,41] In addition, nociception and behavior related to noxious stimuli are correlated in several studies of humans and monkeys.[42–46] Thus, studying electrical activity of STT cells in anesthetized monkeys provides important information about nociception that can be related to humans.

In anesthetized animals, extracellular action potentials of STT cells are identified by stimulating the STT cell axons that project to the ventropostero-lateral nucleus and the medial nuclei of the thalamus (Fig. 2).[47] The ventropos-terolateral nucleus and possibly the posterior thalamus may play a role in sensory discrimination because projections from these regions terminate pri-

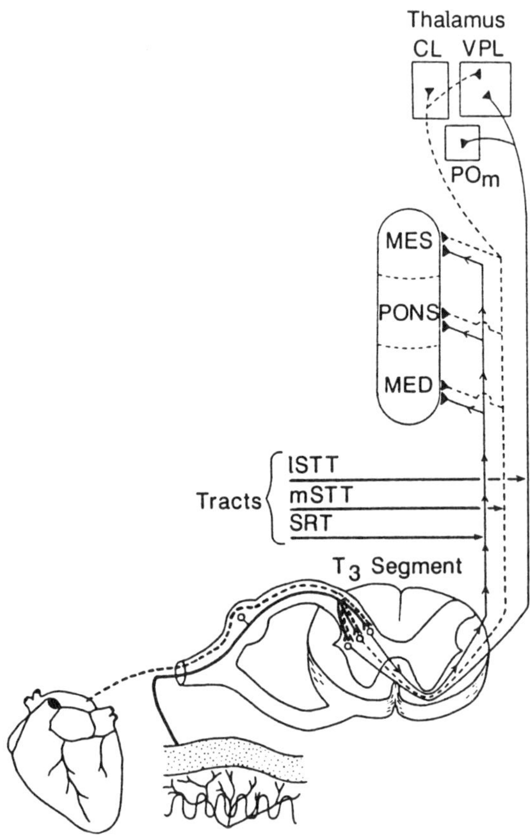

Figure 2. *Schematic diagram illustrating the nociceptive pathways in the spinal cord that project to the brain stem and thalamus. Afferent information arising from the heart (dashed line) and somatic structures (solid line) converge directly or indirectly on cells of origin of the spinothalamic tract (STT). lSTT: lateral STT; mSTT: medial STT; SRT: spinoreticular tract; MES: mesencephalon; MED: medulla; CL: centralis lateralis nucleus of the medial thalamus; VPL: ventroposterolateral nucleus of the thalamus;* PO_M*: medial portion of the posterior thalamus.*

marily in the primary somatosensory cortex. The medial thalamus appears to be involved in the motivational-affective behavior that often is associated with pain because its projections end in the cingulate gyrus and association regions of the cortex.[48–50] Although the SRT is not discussed extensively in this chapter, it can transmit visceral and somatic information into the brain stem reticular formation. The SRT also is involved in aversive drive and pain-related behavior.[51–54] STT cells in the upper thoracic segments of the spinal cord are excited by myelinated and unmyelinated sympathetic afferent fibers arising from the cardiopulmonary region.[47,55,56] Approximately half the population of STT cells is excited by both myelinated and unmyelinated afferent fibers that are activated electrically by stimulation across the left stellate ganglion, but the other half is excited only by myelinated fibers. Most STT cells receive both visceral and somatic input.

Angina pectoris often is perceived as deep, aching pain that is referred to overlying somatic structures. Our experimental studies provide a neurophysiological basis for this clinical observation. STT cells that are excited by sympathetic afferent input have somatic receptive fields in proximal structures that are excited predominately by noxious muscle pinch.[57] In contrast, STT cells with distal somatic receptive fields in the hand and lower forearm receive very little sympathetic afferent input and respond primarily to noxious cutaneous stimulation. Since deep, aching pain sensations usually originate from muscle,[58] the characteristic pain of angina pectoris may occur because STT cells receiving primarily muscle and visceral input produce a unique pattern of activity that is interpreted as deep, aching pain. The somatic receptive fields of STT cells that receive convergent sympathetic afferent input usually are restricted to the ipsilateral chest and forelimb and do not cross the midline (Fig. 3A).[47] A population of cells that project to the medial thalamus, however, often have receptive fields that are bilateral or are large and unilateral (Fig. 3B). Thus, most somatic fields are found in the proximal dermatomes overlying the heart. The location of these fields is similar to the areas of pain referral that are experienced by patients with angina pectoris.[59–65] These findings support and extend the convergence-projection theory of Ruch,[66] who proposed that nociceptive somatic and visceral afferents converge on the same neuron at some point in the sensory pathway to produce referred pain associated with visceral organs.

Anginal pain referred to somatic structures most likely occurs when chemosensitive and mechanosensitive cardiac receptors of sympathetic afferents are excited during ischemic episodes. It is important to examine the effects of natural stimulation of cardiac receptors to understand how STT cells respond to activation of sympathetic afferent fibers during ischemic episodes associated with coronary artery occlusion. Coronary artery occlusion activates STT cells during ischemic events in one of at least four different patterns.[67] These patterns include STT cells whose activity

1. increases during the ischemic phase of the coronary artery occlusion;
2. increases at the onset of occlusion, adapts, and then increases again as ischemic symptoms develop;

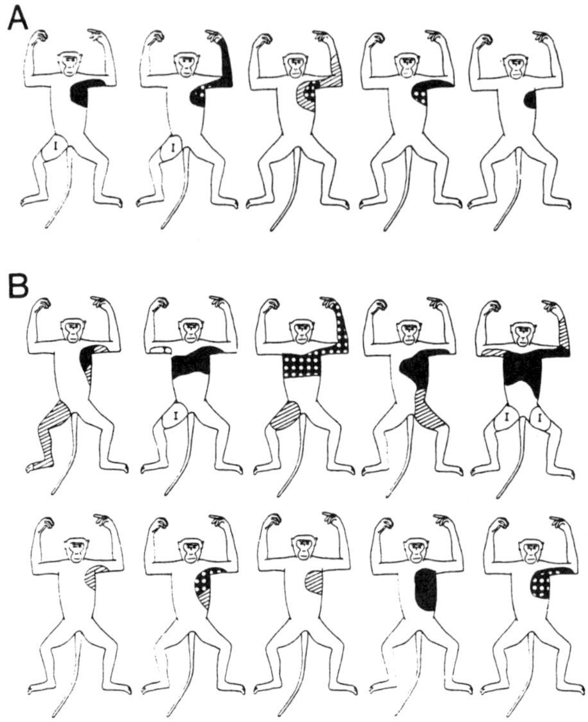

Figure 3. *Locations of somatic receptive fields of STT cells in the T_2–T_5 segments of the spinal cord that project to the ventroposterolateral nucleus of the thalamus (lateral spinothalamic tract) (A) and to the medial thalamus (medial spinothalamic tract) (B). Black areas: input from skin and muscle; white dots: excitatory hair field overlaying skin and muscle field; striped area: response to muscle only; white triangles: inhibitory input caused by hair movement; I: inhibitory receptive field from skin or muscle. Reproduced with permission from Cervero F, Foreman RD: Sensory innervation of the viscera. In AD Loewy, KM Spyer (eds): Central Regulation of Autonomic Functions. New York, NY, Oxford University Press, 1990, p. 116.*

3. increases rapidly at the onset or the release of the occlusion and adapts or remains elevated throughout the occlusion; and
4. does not change during the occlusion period.

Cells that respond immediately to coronary artery occlusion (patterns two and three) are most likely responding to mechanical changes caused by the occlusion. The coronary artery is occluded by a suture that is passed around the artery and is pulled through a plastic tube. This response is considered innocuous. For cells that respond during the ischemic phase, activity usually increases approximately 13 seconds after the onset of the occlusion. Increased activity often is associated with changes in the electrocardiogram and with falls in systemic blood pressure, left ventricular pressure, and contractility. Activity of STT cells during the ischemic episode is more likely to increase if cells are excited by A-δ and C sympathetic afferent fibers than if cells are excited only by A-δ sympathetic afferent fibers. These observations lead to the suggestion that C-fibers are important for an STT cell response to myocardial ischemia.

Injection of noxious chemicals into the coronary circulation provides another method for activating receptors of the heart that increase the discharge rate of sympathetic afferent fibers. Bradykinin has been used in STT studies to activate cardiac receptors. Bradykinin produces pain in animals and humans,[68,69] strongly activates muscle afferent fibers,[70] and is found in increased amounts in the effluent of the coronary sinus following coronary artery occlusion.[71] Bradykinin injected into the left atrium of the heart increases activity in approximately 75% of upper thoracic STT cells approximately 15 seconds after bradykinin is injected.[56,72] Control experiments demonstrate that receptors of the heart are activated because bradykinin enters the coronary circulation.[72] The latency of onset of cell excitation correlates closely with the response time necessary for bradykinin to increase activity of single unit recordings from sympathetic afferent fibers.[73]

Bradykinin is not the only chemical that can activate STT cells during ischemia of the myocardium. It is possible that prostaglandins may be a necessary intermediary step to activate receptors and thus increase the discharge rate of STT cells.[74,75] This intermediate step might explain the long latency before bradykinin increases discharge rate of cells. Adenosine may be another chemical that produces pain during myocardial ischemia.[76,77] Further studies using chemicals or combinations of chemicals that are involved in the ischemic response need to be done to determine the chemical mediators that are necessary in the production of angina pectoris. Nevertheless, it is evident that angina pectoris can result from chemicals that are released during ischemic episodes and excite cardiac receptors of the afferent fibers.

Vagal Afferents and the Spinothalamic Tract Cells

The ability of vagal stimulation to inhibit cardiovascular responses and the effects of noxious stimulation suggest the possibility that vagal stimulation also inhibits STT cells excited by input from sympathetic afferents whose receptors are located in the heart. As described in the previous section, intracardiac injections of bradykinin strongly excite STT cells located in upper thoracic segments of the spinal cord. Stimulation of the left thoracic vagus markedly inhibits STT cell activity following bradykinin injection (Fig. 4A). Transection of the cervical vagi abolishes suppression of STT cell activity during stimulation of the left thoracic vagus (Fig. 4B). These results support the hypothesis that activation of afferent fibers traveling in the vagus can suppress potentially noxious sympathetic cardiac afferent input that activates STT cells in upper thoracic segments.

The concept that activation of vagal afferents inhibits activity of STT cells so as to suppress responses to noxious somatic stimuli was tested by applying a noxious pinch to the somatic receptive field that excites the STT cell being studied (Fig. 5A). During the noxious stimulus, electrical stimulation of the

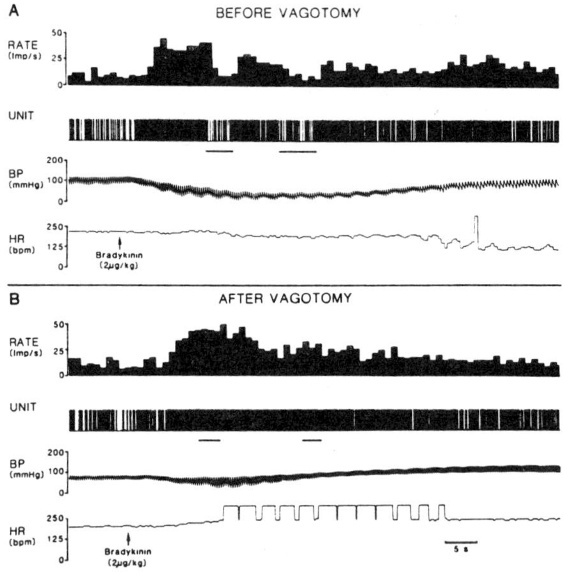

Figure 4. *Electrical stimulation of left thoracic vagus reduces STT cell activity that results from a potentially noxious visceral stimulus. Each panel shows the response of the same STT cell to an intracardiac injection of bradykinin before (A) and after (B) bilateral cervical vagotomy. Stimulation of the vagus (6.9 V, 2 msec, 20 Hz) occurs during period shown by bars below second trace in each panel. Tracings in each panel from top to bottom are rate of cell discharge (Rate), output of the window discriminator where each deflection represents one extracellular action potential (Unit), blood pressure (BP), and heart rate (HR). Reproduced by permission of the American Heart Association, Inc. from Ammons WS, Blair RW, Foreman RD: Vagal afferent inhibition of spinothalamic cell responses to sympathetic afferents and bradykinin in the monkey. Circ Res 53:607, 1983.*

left thoracic vagus markedly suppresses STT cell activity. Vagal stimulation significantly reduces the activity of the population of upper thoracic STT cells analyzed in this study (Fig. 5B). The ability of vagal activity to suppress somatic input to the STT may provide one explanation for the higher threshold of pain in patients with silent ischemia, as discussed in the section below entitled "Vagal Afferents and Silent Ischemia."

Is suppression of cell activity by vagal afferents specifically targeted for STT cells in the thoracic spinal cord or is there a generalized suppression of cells in all segments of the spinal cord? Studies showed that spontaneous and evoked activities of STT cells at the lower cervical,[20] thoracic,[6,20] and lumbosacral[19] segments of the spinal cord were suppressed (Fig. 6). Similar findings also were observed in lumbosacral spinal neurons and STT cells of the rat.[21,23] We also found that vagal stimulation suppressed evoked activity arising from other visceral organs, such as the urinary bladder.[78] Thus, we conclude that vagal afferent stimulation causes a general inhibitory effect at most levels of the spinal cord on neurons that transmit nociceptive information to the thalamus and then to areas involved with pain perception.

Does this suppression of STT cell activity originate from vagal afferents of

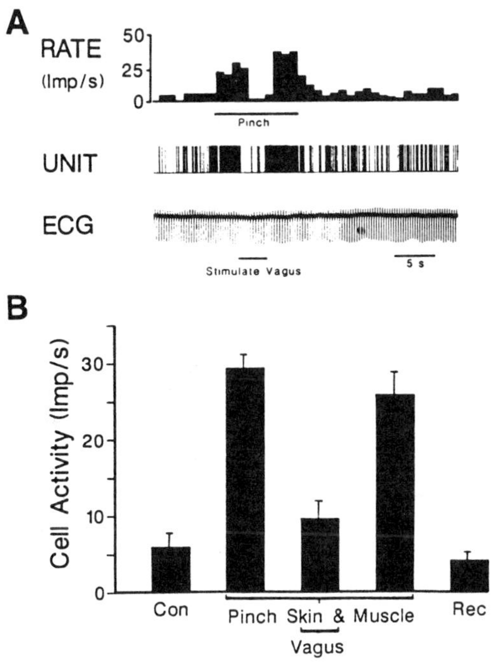

Figure 5. *Vagal stimulation suppresses activity of STT cells that are increased when a noxious pinch is applied to the somatic receptive field. In panel A, line below top trace indicates skin over the left chest is pinched. Line below the ECG represents period of thoracic vagal stimulation. Graph of panel B shows effects of vagal stimulation while recording responses of 21 STT cells to noxious somatic pinch of skin or skin and muscle. Solid bar under pinch skin and muscle shows response of cells to a maintained pinch. During this maintained pinch, the vagus was stimulated. Second and fourth bars represent cell activity just before and after the vagal stimulation occurs. Con: control activity just before any stimulus was applied; Rec: cell activity after the stimulus period ended.*

the cardiopulmonary region? This issue is addressed in two ways. First, electrical stimulation of the thoracic vagus or cervical vagus suppresses activity of primate STT cells in the thoracic and lumbosacral region. Stimulation of the vagus between the heart and diaphragm, however, does not produce significant inhibition (Fig. 7).[6,19] This observation suggests that inhibition is produced by afferent fibers arising from the cardiopulmonary region. Second, the effect of left thoracic vagal stimulation is compared to stimulation of the cardiac branch of the vagus.[7] Electrical stimulation of the cardiac branch of the vagus reduces the discharge rate of STT cells similar to the inhibition observed for thoracic vagal stimulation. Thus, these results support the idea that vagal afferent fibers from the cardiopulmonary region and probably from the heart are critical for producing suppression of STT cell activity.

Although our studies show that stimulation of the abdominal vagus does not affect spontaneous or evoked activity of STT cells, these results do not agree with findings that have been reported in the rat.[79] In rats, electrical

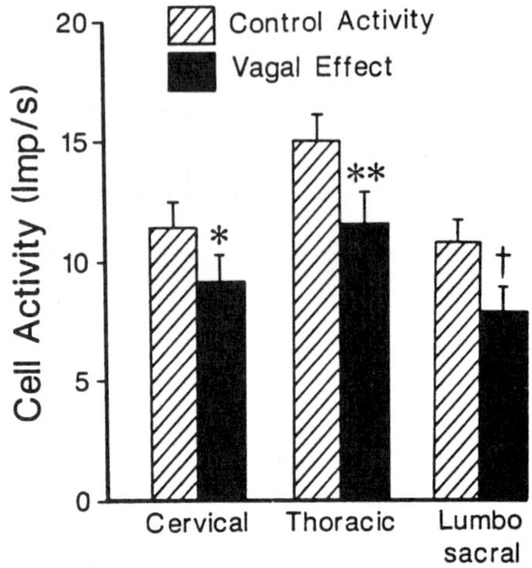

Figure 6. *Comparison of effects of electrical stimulation of the vagus above the heart on the spontaneous activity of STT cells in the cervical, thoracic, and lumbosacral segments. Control activity is measured just before the vagus is stimulated. Solid bars show average activity in all cells during vagal stimulation. Cells that increased, decreased, or did not change activity were included in this analysis. (Paired t test; *, $P<0.005$; **, $P<0.002$; †P, <0.001.)*

stimulation of abdominal vagal afferent fibers inhibits the tail-flick reflex. There is a possibility that there may be a difference in the species studied, the anesthetic used, or the parameters measured.

The predominant effect of electrical stimulation of thoracic vagal afferent fibers is inhibition of STT cell activity. Approximately 60% of STT cells are suppressed during left thoracic vagal stimulation.[6] Approximately 10% of the cells studied, however, are excited or are excited and then inhibited. The remainder of the cells do not respond to vagal stimulation. When responses of all cells tested for vagal stimulation are compared to spontaneous activity (control), vagal stimulation significantly decreases overall cell activity. These observations differ somewhat from observations made in rats,[21,23] in which a larger percentage of STT cells and spinal neurons were facilitated during cervical vagal stimulation. These studies reported that low intensities of stimulation during a noxious stimulus facilitated the activity of approximately 25% of the cells, and that higher stimulus intensities inhibited the noxious responses.[21,23] We routinely have not stimulated at lower stimulus intensities; therefore, it is possible that we may have missed this facilitatory response. There also is a possibility that stimulation of the cervical vagus may activate nonvagal fibers that produce facilitation.[9] We also have noted occasionally that left thoracic vagal stimulation after cervical vagotomy has excited an STT cell that was inhibited before vagotomy. This observation raises the possibility that facilitation might be elicited from pathways other than the vagus nerve. In summary, we believe the predominant effect of vagal stimulation is suppression of somatic and cardiac input to STT cells, which provides a mechanism for increasing pain threshold and decreasing pain sensitivity.

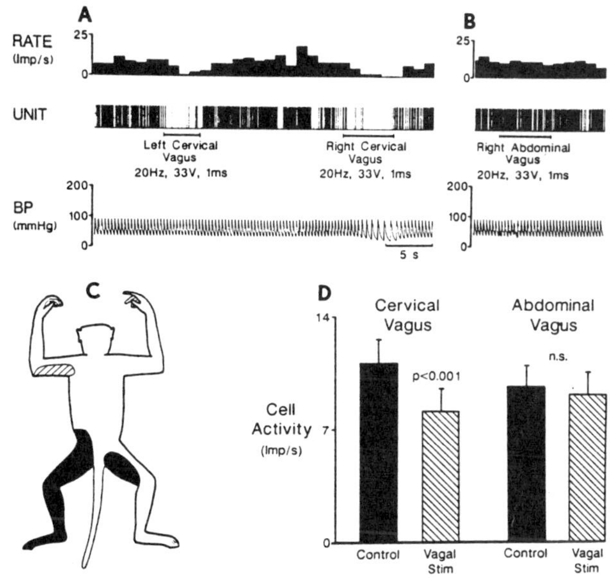

Figure 7. *Effects of stimulation of the cervical vagus above the heart and of abdominal vagal afferent fibers below the heart on the activity of STT cells in the lumbosacral spinal cord. The cervical vagus contains both the thoracic and abdominal afferents. A: Effects of electrically stimulating right and left cervical vagus. B: Effect of electrically stimulating right abdominal vagus. In A and B, top trace shows rate of cell discharge in impulses per second (imp/s) averaged over 1 s; middle trace shows deflection (Unit) from window discriminator each time the STT cell discharges. Top trace is delayed 1 s compared with unit trace. Bottom trace shows arterial blood pressure (BP). C: Somatic receptive field for this neuron. Pinch of black areas excites cell; pinch of the striped area inhibits cell. D: Summary of effects of electrical stimulation of cervical and abdominal vagal afferent fibers. Solid bars, average activity in all STT cells tested before vagal stimulation (control); striped bars, average activity of STT cells during vagal stimulation. Cervical vagus significantly reduces STT activity. In contrast, abdominal vagal afferent stimulation does not significantly affect activity. Cells that increase, decrease, or do not change their spontaneous activity are included in the analysis. Reproduced with permission from Hobbs SF, Oh UT, Chandler MJ, et al: Cardiac and abdominal vagal afferent inhibition of primate T9–S1 spinothalamic cells. Am J Physiol 257:R891, 1989.*

Central Integration and Descending Pathways

This section discusses possible supraspinal pathways that may be involved in suppression of STT cell activity by vagal stimulation. Based on anatomical, behavioral, and physiological evidence, we propose that the parabrachial subcoeruleus/locus coeruleus region of the pons may be one of the important relays for producing vagal suppression of STT cells.

Cell bodies of vagal afferent fibers are located primarily in the nodose ganglion. Most of the axons of these cell bodies terminate in the nucleus tractus solitarius (NTS) of the medulla,[80] but the heaviest site of termination is found in the caudal end of this nucleus (Fig. 8A). Physiological evidence in the rat suggests that vagal suppression of activity of spinal neurons is transmitted

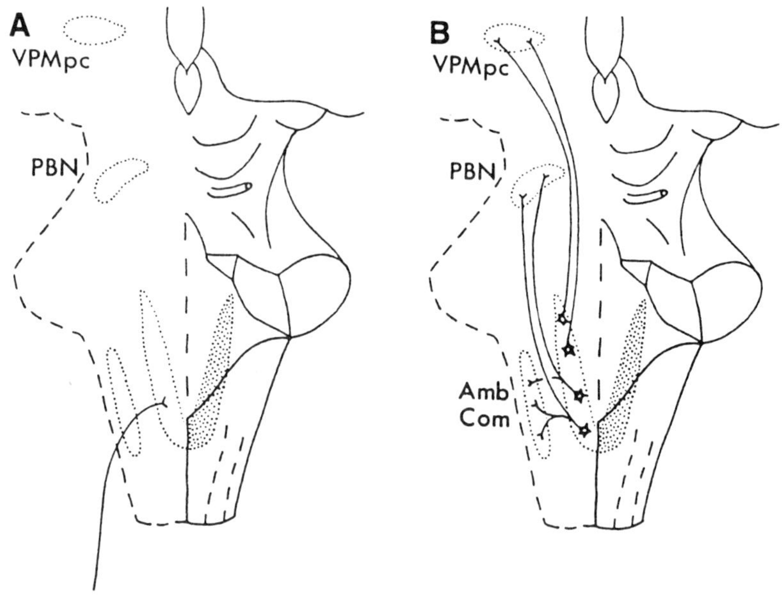

Figure 8. *Schematic diagram of the dorsal view of a monkey's brain stem. Panel A shows a composite of vagal afferent fibers entering brain stem and terminating primarily in the caudal aspect of the NTS. Panel B shows representative cell bodies that project from the NTS to the parabrachial nuclei and other brain regions. Amb Com: ambiguous complex; PBN: parabrachial nuclei; VPMpc: paracellular region of the ventroposteromedial nucleus of the thalamus. Modified with permission from Beckstead RM, Morse JR, Norgren R: The nucleus of the solitary tract in the monkey: Projections to the thalamus and brainstem nuclei. J Comp Neur 190:276, 1980.*

through the NTS.[81] A significant number of afferent fibers also cross over to the contralateral NTS.

Anatomical studies in the monkey show that, in the caudal part of the NTS, neurons send a major projection of fibers to the medial and lateral parabrachial nuclei (Fig. 8B).[82] A population of cells that compose the subcoeruleus-parabrachial (SC-PB) region then sends axons to the spinal cord.[83–86] Thus, the anatomical substrate for carrying information from the vagus to the SC-PB region and then to STT cells is present.

Behavorial and pharmacological studies support the possibility that the SC-PB is important for modulation of nociceptive transmission in the spinal cord. Electrolytic destruction of the medial parabrachial nucleus does not alter basal nociceptor thresholds, but does attenuate morphine analgesia as assessed by tail-flick or hot-plate tests.[87] In addition, microinjections of the muscarinic antagonist carbachol in an area dorsal or ventral to the brachium conjunctivum in the vicinity of the SC-PB region markedly suppresses nociceptive responses.[88,89]

Electrophysiological studies also support the notion that the SC-PB region is important for producing antinociception during vagal afferent stimulation.

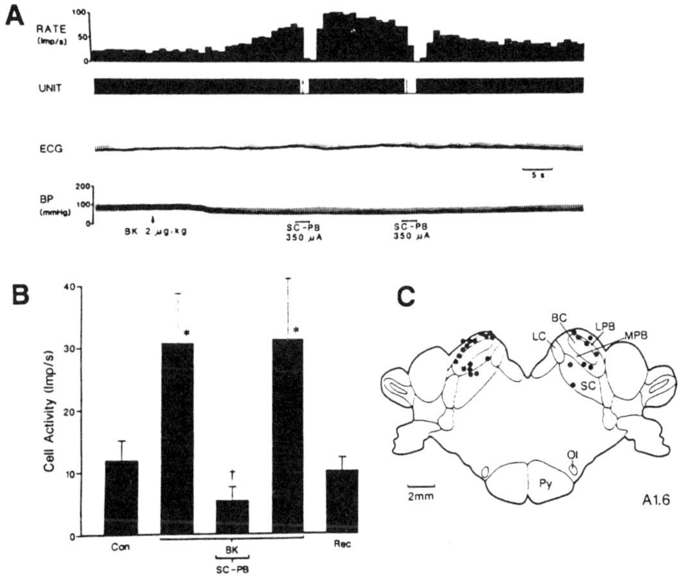

Figure 9. *Electrical stimulation of the subcoeruleus parabrachial (SC-PB) region suppresses activity of STT cells. In panel A, electrical stimulation of this region reduces activity of a STT cell that increased its discharge rate in response to an intracardiac injection of bradykinin (BK). Panel B is a graph showing a summary of STT cells (n = 8) to BK injections and SC-PB stimulation. Line under the second to fourth bar indicates that responses to BK are maintained during this period. After cell activity has increased its activity, the effects of SC-PB stimulation is shown (second line under third bar). Increased cell activity caused by BK is significantly greater than control (*, P<0.05). SC-PB stimulation significantly reduces cell activity below BK values (+, P<0.05 versus BK). Panel C shows stimulation sites marked by black dots of one brain stem section. The left side is ipsilateral to recorded STT cells. BC: brachium conjunctivum; LPB: lateral parabrachial nucleus; MPB: medial parabrachial nucleus; SC: nucleus subcoeruleus; LC: nucleus locus coeruleus; Py: pyramid; OI: inferior olivary nucleus. Modified with permission from Brennan TJ, Oh UT, Giradot M-N, et al: Inhibition of cardiopulmonary input to thoracic spinothalamic tract cells by stimulation of the subcoeruleus-parabrachial region in the primate. J Autonom Nerv Sys 18:66, 1987.*

Electrical stimulation of ipsilateral and contralateral sites in the SC-PB region suppresses the increased STT cell activity following intracardiac injections of bradykinin (Fig. 9)[90] and during noxious stimulation of the somatic receptive fields.[91] Furthermore, bilateral injection of ibotenic acid, a selective neurotoxin for cell bodies, into the locus coeruleus/subcoeruleus region significantly attenuates the suppression of nociceptive spinal activity when the vagus is stimulated in the rat (Fig. 10).[81] These studies suggest that neurons in the locus coeruleus, subcoeruleus, and parabrachial region may be important for descending modulation of pain when the vagal afferents are excited.

Other nuclei that may be involved in suppression of cell activity during vagal stimulation include the nucleus raphe magnus and rostral ventrolateral medulla.[81,92–95] These studies are not discussed here because the anatomical connections between vagal afferents and descending inhibitory pathways from

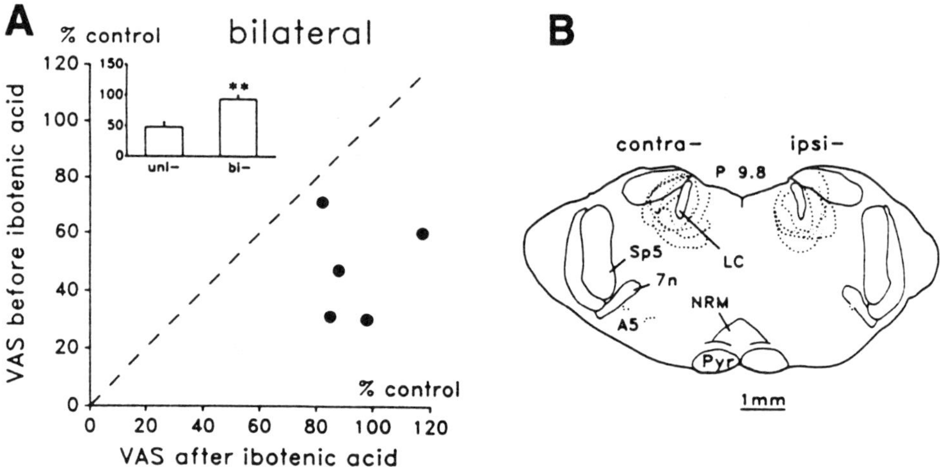

Figure 10. *Effects of disrupting cell activity in the dorsolateral pons with microinjections of ibotenic acid on responses of spinal neurons to electrical stimulation of the vagus nerve. Panel A shows effects of vagal stimulation at the same intensity on spinal neurons that responded to heating of the skin before and after ibotenic acid is microinjected bilaterally into the dorsolateral pons. The x and y axes are expressed as a percentage of the control response to heating, total number of impulses in 22 s. Inset in A illustrates mean data after unilateral and bilateral microinjections of ibotenic acid. Dotted lines in panel B show extent of lesions produced by ibotenic acid. A5: cell group; contra-: contralateral to spinal recording site; P 9.8: brain stem section 9.8 mm posterior to the bregma in the rat; LC: locus coeruleus; ipsi-: ipsilateral to spinal recording site; NRM: nucleus raphe magnus; Pyr: pyramidal tract; 7n: facial nerve; Sp5: spinal trigeminal nucleus. Reproduced with permission from Ren K, Randich A, Gebhart GF: Electrical stimulation of cervical vagal afferents. I. Central relays for modulation of spinal nociceptive transmission. J Neurophysiol 64:1104, 1990.*

these nuclei have not been defined. Additional central areas may be identified as research continues to define the neural mechanisms underlying vagal suppression of spinal neuronal activity.

Vagal Afferents and Silent Ischemia

Clinical Description

Silent myocardial ischemia is a transient imbalance in myocardial oxygen supply and demand that results in a sequence of metabolic, mechanical, hemodynamic, and electrocardiographic events that can be documented objectively.[24] This sequence of events occurs in the absence of chest pain or the usual angina equivalents such as arm or jaw pain and numbness. Patients are classified as symptomatic if they experience angina pectoris during myocardial ischemia and classified as asymptomatic if they have episodes of ischemia without the associated pain. Cohn[96] has classified silent myocardial ischemia into three types: type I is the condition that may occur in patients who are asymptomatic and have no history of myocardial infarction or angina pectoris; type II is found in asymptomatic patients who have had myocardial infarction; and type III is found in patients who experience angina pectoris but who also experience episodes of silent myocardial ischemia. Detection, prevalence, and prognosis of silent myocardial ischemia varies according to patient type. Approximately 60% to 80% of all ischemic events are asymptomatic.[24] At times, ischemic events are prolonged and may last up to 40 minutes. Silent myocardial ischemia generally is not associated with physical activity or increased myocardial oxygen demand. This ischemia has independent prognostic significance and may persist despite the absence of angina pectoris.[24]

Clinical Correlations of Vagal Afferents and Silent Ischemia

At least three separate theories have been proposed to explain why angina pectoris is not expressed during episodes of significant myocardial ischemia.[24] The three theories are: global deficiency in pain perception; anatomical changes in pain receptors and nerves; and quantitative theory of silent myocardial ischemia, which suggests that myocardial ischemia is quantitatively less when it is associated with silent ischemia than when it is associated with angina pectoris. Although all three theories may explain silent myocardial ischemia, the mechanisms related to global deficiency in pain perception are addressed in this section.

Myocardial ischemia activates both sympathetic and vagal afferent fibers. An imbalance in the activity of these afferent fibers may lead to angina pectoris or silent ischemia, depending on the afferent fibers that are stimulated more intensely. This imbalance may occur because sympathetic and vagal afferent fibers have different densities of receptors in different regions of the heart. Vagal afferents are more pronounced in the inferior-posterior wall of the left ventricle.[97,98] This idea is supported by hemodynamic studies that show that myocardial infarction of the inferior wall of the ventricle often results in bradycardia and hypotension, responses that usually are associated with activation of vagal reflexes.[99,100] In contrast, anterior myocardial infarction results more often in tachycardia and hypertension, responses that often are associated with activation of sympathetic reflexes.[99,100] Experimental occlusion of the left circumflex artery more effectively evokes vagal reflexes than does occlusion of the left anterior descending artery.[101] Since activation of sympathetic afferent fibers significantly increases activity of the STT cells and activation of vagal afferents can suppress this activity, the distribution of vagal and sympathetic afferent fibers to the heart may provide a possible neural basis for episodes of angina pectoris or silent myocardial ischemia.

Preferential distribution of vagal afferent fibers and vagal reflexes to the inferior-posterior regions of the left ventricle raises the possibility that patients who experience ischemia in the inferior-posterior regions of the left ventricle are more likely to have silent myocardial ischemia. Blood supply to this region of the heart originates from the right coronary artery and from the left circumflex coronary artery. The location of coronary stenosis and left ventricular wall motion abnormalities have been compared in two groups of patients with one-vessel disease to determine if the site of an ischemic event is related to ischemic pain perception.[102] Both groups of patients exhibit reproducible objective signs of myocardial ischemia when they perform exercise tests, but one group of patients experiences angina pectoris and another group has silent myocardial ischemia (i.e., asymptomatic). Abnormalities in left ventricular wall movement localized to the posterobasal or diaphragmatic regions are related significantly to patients with silent myocardial ischemia (Fig. 11). Thus, asymptomatic patients more frequently have right coronary artery stenosis or left circumflex stenosis, whereas patients who experience angina pectoris more often have stenosis of the left anterior descending artery.

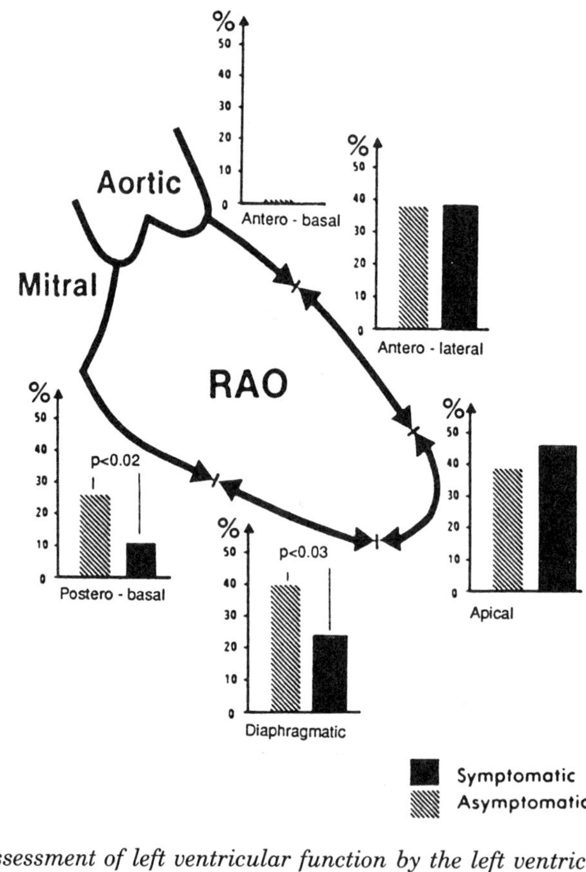

Figure 11. *Assessment of left ventricular function by the left ventriculogram in right anterior oblique (RAO) projections in patients with silent myocardial ischemia and symptomatic myocardial ischemia. Circumference of the left ventricle was divided into five segments. Graphs represent frequency (in percent) of abnormal wall motion in different segments in patients with silent myocardial ischemia (hatched bars) and with angina pectoris (solid bars). Modified with permission from Droste C, Greenlee MW, Ruf G, et al: Localization of a coronary stenosis, left ventricular function, and pain perception during myocardial ischemia in patients with one-vessel disease. J Cardiovasc Electrophysiol 2:S68, 1991.*

Based on these findings, it is proposed that myocardial ischemia localized in the inferior-posterior region of the heart tends to be asymptomatic because vagal afferent fibers are activated preferentially.[102] Our findings that vagal stimulation suppresses STT cell activity that is increased during excitation of sympathetic afferents from the heart support these observations.

A general inability to perceive somatic pain also may explain why patients are asymptomatic during episodes of myocardial ischemia. Somatic pain perception has been studied in patients with angina pectoris and with silent myocardial ischemia. Both groups exhibit significant ST segment depression during exercise stress testing.[25,77,103–106] Altered pain perception most likely is not due to destruction of specific myocardial nociceptive pathways because frequency of prior infarction, extent of multivessel coronary disease, and diseases such as diabetes and alcoholism that alter nociceptive capabilities are similar for both groups of patients. Different types of nociceptive modalities including electric shock, cold pressor stimulation, and tourniquet-induced forearm ischemia reveal that patients with silent myocardial ischemia experience a higher pain threshold and greater tolerance for these types of somatic pain than those with angina pectoris (Fig. 12). Our finding that the vagus

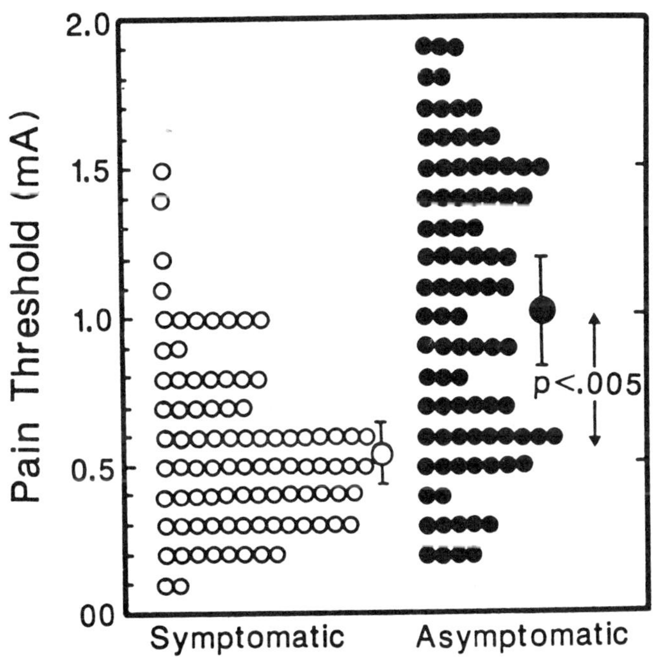

Figure 12. *Effects of electrical pain test on pain threshold in patients symptomatic and asymptomatic for pain associated with myocardial ischemia. Mean values + 1 SE and distribution of individual values on electrical pain test. Symptomatic patients (open circles) have a mean pain threshold of 0.55 mA. In contrast, asymptomatic patients have a significantly higher mean pain threshold of 1.0 mA. Reproduced with permission from Droste C, Greenlee MW, Roskamm H: A defective angina pectoris pain warning system: Experimental findings of ischemic and electrical pain test. Pain 26:199, 1986.*

suppresses activity arising from somatic structures supports the possibility that increased vagal activity may lead to higher pain thresholds and greater pain tolerance. Since asymptomatic patients can demonstrate decreased pain sensitivity even when there is no myocardial ischemic episode, tonic vagal activity may generally suppress STT cell activity. This aspect of the puzzle has not been clarified experimentally.

Conceptual Description of Physiological and Clinical Mechanisms

Based on physiological and clinical studies, we propose a concept to describe how vagal afferents may play a role in patients who experience silent myocardial ischemia. This section summarizes information described in the previous sections. Figure 13 enhances this description. Myocardial ischemia of the inferior-posterior wall of the left ventricle predominately activates mechanosensitive and chemosensitive receptors of vagal afferents. At the same time, sympathetic afferent fibers from this region are also excited. Action potentials in vagal afferent fibers are transmitted through the nodose ganglion to

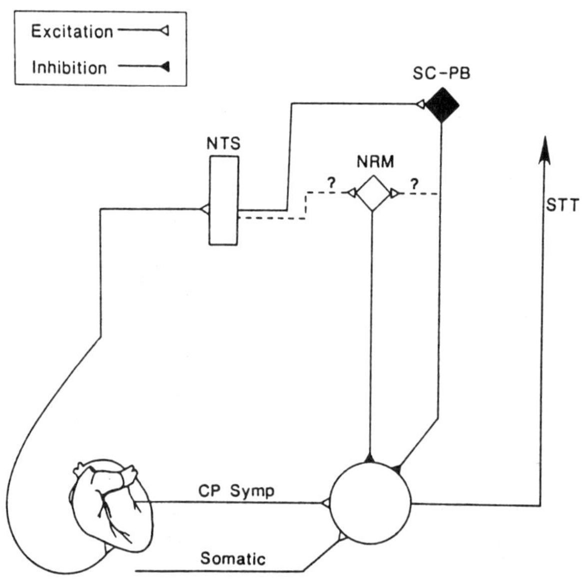

Figure 13. *A summary diagram showing possible connections of afferent input and ascending and descending pathways. The filled diamond emphasizes a likely site for integration of vagal inhibition. Continuous lines represent known pathways and interrupted lines represent hypothetical or indirect pathways. Connections between input and representative cell nucleus or region may be monosynaptic or polysynaptic. Inhibition from descending pathways may be presynaptic or postsynaptic. CP Symp: cardiopulmonary sympathetic afferent fibers; NTS: nucleus tractus solitarius; NRM: nucleus raphe magnus; Somatic: somatic afferent fibers; STT: spinothalamic tract system; SC-PB: subcoeruleus-parabrachial region.*

terminal axons that are located in the caudal pole of the NTS. These terminal axons then make excitatory synaptic connections with cell bodies of the NTS whose axons project to the SC-PB/locus coeruleus region and synapse with cells located in this region. These axons project down the spinal cord and either directly or indirectly suppress the activity of STT cells that are activated by the increased impulses that are transmitted in sympathetic afferent fibers and somatic afferent fibers. Thus, the increased activity of STT cells is suppressed indirectly by activation of the vagal afferent fibers. As a result of suppression of STT cell activity, angina pectoris associated with myocardial ischemia is ameliorated.

Acknowledgments: We thank Angela Evans for her helpful comments about the chapter. We also gratefully acknowledge Charlene Smith for typing the chapter, Diana Holston for technical assistance, and Tammi Williams for the illustrations and photography.

References

1. Kezdi P, Kordenate RK, Misra SN: Reflex inhibitory effects of vagal afferents in experimental myocardial infarction. Am J Cardiol 33:853, 1974.
2. Lombardi F, Casalone C, Della Bella P, et al: Global versus regional myocardial ischaemia: Differences in cardiovascular and sympathetic responses in cats. Cardiovasc Res 18:14, 1984.
3. Schwartz PJ, Pagani M, Lombardi F, et al: A cardiocardiac sympathovagal reflex in the cat. Circ Res 32:215, 1973.
4. Thames MD, Abboud FM: Inhibition of renal sympathetic nerve activity during myocardial ischemia mediated by left ventricular receptors with vagal afferents in dogs. J Clin Invest 63:395, 1979.
5. Thoren PN, Donald DE, Shepherd JT: Role of heart and lung receptors with nonmedullated vagal afferents in circulatory control. Circ Res 38:2, 1976.
6. Ammons WS, Blair RW, Foreman RD: Vagal afferent inhibition of primate T_1–T_5 spinothalamic neurons. J Neurophysiol 50:926, 1983.
7. Ammons WS, Blair RW, Foreman RD: Vagal afferent inhibition of spinothalamic cell responses to sympathetic afferents and bradykinin in the monkey. Circ Res 53:603, 1983.
8. Maixner W, Randich A: Role of the right vagal nerve trunk in antinociception. Brain Res 298:374, 1984.
9. Maixner W, Bossut DF, Whitsel EA: Evaluation of vagal afferent modulation of the digastric reflex in cats. Brain Res 560:55–62, 1991.
10. Foreman RD: Organization of the spinothalamic tract as a relay for cardiopulmonary sympathetic afferent fiber activity. In D Ottoson, H Autrum, ER Perl, et al (eds): Progress in Sensory Physiology. Vol. 9. Heidelberg, Springer-Verlag, 1989, pp. 1–51.
11. Randich A, Thurston CL: Antinociceptive states and hypertension. J Cardiovasc Electrophysiol 2:S54, 1991.
12. Zamir N, Segal M: Hypertension-induced analgesia: Changes in pain sensitivity in experimental hypertensive rats. Brain Res 160:170, 1979.
13. Maixner W, Touw KB, Brody MJ, et al: Factors regulating the altered pain perception in the spontaneously hypertensive rat. Brain Res 237:137, 1982.
14. Zamir N, Shuber E: Altered pain perception in hypertensive humans. Brain Res 201:471, 1980.
15. Ghione S, Rosa C, Panattoni E, et al: Comparison of sensory and pain threshold in

tooth pulp stimulation in normotensive man and essential hypertension. J Hypertens 3:S113, 1985.

16. Ghione S, Rosa C, Mezzasalma L, et al: Arterial hypertension is associated with hypalgesia in humans. Hypertension 12:491, 1988.
17. Rosa C, Ghione S, Panattoni E, et al: Comparison of pain perception in normotensives and borderline hypertensives by means of a tooth pulp-stimulation test. J Cardiovasc Pharmacol 8:S125, 1986.
18. Thies R, Foreman RD: Inhibition and excitation of thoracic spinoreticular neurons by electrical stimulation of vagal afferent nerves. Exp Neurol 82:1, 1983.
19. Hobbs SF, Oh UT, Chandler MJ, et al: Cardiac and abdominal vagal afferent inhibition of primate T9-S1 spinothalamic cells. Am J Physiol 257:R889, 1989.
20. Chandler MJ, Hobbs SF, Bolser DC, et al: Effects of vagal afferent stimulation on cervical spinothalamic tract neurons in monkeys. Pain 44:81, 1991.
21. Ren K, Randich A, Gebhart GF: Effects of electrical stimulation of vagal afferents on spinothalamic tract cells in the rat. Pain 44:311, 1991.
22. Thies R, Foreman RD: Descending inhibition of spinal neurons in the cardiopulmonary region by electrical stimulation of vagal afferent nerves. Brain Res 207:178, 1981.
23. Ren K, Randich A, Gebhart GF: Vagal afferent modulation of spinal nociceptive transmission in the rat. J Neurophysiol 62:401–415, 1989.
24. Assey ME: The recognition and treatment of silent myocardial ischemia. In JW Hurst (ed): The Heart, Arteries and Veins. New York, NY, McGraw-Hill Information Services Company, 1990, p. 1079.
25. Droste C, Greenlee MW, Roskamm H: A defective angina pectoris pain warning system: Experimental findings of ischemic and electrical pain test. Pain 26:199, 1986.
26. Foreman RD: Spinal substrates of visceral pain. In TL Yaksh (ed): Spinal Afferent Processing. New York, NY, Plenum Publishing Corporation, 1986, p. 271.
27. Coleridge JCG, Hemingway A, Holmes RL, et al: The location of atrial receptors in the dog: A physiological and histological study. J Physiol (Lond) 136:174, 1957.
28. Paintal AS: Vagal sensory receptors and their reflex effects. Physiol Rev 53:159, 1973.
29. Thoren P: Role of cardiac vagal C-fibers in cardiovascular control. Rev Physiol Biochem Pharmacol 86:1, 1979.
30. Coleridge HM, Coleridge JCG, Kidd C: Cardiac receptors in the dog with particular reference to two types of endings in the ventricular wall. J Physiol (Lond) 174:323, 1964.
31. Donald DE, Shepherd JT: Reflexes from the heart and lungs: Physiological curiosities or important regulatory mechanisms. Cardiovasc Res 12:449, 1978.
32. Baker DG, Coleridge HM, Coleridge JCG: Vagal afferent C fibers from the ventricle. In R Hainsworth, C Kidd, RJ Linden (eds): Cardiac Receptors. Cambridge, Cambridge University Press, 1979, pp. 117–137.
33. Muers MF, Sleight P: Action potentials from ventricular mechanoreceptors stimulated by occlusion of the coronary sinus in the dog. J Physiol (Lond) 221:283, 1972.
34. Sleight P, Widdicombe JG: Action potentials in fibres from receptors in the epicardium and myocardium of the dog's left ventricle. J Physiol (Lond) 181:235, 1965.
35. Thoren PN: Characteristics of left ventricular receptors with nonmedullated vagal afferents in cats. Circ Res 40:415, 1977.
36. Kaufman MP, Baker DG, Coleridge HM, et al: Stimulation by bradykinin of afferent vagal C-fibers with chemosensitive endings in the heart and aorta of the dog. Circ Res 46:476, 1980.
37. Oberg B, Thoren P: Circulatory responses to stimulation of medullated and non-medullated afferents in the cardiac nerve of the cat. Acta Physiol Scand 87:121, 1972.

38. Thoren PN: Activation of left ventricular receptors with nonmedullated vagal afferent fibers during occlusion of a coronary artery in the cat. Am J Cardiol 37:1046, 1976.
39. Willis WD Jr: The Pain System: The Neural Basis of Nociceptive Transmission in the Mammalian Nervous System. Basel, Karger, 1985, p. 145.
40. Hoffman DS, Dubnar R, Hayes RL, et al: Neuronal activity in medullary dorsal horn of awake monkeys trained in the thermal discrimination task. I. Responses to innocuous and noxious thermal stimuli. J Neurophysiol 46:409, 1981.
41. Willis WD, Coggeshall RE: Sensory mechanisms of the spinal cord. New York, NY, Plenum Press, 1978, p. 485.
42. Dubner R, Price DD, Beitel RE, et al: Peripheral neural correlates of behavior in monkey and human related to sensory-discriminative aspects of pain. In DJ Anderson, B
Matthews (eds): Pain in the Trigeminal Region. Amsterdam, Elsevier, 1977, p. 57.
43. Gybels J, Handwerker HO, Van Hees J: A comparison between the discharges of human nociceptive nerve fibres and the subject's ratings of his sensations. J Physiol (Lond) 292:193, 1979.
44. LaMotte RH, Campbell JN: Comparison of responses of warm and nociceptive C-fiber afferents in monkey with human judgments of thermal pain. J Neurophysiol 41:509, 1978.
45. Torebjork HE, Hallin RG: Identification of afferent C units in intact human skin nerves. Brain Res 67:387, 1974.
46. Van Hees J, Gybels JM: C nociceptor activity in human nerve during painful and nonpainful skin stimulation. J Neurol Neurosurg Psychiatry 44:600, 1981.
47. Ammons WS, Girardot M-N, Foreman RD: T_2–T_5 spinothalamic neurons projecting to medial thalamus with viscerosomatic input. J Neurophysiol 54:73, 1985.
48. Melzack R, Wall PD: The Challenge of Pain. New York, NY, Basic Books Inc, 1982.
49. Price DD, Dubner R: Neurons that subserve the sensory-discriminative aspects of pain. Pain 3:307, 1977.
50. Melzack R, Casey KL: Sensory, motivational and central control determinants of pain. In D Kenshalo (ed): The Skin Senses. Springfield, IL, Charles C Thomas, 1968, p. 423.
51. Casey KL, Keene JJ, Morrow T: Bulboreticular and medial thalamic unit activity in relation to aversive behavior and pain. In JJ Bonica (ed): Pain. New York, NY, Raven Press, 1974, p. 197.
52. Foreman RD, Blair RW, Weber RN: Viscerosomatic convergence onto T_2–T_4 spinoreticular, spinoreticular-spinothalamic and spinothalamic tract neurons in the cat. Exp Neurol 85:597–619, 1984.
53. Haber LH, Moore BD, Willis WD: Electrophysiological response properties of spinoreticular neurons in the monkey. J Comp Neurol 207:75, 1982.
54. Kevetter GA, Haber LH, Yezierski RP, et al: Cells of origin of the spinoreticular tract in the monkey. J Comp Neurol 207:61, 1982.
55. Blair RW, Weber RN, Foreman RD: Characteristics of primate spinothalamic tract neurons receiving viscerosomatic convergent inputs in T_3–T_5 segments. J Neurophysiol 46:797, 1981.
56. Ammons WS, Girardot M-N, Foreman RD: Effects of intracardiac bradykinin on T_2–T_5 medial spinothalamic cells. Am J Physiol 249:R147, 1985.
57. Hobbs SF, Chandler MJ, Bolser DC, et al: Segmental organization of visceral and somatic input onto C_3-T_6 spinothalamic tract cells of the monkey. J Neurophysiol 68:1575, 1992.
58. Lewis T: Pain. New York, NY, Macmillan, 1942.
59. Boucek RJ, Morales AR, Romanell R, et al: Coronary Artery Disease. Baltimore, MD, Williams & Wilkins Co, 1984.
60. Christi LG, Conti CR: Systematic approach to evaluation of angina-like chest pain: Pathophysiology and clinical testing with emphasis on objective documentation of myocardial ischemia. Am Heart J 102:897, 1981.

61. Hammermeister KE, Bonica JJ: Cardiac and aortic pain. In JJ Bonica (ed): The Management of Pain. Philadelphia, PA, Lea & Febiger, 1990, p. 1001.
62. Harrison TR, Reeves RJ, Joseph T: Principles and Problems of Ischemic Heart Disease. Chicago, IL, Year Book Medical Publishers, 1968, p. 197.
63. Miller HR: Angina Pectoris: Nerve Pathways, Physiology, Symptomatology and Treatment. Baltimore, MD, Williams & Wilkins Co, 1939, p. 86.
64. Procacci P, Zoppi M: Heart pain. In PD Wall, R Melzack (eds): Textbook of Pain. Edinburgh, Churchill Livingstone, 1989, p. 410.
65. Sampson JJ, Cheitlin MD: Pathophysiology and differential diagnosis of cardiac pain. Prog Cardiovasc Dis 23:507, 1971.
66. Ruch TC: Pathophysiology of pain. In TC Ruch, HD Patton, JW Woodbury, et al (eds): Neurophysiology. Philadelphia, PA, WB Saunders Co, 1961, pp. 350–368.
67. Blair RW, Ammons WS, Foreman RD: Responses of thoracic spinothalamic and spinoreticular cells to coronary artery occlusion. J Neurophysiol 51:636, 1984.
68. Chahl LA, Kirk EJ: Toxins which produce pain. Pain 1:3–49, 1975.
69. Chen HJ, Huang TF: Comparative study on pain responses to intraarterial (coronary and femoral) and intraperitoneal injection of algesic agents in dogs. Chin J Physiol 20:173–181, 1969.
70. Foreman RD, Schmidt RF, Willis WD: Effects of mechanical and chemical stimulation of fine muscle afferents upon primate spinothalamic tract cells. J Physiol (Lond) 286:215, 1979.
71. Hashimoto K, Hirose M, Furukawa S, et al: Changes in hemodynamics and bradykinin concentration in coronary sinus blood in experimental coronary artery occlusion. Jpn Heart J 18:679, 1977.
72. Blair RW, Weber RN, Foreman RD: Responses of thoracic spinothalamic neurons to intracardiac injection of bradykinin in the monkey. Circ Res 51:83, 1982.
73. Lombardi F, Della Bella P, Casati R, et al: Effects of intracoronary administration of bradykinin on the impulse activity of afferent sympathetic unmyelinated fibers with left ventricular endings in the cat. Circ Res 48:69, 1981.
74. Needleman P: The synthesis and function of prostaglandins in the heart. Fed Proc 35:2376, 1976.
75. Nerdrum T, Baker DG, Coleridge HM, et al: Interaction of bradykinin and prostaglandin E on cardiac pressor reflex and sympathetic afferents. Am J Physiol 250:R815, 1986.
76. Sylven C: Angina pectoris. Clinical characteristics, neurophysiological and molecular mechanisms. Pain 36:145, 1989.
77. Crea F, Pupita G, Galassi AR, et al: Role of adenosine in pathogenesis of anginal pain. Circulation 81:164, 1990.
78. Brennan TJ, Oh UT, Hobbs SF, et al: Urinary bladder and hindlimb afferent input inhibits activity of primate T_2–T_5 spinothalamic tract neurons. J Neurophys 61:573–588, 1989.
79. Thurston L, Randich A: Acute increases in arterial blood pressure produced by occlusion of the abdominal aorta induces antinociception: Peripheral and central substrates. Brain Res 519:12, 1990.
80. Beckstead RM, Norgren R: An autoradiographic examination of the central distribution of the trigeminal, facial, glossopharyngeal, and vagal nerves in the monkey. J Comp Neurol 184:455, 1979.
81. Ren K, Randich A, Gebhart GF: Electrical stimulation of cervical vagal afferents. I. Central relays for modulation of spinal nociceptive transmission. J Neurophysiol 64:1098–1114, 1990.
82. Beckstead RM, Morse JR, Norgren R: The nucleus of the solitary tract in the monkey: Projections to the thalamus and brainstem nuclei. J Comp Neur 190:259, 1980.
83. Hancock MB, Fougerousse CL: Spinal projections from the nucleus locus coeruleus and nucleus subcoeruleus in the cat and monkey as demonstrated by the retrograde transport of horseradish peroxidase. Brain Res Bull 1:229, 1976.

84. Takeuchi Y, Uemura M, Matsuda K, et al: Parabrachial nucleus neurons projecting to the lower brainstem and the spinal cord. A study in the cat by the Fink-Heimer and the horseradish peroxidase methods. Exp Neurol 70:403, 1980.
85. Westlund KN, Bowker RM, Ziegler MG, et al: Origins and terminations of descending noradrenergic projections to the spinal cord of the monkey. Brain Res 292:1, 1984.
86. Westlund KN, Coulter JD: Descending projections of the locus coeruleus and subcoeruleus/medial parabrachial nuclei in the monkey: Axonal transport studies and dopamine-b-hydroxylase neurocytochemistry. Brain Res 2:235, 1980.
87. Hammond DL, Proudfit HK: Effects of locus coeruleus lesions on morphine-induced antinociception. Brain Res 188:79, 1980.
88. Katayama Y, Watkins LR, Becker DP, et al: Evidence for involvement of cholinoceptive cells of the parabrachial region in environmentally induced nociceptive suppression in the cat. Brain Res 229:348, 1984.
89. Katayama Y, Watkins LR, Becker DP, et al: Non-opiate analgesia induced by carbacol microinjection into the pontine parabrachial region of the cat. Brain Res 296:262, 1984.
90. Brennan TJ, Oh UT, Girardot M-N, et al: Inhibition of cardiopulmonary input to thoracic spinothalamic tract cells by stimulation of the subcoeruleus-parabrachial region in the primate. J Auton Nerv Syst 18:61, 1987.
91. Girardot M-N, Brennan TJ, Ammons WS, et al: Effects of stimulating the subcoeruleus-parabrachial region on the non-noxious and noxious responses of T_2–T_4 spinothalamic tract neurons in the primate. Brain Res 409:19, 1987.
92. Ammons WS, Blair RW, Foreman RD: Raphe magnus inhibition of primate T_1–T_4 spinothalamic cells with cardiopulmonary visceral input. Pain 20:247–260, 1984.
93. Randich A, Ren K, Gebhart GF: Electrical stimulation of cervical vagal afferents. II. Central relays for behavioral antinociception and arterial blood pressure decreases. J Neurophysiol 64:1115–1124, 1990.
94. Randich A, Aicher SA: Medullary substrates mediating antinociception produced by electrical stimulation of the vagus. Brain Res 445:68–76, 1988.
95. Ren K, Randich A, Gebhart GF: Modulation of spinal nociceptive transmission from nuclei tractus solitarii: A relay for effects of vagal afferent stimulation. J Neurophysiol 63:971–986, 1990.
96. Cohn PF: Silent myocardial ischemia: Classification, prevalence and prognosis. Am J Med 79:2, 1985.
97. Walker JL, Thames MD, Abboud FM, et al: Preferential distribution of inhibitory cardiac receptors in left ventricle of the dog. Am J Physiol 235:H188, 1978.
98. Felder RB, Thames MD: Interaction between cardiac receptors and sinoaortic baroreceptors in the control of efferent cardiac sympathetic nerve activity during myocardial ischemia in dogs. Circ Res 45:728, 1979.
99. Webb SW, Adgey AA, Pantridge JF: Autonomic disturbances at onset of acute myocardial infarction. Br Med J 3:89, 1972.
100. Randall DC, Hasson DM, Brady JV: Acute cardiovascular consequences of anterior descending coronary artery occlusion in unanesthetized monkey. Proc Soc Exp Biol Med 58:135, 1978.
101. Thames MD, Klopfenstein HS, Abboud FM, et al: Preferential distribution of inhibitory cardiac receptors with vagal afferents to the inferoposterior wall of the left ventricle activated during coronary occlusion in the dog. Circ Res 43:512, 1978.
102. Droste C, Greenlee MW, Ruf G, et al: Localization of a coronary stenosis, left ventricular function, and pain perception during myocardial ischemia in patients with one-vessel disease. J Cardiovasc Electrophysiol 2:S68, 1991.
103. Droste C, Roskamm H: Experimental pain measurement in patients with asymptomatic myocardial ischaemia. J Am Coll Cardiol 1:940, 1983.
104. Glazier JJ, Chierchia S, Brown MJ, et al: Importance of generalized defective perception of painful stimuli as a cause of silent myocardial ischemia in chronic stable angina pectoris. Am J Cardiol 58:667, 1986.

105. Falcone C, Sconocchia R, Guasti L, et al: Dental pain threshold and angina pectoris in patients with coronary artery disease. J Am Coll Cardiol 12:348, 1988.
106. Pedersen F, Pietersen A, Madsen JK, et al: Elevated pain threshold in patients with effort-induced angina pectoris and asymptomatic myocardial ischemia during exercise test. Clin Cardiol 12:639, 1989.

CHAPTER 23

Mechanisms of Arterial Baroreflex Control

M.D. Thames, M.E. Dibner-Dunlap, M.L. Smith

The arterial baroreflexes exert important control on vagal outflow to the heart. As described in Chs. 13 and 14, the parasympathetic influences on the heart are most evident in the cardiac rate and atrioventricular (AV) conduction, with much more modest effects on ventricular function. In this chapter, the emphasis is placed on the control of vagal outflow to the sinoatrial (SA) node by arterial baroreflexes. This area is the one most heavily investigated both in animal models and in humans, and about which the most is known. The goal of this chapter is to provide an understanding of baroreflex control of the SA node under both normal circumstances and in pathophysiological states.

Arterial Baroreceptors

The determinants of arterial baroreceptor discharge and of the reflex effects they mediate have been extensively reviewed previously.[1,2] The afferent limbs of the arterial baroreflex originate in the carotid sinus and aortic arch. Sensory endings that are sensitive to stretch are located at these sites, and these endings increase their discharge frequency as pressure is raised and reduce their discharge frequency as pressure is lowered. The sensory information from these endings traverses the glossopharyngeal nerve in the case of the carotid sinus baroreceptors and traverses the aortic depressor and vagal nerves in the case of the aortic arch baroreceptors. After entering the brain stem, these primary afferent neurons pass to the nucleus tractus solitarius (NTS), wherein they synapse with second-order neurons in the arterial baroreflex pathway.[3] From this location, there are projections to many areas of the brain, including the hypothalamus, portions of the midbrain, and the caudal and rostral ventrolateral medulla, which are all important sites in autonomic control. Included among these central projections are ties from the NTS to the

Supported by HL30506 and by funds from the Department of Veterans Affairs.
From *Vagal Control of the Heart: Experimental Basis and Clinical Implications* edited by MN Levy, PJ Schwartz © 1994, Futura Publishing Co. Inc., Armonk, NY.

nucleus ambiguus (NA), which is the principal location of preganglionic parasympathetic nerves (vagal efferent fibers). The activity of these preganglionic vagal fibers is under the influence of muscarinic cholinergic mechanisms, which tonically inhibit the activity of these fibers. Low doses of atropine that have little effect on peripheral muscarinic receptors (mAChRs) block the central cholinergic receptors sufficiently to reduce this inhibition and cause increases in efferent vagal activity to the SA node.[4] These vagal fibers then pass to the heart via the tenth cranial nerve, where they synapse with cell bodies in the cardiac ganglia. Postganglionic cells then provide fibers that innervate the SA and AV nodes, the atria, and the ventricles.

There are two types of afferent fibers that subserve arterial baroreceptors. One group of fibers is myelinated (A- and A-delta-fibers) with conduction velocities in excess of 2.5 milliseconds, whereas the other group is subserved by unmyelinated C-fibers that have a conduction velocity of less than 2.5 milliseconds.[2,5] The A-fiber baroreceptors are much more sensitive to the dynamic component of the stimulus (the pressure pulse), whereas the C-fibers are more responsive to changes in the static component of the stimulus (the prevailing level of arterial pressure) to these endings.[2] Activation of either group of afferent fibers, however, results in reflex vagal activation and cardiac slowing.[6] The effects on vagal outflow of the C-fiber baroreceptors are much greater than the influence of myelinated baroreceptor afferents.

The discharge of carotid and aortic baroreceptors is modulated by neural and humoral factors. For example, several studies have shown that the discharge of the carotid sinus baroreceptors is influenced by the prevailing level of sympathetic nerve activity (SNA) passing to the carotid sinus region.[7] Inhibition of SNA reduces the sensitivity of carotid baroreceptors, whereas increases in SNA to this region have the opposite effect. Arterial baroreceptor stimulation activates vagal efferent activity and inhibits sympathetic outflow to the heart and peripheral circulation. Reduced baroreceptor input has the opposite effect. Therefore, these modulating influences on baroreceptor discharge may be important in determining the net reflex responses to a particular stimulus.

When arterial baroreceptor activity is altered, there are changes in vagal outflow to the heart and in sympathetic outflow to the heart and peripheral circulation. These changes often occur at the same time, so it may be difficult to differentiate the effects on the heart that are mediated by vagal mechanisms from those mediated by sympathetic mechanisms. As part of this review, we will try to assess the relative roles of sympathetic and parasympathetic mechanisms in control of the SA node via the baroreflexes.

Studies on Arterial Baroreflex Control of Heart Rate in Animals

Baroreflex control of heart rate has been studied by a variety of different methods. These methods include the administration of vasoactive drugs to raise and lower arterial pressure and, thereby, alter the stimulus to the arterial baroreceptors. The methods also include alterations in sensory input induced by electrical stimulation of baroreceptor afferent fibers and by vascular isolation of the carotid sinus and aortic arch baroreceptive areas for independent control of the stimulus to these regions. New methods have been developed for studying baroreflex control of SA node rate in conscious animals. These methods are discussed in relationship to the findings obtained from these experiments. In addition, techniques that have been developed for evaluation of baroreflex control of SA node function in humans also have been applied to animals.

When the activity of the arterial baroreceptors is increased, such as occurs during administration of substances that raise arterial pressure, there is reflex SA node slowing. This occurrence has been known since the 19th century, when Cyon and Ludwig showed that electrical stimulation of the carotid sinus nerve resulted in reflex cardiac slowing.[8] One area of controversy regarding the mechanism of this cardiac slowing has been the relative contribution of vagal and sympathetic mechanisms to its mediation. Various studies have indicated a preponderance of vagal effects over the sympathetic effects in the mediation of this cardiac slowing. The consensus is that the bradycardia accompanying increased baroreceptor discharge is mediated principally by increases in efferent vagal activity rather than by withdrawal of sympathetic activity. Administration of mAChR antagonists, such as atropine, essentially abolishes the bradycardia that accompanies increased baroreceptor stimulation.[9] In contrast, baroreflex slowing appears to be unaffected or even enhanced after β-adrenergic blockade with propranolol.[9]

The arterial baroreflex control of vagal outflow to the heart appears to result from the algebraic summation of the effects of carotid and aortic baroreflexes.[10,11] This finding stands in contrast to the control of sympathetic outflow to the heart and peripheral circulation by the carotid and aortic baroreceptors. Such control appears to be redundant. In experimental animals, denervation of either carotid or aortic baroreceptors reduces the baroreflex bradycardia that results from increases in arterial pressure. Thus, the control of vagal preganglionic parasympathetic nerves by carotid and aortic baroreceptors is not redundant.

The evidence that suggests a preponderant effect of vagal mechanisms on baroreflex-induced changes in heart rate results from studies in which bolus injections of vasopressor and vasodepressor substances cause rapid changes in arterial pressure. The responses differed slightly when arterial pressure is varied as a slow ramp or as small, step changes in arterial pressure. Under these circumstances, the contribution of the sympathetic nerves to heart rate control becomes larger.[12] Figure 1 depicts the relative contribution of parasympathetic and sympathetic effects to the heart rate response to blood pressure changes. In addition, there may be important species differences in the relative contribution of vagal and sympathetic mechanisms in heart rate control during stimulation of baroreflexes. In animals with low basal vagal tone, such as rats and rabbits, sympathetic mechanisms may play a more significant role.

There is convincing evidence that vagal nerves influence cardiac performance. In addition, data from anesthetized animals suggest that the arterial

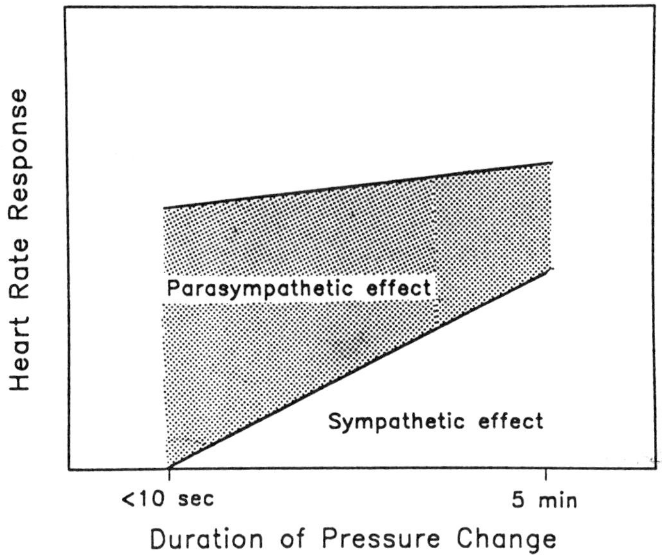

Figure 1. *Schematic representation of the relative contribution of parasympathetic and sympathetic effects on the heart rate response to a change in arterial pressure. Pressure changes of short duration (<10 sec) are exclusively mediated by parasympathetic effects. Pressure changes of longer duration are mediated by a combination of parasympathetic and sympathetic effects. Adapted with permission from Chen RYZ, Fan FC, Schuessler GB, et al: Baroreflex control of heart rate in humans during nitroprusside-induced hypotension. Am J Physiol 243:R18–R24, 1982.*

baroreflexes can alter cardiac contractility. Whether vagal mechanisms contribute importantly to this effect is not clearly established. Moreover, baroreflex control of ventricular function in conscious animals appears to be very small and of uncertain physiological significance.[13]

Stephenson and Donald[14] developed an elegant technique to study the reversible vascular isolation of the carotid sinuses in conscious dogs. This technique has permitted the investigation of reflexes from the isolated carotid sinuses of intact and vagotomized conscious dogs[15] and has allowed the subsequent investigation of the role of arterial baroreflexes in circulatory control during exercise.[16–18] Stephenson and Donald[15] found that large, step increases in sinus pressure from 50 mm Hg to various higher levels resulted in large initial bradycardia and hypotension that then reverted in the steady state to very modest bradycardia and moderate decreases in arterial pressure. Anesthesia shifted the responses to a higher basal mean arterial pressure (MAP) and heart rate, but did not impair the gain of the carotid sinus baroreceptor reflex.[15] Vagotomy changed the operating point for control of blood pressure toward the saturation end of the arterial baroreflex, whereas it shifted the operating point for heart rate from threshold to the mid-range of the stimulus versus response relationship.

Using this approach, Walgenbach and Donald[16] subsequently investigated the ability of the carotid baroreceptors to regulate arterial pressure during graded exercise in the chronic absence of the aortic baroreflex. They found that the relationship of arterial pressure to workload was steeper when carotid sinuses were vascularly isolated from the circulation and thus prevented from detecting the increases in arterial pressure that occurred with exercise. At the heaviest workload, MAP was much higher when the carotid sinuses were not permitted to regulate arterial blood pressure. They concluded that, because the blood flow to the exercising muscle was the same whether or not the carotid sinuses were isolated, the large increase in pressure during severe exercise with the sinuses isolated must be due to a marked constriction in resistance vessels in the nonexercising beds. There was little effect of the isolation of the carotid sinuses on the heart rate responses to exercise. This result suggests that the effects of central command and of muscle metaboreflexes on heart rate must be predominant over the influence of the carotid baroreceptor reflex on heart rate control during exercise.

Studies in Humans

Although it has long been known that increases in blood pressure or local massage of the carotid sinus regions result in baroreflex slowing of the heart in humans, the most widely used method for studying baroreflex control of heart rate was established by Smyth et al.[19] These investigators showed that there was a linear correlation between the RR interval and the systolic blood pressure of the preceding beat when pressure was elevated with bolus administration of phenylephrine. The slope of this relationship was identified as the "baroreflex sensitivity." This method has been used widely to study baroreflex control of the SA node in normal subjects and in a variety of pathological states, some of which are discussed below. This technique alters the stimulus to both carotid and aortic baroreceptors.

Another method for studying baroreflex control of sinus rate uses a collar that is applied to the neck and to which suction and pressure can be applied so as to change the carotid sinus transmural pressure.[20] Application of suction increases transmural pressure, whereas increasing pressure inside this collar reduces transmural pressure. These two stimuli respectively increase and decrease carotid sinus baroreceptor discharge. This method permits selective alterations in the stimulus to the carotid baroreceptors. Interpretation of experiments using this methodology must be made with caution, because reflex responses provoked by altered carotid baroreceptor input change aortic pressure and aortic baroreceptor discharge. Such responses oppose the effects of the carotid baroreceptors. Thus, the early heart rate responses occur with little modulation by aortic baroreceptor input. When the suction is maintained, however, the modulating influence of the aortic baroreflex comes into play. In the remainder of this section, insights into baroreflex control obtained with both bolus phenylephrine injections as well as with the neck collar are reviewed. These studies address issues in normal humans.

In a series of experiments using the phenylephrine technique, Sleight and his colleagues[19,21,22] have obtained substantial insight into the cardiac baroreflex. They found, for example, that increasing age resulted in depression of baroreflex sensitivity.[21] They also found that upright posture and exercise reduced baroreflex sensitivity.[22] With regard to exercise, they found that reflex heart rate changes induced by sudden changes of arterial pressure were predominantly parasympathetic. The responses diminished during exercise together with the decrease of parasympathetic tone.[23] They found that baroreflex sensitivity was augmented during sleep and was actually highest during dreaming.[19] Although these studies are of great interest, they are relatively descriptive in nature and provide little insight as to the mechanism for alterations in reflex control during ageing or during exercise.

Several other investigators have attempted to assess the relative contribution of vagal and sympathetic mechanisms to heart rate control in such circumstances as exercise. Robinson and colleagues[24] found that the relative contribution of vagal and sympathetic mechanisms to control of the SA node depended on the tonic levels of activity in these two efferent limbs of the autonomic nervous system. In subjects with high vagal tone, the vagal efferent limb was predominant in heart rate control. During circumstances such as exercise, in which vagal control is low and sympathetic tone is high, heart rate control was mediated principally by the sympathetic efferent limb. Chen and colleagues[25] found in lightly-anesthetized humans that sodium nitroprusside-induced baroreflex-mediated changes in heart rate were mediated initially by vagal mechanisms, but that the more persistent responses were mediated by sympathetic mechanisms (Fig. 1). Finally, Pickering and colleagues[26] found that heart rate responses to rising and falling arterial pressures were asymmetrical in humans. The cardiac slowing that occurs with increasing pressure was significantly greater than was the tachycardia that resulted from equivalent decreases in pressure.[26]

Although it appears that carotid and aortic baroreflexes contribute nearly equally to vagal control of the SA node in animals, there appears to be an unequal influence of carotid and aortic baroreceptors in humans. Ferguson and colleagues[27] studied the contribution of carotid and extracarotid baroreceptors in the control of heart rate in normal humans. They found that extracarotid (presumably aortic) and carotid baroreflexes both participated in the control of heart rate in humans. Extracarotid (aortic) baroreflexes, however, appeared to have the greater role in control of heart rate during dynamic increases in arterial pressure. This finding was unexpected and remains to be confirmed by other investigators. The novel technique they used capitalized on the neck collar approach to control carotid baroreceptor input at a time that systemic arterial pressure was being changed with vasoactive substances to alter both carotid and aortic baroreceptor input.

More than any other individual, Eckberg[20] has used the method of neck suction and neck pressure to study responses to selective activation or unloading of carotid baroreceptors. He and his coworkers have provided important insights into carotid baroreflex function.[20] Eckberg detected that the maximum SA node inhibition occurred when the stimuli were delivered about 0.75 seconds before the anticipated appearance of the subsequent P wave.[28] The time from the onset of baroreceptor stimulation until the earliest occurrence of pulse interval prolongation averaged 0.24 seconds. Pulse interval prolongation was proportional to baroreceptor stimulus strength and duration. By using this technique, this study demonstrated the critical nature of the timing of baroreceptor stimulation.

Eckberg and colleagues[29] also demonstrated that upright posture enhances baroreflex sensitivity, but that this effect was masked by β-adrenergic stimulation. β-adrenergic blockade alone augmented baroreflex sensitivity in the resting supine state. His findings may help to explain the diminished baroreflex sensitivity observed during upright posture by the Oxford group.[29] In 1977, Eckberg[30] reported the importance of stimulus intensity, duration, and rate of pressure change on carotid baroreflex-mediated responses. SA node responses were found to be proportional to the first derivative (dP/dt) of the arterial pressure pulse. Carotid baroreflex responses were linear over a wide range that extended beyond the normal range for human systolic arterial pressures[31] (see Fig. 2). Saturation of the carotid baroreceptor cardiac reflex occurred at transmural distending pressures of about 160 mm Hg and operational pressure (resting arterial pressure) was near the threshold (Fig. 2). The carotid baroreflex responses were highly reproducible over time.

In a companion paper, Eckberg[32] demonstrated that application of prolonged neck suction resulted in adaptation of the human carotid baroreceptor cardiac reflex. This adaptation was not altered by β-adrenergic blockade. It is not clear how much of this adaptation resulted from adaptation of the carotid baroreceptors, to the modulating influence of the aortic baroreflex, or both.

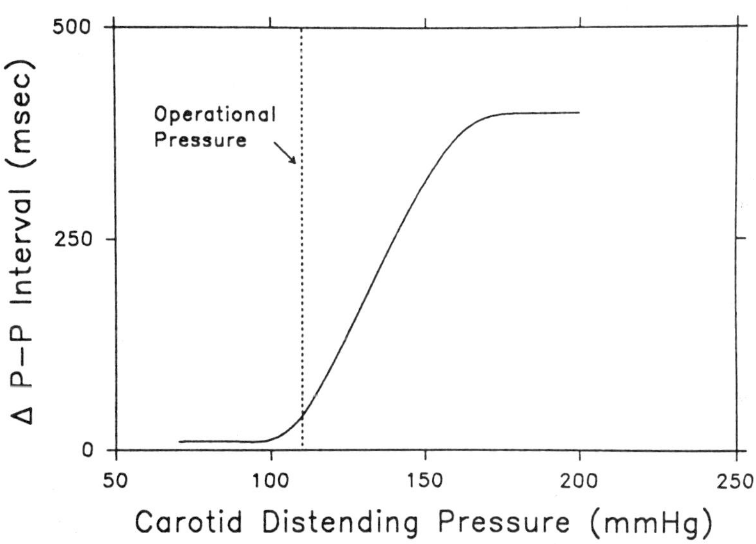

Figure 2. *Illustration of the sigmoid stimulus-response relation between carotid distending pressure and P-P interval in humans derived from brief neck suction of variable pressures superimposed on a neck pressure of 40 mm Hg. The dotted line indicates the operational (baseline) systolic pressure and demonstrates that the carotid baroreflex functions near the threshold. Adapted with permission from Eckberg DL: Nonlinearities of the human carotid baroreceptor-cardiac reflex. Circ Res 47:208–216, 1980.*

Finally, Fritsch and colleagues[33] were able to demonstrate rapid resetting of the carotid baroreceptor cardiac reflex in humans as early as 25 minutes after the onset of sustained arterial pressure changes. Many of these observations made by Eckberg and colleagues confirmed the marked similarities in baroreceptor cardiac reflexes between humans and experimental animals.

Modulation of Arterial Baroreflexes by Other Reflexes

The interactions between the arterial baroreflexes and other cardiovascular reflexes are important in altering the vagal control of the heart. The interaction between cardiac mechanoreflexes and chemoreflexes with the arterial baroreflexes has been most extensively investigated. In animals, increasing the blood volume activates atrial receptors and results in reflex tachycardia. This tachycardia occurs in conscious animals despite the increase in arterial pressure that accompanies this volume expansion.[34] This response is the classic Bainbridge reflex, and the efferent mechanisms that mediate these responses are controversial. Linden and colleagues[35] have suggested that this response was due to a selective effect of atrial receptors on sympathetic outflow to the SA node. Edis and colleagues suggested,[36] however, that the responses depended on the prevailing influence of the two efferent limbs of the autonomic nervous system. In animals with high-resting vagal tone, vagal withdrawal mediates the tachycardia, whereas in animals with little resting vagal tone, increases in sympathetic activity account for the tachycardia.

It is interesting that tachycardia occurs during volume expansion in animals, because the same stimulus activates sensory receptors in the ventricles.[37] Increased activity in these receptors results in sympathetic withdrawal and vagal activation.[37] The atrial receptor mechanism described above is mediated by sensory receptors with myelinated afferent fibers, whereas those in the ventricles are mediated principally by C-fiber afferents.[37] A group of sensory endings in the left ventricle appears to be relatively insensitive to mechanical stimuli, but respond to various chemical stimuli. These chemosensitive endings[38] are activated by certain natural substances, including bradykinin and prostaglandins. Intracoronary administration of prostaglandins results in reflex bradycardia and reduces the sensitivity of the arterial baroreflex control of heart rate.[39] These responses are due to a central interaction between cardiac reflexes and arterial baroreflexes.

Afferent input from cardiopulmonary mechanoreceptors also appears to modulate arterial baroreflex control of heart rate and vascular resistance in animals and humans. Increases in central venous pressure decrease arterial baroreflex gain, whereas decreases in central venous pressure augment baroreflex gain.[40–43]

Another important mechanism for modulation of arterial baroreflex control of heart rate is related to respiration. During inspiration, mechanoreceptors in the lung are stimulated and activate the lung inflation reflex. In addition, central mechanisms diminish vagal activity during inspiration, and vagal tone returns during exhalation. This action is more widely recognized as respiratory sinus arrhythmia. Baroreceptor stimuli are much more effective in inducing cardiac slowing when they are delivered during exhalation than during inspiration.[28]

Effects of Pathophysiological States on Baroreflex Control

Arterial baroreflex control of heart rate is impaired in virtually every experimental model of hypertension as well as in humans with essential hypertension. In experimental models of hypertension, baroreflex control of the SA node has been shown to be impaired in renal hypertension, desoxycorticosterone acetate (DOCA)/salt hypertension, and spontaneously-hypertensive rats.

The abnormality of heart rate control in experimental animals appears to be due mainly to impairment in the baroreflex regulation of the vagal limb of the baroreflex. In conscious dogs with renal hypertension, propranolol had no significant effect on baroreflex control of the SA node, whereas atropine largely abolished the SA node responses to phenylephrine-induced increases and nitroprusside-induced decreases in arterial pressure.[44] Moreover, the abnormalities in reflex control were apparent during increases, but not during decreases, in arterial pressure. Since the cardiac slowing that occurs during increases in arterial pressure is due mainly to activation of efferent vagal mechanisms and because such responses are abolished by atropine in both normotensive and hypertensive animals, it seems likely that vagal mechanisms are largely responsible for the cardiac slowing during increases in arterial pressure and that these vagal responses are impaired in hypertension.

A similar abnormality has been observed in rabbits with renal hypertension. In the one kidney, one wrap model, the baroreflex control of heart rate became abnormal even before baroreflex control of sympathetic nerve activity was impaired.[11] It appeared that the redundancy between carotid and aortic baroreceptors in the control of sympathetic outflow was sufficient to compensate for impairment in the afferent limb of the baroreflex. There was no such redundancy, however, in the control of vagal outflow and, therefore, there was no compensation for the impairment in the afferent limb of the baroreflex. There also may be central neural abnormalities in heart rate control in experimental hypertension.

Humans with essential hypertension have impaired baroreflex control of heart rate.[45] Again, this occurrence may be due largely to impairment of the vagal efferent component of the baroreflex. As in animals, such abnormalities are most prominent during increases in arterial pressure and less evident during decreases in arterial pressure. The neck collar technique[46] has shown that carotid sinus baroreflex control of the SA node is impaired in humans with essential hypertension.

In experimental models of hypertension and in humans with essential hypertension, it remains largely unknown whether the abnormalities reside, solely in the afferent limb of the baroreflex or whether they may also be present in the central neural component of this reflex.

Congestive Heart Failure

The arterial baroreflex control of heart rate is impaired in humans with congestive heart failure (CHF)[47] as well as in experimental animal models with high- and low-output CHF. In humans, most arterial baroreflex slowing is vagally mediated. Thus, impaired slowing in response to increases in arterial pressure has been attributed largely to impaired activation of efferent vagal mechanisms. Impairment of heart rate control by arterial baroreflexes has been demonstrated in a model of high-output CHF induced by creation of an aortocaval fistula,[48] and in a low-output model of heart failure induced by rapid ventricular pacing.[49] The mechanism for these abnormalities is not entirely clear. Studies in anesthetized[49] and conscious[50] dogs suggest that, in the rapid ventricular pacing model, there may be abnormalities in the reflex control of the sympathetic component of the baroreflex. Such abnormalities may contribute importantly to the defective heart rate control observed in this model.[49]

Efforts have been made to investigate the effects of reversal of heart failure on the baroreflex control of the SA node. Occlusion of the aortocaval fistula in dogs with high-output CHF resulted in some reversal, but not in total resolution of these abnormalities.[51] In humans, cardiac transplantation resulted in rapid return of the baroreflex control of the recipient SA node to normal levels.[52] A similar rapid reversal is observed in the rapid ventricular pacing model of heart failure in dogs (unpublished observations). These observations are important because they indicate that the baroreflex abnormalities observed in heart failure probably do not result from structural abnormalities, but are more likely due to functional abnormalities related to the neurohumoral excitatory state in heart failure.

References

1. Kirchheim H: Systemic arterial baroreceptor reflexes. Physiol Rev 56:100–176, 1976.
2. Brown AM: Receptors under pressure: An update on baroreceptors. Circ Res 46:1–10, 1980.
3. Spyer KM: The neural organization and control of the baroreflex. Rev Physiol Biochem Pharmacol 88:24–124, 1981.
4. Katona PG, Lipson D, Dauchot PJ: Opposing peripheral and central effects of atropine on parasympathetic cardiac control. Am J Physiol 232:H146–H151, 1977.
5. Fidone SJ, Sato A: A study of chemoreceptor and baroreceptor A- and C-fibers in the cat carotid sinus nerve. J Physiol (Lond) 205:527–548, 1969.
6. Kardon MB, Peterson DF, Bishop VS: Reflex heart rate control via specific aortic nerve afferents in the rabbit. Circ Res 37:41–47, 1975.
7. Felder RB, Heesch CM, Thames MD: Reflex modulation of carotid sinus barore-

ceptor activity in the dog. Am J Physiol 244 (Heart Circ Physiol 13):H437–H443, 1983.

8. Cyon E, Ludwig C: Die reflexe eines der sensiblen nerven des herzens auf die motorischen der blutgefusse. Ber Saeschs Ges Akad Wissenschaften 18:307–329, 1866.
9. Thames MD, Kontos HA: Mechanism of baroreceptor induced changes in heart rate. Am J Physiol 218:251–256, 1970.
10. Guo GB, Thames MD, Abboud FM: Differential control of heart rate and hind limb resistance by carotid, aortic, and cardiopulmonary baroreflexes in rabbits. Circ Res 50:554–565, 1982.
11. Guo GB, Thames MD, Abboud FM: Arterial baroreflexes in renal hypertensive rabbits: Selectivity and redundancy of baroreceptor influence on heart rate, vascular resistance, and lumbar sympathetic nerve activity. Circ Res 53:223, 1983.
12. Coleman TG: Arterial baroreflex control of heart rate in the conscious rat. Am J Physiol 238 (Heart Circ Physiol 7):H515–H520, 1980.
13. Vatner SF, Higgins CB, Franklin D, et al: Extent of carotid sinus regulation of the myocardial contractile state in conscious dogs. J Clin Invest 51:995–1008, 1977.
14. Stephenson RB, Donald DE: Reversible vascular isolation of carotid sinuses in conscious dogs. Am J Physiol 238 (Heart Circ Physiol 7):H809–814, 1980.
15. Stephenson RB, Donald DE: Reflexes from isolated carotid sinuses of intact and vagotomized conscious dogs. Am J Physiol 238 (Heart Circ Physiol 7):H815–H822, 1980.
16. Walgenbach SC, Donald DE: Inhibition by carotid baroreflex of exercise-induced increases in arterial pressure. Circ Res 52:253–262, 1983.
17. Walgenbach SC, Donald DE: Cardiopulmonary reflexes and arterial pressure during rest and exercise in dogs. Am J Physiol 244 (Heart Circ Physiol 13):H362–H369, 1983.
18. Daskalopoulos DA, Shepherd JT, Walgenbach SC: Cardiopulmonary reflexes and blood pressure in exercising sinoaortic-denervated dogs. J Appl Physiol 57:1417–1421, 1984.
19. Smyth HS, Sleight P, Pickering GW: Reflex regulation of arterial pressure during sleep in man. A quantitative method of assessing baroreflex sensitivity. Circ Res 24:109–121, 1969.
20. Eckberg DL, Cavanagh MS, Mark AL, et al: A simplified neck suction device for activation of carotid baroreceptors. J Lab Clin Med 85:167–173, 1975.
21. Gribbin B, Pickering TG, Sleight P, et al: Effect of age and high blood pressure on baroreflex sensitivity in man. Circ Res 29:424–431, 1971.
22. Pickering TG, Gribbin B, Petersen ES, et al: Comparison of the effects of exercise and posture on the baroreflex in man. Circ Res 5:582–586, 1971.
23. Bristow JD, Brown EB, Cunningham DJ, et al: Changes in the baroreceptor–cardiac reflex in exercise. J Physiol (Lond) 201:106–107, 1969.
24. Robinson BF, Epstein SE, Beiser GD, et al: Control of heart rate by the autonomic nervous system. Studies in man on the interrelation between baroreceptor mechanisms and exercise. Circ Res 19:400–411, 1966.
25. Chen RYZ, Fan FC, Schuessler GB, et al: Baroreflex control of heart rate in humans during nitroprusside-induced hypotension. Am J Physiol 243:R18–R24, 1982.
26. Pickering TG, Gribbin B, Sleight P: Comparison of the reflex heart rate response to rising and falling arterial pressure in man. Cardiovasc Res 6:277–283, 1972.
27. Ferguson DW, Abboud FM, Mark AL: Relative contribution of aortic and carotid baroreflexes to heart rate control in man during steady state and dynamic increases in arterial pressure. J Clin Invest 76:2265–2274, 1985.
28. Eckberg DL: Temporal response patterns of the human sinus node to brief carotid baroreceptor stimuli. J Physiol (Lond) 258:769–782, 1976.
29. Eckberg DL, Abboud FM, Mark AL: Modulation of carotid baroreflex responsiveness in man: Effects of posture and propranolol. J Appl Physiol 41:383–387, 1976.
30. Eckberg DL: Baroreflex inhibition of the human sinus node: Importance of stimulus

intensity, duration, and rate of pressure change. J Physiol (Lond) 269:561–577, 1977.

31. Eckberg DL: Nonlinearities of the human carotid baroreceptor-cardiac reflex. Circ Res 47:208–216, 1980.
32. Eckberg DL: Adaptation of the human carotid baroreceptor-cardiac reflex. J Physiol (Lond) 269:579–589, 1977.
33. Fritsch JM, Rea RF, Eckberg DL: Carotid baroreflex resetting during drug-induced arterial pressure changes in humans. Am J Physiol 256:R549–R553, 1989.
34. Vatner SF, Bottcher DH, Heyndrick GR, et al: Reduced baroreflex sensitivity with volume loading in conscious dogs. Circ Res 37:236–242, 1975.
35. Linden RJ: Reflexes from the heart. Prog Cardiovasc Dis 18:201–222, 1975.
36. Edis AJ, Donald DE, Shepherd JT: Cardiovascular reflexes from stretch of pulmonary vein-atrial junctions in the dog. Circ Res 27:1091–1100, 1970.
37. Bishop VS, Malliani A, Thoren P: Cardiac mechanoreceptors. In JT Shepherd, FM Abboud (eds): Handbook of Physiology: Peripheral Circulation and Organ Blood Flow. Vol. III, Part 2. Baltimore, MD, Williams and Wilkins, 1983, pp. 497–555.
38. Baker DG, Coleridge HM, Coleridge JCG: Vagal afferent C fibers from the ventricle. In R Hainsworth, C Kidd, RJ Linden (eds): Cardiac Receptors. Cambridge, U.K., Cambridge University Press, 1979, pp. 117–137.
39. Hintze TH: Reflex regulation of the circulation after stimulation of cardiac receptors by prostaglandins. Fed Proc 46:73–80, 1987.
40. Billman GE, Dickey DT, Teoh KK, et al: Effects of central venous blood volume shifts on arterial baroreflex control of heart rate. Am J Physiol 241:H571–H575, 1981.
41. Pawelczyk JA, Raven PB: Reductions in central venous pressure improve carotid baroreflex responses in conscious men. Am J Physiol 257:H1389–H1395, 1989.
42. Vatner SR, Boettcher DH, Heyndrick GR, et al: Reduced baroreflex sensitivity with volume loading in conscious dogs. Circ Res 37:236–242, 1975.
43. Victor RG, Mark AL: Interaction of cardiopulmonary and carotid baroreflex control of vascular resistance in humans. J Clin Invest 76:1592–1598, 1985.
44. Thames MD, Eastham CL, Marcus ML: Baroreflex control of heart interval in conscious renal hypertensive dogs. Am J Physiol 241:H332–H336, 1981.
45. Bristow JD, Honour AJ, Pickering GW, et al: Diminished baroreflex sensitivity in high blood pressure. Circulation 39:48–54, 1969.
46. Mancia G, Ludbrook J, Ferrari A, et al: Baroreceptor reflexes in human hypertension. Circ Res 43:170–177, 1978.
47. Eckberg DL, Drabinsky M, Braunwald E: Defective cardiac parasympathetic control in patients with heart disease. N Engl J Med 285:877–883, 1971.
48. White CW: Abnormalities in baroreflex control of heart rate in canine heart failure. Am J Physiol 240:H793–H799, 1981.
49. Dibner-Dunlap ME, Thames MD: Reflex control of renal sympathetic nerve activity is preserved in heart failure despite reduced arterial baroreceptor sensitivity. Circ Res 65:1526–1535, 1989.
50. Chen JS, Wang W, Bartholet T, et al: Analysis of baroreflex control of heart rate in conscious dogs with pacing-induced heart failure. Circulation 83:260–267, 1991.
51. White CW: Reversibility of abnormal arterial baroreflex control of heart rate in heart failure. Am J Physiol 241:H778–H782, 1981.
52. Ellenbogen KA, Mohanty PK, Szentpetery S, et al: Baroreflex abnormalities in heart failure: Reversal after orthotopic cardiac transplantation. Circulation 79:51–58, 1989.

CHAPTER 24

Baroreflexes in Health and Disease

V.K. Somers, F.M. Abboud

Arterial baroreceptor perturbations elicit reflex changes in sympathetic and vagal activity. These reflex changes serve to buffer the blood pressure change so as to maintain circulatory homeostasis.

Baroreflex responses primarily affect heart rate, vascular resistance, and the renin angiotensin system. In the intact human, the baroreflex is part of an interactive unit. It influences (and is influenced by) other cardiovascular reflexes such as the chemoreceptor reflex and the cardiopulmonary reflex, and are affected by respiration via the pulmonary afferents as well as by humoral agents such as vasopressin and angiotensin II.

Arterial baroreflexes modulate not only heart rate but also heart rate variability. Baroreflex-mediated vagal activation may also affect atrioventricular (AV) nodal conduction and myocardial contractility. Baroreflex function (and abnormalities thereof) are important in both physiological and pathological conditions. Baroreflex abnormalities may occur in one or more of the afferent, central, efferent, or end-organ components. In humans, analysis of the integrity of the baroreflex-mediated vagal control of the heart is, for the most part, limited to measurements of baseline heart rate, heart rate variability, and heart rate responses to blood pressure changes. Concomitant changes in cardiac sympathetic activity significantly influence these variables. More recently, power spectral analysis of heart rate over time has allowed simultaneous evaluation of both sympathetic and vagal influences on subtle systematic oscillations in heart rate (see also Part V). The sympathetic-linked, low-frequency oscillation occurs at about 0.1 Hz, and is reduced by β blockade. The parasympathetic-linked, high-frequency oscillation occurs at about 0.4 Hz, is closely related to breathing, and is blocked by atropine.

This chapter focuses on the role of the arterial baroreflex in regulating vagal control of the heart in both health and disease in humans. Baroreflex physiology and reflex interactions are examined in detail in other reviews and is discussed only briefly here.

From *Vagal Control of the Heart: Experimental Basis and Clinical Implications* edited by MN Levy, PJ Schwartz © 1994, Futura Publishing Co. Inc., Armonk, NY.

Physiology of the Arterial Baroreflex in Humans

Relative Contributions of Carotid and Aortic Baroreflexes

Arterial baroreflex afferents arise from the aortic and carotid sinus regions. Studies of the relative contributions of each of these receptor regions to steady state and dynamic changes in blood pressure in humans suggest that the aortic baroreceptors exert a slightly greater influence on heart rate control than do the carotid baroreceptors.[1,2] Nevertheless, both aortic and carotid baroreflexes are important in maintaining optimal baroreflex heart rate control. Denervation of either set of baroreflexes impairs the heart rate responses to changes in blood pressure in animals.[3] In contrast, sympathetic responses after selective denervation are, for the most part, preserved. These experiments suggest two important concepts. First, there is a redundancy in baroreflex-mediated sympathetic, but not vagal, responses to blood pressure fluctuations. Second, impaired baroreflex regulation of heart rate does not necessarily imply impaired regulation of vascular responses.

Arterial Baroreflex Interactions

Baroreflex responses derive from interactions between multiple reflex inputs, and are often substantially different from the responses seen when the baroreflex is studied in isolation. Animal studies have shown significant interplay between the baroreflexes and the cardiopulmonary reflexes, the chemoreflexes, and the somatic pressor reflex. These interactions may selectively influence some, but not other, efferent responses. For example, neck suction (baroreflex activation) selectively inhibits the heart rate and splanchnic vascular responses, but not the forearm vascular response to lower body suction.[4]

Other interactions, such as those that occur during breathing and mental stress, also modulate baroreflex efferent responses. Heart rate responses to both neck pressure and neck suction are far more pronounced during expiration than during inspiration.[5,6] Baroreflex parasympathetic modulation by respiration is discussed in detail by Spyer[7] (see also Ch. 5). In brief, respiratory gating at the preganglionic cardiac vagal motor neuron is mediated by both the central respiratory rhythm generator and by lung inflation. Both of these mechanisms are normally in phase, resulting in sinus arrhythmia. Cortical arousal also modulates the baroreflex response. Baroreflex activation by phenylephrine infusion does not eliminate the tachycardia and sympathetic activation induced by mental stress.[8] Thus, such factors as hyperventilation and arousal may affect the heart rate response to baroreflex perturbations.

Lastly, humoral factors, such as vasopressin, angiotensin II, and epinephrine, modify the baroreflex. Vasopressin augments the baroreflex-mediated bradycardia both by sensitizing the baroreflex afferents and by a central mechanism.[4] Angiotensin II acts centrally to attenuate the reflex bradycardia during baroreflex activation.[9] Epinephrine facilitates norepinephrine (NE) release at the nerve terminal.

Thus, the baroreflex is modulated by humoral substances and by other reflexes. These interactions may occur at the afferent, central, or end-organ level.[10] Recognition of potential interactions is important for proper understanding of reflex responses in complex disease states, such as heart failure, in which multiple afferent inputs and humoral mediators are involved.

Baroreflexes in Health

During Exercise

During both dynamic and isometric exercise, there are simultaneous increases in blood pressure and heart rate, and vasoconstriction occurs in the nonexercising muscle and other vascular beds. Therefore, the expected cardiovascular response arising from baroreflex activation by the increase in blood pressure is overridden, and the baroreflex does not inhibit the sympathetic drive induced by exercise. The weight of evidence, though not unequivocal, suggests that the baroreflexes continue to function during both dynamic and isometric exercise. They operate, however, at a higher baseline level of blood pressure and heart rate, and appear to have less gain than they do during rest. Bristow et al,[11] using the heart rate response to phenylephrine, showed that within five seconds of the onset of dynamic exercise, the sensitivity of baroreflex control of heart rate decreased. Reflex sensitivity decreased progressively with increasing exercise. Sleight et al[12] have reported an inverse relationship between baroreflex sensitivity and the rise in blood pressure and NE levels during exercise.

Simulated exercise in anesthetized animals (by electrical stimulation of ventral spinal nerve roots), however, does not alter the bradycardic response to a rise in blood pressure.[13] Hyperventilation or reflex interactions during exercise may inhibit the bradycardic response to arterial baroreceptor activation, perhaps by central actions on vagal cardiac inhibitory neurons. Alternatively, the apparent reduction in the baroreflex gain may reflect appropriate baroreflex resetting to higher blood pressure and heart rate levels. The importance of the baroreflex during exercise may lie in the prevention of excessive heart rate fluctuations, thus providing myocardial protection, rather than in the reduction of blood pressure during exercise.

After Exercise

Blood pressure falls significantly after exercise, and in the second half-hour after exercise, it is markedly lower than before exercise.[14] Faris et al[15] reported that baroreflex gain in rabbits, was markedly reduced immediately after exercise. Somers et al,[16] using the heart period response to bolus injections of phenylephrine before and at various intervals after maximal voluntary exercise, have shown that baroreflex control of heart period is suppressed 10 minutes after exercise. It recovers within 20 minutes, however, and the gain of the baroreflex is significantly greater at 40 and 60 minutes after exercise than it is before exercise. Similarly, Bennett et al[17] have reported that, at 30 and 60 minutes after exercise, lower body suction elicited greater increases in heart rate and forearm vascular resistance (FVR) than it did before exercise.

Increased baroreflex gain after exercise may be mediated by sensitization of baroreflex afferents, either due to the pulsatile pressure during exercise or possibly by humoral factors. Central resetting of baroreflexes by the higher blood pressure levels during exercise may be involved. Increased circulatory catecholamines present immediately after exercise may mask the increased baroreflex gain, which only becomes apparent later in the postexercise period.

Endurance Training

Bristow et al[18] and Eckberg[19] have shown a positive correlation between RR interval and baroreflex sensitivity. These results suggest that people with more sensitive baroreflexes have slower heart rates, and vice versa. Also, their RR intervals are more variable. Endurance training slows heart rate and lowers blood pressure in normal[20] and hypertensive humans.[21] In hypertensive humans, endurance training also increases baroreflex gain. RR variability is also increased, especially during sleep (Fig. 1).[21] Thus, the bradycardia and lower blood pressures that result from endurance training may in part be mediated by an increase in baroreflex sensitivity.[22–24]

Changes in baroreflex gain, RR interval, and RR variability with endurance training may have implications for both the pathophysiology and the consequences of hypertension. Hypertensive patients have an impaired baroreflex control of heart rate,[25,26] and reduced RR range and variability.[26] Early hypertension may be associated with a hyperdynamic state,[27] in which the higher blood pressure levels are accompanied by increased heart rate and cardiac output.

An increased baroreflex gain may have cardioprotective effects. Billman et al[28] showed that, in the period after a myocardial infarction, dogs with more sensitive baroreflexes are resistant to ventricular fibrillation. A subsequent study showed that physical training of these susceptible dogs not only increased baroreflex sensitivity but also protected these dogs against exercise-induced ventricular arrhythmias, including ventricular fibrillation.[29] A correlate derived from studies in humans is that a low baroreflex sensitivity after the first myocardial infarction is associated with a high risk of sudden death.[30]

Baroreflex vagal activity may also affect cardiovascular morbidity and mortality by way of heart rate and of heart rate variability. Coronary arteries are subject to unique flow profiles, with blood flow varying during isovolumic

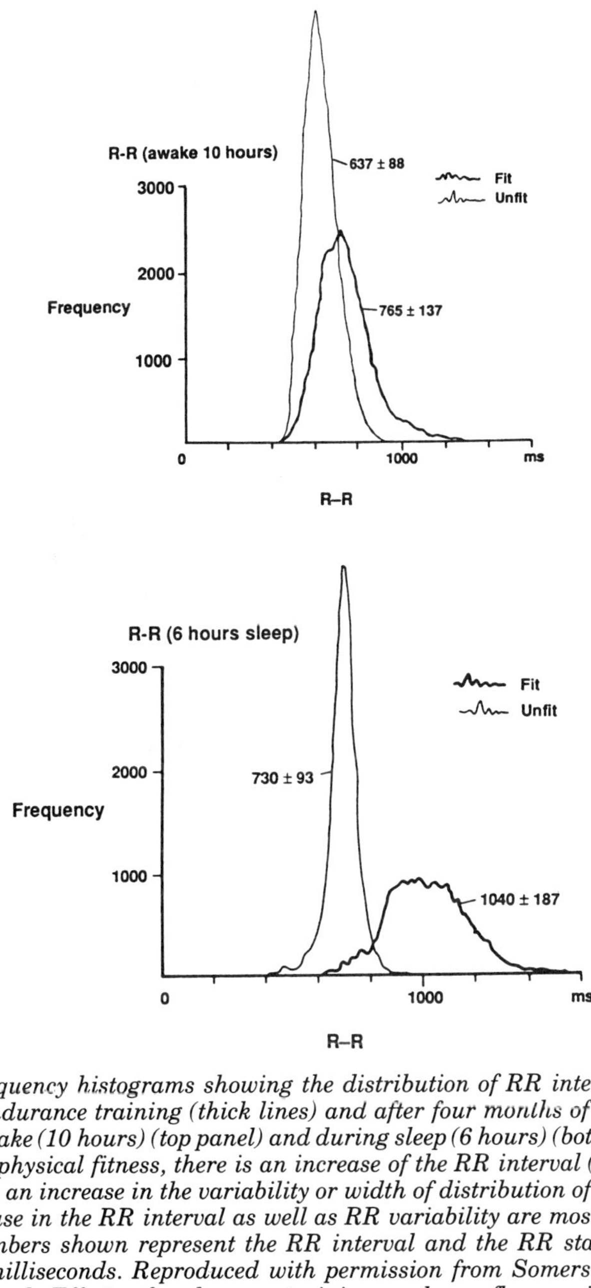

Figure 1. *Frequency histograms showing the distribution of RR intervals in a single subject after endurance training (thick lines) and after four months of detraining (thin lines) when awake (10 hours) (top panel) and during sleep (6 hours) (bottom panel). With an increase in physical fitness, there is an increase of the RR interval (slowing of heart rate) as well as an increase in the variability or width of distribution of the RR interval. Both the increase in the RR interval as well as RR variability are most marked during sleep. The numbers shown represent the RR interval and the RR standard deviation measured in milliseconds. Reproduced with permission from Somers VK, Conway J, Johnston J, et al: Effects of endurance training on baroreflex sensitivity and blood pressure in borderline hypertension. Lancet 337:1363–1368, 1991. Copyright © by The Lancet Ltd.*

cardiac contraction, peak systolic pressure, end systole, isovolumic relaxation, and end diastole.[31] Beere et al[31] proposed that shear stress associated with this unique pulsatile flow profile may explain the predisposition of coronary arteries to plaque deposition, and that faster heart rates would amplify atherogenesis. They tested this hypothesis in monkeys that were fed an atherogenic diet and whose heart rates were lowered by sinoatrial (SA) node ablation. Monkeys with slow heart rates had less than half the coronary atherosclerosis that occurred in monkeys with faster heart rates. These results were independent of blood pressure, lipids, or body weight. Increased baroreflex gain is also associated with increased heart rate variability. Kleiger et al[32] reported an inverse correlation between heart rate variability and mortality after myocardial infarction.

During Sleep

Sleep is divided, on the basis of the electroencephalogram and electromyogram, into rapid eye movement (REM) (or desynchronized) sleep and non-REM (or synchronized) sleep.[33] Non-REM sleep is further subdivided into progressively deepening states, classified as I, II, III, and IV. In humans, during progressively deepening stages of non-REM sleep, blood pressure, heart rate, and sympathetic nerve activity decline.[34,35] By contrast, during REM, there is an increase in heart rate and sympathetic activity, with marked fluctuations in respiration and blood pressure. The role of the baroreflex in mediating these changes in humans is unclear. Attempts to lower blood pressure with nitroprusside in awake humans to levels similar to those seen in Stage IV sleep result in tachycardia and sympathetic excitation.[35] In contrast, bradycardia and decreased sympathetic activity accompanies the hypotension of Stage IV sleep.[35] Thus, the baroreflex is significantly reset during sleep; the reset baroreflex permits heart rate slowing despite blood pressure reduction.

Spectral analysis of 24-hour heart rate and intra-arterial blood pressure measurements suggest an increased baroreflex gain during the nighttime hours. The high-frequency component of power spectral analysis of heart rate variability is increased during sleep. This finding indicates an increased vagal tone.[36] Specific studies of the baroreflex in humans during sleep show that the set point of the reflex is diminished to a lower pressure during non-REM sleep.[37,38] The changes in baroreflex gain are not clear. Smyth et al[37] suggested that the gain of the baroreflex control of heart rate was increased, although a subsequent study[38] did not confirm these findings. Conway et al[39] reported lower blood pressure and increased baroreflex gain during sleep in humans.

Studies of sympathetic activity and heart rate during sleep indicate distinct differences between light and deep non-REM sleep and between REM and non-REM sleep.[34,35] Thus, a clear understanding of the baroreflexes during sleep can only be obtained by specific study of the reflex during each of the different sleep stages. These data are presently not available.

Arousal and Mental Stress

Conway et al[39] measured baroreflex gain during sleep, quiet wakefulness, reading, and verbal mental arithmetic. With progressive increases in mental arousal, baroreflex gain decreased and blood pressure increased, with baroreflex gain (measured by bolus injections of intravenous phenylephrine) being most reduced during mental arithmetic. As a corollary to this, Anderson et al[8] studied the effects of mental arithmetic on heart rate before and during a phenylephrine infusion. Despite the higher baseline blood pressure and slower heart rate during phenylephrine administration, heart rate increases with mental stress were not detectably affected by the phenylephrine. Thus, heart rate responses to baroreflex activation are attentuated during mental stress, and baroreflex activation does not prevent the heart rate response to mental stress.

Ageing

The incidence of hypertension and orthostatic hypotension is increased in the elderly.[40,41] Orthostatic hypotension is also a significant cause of morbidity and mortality, since it leads to injury from syncope and falls.[41,42] Orthostatic hypotension alone affects 20% of medical outpatients over 65 years of age and affects 30% of outpatients over 75 years of age.[41] Impairment of baroreflex mechanisms with advancing age may contribute to both of these problems. Heart rate responses to blood pressure changes are significantly reduced in elderly people.[25,43]

Studies in animals have attempted to clarify the site of the defect. The baroreflex control of heart rate is clearly defective in older animals.[44–47] This defect is not explained by impaired SA node responses to vagal stimulation. The responses are, in fact, enhanced, probably as a consequence of receptor upregulation secondary to decreased tonic vagal efferent activity.[46]

A decreased sensitivity of baroreceptor afferents to changes in arterial pressure has been demonstrated in older rats.[44,48] Attenuated blood pressure changes with aortic depressor nerve stimulation in older rats has also suggested the presence of impaired central mediation of the baroreflex.[45,49] Hajduczok et al[50] have demonstrated rapid adaptation and loss of reflex inhibition of renal sympathetic nerve activity (RSNA) over time during sustained increases in carotid sinus pressure in older dogs. The escape of sympathetic inhibition could not be explained by a decline of afferent input. Hence, this adaptation may occur at a central level (Fig. 2). Thus, ageing is clearly associated with impaired baroreflex control of heart rate. This impairment may occur centrally. The mechanism of the impairment is not known, although Tanabe and Bunag[51] have demonstrated that lesioning of the hypothalamus corrects the reduction in baroreflex sensitivity associated with ageing.

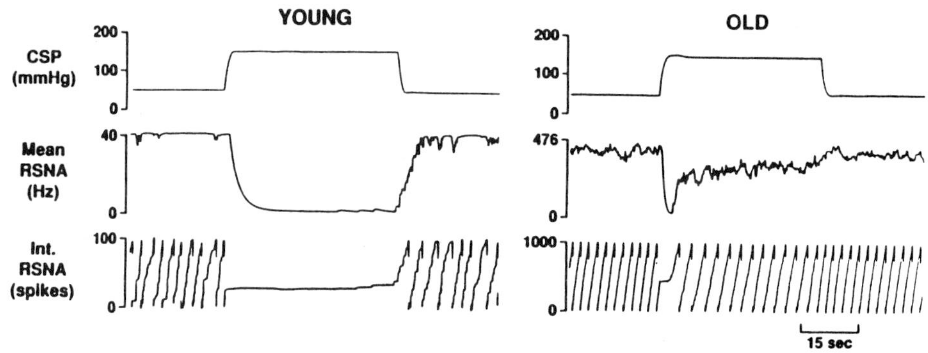

Figure 2. *Recordings of isolated carotid sinus pressure (CSP) and renal sympathetic nerve activity (RSNA) in a young (left) and old (right) dog, showing that baroreflex inhibition of RSNA is sustained in the young, but not the old, dog due to adaptation of the baroreflex with ageing. Reproduced with permission from Hajduczok G, Chapleau MW, Abboud FM: Rapid adaptation of central pathways explains the suppressed baroreflex with aging. Neurobiol Aging 12:601–604, 1991.*

Baroreflexes in Disease

Hypertension

Baroreflex control of heart rate is impaired in patients with established hypertension. Although the baroreflex retains the ability to buffer blood pressure increases, it acts at a higher set point,[18] and the sensitivity of the reflex (as measured by the prolongation of the RR interval in response to intravenous phenylephrine) decreases, independent of the effect of age.[25] The sensitivity of the reflex is negatively correlated with the blood pressure level.[18,52,53] There is also anecdotal evidence that suggests that hypertension occurs in man after surgical denervation of the carotid sinus.[54]

A greater baroreflex sensitivity is associated with an increase in the variability and range of heart rate and a reduction in the variability and range of blood pressure.[52,55] Thus, humans with more sensitive baroreflexes may be able to control blood pressure more tightly over 24 hours by greater variations in heart rate.

Although baroreflex control of heart rate is impaired even in early hypertension, evidence from both animal and human studies indicates that the sympathetic and vascular responses are preserved.[56–58] Thus, earlier hypotheses suggesting that baroreflex impairment may serve to initiate hypertension are likely to be incorrect.

The selective impairment of the heart rate (but not the vascular) responses in early hypertension may be explained by redundancy in the baroreflex control of vascular resistance.[3] In studies in rabbits that experienced six weeks of renal hypertension, Guo and Thames[59] reported preserved baroreflex control of lumbar sympathetic activity, but impaired control of heart rate, probably due to an impairment of the afferent limb of the baroreflex (see also Ch. 23). In chronic (four months) renal hypertensive rabbits, however, both vascular and heart rate responses are impaired, both during arterial pressure changes and during electrical stimulation of baroreflex afferents. These findings suggest central impairment of the baroreflex.[60] Thus, in early hypertension, redundancy in baroreflex control of vascular resistance, but not of heart rate, allows impaired baroreflex afferents to manifest as a selective impairment of the heart rate response to blood pressure changes. In chronic hypertension, both vascular and heart rate responses are impaired, probably via a central mechanism. In studies of the cardiac responsiveness to efferent vagal stimulation and to methacholine in rats, Ferrari et al[61] have demonstrated an exaggerated bradycardia in established hypertensive rats, as compared to early hypertensive and normotensive rats (Fig. 3). These results suggest, first, that the impaired baroreceptor-heart rate reflex cannot be explained by depressed end-organ responsiveness and, second, the excessive sensitivity to cardiac vagal efferent stimulation in hypertensive rats may be secondary to upregulation of cardiac muscarinic receptors (mAChRs) consequent upon the chronically reduced vagal tone in hypertension.

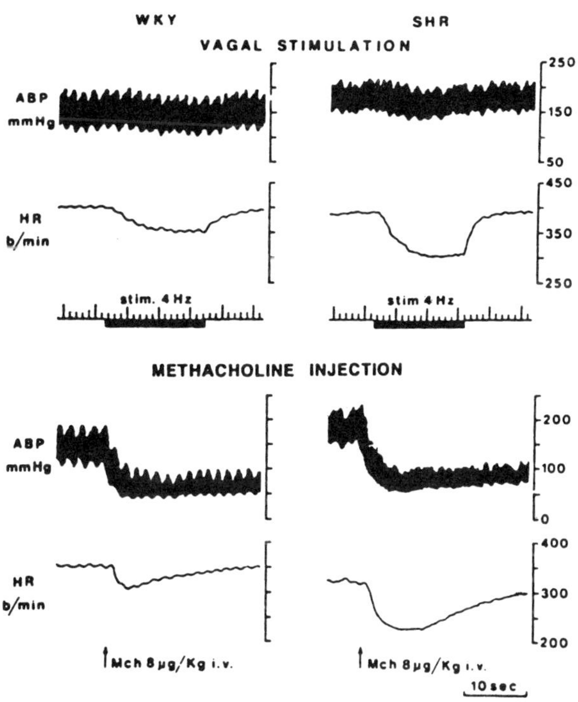

Figure 3. *Recordings of the bradycardic responses to electrical vagal stimulation (top panel) and to methacholine (Mch) injection (bottom panel) in 12-week-old Wistar-Kyoto (WKY) rat and spontaneously hypertensive rat (SHR). Both stimuli elicit greater bradycardic responses in the hypertensive animals, suggesting that SA node sensitivity to vagal stimulation is enhanced rather than impaired, possibly because of a reduction of tonic cardiac vagal activity in hypertension. Reproduced by permission of the American Heart Association, Inc. from Ferrari AU, Daffonchio A, Franzelli C, et al: Cardiac parasympathetic hyperresponsiveness in spontaneously hypertensive rats. Hypertension 19:653–657, 1992.*

Humoral factors (such as renin-angiotensin) may modulate the decreased baroreflex-heart rate gain in hypertension. The reduction in heart rate induced by blood pressure elevation from angiotensin II infusion in humans is significantly less than that seen with equivalent blood pressure elevations evoked by phenylephrine.[62] This finding suggests that angiotensin II inhibits the baroreflex control of heart rate. In addition, acute angiotensin-converting enzyme inhibition in hypertensive humans enhances the baroreflex-mediated parasympathetic responsiveness.[63] Guo and Abboud,[9] in studies in rabbits, concluded that angiotensin II acts centrally to selectively impair baroreflex heart rate responses to increases, but not to decreases, in blood pressure.

Heart Failure

Studies in patients with heart failure have shown that the relationship of the RR interval to the systolic pressure is impaired.[64] Animal studies in models of heart failure confirm that this impairment applies to both increases and decreases in blood pressure.[65] Studies of heart rate variability confirm the existence of impaired regulation in heart failure patients. Dogs with heart failure appear to have a high-resting sympathetic tone and a low-resting vagal tone.[66] These findings are consistent with impaired baroreflex regulation.

The site of this impairment may be at the afferent receptor level. Dibner-Dunlap and Thames[67] have shown that aortic baroreceptor discharge is depressed in dogs with pacing-induced heart failure (see also Ch. 23). Similar data were obtained by Wang et al,[68] who suggested that this abnormality may be explained by an augmentation of Na^+K^+-ATPase activity in the carotid sinus baroreceptor, because cardiac glycosides (ouabain) shifted the pressure-discharge curve towards normal.

Humoral factors (renin, angiotensin, atrial natriuretic factor, and vasopressin) that are increased in heart failure may contribute to the baroreflex impairment. Interactions with other cardiovascular reflexes (cardiopulmonary and ventricular receptors) may also be implicated. Central processing of the afferent signal or the efferent vagal limb may be impaired because there is a selective preservation of baroreflex control of efferent renal sympathetic activity in dogs with pacing-induced heart failure.[69,70] White[71] has shown that the heart rate response to direct vagal nerve stimulation was diminished in dogs with heart failure. These animals also had a depressed SA node responsiveness to cholinergic stimuli, which indicated a defective vagal efferent limb of the baroreflex.

Interestingly, in heart failure patients treated successfully with orthotopic heart transplantation, there is no evidence of impairment of the heart rate response to phenylephrine in the recipient atrium (measured by intracardiac electrograms). The baroreflex sensitivity is similar to that in normal controls.[72] In this cross-sectional study, nontransplanted patients with heart failure had markedly depressed baroreflex slopes (Fig. 4). Three patients with heart failure had baroreflex measurements taken before and after transplantation, and it was found that the baroreflex gain increased substantially after cardiac transplantation (Fig. 5). Subjects were studied within two weeks to four years after

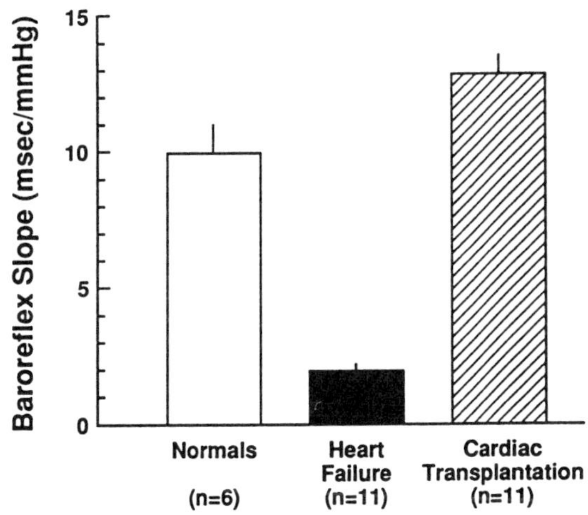

Figure 4. *Bar graph of baroreflex slopes in normal subjects, heart failure patients, and patients with heart failure after cardiac transplantation. Baroreflex slopes in normal and cardiac transplant patients were not significantly different from each other, but were significantly greater than those in heart failure patients. Reproduced by permission of the American Heart Association, Inc. from Ellenbogen KA, Mohanty PK, Szentpetery S, et al: Arterial baroreflex abnormalities in heart failure: Reversal after orthotopic cardiac transplantation. Circulation 79:51–58, 1989.*

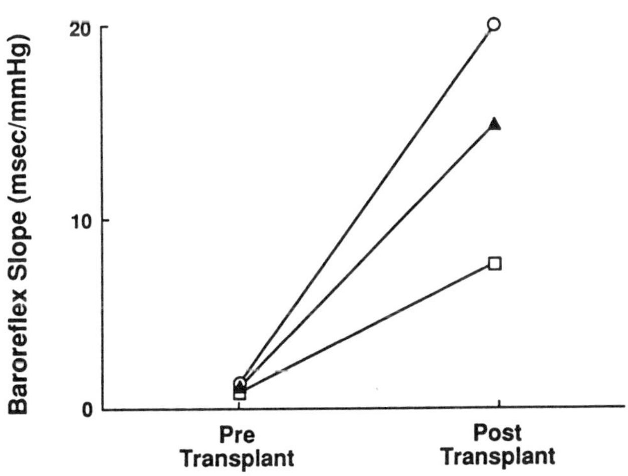

Figure 5. *Changes in baroreflex sensitivity before and after cardiac transplantation in three patients with heart failure. Reproduced by permission of the American Heart Association, Inc. from Ellenbogen KA, Mohanty PK, Szentpetery S, et al: Arterial baroreflex abnormalities in heart failure: Reversal after orthotopic cardiac transplantation. Circulation 79:51–58, 1989.*

transplantation. Thus, neurohumoral factors, rather than structural abnormalities, may be responsible for the baroreflex impairment in heart failure.

In summary, heart failure in humans and animals is associated with impairment of the baroreflex. This impairment may be mediated by afferent, central, efferent, and humoral factors. Baroreflex sensitivity normalizes after cardiac transplantation, which confirms that the reflex impairment is functional rather than structural.

Diabetes

Diabetes is associated with a greatly increased mortality and morbidity. Cardiovascular reflexes are abnormal in diabetic patients, even before any symptoms of peripheral autonomic neuropathy appear.[73,74] Thus, cardiac dysautonomia arising from diabetes may be a very early and common defect, and may contribute to the increased cardiovascular attrition in these patients.

Indeed, mortality and autonomic neuropathy are highly correlated in diabetic patients. In a prospective five-year study of 73 diabetic patients with possible autonomic neuropathy, Ewing et al[75] found that 26 of the 73 patients died in the period of follow-up (Fig. 6). Twenty-one of these 26 patients had abnormal cardiovascular reflexes at first testing. In patients with autonomic symptoms and abnormal autonomic function, the calculated mortality rate was markedly increased to 56% at five years. Of the 21 patients with evidence of autonomic dysfunction who died, half died of renal failure. The other half died of causes possibly related to autonomic neuropathy. Six of these patients died suddenly. Hence, the sudden death of these patients may have been related to cardiac parasympathetic dysautonomia.

Watkins and Mackay[76] studied the incidence of cardiac denervation in patients with diabetes. They used the heart rate variation with deep breathing as an index of the integrity of parasympathetic control of the heart. They studied 54 normal subjects, 143 diabetics without neuropathy, 93 diabetics with peripheral neuropathy but without clinical evidence of autonomic neuropathy, and 64 patients with clinical evidence of autonomic neuropathy and peripheral neuropathy. About 7% of the diabetics without any other evidence of neuropathy showed some evidence of abnormal parasympathetic control of the heart. Twenty-nine percent of the patients with peripheral neuropathy showed this abnormality, and 84% of those patients with autonomic neuropathy also had an abnormal heart rate variation with breathing. Therefore, the absence of peripheral neuropathy does not necessarily imply an intact autonomic control of the circulation.

In a study of 10 young diabetics without symptoms of autonomic neuropathy and 12 age-matched controls, Eckberg et al[77] reported subnormal RR variability and attenuated changes in RR interval in response to changes in blood pressure in the diabetic subjects. Assessment of heart rate variability by power spectral analysis has confirmed the presence of diminished RR variance in patients with uncomplicated diabetes.[78–80]

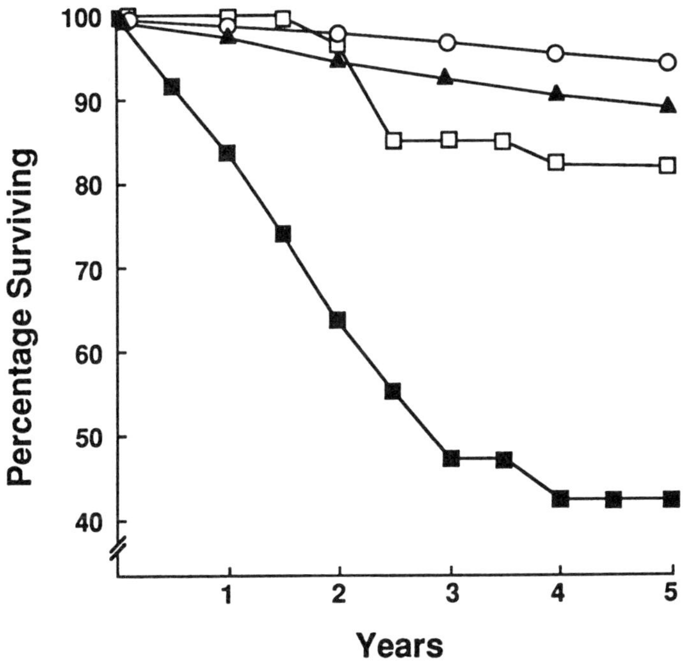

Figure 6. *Five-year survival curves for age- and sex-matched general population (expected) (open circles), diabetic population (expected) (closed triangles), 33 diabetic patients with normal (open squares), and 40 diabetic patients with abnormal autonomic function tests (closed squares), indicating the increased mortality in diabetic patients with significant dysautonomia. Reproduced with permission of Oxford Univesity Press from Ewing DJ, Campbell IW, Clarke BF: The natural history of diabetic autonomic neuropathy. Q J Med 49(193):95, 1980.*

The location of the autonomic defect in diabetic patients is unclear. The defect may be located within the afferent and/or the efferent limbs of the reflex arc. Bennett et al[81] found that cardiac responses to hypotension were intact, but responses to hypertension were suppressed in diabetic patients.

Bennett et al[82,83] have also reported that diabetics with decreased RR variability at rest may still exhibit substantial RR variability during sleep and during face immersion. These findings, as well as those of Eckberg et al,[77] that suggested that the baseline RR standard deviation does not predict the RR response to blood pressure changes may argue against the presence of a significant vagal efferent defect.

Eckberg et al[77] suggested that the defect may lie at the central processing level. Diabetic patients with abnormal regulation of baseline and reflex RR intervals also had prolonged brain stem auditory-evoked potentials. This finding indicates the presence of central neural abnormalities in diabetes,[84] but does not establish any causal relationship.

In studies of diabetic rabbits, McDowell et al[85,86] have reported a selective defect in baroreflex-mediated parasympathetic activation. Neither afferent input nor reflex renal sympathetic responses was impaired. This finding again suggests that the defect may lie at the central level.

Central processing may also be influenced by interactions between the baroreflex and other cardiovascular afferent inputs. For example, cardiac afferents may be impaired in diabetes. Studies on diabetic dogs showed significant changes in myocardial stiffness over a period of one year.[87] The stiffness was associated with accumulation of glycoproteins and lipids in the myocardium and was not reversed by insulin treatment.[88] This decreased cardiac compliance may impair the cardiac baroreflex afferents, which consist mainly of stretch receptors.

Diabetes appears to be associated with both sympathetic and vagal dysautonomia. Selective vagal dysfunction occurs early in diabetes. It may be mediated in part by central mechanisms, and it could be implicated in sudden death in diabetic patients.

Carotid Sinus Hypersensitivity

In 1930, Roskam[89] reported the association of recurrent syncope with hypotension and bradycardia and suggested that this occurrence may be due to a hypersensitive carotid sinus reflex. Weiss and Baker[90] subsequently demonstrated that, in 15 cases, unconsciousness and convulsions could be induced by exerting pressure over one carotid sinus. They suggested that the carotid sinus mechanism was abnormally sensitive.

The syndrome of carotid sinus hypersensitivity, once thought to be a variant of the sick sinus syndrome, is now recognized as an entity in its own right. The syndrome increases with age (usually in patients over 50), is more common in males, may be associated with resting sinus bradycardia and aortic stenosis,[91] and may be evoked primarily by right carotid sinus massage.

The syndrome has been classified as cardioinhibitory (in which carotid sinus massage induces asystole for >3 seconds) (Fig. 7), vasodepressor (in which systolic blood pressure falls by >50 mm Hg without significant fall in heart rate), and mixed (in which cardioinhibitory and vasodepressor effects occur together).[92] The mixed type is most common, and the pure vasodepressor type is rare.

Diagnosis may be made by massage of each carotid sinus for about 15 seconds, with a positive test indicated by asystole, sinus arrest, or complete heart block lasting >3 seconds, with or without symptoms typical of a spontaneous attack (Fig. 7).[93]

There is a significant incidence (28%) of carotid sinus hypersensitivity in patients with unexplained syncope.[94] Diagnosis is important, as the syndrome (especially the cardioinhibitory type) is eminently treatable. Trout et al[95] have reported good results from carotid sinus denervation. Patients with significant cardioinhibition benefit from dual-chamber pacing. Single-chamber (VVI)

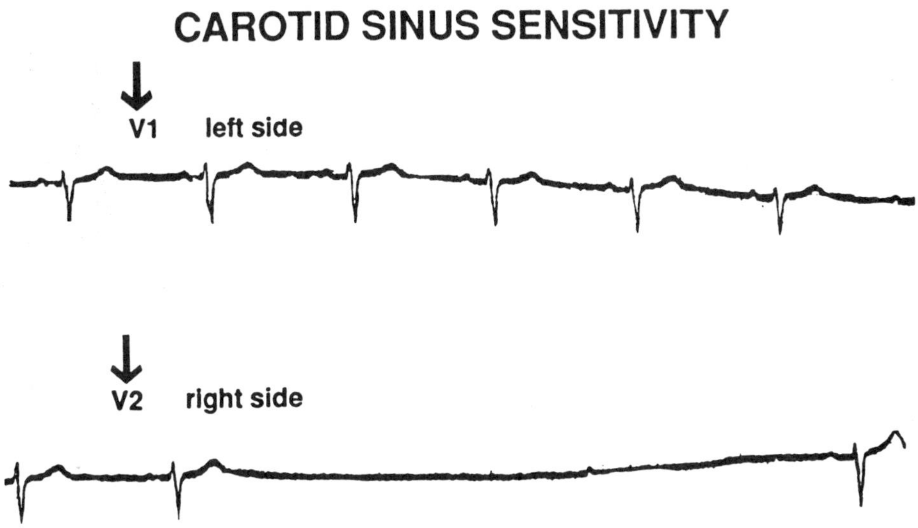

Figure 7. *EKG tracing showing period of asystole after stimulation of the right, but not the left, carotid sinus. Reproduced with permission from Trout HH, Brown LL, Thompson JE: Carotid sinus syndrome: Treatment by carotid sinus denervation. Ann Surg 189(5):575, 1979.*

pacing may augment the vasodepressor component, and dual-chamber pacing (DVI) is the optimal pacing mode.[96]

The underlying defect in the carotid sinus syndrome is unclear. Patients with the syndrome exhibit an exaggerated bradycardic response to intravenous phenylephrine injection.[97] There does not appear to be any characteristic histologic abnormality in the carotid sinuses of these patients.[98] Baig et al[99] have hypothesized that the defect may be at the central processing level.

Clinical Aspects of Ventricular Receptors

A detailed discussion of ventricular mechanoreceptors and their clinical consequences is beyond the scope of this chapter and is reviewed elsewhere.[100] In brief, nerve endings in the ventricle may be activated mechanically (by cardiac distension or contraction) or chemically (by veratridine or nicotine). Activation induces hypotension and bradycardia (Bezold-Jarisch reflex). This reflex may contribute to hypotension, bradycardia, and syncope in a number of clinical conditions, including aortic stenosis, vasovagal syncope, coronary arteriography,[101] and inferoposterior myocardial infarction. Syncopal responses to drugs such as nitroglycerin and isoproterenol[102,103] may also be mediated via this mechanism, as may the paradoxical bradycardia during nitroprusside-induced hypotension in patients with preeclampsia (a syndrome itself associated with arterial baroreflex impairment) (Fig. 8).[104]

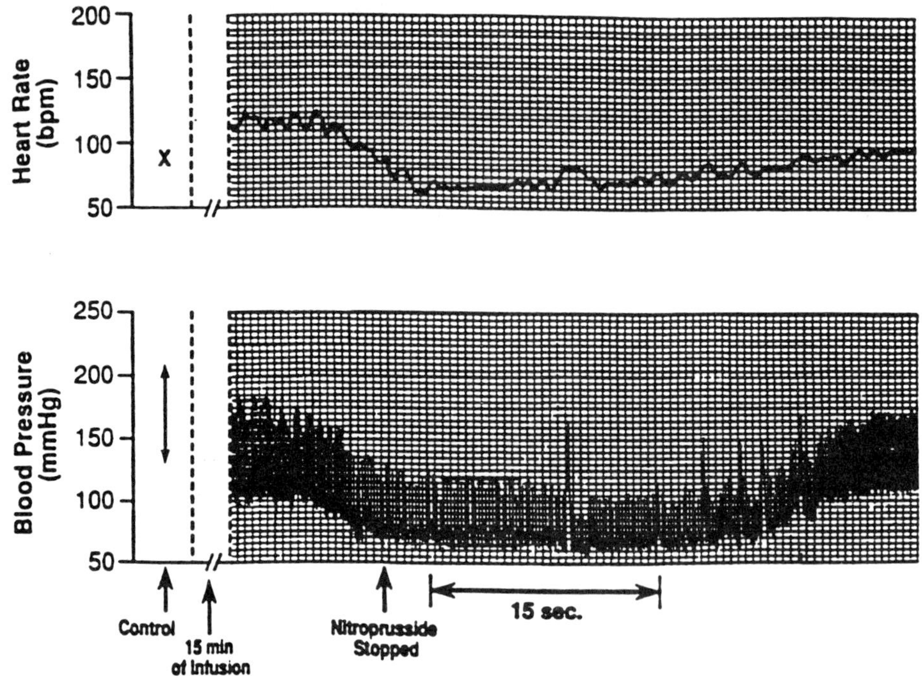

Figure 8. *Recording showing time-course of hypotension and bradycardia in a patient with preeclampsia during an infusion of nitroprusside. There is a paradoxical bradycardia accompanying the hypotension. Reproduced by permission of the American Heart Association, Inc. from Wasserstrum N: Nitroprusside in preeclampsia: Circulatory distress and paradoxical bradycardia. Hypertension 18:79, 1991.*

Conclusion

Baroreflex modulation of heart rate contributes significantly to circulatory control in normal humans. Impairment of the baroreflex may be involved in the maintenance of circulatory disorders. There is unequivocal evidence for the existence of baroreflex abnormalities in the disorders described, as well as indications that these abnormalities may have prognostic implications.

The precise neurohumoral, biochemical, and molecular mechanisms that underlie the parasympathetic reflex abnormality in different disease states have yet to be clarified, primarily because of limitations with regard to animal models of human disease, and the lack of methods for accurate study of all components of the reflex arc in humans.

Acknowledgment: The authors would like to express appreciation to Ms. Nancy Stamp for expert typing of this manuscript.

References

1. Mancia G, Ferrari A, Gregorini L, et al: Circulatory reflexes from carotid and extracarotid baroreceptor areas in man. Circ Res 41:309, 1977.
2. Ferguson DW, Abboud FM, Mark AL: Relative contribution of aortic and carotid baroreflexes in heart rate control in man during steady state and dynamic increases in arterial pressure. J Clin Invest 76:2265, 1985.
3. Guo GB, Thames MD, Abboud FM: Differential baroreflex control of heart rate and vascular resistance in rabbits. Relative role of carotid, aortic, and cardiopulmonary baroreceptors. Circ Res 50:554, 1982.
4. Abboud FM: Interaction of cardiovascular reflexes in humans. In B Lown, A Malliani, M Prosdocimi (eds): Neural Mechanisms and Cardiovascular Disease. Padova, Liviana Press, 1986, p. 73.
5. Eckberg DL, Orshan CR: Respiratory and baroreceptor reflex interactions in man. J Clin Invest 59:780, 1977.
6. Trzebski A, Raczkowska M, Kubin L: Carotid baroreceptor reflex in man, its modulation over the respiratory cycle. Acta Neurobiol Exp 40:807, 1980.
7. Spyer KM: Neural organization and control of the baroreceptor reflex. Rev Physiol Biochem Pharmacol 88:23–124, 1981.
8. Anderson EA, Sinkey CA, Mark AL: Mental stress increases sympathetic nerve activity during sustained baroreceptor stimulation in humans. Hypertension 17 (suppl III):III43, 1991.
9. Guo GB, Abboud FM: Angiotensin II attenuates baroreflex control of heart rate and sympathetic activity. Am J Physiol 246:H80, 1984.
10. Abboud FM, Thames MD: Interaction of cardiovascular reflexes in circulatory control. In JT Shepherd, FM Abboud (eds): Handbook of Physiology. Section 3: The Cardiovascular System. Bethesda, MD, American Physiological Society, 1984, p. 675.
11. Bristow JD, Brown EB, Cunningham DJC, et al: Effect of bicycling on the baroreflex regulation of pulse interval. Circ Res 28:582, 1971.
12. Sleight P, Floras JS, Hassan MO, et al: Baroreflex control of blood pressure and plasma noradrenaline during exercise in essential hypertension. Clin Sci 57:169S, 1979.
13. Streatfield KA, Davison NS, McCloskey DI: Muscular reflex and baroreflex influences on heart rate during isometric contractions. Cardiovasc Res 11:87, 1977.
14. Somers VK, Conway J, Coats A, et al: Post-exercise hypotension is not sustained in normal and hypertensive humans. Hypertension 18:211, 1991.
15. Faris IB, Jamieson GG, Ludbrook J: Effect of exercise on gain of the carotid-sinus reflex in rabbits. Clin Sci 63:115, 1982.
16. Somers VK, Conway J, LeWinter M, et al: The role of baroreflex sensitivity in post-exercise hypotension? J Hypertens 3(suppl 3):S129, 1985.
17. Bennett T, Wilcox RG, MacDonald IA: Post-exercise reduction of blood pressure in hypertensive men is not due to acute impairment of baroreflex function. Clin Sci 67:97, 1984.
18. Bristow JD, Honour AJ, Pickering GW, et al: Diminished baroreflex sensitivity in high blood pressure. Circulation 39:48, 1969.
19. Eckberg DL: Transfer characteristics of the human carotid baroreceptor reflex. J Physiol (Lond) 269:561, 1977.
20. Somers VK, Conway J, Sleight P: The effect of physical training on home blood pressure measurements in normal subjects. J Hypertens 4(suppl 6): S657, 1986.
21. Somers VK, Conway J, Johnston J, et al: Effects of endurance training on baroreflex sensitivity and blood pressure in borderline hypertension. Lancet 337:1363, 1991.

22. Clausen JP: Circulatory adjustments to dynamic exercise and effect of physical training in normal subjects and in patients with coronary artery disease. Prog Cardiovasc Dis 18:459, 1976.
23. Blomqvist CG, Saltin B: Cardiovascular adaptation to physical training. Annu Rev Physiol 45:169, 1983.
24. McMahon M, Palmer RM: Exercise and hypertension. Med Clin North Am 69:57, 1985.
25. Gribbin R, Pickering TG, Sleight P, et al: The effect of age and high blood pressure on baroreflex sensitivity in man. Circ Res 29:424, 1971.
26. Conway J: Hemodynamic aspects of essential hypertension in humans. Physiol Rev 64:617, 1984.
27. Julius S, Esler M: Autonomic nervous cardiovascular regulation in borderline hypertension. Am J Cardiol 36:685, 1975.
28. Billman GE, Schwartz PJ, Stone HL: Baroreceptor reflex control of heart rate. A predictor of sudden cardiac death. Circulation 66:874, 1982.
29. Billman GE, Schwartz PJ, Stone HL: The effects of daily exercise on susceptibility to sudden cardiac death. Circulation 69:1182, 1984.
30. La Rovere MT, Speechia G, Mortara A, et al: Baroreflex sensitivity, clinical correlates, and cardiovascular mortality among patients with a first myocardial infarction. A prospective study. Circulation 78:816, 1988.
31. Beere PA, Glagov S, Zarins CK: Retarding effect of lowered heart rate on coronary atherosclerosis. Science 226:180, 1984.
32. Kleiger RE, Miller JP, Bigger JT Jr, et al: Heart rate variability: A variable predicting mortality following acute myocardial infarction. Am J Cardiol 59:256, 1987.
33. Mancia G, Zanchetti A: Cardiovascular regulation during sleep. In J Oren, CD Barnes (eds): Physiology in Sleep. New York, NY, Academic Press, 1980, p. 2.
34. Hornyak M, Cejnar M, Elam M, et al: Sympathetic muscle nerve activity during sleep in man. Brain 114:1281, 1991.
35. Somers VK, Dyken ME, Mark AL, et al: Sympathetic-nerve activity during sleep in normal subjects. N Engl J Med 328:303, 1993.
36. Furlan R, Guzzette S, Crivellaro W, et al: Continuous 24-hour assessment of the neural regulation of systemic arterial pressure and RR variabilities in ambulant subjects. Circulation 81:537, 1990.
37. Smyth HS, Sleight P, Pickering GW: Reflex regulation of arterial pressure during sleep in man: A quantitative method of assessing baroreflex sensitivity. Circ Res 24:109, 1969.
38. Bristow JD, Honour AJ, Pickering TG, et al: Cardiovascular and respiratory changes during sleep in normal and hypertensive subjects. Cardiovasc Res 3:476, 1969.
39. Conway J, Boon N, Jones JV, et al: Involvement of the baroreceptor reflexes in the changes in blood pressure with sleep and mental arousal. Hypertension 5:746, 1983.
40. Landahl S, Bengtsson C, Sigurdsson JA, et al: Age-related changes in blood pressure. Hypertension 8:1044, 1986.
41. Lipsitz LA: Orthostatic hypotension in the elderly. N Engl J Med 321:952, 1989.
42. Sehested P, Severin-Neilsen T: Falls by hospitalized elderly patients: Causes and prevention. Geriatrics 34:101, 1979.
43. Shimada K, Kitazumi T, Sadakane N, et al: Age related changes in baroreflex function, plasma norepinephrine and blood pressure. Hypertension 7:113, 1985.
44. Rothbaum DA, Shaw DJ, Angell CS, et al: Age differences in the baroreceptor response of rats. J Gerontol 29:488, 1974.
45. Tanabe S, Bunag RD: Age-related central and baroreceptor impairment in female Sprague-Dawley rats. Am J Physiol 256:H1399, 1989.
46. Ferrari AU, Daffonchio A, Mancia G: Alterations in cardiac parasympathetic function in aged rats. Am J Physiol 260:H647, 1991.

47. Hajduczok G, Chapleau MW, Johnson SL, et al: Increase in sympathetic activity with age. I. Role of impairment of arterial baroreflexes. Am J Physiol 260:H1113, 1991.
48. Andresen MC: Short- and long-term determinants of baroreceptor function in aged normotensive and spontaneously hypertensive rats. Circ Res 54:750, 1984.
49. Ma S, Chapleau MW, Abboud FM: Defect in central mediation of the baroreflex with aging. FASEB J 6:A951, 1992.
50. Hajduczok G, Chapleau MW, Abboud FM: Rapid adaptation of central pathways explains the suppressed baroreflex with aging. Neurobiol Aging 12:601, 1991.
51. Tanabe S, Baunag RD: Aging escalates baroreceptor reflex suppression by the posterior hypothalamus in rats. Hypertension 17:80, 1991.
52. Conway J, Boon N, Davies C, et al: Neural and humoral mechanisms involved in blood pressure variability. J Hypertens 2:203, 1984.
53. Welch K, Ward A, Hanson P: Exercise blood pressure and baroreflex function in borderline hypertensive and normotensive young men. Clin Sci 68:631, 1985.
54. Pickering TG, Sleight P: Baroreceptors and hypertension. In W de Jong, AP Provoost, AP Shapiro (eds): Progress in Brain Research: Hypertension and Brain Mechanisms. Amsterdam, Elsevier, 1977, pp. 43–60.
55. Mancia G, Parati G, Pomidossi G, et al: Arterial baroreflexes and blood pressure and heart rate variabilities in humans. Hypertension 8:147, 1986.
56. Mancia G, Ferrari L, Gregorini G, et al: Control of blood pressure by carotid sinus baroreceptors in human beings. Am J Cardiol 44:895, 1979.
57. Guo GB, Thames MD, Abboud FM: Impaired control of vascular resistance after denervation of either carotid or aortic baroreceptors in hypertension. Clin Res 29:201A, 1981. Abstract.
58. Rea RF, Hamdan M: Baroreflex control of muscle sympathetic nerve activity in borderline hypertension. Circulation 82:856, 1990.
59. Guo GB, Thames MD: Abnormal baroreflex control in renal hypertension is due to abnormal baroreceptors. Am J Physiol 245:H420, 1983.
60. Guo GB, Abboud FM: Impaired central mediation of the arterial baroreflex in chronic renal hypertension. Am J Physiol 246:H720, 1984.
61. Ferrari AU, Daffonchio A, Franzelli C, et al: Cardiac parasympathetic hyperresponsiveness in spontaneously hypertensive rats. Hypertension 19:653, 1992.
62. Matsukawa T, Totoh E, Miyajima E, et al: Angiotensin II inhibits baroreflex control of muscle sympathetic nerve activity and the heart rate in patients with essential hypertension. J Hypertens 6(suppl 4):S501, 1988.
63. Zanchetti A: The clinical role of angiotensin converting enzyme inhibitors in antihypertensive therapy in the 1990s. J Hypertens 7(suppl 5):S37, 1989.
64. Eckberg DL, Drabinsky M, Braunwald E: Defective cardiac parasympathetic control in patients with heart disease. N Engl J Med 285:877, 1971.
65. Vatner SF, Higgins CB, Braunwald E: Sympathetic and parasympathetic components of reflex tachycardia induced by hypotension in conscious dogs with and without heart failure. Cardiovasc Res 8:153, 1974.
66. Chen J-S, Wang W, Bartholet T, et al: Analysis of baroreflex control of heart rate in conscious dogs with pacing-induced heart failure. Circulation 83:260, 1991.
67. Dibner-Dunlap ME, Thames MD: Arterial baroreflex control of renal sympathetic nerve activity is preserved in heart failure. Circulation 78:II-365, 1988. Abstract.
68. Wang W, Chen J-S, Zucker IH: Carotid sinus baroreceptor sensitivity in experimental heart failure. Circulation 81:1959, 1990.
69. Dibner-Dunlap ME, Thames MD: Baroreflex control of renal sympathetic nerve activity is preserved in heart failure despite reduced arterial baroreceptor sensitivity. Circ Res 65:1526, 1989.
70. Wang W, Chen J-S, Zucker IH: Carotid sinus baroreceptor reflex in dogs with experimental heart failure. Circ Res 68:1294, 1991.
71. White CW: Abnormalities in baroreflex control of heart rate in canine heart failure. Am J Physiol 240:H793, 1981.

72. Ellenbogen KA, Mohanty PK, Szentpetery S, et al: Arterial baroreflex abnormalities in heart failure: Reversal after orthotopic cardiac transplantation. Circulation 79:51, 1989.
73. Ewing DJ: Cardiovascular reflexes and autonomic neuropathy. Clin Sci Mol Med 55:321, 1978.
74. Clarke BF, Ewing DJ, Campbell IW: Diabetic autonomic neuropathy. Diabetologia 17:195, 1979.
75. Ewing DJ, Campbell IW, Clarke BF: The natural history of diabetic autonomic neuropathy. Q J Med 49:95, 1980.
76. Watkins PJ, Mackay JD: Cardiac denervation in diabetic neuropathy. Ann Intern Med 92(Part 2):304, 1980.
77. Eckberg DL, Harkins SW, Fritsch JM, et al: Baroreflex control of plasma norepinephrine and heart period in healthy subjects and diabetic patients. J Clin Invest 78:366, 1986.
78. Kitney RI, Byrne S, Edmonds ME, et al: Heart rate variability in the assessment of autonomic diabetic neuropathy. Automedica 4:144, 1982.
79. Lishner M, Akselrod S, Mor Avi V, et al: Spectral analysis of heart rate fluctuations. A non-invasive, sensitive method for the early diagnosis of autonomic neuropathy in diabetes mellitus. J Auton Nerv Syst 19:987, 1991.
80. Pagani M, Malfatto G, Pierini S, et al: Spectral analysis of heart rate variability in the assessment of autonomic diabetic neuropathy. J Auton Nerv Syst 23:143, 1988.
81. Bennett T, Hosking DJ, Hampton JR: Baroreflex sensitivity and responses to the Valsalva manoeuvre in subjects with diabetes mellitus. J Neurol Neurosurg Psychiatry 39:178, 1976.
82. Bennett T, Fentem PH, Fitton D, et al: Assessment of vagal control of the heart in diabetes. Measures of R-R interval variation under different conditions. Br Heart J 39:25, 1977.
83. Bennett T, Farquhar IK, Hosking DJ, et al: Assessment of methods for estimating autonomic nervous control of the heart in patients with diabetes mellitus. Diabetes 27:1167, 1978.
84. Donald MW, Erdahl DLW, Surridge DHC, et al: Functional correlates of reduced central conduction velocity in diabetic subjects. Diabetes 33:627, 1984.
85. McDowell TS, Chapleau MW, Hajduczok G, et al: Selective impairment of parasympathetic control of heart rate in conscious diabetic rabbits. FASEB J 4:A285, 1990.
86. McDowell TS, Chapleau MW, Hajduczok G, et al: Site of baroreflex dysfunction in diabetes. Circulation 82:III-335, 1990.
87. Regan TJ, Ettinger PO, Khan MI, et al: Altered myocardial function and metabolism in chronic diabetes mellitus without ischemia in dogs. Circ Res 35:222, 1974.
88. Regan TJ, Wu CF, Yeh CK, et al: Myocardial composition and function in diabetes. The effects of chronic insulin use. Circ Res 49:1268, 1981.
89. Roskam J: Un syndrome nouveau. Syncopes cardiaques graves et syncopes repetees par hyperreflexivite sino-carotidienne. Presse Med 38:590, 1930.
90. Weiss S, Baker JP: The carotid sinus reflex in health and disease: Its role in the causation of fainting and convulsions. Medicine 12:297, 1993.
91. Hartzler GO, Maloney JD: Cardioinhibitory carotid sinus hypersensitivity. Arch Intern Med 137:727, 1977.
92. Lown B, Levine SA: The carotid sinus: Clinical value of its stimulation. Circulation 23:766, 1961.
93. Morley CA: A study of the mechanism of carotid sinus hypersensitivity and the treatment of carotid sinus syndrome. Oxford, University of Oxford, 1985, p. 23. Thesis.
94. Huang SKS, Ezri JD, Hauser RG, et al: Carotid sinus hypersensitivity in patients with unexplained syncope: Clinical, electrophysiologic, and long-term follow-up observations. Am Heart J 116:989, 1988.
95. Trout HH, Brown LL, Thompson JE: Carotid sinus syndrome: Treatment by carotid sinus denervation. Ann Surg 189:575, 1979.

96. Madigan NP, Flaker GC, Curtis JJ, et al: Carotid sinus hypersensitivity: Beneficial effects of dual-chamber pacing. Am J Cardiol 53:1034, 1984.
97. Morley CA, Dehn TCB, Perrins EJ, et al: Baroreflex sensitivity measured by the phenylephrine pressor test in patients with carotid sinus and sick sinus syndromes. Cardiovasc Res 18:752, 1984.
98. Beaujean MA, Boland J, Bodson L: The therapeutic approach of the carotid sinus hyperreflexivity (Roskams disease). In C Meere (ed): Proceedings of the VIth World Symposium on Cardiac Pacing. Montreal, Laplante & Languein, 1979, Chapter 13.
99. Baig W, Kaye GC, Perrins EJ: Hypothesis: Can central neuropeptides be implicated in carotid sinus reflex hypersensitivity? Med Hypotheses 28:235, 1989.
100. Abboud FM: Ventricular syncope. Is the heart a sensory organ? N Engl J Med 320:390, 1989.
101. Eckberg DL, White CW, Kioschos JM, et al: Mechanisms mediating bradycardia during coronary arteriography. J Clin Invest 54:1455, 1974.
102. Waxman MB, Yao L, Camerson DA, et al: Isoproterenol induction of vasodepressor-type reaction in vasodepressor-prone persons. Am J Cardiol 63:58, 1989.
103. Almquist A, Goldenberg IF, Milstein S, et al: Provocation of bradycardia and hypotension by isoproterenol and upright posture in patients with unexplained syncope. N Engl J Med 320:346, 1989.
104. Wasserstrum N: Nitroprusside in preeclampsia: Circulatory distress and paradoxical bradycardia. Hypertension 18:79, 1991.

CHAPTER 25

Chemoreflex Control of Cardiac Vagal Activity

V.K. Somers, F.M. Abboud

The arterial chemoreceptors are located in the carotid bodies (at the bifurcation of the common carotid artery) and the aortic bodies (situated along the aortic arch). Chemoreflex responses to hypoxia in humans are mediated mainly by stimulation of receptors in the carotid bodies. Hypercapnia and acidosis also elicit increases in chemoreceptor afferent discharge, and these conditions potentiate the effects of hypoxia.[1–4]

The predominant responses to chemoreflex activation are increases in ventilation and selective, sympathetically-mediated vasoconstriction, as well as vagally-mediated bradycardia. These three responses interact with each other, so that in the intact animal exposed to hypoxia, the predominant response is hyperventilation, with accompanying tachycardia rather than chemoreflex-mediated bradycardia. Other responses include neurogenic vasodilation in coronary (cholinergic vasodilation)[5] and cutaneous (noncholinergic vasodilation) vessels[6] and nonneurogenic cerebral vasodilation. Thus, there is great selectivity in reflex responses to chemoreceptor stimulation. Studies of the chemoreflex, especially in humans, have focused mainly on the ventilatory and vasoconstrictor responses. The vagal response to chemoreflex activation, however, has received limited attention, especially with regard to its role in disease states.[7] This chapter examines the effects of chemoreflex activation, with emphasis on cardiac vagal responses. The clinical significance of chemoreflex-mediated vagal activation and the importance of chemoreflex interactions with other reflexes are discussed. Hypotheses that implicate the chemoreflex as well as chemoreflex-baroreflex interactions in several disease states are also proposed.

Chemoreflex Responses to Hypoxia

The intact animal responds to hypoxia by chemoreflex-mediated increases in ventilation. Perfusion of vital organs such as the heart and brain is maintained by chemoreflex-induced sympathetic vasoconstriction in nonessential vascular

From *Vagal Control of the Heart: Experimental Basis and Clinical Implications* edited by MN Levy, PJ Schwartz © 1994, Futura Publishing Co. Inc., Armonk, NY.

beds such as the muscle, splanchnic, and renal vascular beds.[8] This sympathetic vasoconstriction occurs in opposition to the direct vasodilator action of hypoxia. Although heart rate usually increases during hypoxia, the primary reflex response to hypoxia is bradycardia, due to increased vagal efferent activity.[9] This bradycardia becomes evident only when the ventilatory response to hypoxia is eliminated; that is, during apnea. Apnea also potentiates the sympathetic response to hypoxia.[10,11] Thus, ventilatory, sympathetic, and vagal responses to chemoreflex activation interact with each other so that the ventilatory response attenuates the sympathetic and vagal responses. This ventilatory inhibition of autonomic activity is mediated by central inhibition of the cardiac vagal motoneuron (CVM) by central inspiratory neuronal activity, as well as by vagal afferents from thoracic stretch receptors.[12] Reduction in carbon dioxide tension during hyperventilation may also partially buffer the chemoreflex response to hypoxia. The bradycardic response, therefore, is evident only with elimination of the ventilatory response, for example, during apnea.

Chemoreflex-mediated cardiac vagal activation may also induce coronary vasodilation. Hackett et al,[5] in studies in anesthetized dogs, reported that stimulation of arterial chemoreceptors with nicotine or cyanide, as well as carotid sinus nerve stimulation, caused abrupt and sustained coronary vasodilation (Fig. 1). Vagotomy and atropine attenuated this response. This attenua-

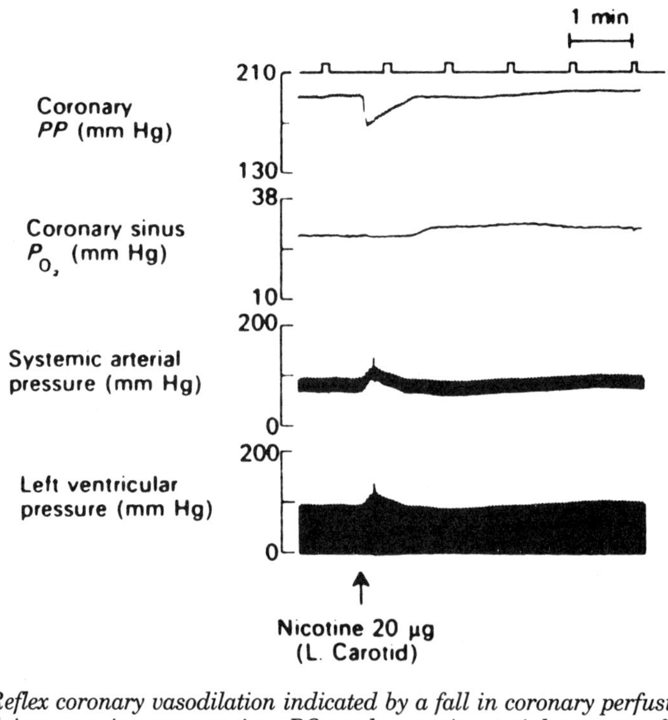

Figure 1. *Reflex coronary vasodilation indicated by a fall in coronary perfusion pressure together with increases in coronary sinus PO_2 and systemic arterial pressure after chemoreflex activation by injection of nicotine into the left carotid. Reproduced by permission of the American Heart Association, Inc. from Hackett JG, Abboud FM, Mark AL, et al: Coronary vascular responses to stimulation of chemoreceptors and baroreceptors. Evidence for reflex activation of vagal cholinergic innervation. Circ Res 31:8–17, 1972.*

tion indicates that vagal cholinergic vasodilation was, at least, partly involved. Vatner and McRitchie,[13] in studies in conscious dogs, subsequently reported that chemoreflex-induced coronary vasodilation is mediated by both reflex vagal cholinergic vasodilation (minor component) and by withdrawal of α-adrenergic vasoconstriction secondary to an increase in ventilation (major component).

Chemoreflex Interactions

Chemoreflex-mediated cardiac vagal activation in the intact human is profoundly influenced by other reflex inputs in addition to ventilation, as discussed earlier. Recognition of these interactions is important in the proper understanding of chemoreflex vagal control in both physiological and pathophysiological states. Some of these interactions are discussed in detail in an excellent review by de Burgh Daly et al.[7]

Humoral factors such as hypercapnia and acidosis potentiate chemoreceptor afferent discharge. In animal studies, hypercapnia potentiated the pressor response to hypoxia.[14,15] In studies in humans, combined hypoxia and hypercapnia resulted in synergistic increases in both minute ventilation and sympathetic activation.[11,16] It is likely, but not proven, that a similar potentiation applies to the bradycardic response to chemoreceptor stimulation.

The arterial baroreceptors (see Chs. 23 and 24) interact closely with the chemoreflex. Arterial baroreceptor activation (increased blood pressure) inhibits both ventilatory and vasoconstrictor responses to chemoreflex activation in dogs. Baroreceptor deactivation potentiates these responses.[17,18] In humans, baroreflex activation selectively eliminates sympathetic responses to hypoxia, but not hypercapnia. Little data are available on baroreflex influences on chemoreflex-mediated bradycardia.[19] One would expect that simultaneous activation of both baroreflexes and chemoreflexes would increase the bradycardia induced by the chemoreflex. Studies[19] of a mildly hypertensive, but otherwise normal subject, who manifested marked bradycardia and asystole during hypoxia and apnea (Fig. 2), however, showed that baroreflex activation (by neck suction or phenylephrine) significantly attenuated the bradycardia during apnea (Fig. 3). Thus, preliminary data confirm that the baroreflexes inhibit not only the sympathetic, but also the parasympathetic responses to chemoreflex activation. The clinical significance of this interaction is discussed later.

Carotid chemoreceptors also interact with afferents arising from the face and upper airways.[7] In studies in dogs, Angell-James and de Burgh Daly[20] demonstrated that simultaneous stimulation of the laryngeal and carotid body afferents resulted in apnea and marked bradycardia. The bradycardic effect of this interaction was blocked by atropine. Similar results were obtained in studies in monkeys, where laryngeal stimulation during chemoreflex activation again resulted in apnea, increased peripheral vasoconstriction, and bradycardia (Fig. 4).[21] Thus, these afferents inhibit the ventilatory response to chemoreflex activation, but potentiate the autonomic response, and thus result in the diving response (apnea, bradycardia, and selective vasoconstriction), which is explored in greater detail below.

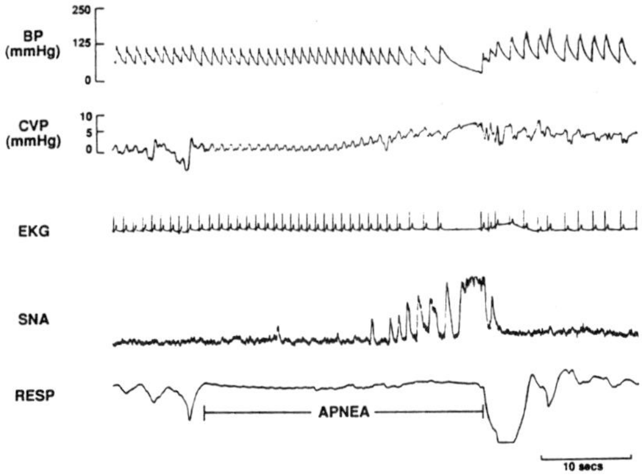

Figure 2. *Changes in blood pressure (BP), central venous pressure (CVP), the electrocardiogram (EKG), and sympathetic nerve activity (SNA), in a mildly hypertensive patient on no medications during voluntary end-expiratory apnea. Chemoreflex stimulation by hypoxia, together with elimination of thoracic afferents during apnea, resulted in increases in both sympathetic nerve discharge to muscle blood vessels and in cardiac vagal activity, resulting in profound bradycardia. These responses were potentiated by exposing the subject to hypoxia, but not hypercapnia. The bradycardia was eliminated by atropine. Reproduced with permission from Somers VK, Dyken ME, Mark AL, et al: Parasympathetic hyperresponsiveness and bradyarrhythmias during apnoea in hypertension. Clin Auton Res 2:171–176, 1992.*

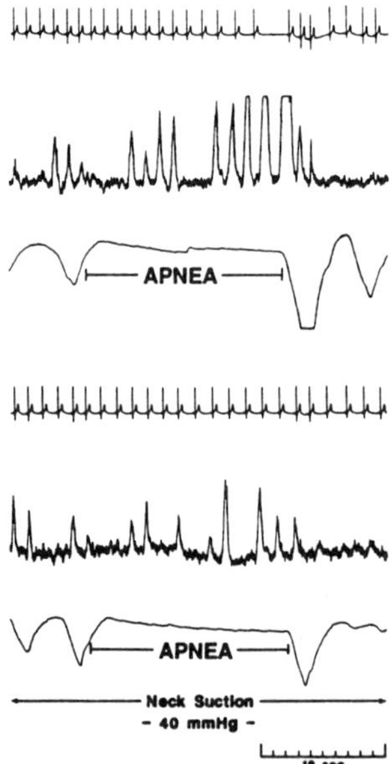

Figure 3. *Recordings of the EKG and SNA during voluntary end-expiratory apnea in the same subject as shown in Figure 2. The upper figure shows sympathetic and cardiac vagal activation in response to apnea. These responses were potentiated by hypoxia. The lower figure shows that baroreflex activation by neck suction not only attenuated the sympathetic response to apnea, but also attenuated the cardiac vagal response. Reproduced with permission from Somers VK, Dyken ME, Mark AL, et al: Parasympathetic hyperresponsiveness and bradyarrhythmias during apnoea in hypertension. Clin Auton Res 2:171–176, 1992.*

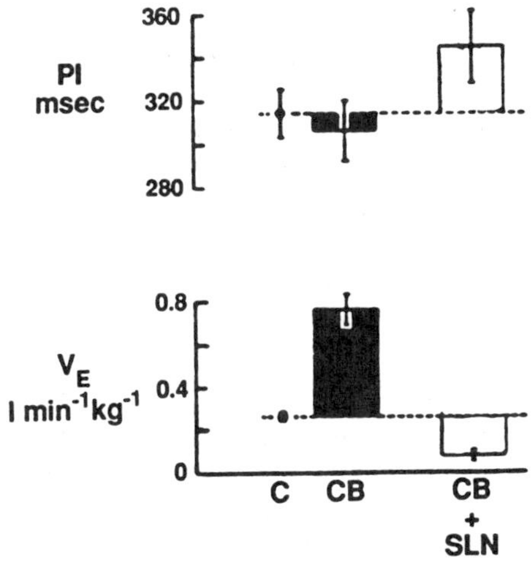

Figure 4. *Measurements of pulse interval (PI) and minute ventilation in the control state (C), during carotid body chemoreceptor stimulation by hypoxic hypercapnic blood (CB), and during combined stimulation of carotid body chemoreceptors and electrical stimulation of central cut ends of the superior laryngeal nerve (CB + SLN). Stimulation of the chemoreceptors alone resulted in increased minute ventilation with little change in pulse interval. Simultaneous stimulation of the chemoreceptors and the superior laryngeal nerve resulted in a reduction in minute ventilation and bradycardia, indicating an interaction between the chemoreceptors, the upper airway receptors, and the thoracic afferents. Modified with permission from Daly M de B, Korner PI, Angell-James JE, et al: Cardiovascular–respiratory reflex interactions between carotid bodies and upper-airway receptors in the monkey. Am J Physiol 234:H293–H299, 1978.*

Clinical Implications of Chemoreflex Vagal Activation

Sleep Apnea

Sleep apnea is increasingly recognized as a significant factor in cardiac and vascular morbidity and mortality.[22,23] Patients with sleep apnea are at increased risk for angina, myocardial infarction, ischemic stroke, and hypertension.[24–26] In addition, up to one third of hypertensive patients may also have sleep apnea.[27]

Autonomic responses to sleep apneic episodes may contribute to the cardiac and vascular morbidity. These autonomic responses are complex and include the effects of apnea, hypoxia, and carbon dioxide retention. In patients with obstructive sleep apnea, changes in intrathoracic and intracardiac pressures during the Müller maneuver (inspiration against a closed glottis), also need to be considered.[28,29]

During apneic episodes, hypoxic stimulation of the arterial chemoreceptors induces both sympathetically-mediated peripheral vasoconstriction as well as vagally-mediated bradycardia. Hypoxic stimulation of the chemoreceptors would be potentiated by hypercapnia and respiratory acidosis. Absence of pulmonary inflation minimizes the inhibitory influence of the pulmonary afferents and augments both the sympathetic and vagal responses. In patients with obstructive sleep apnea (as opposed to those with central sleep apnea), however, respiratory drive is maintained and central inspiratory neuronal activity may still partially inhibit the CVMs.

Bradycardia has been noted in central, obstructive, and mixed sleep apneas, and is more manifest with increased duration of apnea and oxyhemoglobin desaturation.[19,26,30,31] Oxygen administration attenuates the bradycardia. In contrast, normal subjects during sleep showed tachycardia, rather than bradycardia, during hypoxic hypercapnia because of preservation of the ventilatory response. Administration of atropine eliminates the bradycardic response to apnea. This effect confirms that this mechanism is a vagal one, rather than a direct effect of hypoxia or hypercapnia on the cardiac conduction system.

Clearly, bradycardia during the apnea would act to decrease myocardial oxygen consumption and prolong diastolic filling time during a period of severe metabolic stress. Sleep apneic episodes are also associated, however, with marked oscillations in blood pressure and sympathetic activity, with surges in both occurring towards the end of the apnea when bradyarrhythmias would be most profound.[32–34] Thus, increased afterload in a milieu of hypoxia, hypercapnia, and acidosis, together with profound bradyarrhythmias and asystole, may trigger abnormal foci of myocardial electrical activity and result in ventricular fibrillation. Ventricular ectopy during sleep is significantly increased during severe oxygen desaturation (to less than 60%).[35] Both cardiac ischemia and catecholamine excess predispose to ventricular fibrillation.[36,37] Hypertensive patients, who are at increased risk for sleep apnea, coronary artery disease, and left ventricular hypertrophy, would be especially susceptible.

Exaggerated vagal responses to apneic episodes may also be counterproductive. Episodes of apnea can induce asystole lasting more than 10 seconds.[19,31] A marked fall in arterial pressure (Fig. 5, upper panel) accompanies this prolonged asystole. Reduced perfusion of coronary and cerebral circulations in an already hypoxic environment may occur repetitively each night (Fig. 5, lower panel), and it could eventually result in ischemia and infarction in patients with underlying coronary or cerebrovascular disease. In patients with diseased cerebrovascular circulations, impaired autoregulation in ischemic areas of the brain could result in a steal phenomenon and, thereby, result in infarction in watershed areas of the brain. This process suggests a hypothesis for the increased incidence of occlusive stroke in sleep apneic patients.[24,25]

Baroreflex-chemoreflex interactions may have important implications in the understanding of exaggerated bradyarrhythmic responses in patients with sleep apnea. Arterial baroreflex activation inhibits the sympathetic,[38] and possibly the parasympathetic,[19] responses to chemoreflex stimulation. Hypertensive patients have an impairment of the baroreflex response[39] as well as a potentiation of the sympathetic[40] and ventilatory[41] responses to hypoxia. Hypertensive patients are also at risk for sleep apnea. Thus, in sleep apneic patients with hypertension and impairment of the baroreflex, the chemoreflex response to hypoxia may be disinhibited, which would permit excessive, and

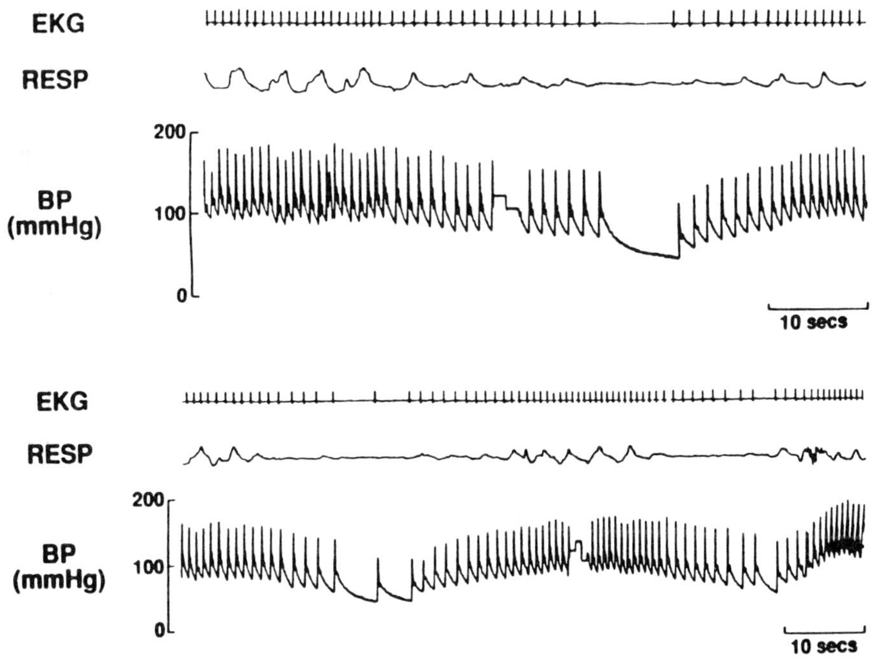

Figure 5. *Bradyarrhythmias during sleep apnea. Upper panel: A period of asystole in association with a reduction in arterial pressure to < 50 mm Hg during an episode of sleep apnea in a hypertensive patient on no medications during REM sleep is shown. Lower panel: Repeated episodes of bradyarrhythmias and hypoperfusion during REM sleep in the same subject are shown. Reproduced with permission from Somers VK, Dyken ME, Mark AL, et al: Parasympathetic hyperresponsiveness and bradyarrhythmias during apnoea in hypertension. Clin Auton Res 2:171–176, 1992.*

potentially lethal, bradyarrhythmic responses to prolonged apneic episodes (Fig. 6). Hypertensive patients with underlying coronary artery disease or left ventricular hypertrophy, who are already at risk for complex ventricular arrhythmias and sudden death,[42,43] may be at especially high risk. Distortion of the upper airways during periods of obstructive apnea may conceivably also potentiate bradycardia via stimulation of the upper airway receptors. There are presently no studies addressing this question.

Chemoreflex-induced cholinergic coronary vasodilation,[5] mediated via the vagi, could help protect against cardiac ischemia during apnea. The significance of this reflex in humans, however, has not been determined. Furthermore, in patients with preexisting coronary artery disease and impaired endothelial function, the vasodilator response to cholinergic stimulation may be absent and the vasoconstrictor response to sympathetic adrenergic stimulation could result in coronary vasoconstriction. Indeed, recent studies confirmed a high incidence of ST depression (suggesting cardiac ischemia) of the electrocardiogram during sleep in patients with sleep apnea.[44] Appropriate treatment of sleep apnea with continuous positive airway pressure resolved the episodes of ST depression. Numerous mechanisms might be involved in cardiac ische-

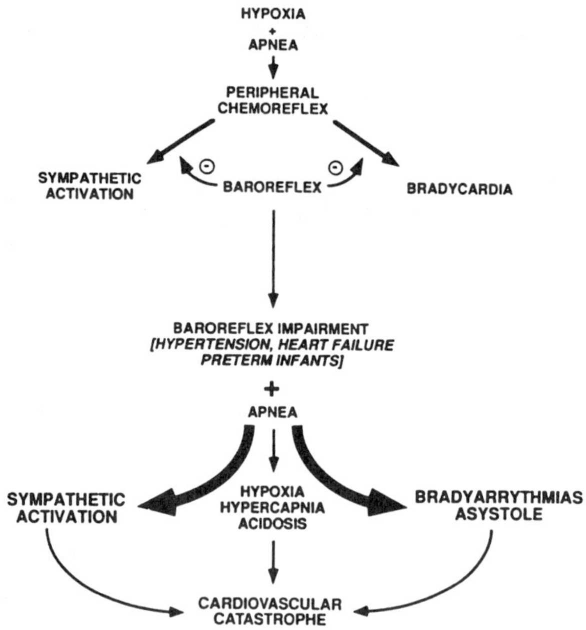

Figure 6. *Schematic indicating proposed mechanisms whereby chemoreflex stimulation in the presence of apnea and baroreflex impairment may result in excessive sympathetic activation to peripheral blood vessels and vagal activation to the heart resulting in cardiovascular catastrophe. Reproduced with permission from Somers VK, Dyken ME, Mark AL, et al: Parasympathetic hyperresponsiveness and bradyarrhythmias during apnoea in hypertension. Clin Auton Res 2:171–176, 1992.*

mia during sleep apnea, however, and there is as yet no evidence that vagal cholinergic mechanisms are impaired in this disorder.

Heart Failure

Heart failure patients are at fivefold greater risk for sudden death than the general population. Heart failure has the highest known risk of sudden death for any subset of patients with chronic cardiovascular disease.[45] About half of all deaths in patients with heart failure are from unexpected cardiac arrest.[46–48]

The mechanism underlying cardiac arrest in heart failure is unclear. Anecdotal reports suggest an association with bradycardia.[49–51] In a report on sudden death in a patient with cardiomyopathy, Bissett et al[52] postulated that a bradycardia-dependent repolarization created a substrate for ventricular fibrillation in the early hours of the morning. Luu et al[53] reviewed electrocardiographic data from 21 cardiac arrests in patients with heart failure. Sinus bradycardia and bradyarrhythmias preceded cardiac arrest in more than half the patients.[53] The cause of the bradycardias was not known.

In patients with severe heart failure, chemoreflex-mediated vagal mechanisms may be implicated. Animals with failing hearts exhibit markedly reduced levels of catecholamine,[54,55] but not acetylcholine (ACh),[56] biosynthesis. Thus, parasympathetic, but not sympathetic, innervation is preserved in heart failure. Heart failure patients are susceptible to periodic or cyclic breathing, known as Cheyne-Stokes respiration, due to a combination of left ventricular failure and depressed sensitivity of the respiratory center to carbon dioxide.[57] Cheyne-Stokes breathing is characterized by a gradual progression in breathing amplitude, from apnea (lasting 10 to 20 seconds) to hyperventilation. During apnea, arterial oxygen levels fall and carbon dioxide levels rise. This combined stimulus triggers hyperventilation and subsequent hypocapnia. Thus, a further period of apnea results. Factors such as sleep, opiates, head injury, and cerebrovascular disease exaggerate Cheyne-Stokes breathing. Oscillations in breathing are also caused by a slow circulation time between the lungs and the central respiratory control mechanism, due to left ventricular failure. This occurrence further prolongs the response time of the system and prevents the achievement of steady state levels of ventilation, oxygen, and carbon dioxide.

We propose two further mechanisms that may potentiate this problem. First, apneic episodes with consequent hypoxia result in reflex pulmonary vasoconstriction, which increases right ventricular afterload and further delays the blood transit time through the pulmonary circulation. Second, hypoxic peripheral chemoreflex stimulation and consequent bradycardia or asystole exacerbates the sluggish blood flow from heart to brain. More importantly, the bradyarrhythmias that precede cardiac arrest, especially those occurring during sleep,[52] may be initiated by chemoreflex cardiac vagal activation induced by the hypoxia and apnea of Cheyne-Stokes breathing.

An additional hypothesis involves the potential role of baroreflex-chemoreflex interactions. Heart failure is associated with marked impairment of cardiac and arterial baroreflexes.[58–60] Activation of baroreceptors inhibits chemoreflex-mediated sympathetic,[38] and probably parasympathetic,[19] responses, as discussed above. Thus, impairment of the baroreflex would permit disinhibition of chemoreflex vagal activation in response to apnea and hypoxia (Fig. 6) and, thus, increase the likelihood of apnea-associated bradyarrhythmias and asystole.

Sudden Infant Death Syndrome

Sudden infant death syndrome (SIDS) occurs in about one in 500 babies.[61] The pathophysiology of this disorder may involve an abnormal regulation of the cardiovascular and respiratory systems. Some premature and term newborn babies are prone to periods of expiratory apnea that last more than 30 seconds and that are associated with hypoxia and bradycardia.[7] Rein et al[62] studied a series of infants with symptomatic bradyarrhythmias associated with apnea and syncope. Some of these infants required implantation of a pacemaker. Sadeh et al[63] have reported that abnormalities in cardiac repolarization may predispose infants to SIDS.

Chemoreflex function is present in both preterm and newborn infants. Thus, chemoreflex excitation by hypoxia occurs during apneic episodes and may be responsible for cardiac slowing in infants. In this regard, two important interactions need to be considered.

First, stimulation of upper airway receptors (for example, by gastroesophageal reflux or upper respiratory infections) may initiate apneas[7] and potentiate chemoreflex-mediated bradycardia.[20,21,64] Second, baroreflex modulation of the chemoreflex response may be inadequate. Baroreflex sensitivity is decreased in the newborn, especially in the preterm period.[65,66] Conversely, the chemoreflexes may be active and responsive.[67,68] Apneic episodes in infants may occur in a milieu of poorly developed autonomic neural integration or baroreflex immaturity and may accentuate the autonomic responses to the apnea-induced chemoreflex excitation. These cardiac vagal and peripheral sympathetic responses could be implicated in cardiac arrhythmias and SIDS (Fig. 6).

Diving Response and Upper Airway Procedures

Apnea, bradycardia, and selective systemic vasoconstriction (excluding the coronary and cerebral vasculature) that occur during facial immersion result from interactions between activation of trigeminal nerve and chemoreceptors, and inactivation of pulmonary afferents.[21,69,70] This combination of reflexes during water immersion maintains cerebral and cardiac perfusion by selective vasodilation and vasoconstriction and minimizes myocardial oxygen consumption by a marked decrease in heart rate. Coronary vasodilation is mediated by both reflex cholinergic vasodilation and by direct effects of hypoxia (the predominant mechanism).[5,8,71] Cerebral resistance vessels dilate in response to direct effects of hypoxia, but they are not influenced by the chemoreflex.[72,73] Studies in humans indicate that simulated diving (breath holding and face immersion) elicited peripheral arterial, arteriolar, and venous constriction, as well as bradycardia.[74] Stimulation of receptors in the face and upper airway (e.g., by water inhalation) reinforces the diving response by further inhibiting breathing and potentiating bradycardia and vasoconstriction.[20,21]

Bradycardia and cardiac arrest can be explained by the combination of upper airway reflexes and chemoreflex activation by hypoxia in other clinical situations, such as tracheal intubation, bronchoscopy, maxillary sinus irrigation, laryngeal packing, dental procedures, and food aspiration.[7] Upper airway suction and discontinuation of mechanical ventilation causes bradycardia in quadriplegic patients if hypoxia occurs (Fig. 7).[75]

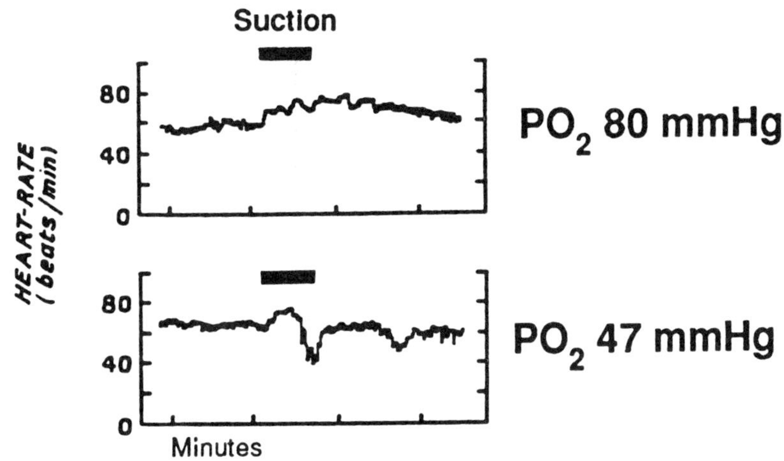

Figure 7. *Measurement of heart rate during tracheal suction in a mechanically ventilated tetraplegic patient at different levels of arterial oxygen tension. The upper panel shows tachycardia during tracheal suction when PO_2 is maintained at 80 mm Hg. When tracheal suction is performed when the subject is hypoxic (PO_2 of 47 mm Hg [lower panel]), bradycardia results, indicating the interaction between the upper airway receptors and the chemoreceptors. Reproduced with permission from Frankel HL, Mathias CJ, Spalding JMK: Mechanisms of reflex cardiac arrest in tetraplegic patients. Lancet II:1183–1185, 1975. Copyright © by The Lancet Ltd.*

Summary and Conclusions

Chemoreflex cardiac vagal control may be implicated in several disease states, especially with regard to mechanisms that initiate bradyarrhythmic cardiac arrest. In contrast to sympathetic responses, however, the vagal responses have received little attention. Several reflex interactions, such as those involving upper airway receptors and the baroreflexes, may, in disease states, potentiate chemoreflex-mediated bradyarrhythmias. Little is known of the contribution of iatrogenic factors, such as sedatives, centrally acting depressants, and drugs that induce cardiac slowing either by direct action on cardiac conduction or by sympathetic inhibition, in these disease states.

Acknowledgment: The authors express their thanks to Kim Nissen for expert typing of this manuscript.

References

1. Eyzaguirre C, Lewin J: Chemoreceptor activity of the carotid body of the cat. J Physiol (Lond) 159:222, 1961.
2. Hornbein TF, Griffo ZJ, Roos A: Quantitation of chemoreceptor activity: Interrelation of hypoxia and hypercapnia. J Neurophysiol 24:561, 1961.

3. Fitzgerald RS, Parks DC: Effect of hypoxia on carotid chemoreceptor response to carbon dioxide in cats. Respir Physiol 12:218, 1971.
4. Eyzaguirre C, Fitzgerald RS, Lahiri S, et al: Arterial chemoreceptors. In JT Shepherd, FM Abboud (eds): Handbook of Physiology. Section 2: The Cardiovascular System, Vol. III. Bethesda, MD, American Physiological Society, 1983, p. 557.
5. Hackett JG, Abboud FM, Mark AL, et al: Coronary vascular responses to stimulation of chemoreceptors and baroreceptors. Evidence for reflex activation of vagal cholinergic innervation. Circ Res 31:8, 1972.
6. Calvelo MG, Abboud FM, Ballard DR, et al: Reflex vascular responses to stimulation of chemoreceptors with nicotine and cyanide. Circ Res 27:259, 1970.
7. Daly M de B, Angell-James JE, Elsner R: Role of carotid-body chemoreceptors and their reflex interactions in bradycardia and cardiac arrest. Lancet 1:764, 1979.
8. Heistad DD, Abboud FM: Circulatory adjustments to hypoxia. Circulation 61:463, 1980.
9. Daly M de B, Scott MJ: An analysis of the primary cardiovascular reflex effects of stimulation of the carotid body chemoreceptors in the dog. J Physiol (Lond) 162:555, 1962.
10. Somers VK, Zavala DC, Mark AL, et al: Influence of ventilation and hypocapnia on sympathetic nerve responses to hypoxia in normal humans. J Appl Physiol 67:2095, 1989.
11. Somers VK, Mark AL, Zavala DC, et al: Contrasting effects of hypoxia and hypercapnia on ventilation and sympathetic activity in humans. J Appl Physiol 67:2101, 1989.
12. Spyer KM: Neural organisation and control of the baroreceptor reflex. Rev Physiol Biochem Pharmacol 88:23, 1981.
13. Vatner SF, McRitchie RJ: Interaction of the chemoreflex and the pulmonary inflation reflex in the regulation of coronary circulation in conscious dogs. Circ Res 37:664, 1975.
14. Pelletier CL: Circulatory responses to graded stimulation of the carotid chemoreceptors in the dog. Circ Res 31:431, 1972.
15. Koehler RC, McDonald BW, Krasney JA: Influence of CO_2 on cardiovascular response to hypoxia in conscious dogs. Am J Physiol 239:H545, 1980.
16. Somers VK, Mark AL, Abboud FM: Sympathetic activation by hypoxia and hypercapnia—implications for sleep apnea. Clin Exp Hypertens, Part A, A10(suppl. 1):413, 1988.
17. Heistad DD, Abboud FM, Mark AL, et al: Interaction of baroreceptor and chemoreceptor reflexes. J Clin Invest 53:1226, 1974.
18. Heistad DD, Abboud FM, Mark AL, et al: Effect of baroreceptor activity on ventilatory response to chemoreceptor stimulation. J Appl Physiol 39:411, 1975.
19. Somers VK, Dyken ME, Mark AL, et al: Parasympathetic hyperresponsiveness and bradyarrhythmias during apnoea in hypertension. Clin Auton Res 2:171, 1992.
20. Angell-James JE, Daly M de B: Some aspects of upper respiratory tract reflexes. Acta Otolaryngol (Stockh) 79:242, 1975.
21. Daly M de B, Korner PI, Angell-James JE, et al: Cardiovascular–respiratory reflex interactions between carotid bodies and upper-airway receptors in the monkey. Am J Physiol 234:H293, 1978.
22. Bliwise DL, Bliwise NG, Partinen M, et al: Sleep apnea and mortality in an aged cohort. Am J Public Health 78:544, 1988.
23. He J, Kryger MH, Zorick FJ, et al: Mortality and apnea index in obstructive sleep apnea: Experience in 385 male patients. Chest 94:9, 1988.
24. Tilkian AR, Guilleminault C, Schroeder JS, et al: Sleep induced apnea syndrome: Relevance of cardiac arrhythmias and their reversal after tracheostomy. Am J Med 63:348, 1977.
25. Palomaki H, Partinen M, Juvela S, et al: Snoring as a risk factor for sleep related brain infarction. Stroke 10:1311, 1989.
26. Shepard JW Jr: Cardiopulmonary consequences of obstructive sleep apnea. Mayo Clin Proc 65:1250, 1990.

27. Lavie P, Ben-Yosef R, Rubin AE: Prevalence of sleep apnea syndrome among patients with essential hypertension. Am Heart J 108:373, 1984.
28. Katenberg C, Olajos M, Morkin E, et al: Effects of changes in airway pressure on the left ventricle and left atrium of dogs. Cardiovasc Res 20:853, 1986.
29. Guzman PA, Maughan WL, Yin FCP, et al: Transeptal pressure gradient with leftward septal displacement during the Mueller manoeuvre in man. Br Heart J 46:667, 1981.
30. Zwillich C, Devlin T, White D, et al: Bradycardia during sleep apnea. Characteristics and mechanism. J Clin Invest 69:1286, 1982.
31. Guilleminault C, Connolly SJ, Winkle RA: Cardiac arrhythmia and conduction disturbances during sleep in 400 patients with sleep apnea syndrome. Am J Cardiol 52:490, 1983.
32. Hedner J, Ejnell H, Sellgren J, et al: Is high and fluctuating muscle nerve sympathetic activity in the sleep apnoea syndrome of pathogenetic importance for the development of hypertension? J Hypertens 6:S529, 1988.
33. Watanabe T, Mano T, Iwase S, et al: Enhanced muscle sympathetic nerve activity during sleep apnea in the elderly. J Auton Nerv Syst 37:223, 1992.
34. Somers VK, Dyken ME, Mark AL, et al: Autonomic and hemodynamic responses during sleep in normal and sleep apneic humans. Clin Res 39:735A, 1991. Abstract.
35. Shepard JW Jr, Garrison MW, Grither DA, et al: Relationship of ventricular ectopy to oxyhemoglobin desaturation in patients with obstructive sleep apnea. Chest 88:335, 1985.
36. Marban E, Robinson SW, Wier WG: Mechanisms of arrhythmogenic delayed and early after depolarizations in ferret papillary muscle. J Clin Invest 78:1185, 1986.
37. Marban E, Kitakaza M, Kusuoka H, et al: Intracellular free calcium concentration measured with ^{19}F NMR spectroscopy in intact ferret hearts. Proc Natl Acad Sci USA 84:6005, 1987.
38. Somers VK, Mark AL, Abboud FM: Interaction of baroreceptor and chemoreceptor control of sympathetic nerve activity in normal humans. J Clin Invest 87:1953, 1991.
39. Bristow JD, Honour AJ, Pickering GW, et al: Diminished baroreflex sensitivity in high blood pressure. Circulation 39:48, 1969.
40. Somers VK, Mark AL, Abboud FM: Potentiation of sympathetic nerve responses to hypoxia in borderline hypertensive subjects. Hypertension 11:608, 1988.
41. Trzebski AM, Tafil M, Zoltowski M, et al: Increased sensitivity of the arterial chemoreceptor drive in young men with mild hypertension. Cardiovasc Res 16:163, 1982.
42. McLenachan JM, Henderson E, Morris KI, et al: Ventricular arrhythmias in patients with hypertensive left ventricular hypertrophy. N Engl J Med 317:787–792, 1987.
43. Kannel WB, Doyle JT, McNamara PM, et al: Precursors of sudden coronary death: Factors related to the incidence of sudden death. Circulation 51:606, 1975.
44. Hanly P, Zuberi N, Alderson M, et al: St segment depression during sleep in patients with obstructive sleep apnea. Am Rev Resp Dis 145:A444, 1992. Abstract.
45. Kannel WB, Plehn JF, Cupples LA: Cardiac failure and sudden death in the Framingham study. Am Heart J 115:869, 1988.
46. Hinkle LE, Thales HT: Clinical classification of sudden cardiac deaths. Circulation 65:457, 1982.
47. Packer M: Sudden unexpected death in patient with congestive heart failure: A second frontier. Circulation 72:681, 1985.
48. Stevenson WG, Stevenson LW, Weiss JN, et al: Inducible ventricular arrhythmias and sudden death during vasodilator therapy of severe heart failure. Am Heart J 116:1447, 1988.
49. Clark MB, Dwyer EM, Greenberg H: Sudden death during ambulatory monitoring. Am J Med 75:801, 1983.
50. Radhakrishnan S, Kaul U, Bahl VK, et al: Sudden bradyarrhythmic death in dilated cardiomyopathy: A case report. PACE 11:1369, 1988.

51. Greenberg HM: Bradycardia at onset of sudden death: Potential mechanisms. Ann NY Acad Sci 427:241, 1984.
52. Bissett JK, Watson JW, Scovil JA, et al: Sudden death in cardiomyopathy: Role of bradycardia-dependent repolarization changes. Am Heart J 99:625, 1980.
53. Luu M, Stevenson WG, Stevenson LW, et al: Diverse mechanisms of unexpected cardiac arrest in advanced heart failure. Circulation 80:1675, 1989.
54. Spann JF JR, Chidsey CA, Pool PE, et al: Mechanisms of norepinephrine depletion in experimental heart failure produced by aortic constriction in the guinea pig. Circ Res 17:312, 1965.
55. DeQuattro V, Nagatsu T, Mendez A, et al: Determinants of cardiac noradrenaline depletion in human congestive failure. Cardiovas Res 7:344, 1973.
56. Roskoski R JR, Schmid PG, Mayer HE, et al: In vitro acetylcholine biosynthesis in normal and failing guinea pig hearts. Circ Res 36:547, 1975.
57. Lange RL, Hecht HH: The mechanism of Cheyne-Stokes respiration. J Clin Invest 41:42, 1962.
58. Eckberg DL, Drabinsky M, Braunwald E: Defective cardiac parasympathetic control in patients with heart disease. N Engl J Med 285:877, 1971.
59. Vatner SF, Higgins CB, Braunwald E: Sympathetic and parasympathetic components of reflex tachycardia induced by hypotension in conscious dogs with and without heart failure. Cardiovasc Res 8:153, 1974.
60. Ellenbogen KA, Mohanty PK, Szentpetery S, et al: Arterial baroreflex abnormalities in heart failure: Reversal after orthotopic cardiac transplantation. Circulation 79:51, 1989.
61. Shannon DC: The sudden infant death syndrome. Clin Chest Med 1:327, 1980.
62. Rein AJJT, Simcha A, Ludomirsky A, et al: Symptomatic sinus bradycardia in infants with structurally normal hearts. J Pediatr 107:724, 1985.
63. Sadeh D, Shannon DC, Abboud S, et al: Altered cardiac repolarization in some victims of sudden infant death syndrome. N Engl J Med 317:1501, 1987.
64. Angell-James JE, Daly M de B: Nasal reflexes. Proc Soc Med 62:1287, 1969.
65. Shinebourne EA, Vapaavuori EK, Williams RL, et al: Development of baroreflex activity in unanesthetized fetal and neonatal lambs. Circ Res 31:710, 1972.
66. Holden K, Morgan JS, Krauss AN, et al: Incomplete baroreceptor responses in newborn infants. Am J Perinatol 2:31, 1985.
67. Purves MJ, Biscoe TJ: Development of chemoreceptor activity. Br Med Bull 22:56, 1966.
68. Blanco CE, Dawes GS, Hanson MA, et al: The response to hypoxia of arterial chemoreceptors in fetal sheep and new-born lambs. J Physiol (Lond) 351:25, 1984.
69. Angell-James JE, Daly M de B: Cardiovascular responses in apnoeic asphyxia: Role of arterial chemoreceptors and the modification of their effects by a pulmonary vagal inflation reflex. J Physiol (Lond) 201:87, 1969.
70. Angell-James JE, Daly M de B: The effects of artificial lung inflation on reflexly induced bradycardia associated with apnoea in the dog. J Physiol (Lond) 274:349, 1978.
71. Abboud FM, Heistad DD, Mark AL, et al: Differential responses of the coronary circulation and other vascular beds to chemoreceptor stimulation. In MJ Purves (ed): The Peripheral Arterial Chemoreceptors. New York, NY, Cambridge University Press, 1975, p. 427.
72. Heistad DD, Marcus ML, Ehrhardt JC, et al: Effect of stimulation of carotid chemoreceptors on total and regional cerebral blood flow. Circ Res 38:20, 1976.
73. Abboud FM: Special characteristics of the cerebral circulation. Fed Proc 40:2296, 1981.
74. Heistad DD, Abboud FM, Eckstein JW: Vasoconstrictor response to simulated diving in man. J Appl Physiol 25:542, 1968.
75. Frankel HL, Mathias CJ, Spalding JMK: Mechanisms of reflex cardiac arrest in tetraplegic patients. Lancet II:1183–1185, 1975.

PART V

Methods for Clinical Assessment of Vagal Activity

CHAPTER 26

Methods for Assessment of Vagal Tone and Reflexes:
Time Domain Measures

J.T. Bigger Jr., J.L. Fleiss

It has been recognized for more than 20 years that parasympathetic dysfunction can occur in patients with heart disease.[1–3] For example, a decrease in the degree of heart rate slowing in response to facial immersion in water at 0°C[4] or after phenylephrine injection[5] has been reported in patients studied during recovery from myocardial infarction. More recently, it has been shown that decreased baroreflex sensitivity in dogs with experimental infarction increases the likelihood of ventricular fibrillation after coronary occlusion during exercise.[6] Preliminary studies in patients recovering from myocardial infarction suggest that decreased baroreflex sensitivity predicts cardiovascular death or nonfatal cardiac arrest.[5] A large longitudinal study of patients recovering from myocardial infarction showed that a frequency domain measure of vagal modulation of heart period, power in the high-frequency band of the heart period power spectrum, predicted death of all causes, cardiovascular death, and arrhythmic death.[7] Time domain measures of vagal modulation of heart period, the root mean square of successive differences and the proportion of differences between successive normal RR intervals >50 milliseconds, had similar predictive value.[8] As a result of the accumulating evidence that the parasympathetic nervous system functions abnormally in some patients with heart disease, an intense interest has developed in measuring vagal tone in various groups of patients with heart disease. The purpose of this chapter is to describe time domain methods for assessing cardiac parasympathetic activity in man.

Supported in part by NIH Grants HL-41552 from the National Heart, Lung, and Blood Institute, Bethesda, MD and RR-00645 from the Research Resources Administration; and by funds from The Milstein Family Foundation, The Dover Foundation, George and Abby O'Neill, Robert Winthrop, and the Shirlee and Henry Benach Foundation, New York, NY.
From *Vagal Control of the Heart: Experimental Basis and Clinical Implications* edited by MN Levy, PJ Schwartz © 1994, Futura Publishing Co. Inc., Armonk, NY.

Tests Based on Respiratory Sinus Arrhythmia

It has been known since the mid–19th century that the vagus nerves mediated sinus arrhythmia and that vagotomy or atropine treatment would abolish sinus arrhythmia.[9] It has been known since the 1930s that a direct interaction of respiratory and cardiovascular medullary centers and reflex mechanisms contribute to respiratory sinus arrhythmia (RSA).[10,11] Katona et al[12] showed, with direct recording of vagus nerve activity, that RSA in chloralose-anesthetized dogs is due to cessation of vagal efferent firing during inspiration. This inhibition of vagal firing by inspiration occurs during normal ventilation, but not during artificial ventilation, and occurs even when vagal tone is increased by inducing arterial hypertension. In a series of ingenious experiments in dogs, Katona and Jih[13] demonstrated that the degree of sinus arrhythmia can be used as a noninvasive quantitative measure of the degree of parasympathetically-mediated heart rate control. They showed that the difference in the maximum and minimum heart period in a respiratory cycle was proportional to the average vagal activity in the cycle. When the vagus nerves in the dogs were temporarily cooled, the average heart period decreased and RSA was abolished (see Fig. 1). Both heart period and sinus arrhythmia returned to control values when the vagus nerves were rewarmed. The change in average heart period during cooling of the vagus nerves was termed parasympathetic control (PC).[13] The same result was obtained when arterial blood pressure was increased or decreased in order to increase or decrease vagal tone; i.e., during altered vagal tone, the respiratory variation in heart period (VHP) still reflected the degree of vagal tone, and the respiratory variation was still abolished by vagal cooling. The relationship between vagal activity and VHP was not altered by cardiac β-adrenergic blockade with propranolol, as previously shown by Wheeler and Watkins.[14] Atropine abolished VHP and, after atropine treatment, the cooling of the vagus nerves had no effect on heart period or variability in heart period over a respiratory cycle.

Both Hirsch and Bishop[15] and Eckberg[16] showed that the frequency of

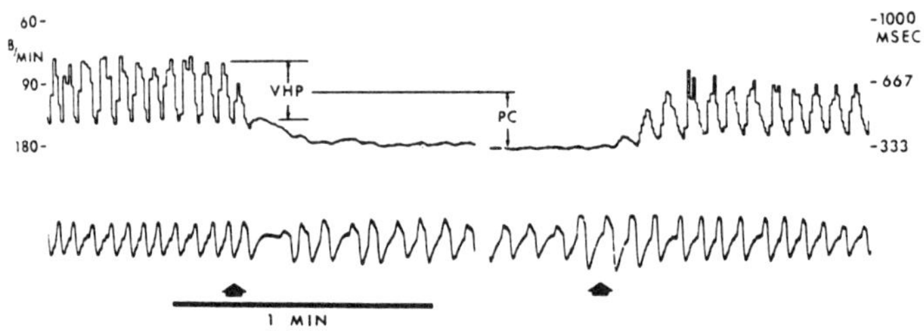

Figure 1. *Effect of bilateral vagal cooling on RSA in the dog. The upper trace shows heart period and the lower one shows ventilation. The vagus nerves were cooled to -5°C between the arrows. The variation in heart period (VHP) was reduced during cooling and the degree of parasympathetic control (PC) of heart period could be measured as the difference between average RR interval before and during bilateral cooling of the vagus nerves. Rewarming the vagus nerves restored the original relationship between ventilation and sinus arrhythmia. Reproduced with permission from Katona PG, Jih F: Respiratory sinus arrhythmia: Noninvasive measure of parasympathetic cardiac control. J Appl Physiol 39:801–805, 1975.*

breathing and tidal volume influenced RSA in normal human subjects. Sinus arrhythmia decreased with increasing frequency of breathing and increased with increasing tidal volume. The effect of breathing frequency on RSA was large. At breathing frequencies of seven breaths/minute or less, RSA was large and constant. As breathing frequency increased above seven breaths/minute, the amplitude of RSA showed a log-linear decrease (see Fig. 2).[15] The effect of tidal volume was small, in that a 50% increase in tidal volume caused only a 15% increase in RSA.[16]

Fouad et al[17] evaluated the method of Katona and Jih[13] in man for the first time. They measured successive normal RR intervals (heart period), respiratory rate, and volume over intervals of at least 30 seconds. They excluded segments of recording that showed artifact or instability in either the ECG or the respiratory recording. The VHP was determined by calculating the difference between the average maximum RR interval and the average minimum RR interval in the window of measurement, e.g., five to eight breaths (see Fig. 3). Parasympathetic control of heart period was defined as the difference in the average RR interval before and after a 0.03 mg/kg dose of atropine (see Fig. 4). There was a strong regression of average VHP on PC (VHP = .216PC-15) and

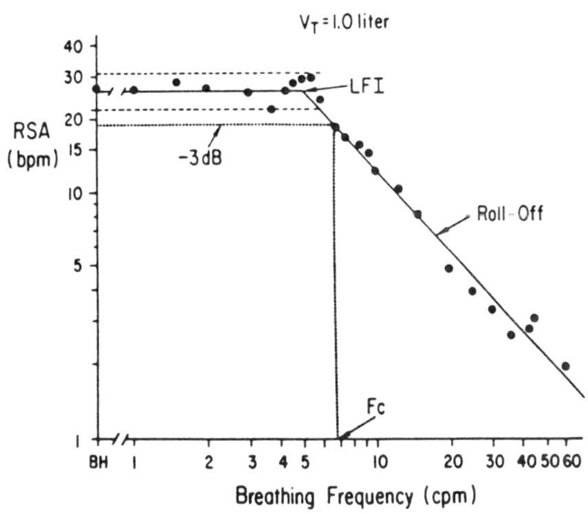

Figure 2. *The relation between RSA and ventilation frequency (log-log plot) obtained with a constant tidal volume (V_T) of 1 L. The solid lines indicate the least-squares regression lines. Dashed lines indicate ±2 SD. LFI: the low-frequency intercept. Dotted lines indicate -3 dB level (0.707 x LFI). Fc indicates the corner frequency. A least-squares regression line was fitted to the data points for breathing frequencies below 6/min. The LFI was the amplitude of RSA at which the regression line intersects the Y axis (28.3 beats/min/L for this subject). A second least-squares regression line was fitted to the data points for breathing frequencies above 6/min. The slope of this line in decibels per decade was the system roll-off (21.6 dB/decade for this subject). In this subject, the two regression lines intersected at 5.0/min. The value of RSA at this intersection was multiplied by 0.707 to obtain the value for RSA that was 3 dB below the LFI and that fell on the roll-off line. The breathing frequency that corresponded to the -3 dB value of RSA was defined as the Fc (here, 6.6 cycles/min). Reproduced with permission from Hirsch JA, Bishop B: Respiratory sinus arrhythmia in humans: How breathing pattern modulates heart rate. J Appl Physiol 241:H620–H629, 1981.*

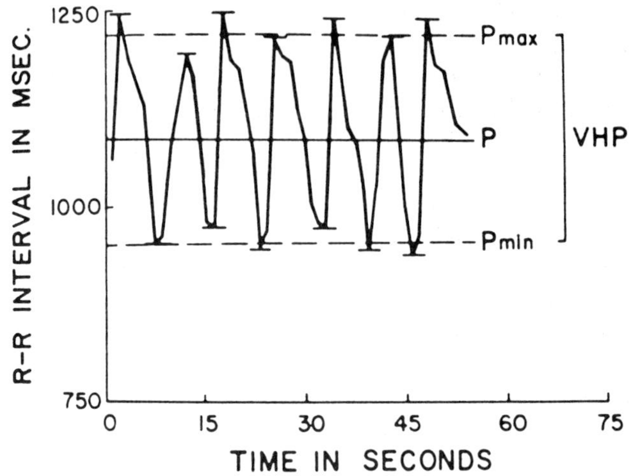

Figure 3. *The method for calculating variation in heart period (VHP) with the multiple breath method. The RR intervals for six respiratory cycles are shown. P: average RR interval; P_{max}: longest RR interval in each respiratory cycle; P_{min}: shortest RR interval in each respiratory cycle; and VHP: average P_{max} - average P_{min} in units of msec. Reproduced with permission from Fouad FM, Tarazi RC, Ferrario CM, et al: Assessment of parasympathetic control of heart rate by a noninvasive method. Am J Physiol 246:H838–H842, 1984.*

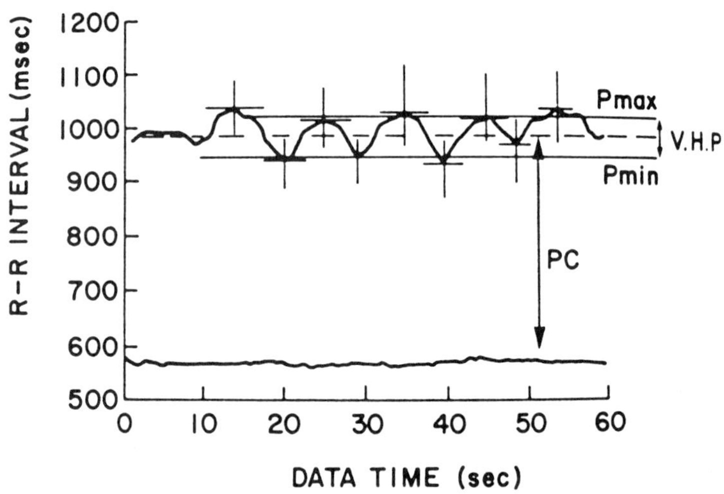

Figure 4. *The method for calculating parasympathetic control (PC) of heart period with the multiple breath method. PC: average RR interval under control conditions—average RR interval after a maximum dose of atropine and VHP: variation in heart period (average P_{max} - average P_{min}). Reproduced with permission from Fouad FM, Tarazi RC, Ferrario CM, et al: Assessment of parasympathetic control of heart rate by a noninvasive method. Am J Physiol 246:H838–H842, 1984.*

the correlation between the two variables was 0.90 (see Fig. 5). It is interesting that resting heart period in supine subjects did not correlate strongly with PC of heart period (r = -0.43). Administration of 10 mg of propranolol intravenously increased the average heart period from 984 milliseconds to 1091 milliseconds. The correlation between the average VHP before and after propranolol was 0.97, and the relationship between average VHP and PC was similar in patients who were given propranolol and in those who were not. Fouad et al[17] concluded that average VHP was an accurate index of parasympathetic activity and was clinically valuable for assessing the vagal tone of the heart. They warned, however, that protocols must be standardized in order to avoid alterations of results by simultaneous changes in sympathetic nervous system activity.

The use of RSA during multiple deep breaths was adapted by Sundkvist et al[18] to a single deep breath method to be used with a conventional ECG machine to assess vagal tone. The patient or subject is asked to conduct a single maximal deep breath with five seconds for inspiration and five seconds for expiration. The shortest RR interval during inspiration (I) and the longest RR interval during expiration (E) are measured and the E:I ratio is calculated. This test has been used to evaluate the autonomic nervous system in patients with diabetes mellitus.[19] Smith[20] computed the E:I ratio in 174 healthy subjects aged 16 to 89 years and used the confidence intervals of the regression to evaluate 134 diabetics aged 15 to 70 years for parasympathetic dysfunction. The relation between the E:I ratio and resting heart rate was not significant, but the E:I ratio decreased significantly with age. Therefore, Smith concluded that age-adjusted normal values should be used to interpret results obtained with E:I ratio.[20]

The difference between maximum and minimum RR interval during a

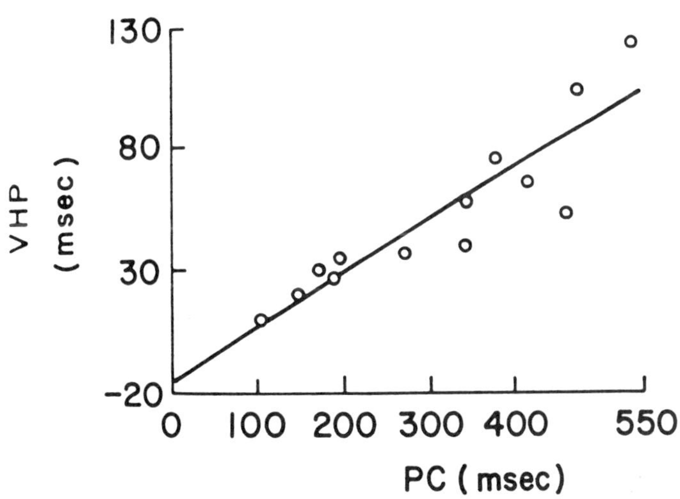

Figure 5. *Correlation between variation in heart period (VHP, see Fig. 3) and parasympathetic control (PC, see Fig. 4). The strong correlation between VHP and PC (r = 0.90) indicates that VHP is a reliable index of PC of heart period in humans. Reproduced with permission from Fouad FM, Tarazi RC, Ferrario CM, et al: Assessment of parasympathetic control of heart rate by a noninvasive method. Am J Physiol 246:H838–H842, 1984.*

single breath or during a period of controlled deep breathing has been used extensively in man to evaluate parasympathetic nervous system function, usually as part of a battery of tests of autonomic function in patients with diabetes mellitus.[21,22] Also, this test has been used in short-term psychological experiments. It has not been used extensively to evaluate either risk or parasympathetic nervous system function in cardiovascular diseases.

Differences in Successive, Normal RR Intervals (NN50 and pNN50)

In 1984, Ewing et al[23] reported that cardiac parasympathetic activity could be estimated in 24-hour ECG recordings by counting the number of positive differences in successive, normal RR intervals (NN intervals) that were >50 milliseconds (NN50 or "RR counts"). They applied this method to 25 normal subjects, average age 37 (range 20 to 65), and to 50 diabetics, 30 with medically-denervated hearts and 20 with normal cardiovascular reflexes. In addition, six patients with cardiac transplants were studied with the method. The following findings linked the counts of NN interval differences >50 milliseconds to parasympathetic activity:

1. the number of counts decreased as a function of age;
2. the number of counts increased at night;
3. the number of counts did not decrease during β-adrenergic blockade; and
4. very low counts and lack of night-day differences in counts were found in patients with diabetic vagal denervation and in patients with heart transplants (surgically-denervated hearts).

These workers also found that NN50 reflected parasympathetic activity much better than mean heart period or heart rate.[23] For example, a comparison of 15

Table 1.
Association Between Age and NN50 in Normal Subjects

	Age (years)		
	<40 (n = 15)	*≥40 (n = 10)*	*P value*
Mean heart rate awake (beats/min)	84	82	n.s.
Mean heart rate asleep (beats/min)	59	61	n.s.
Mean hourly NN50 awake (counts/hr)	243	97	<0.01
Mean hourly NN50 asleep (counts/hr)	443	137	<0.01

HR: heart rate; NN50: positive differences between successive NN intervals >50 msec. Reproduced with permission from Ewing DJ, Neilson JMM, Travis P: New method for assessing cardiac parasympathetic activity using 24-hour electrocardiograms. Br Heart J 52:396–402, 1984.

subjects <40 years of age with 10 subjects >40 years of age showed that, although the mean heart rates were similar, the mean hourly NN50 values were much lower in the older group (Table 1). Bigger et al[24] proposed that the proportion of differences in consecutive, normal RR intervals that were >50 milliseconds (pNN50) in absolute value be used instead of counts of positive differences, because the proportion has better statistical properties and better accounts for differences in heart rate than the count, and because negative differences have the same distribution as positive differences.[23] NN50 and pNN50, however, give similar results in clinical use. Bigger et al[24] showed that patients with low 24-hour heart period variability two weeks after acute myocardial infarction, measured as the standard deviation of all NN intervals over a 24-hour interval (a measure of all sources of variability over the course of a day), also had low values for pNN50.[24]

In 1989, McAreavey et al[25] used NN50 to study 21 patients during the first 24 hours of acute myocardial infarction. Patients were excluded if they had a history of previous myocardial infarction, diabetes, or treatment with β-adrenergic blocking or antihypertensive drugs. Patients with anterior myocardial infarction had significantly lower NN50. This finding suggests that the vagal tone for these patients was lower than that of patients with inferior infarction. The results were discussed in terms of the Bezold-Jarisch reflex[26]; i.e., the higher density of parasympathetic innervation to the posterior and inferior left ventricle and the preponderance of parasympathetically-mediated reflex activity during ischemia of these regions.[27,28] The study by McAreavey et al[25] did not determine how long the difference in vagal tone persisted between acute anterior and inferior myocardial infarction.

Zuanetti et al[29] used NN50 to evaluate the effect of three antiarrhythmic drugs on vagal tone in 56 patients who had stable chronic heart disease and frequent ventricular premature complexes. The three drugs evaluated were amiodarone, flecainide, and propafenone; these drugs decreased NN50 by 8%, 56%, and 64%, respectively. The decreases caused by flecainide and propafenone were statistically significant. The proportions with a substantial decrease in NN50 (>76%) for amiodarone, flecainide, and propafenone were 6%, 22%, and 35%, respectively. The effects of these drugs on NN50 were reversible when treatment was discontinued and were not related to suppression of ventricular arrhythmias. These authors[29] suggested that the decrease in NN50 might have prognostic implications.

Zuanetti et al[29] also showed that in 49 patients who had repeat 24-hour ECG recordings a median of 92 days apart, the values of NN50 correlated well on the two recordings (0.83). Kleiger et al[30] showed that in 14 normal subjects pNN50 was remarkably reproducible when the median time between recordings was 17.5 days.[30] The intraclass correlation coefficient was 0.90 and the standard error of measurement was 4.3. The great stability of NN50 and pNN50 simplifies detection of changes due to disease progression or to drug effects.

Bigger et al[8] showed that low values of pNN50, measured about two weeks after acute myocardial infarction, predicted death over the subsequent three years. When pNN50 was adjusted for age, New York Heart Association functional class, rales in the CCU during the index myocardial infarction, left ventricular ejection fraction, average NN interval in the Holter recording, and the average frequency of ventricular premature complexes, they found that the relationship between pNN50 and all-cause mortality, cardiac death, or arrhythmic death was weak and no longer statistically significant.[8] This finding implies that vagal tone correlates with these other risk predictors that account for much of the association between vagal tone and death.

Bigger et al[24] showed that patients who had low values for the standard deviation of normal RR intervals over a 24-hour period (SDNN) after myocardial infarction also has a low prevalence of sudden large increases ($\geq$200 milliseconds) in NN intervals. The average maximum difference between successive NN intervals was 146$\pm$64 milliseconds (range 80 to 276) in the group with low SDNN compared with 376$\pm$133 milliseconds (range 240 to 600) in the group with high SDNN, a difference that was large and statistically significant ($p < 0.001$). The maximum difference between successive NN intervals was strongly associated with other measures of vagal tone in these patients, e.g., pNN50, root mean square successive difference (rMSSD) and low-frequency power in the heart period power spectrum. Thus the large, sudden increases in NN intervals may result from large packet releases of acetylcholine (ACh) from vagal nerve terminals in the sinoatrial (SA) node region.

These sudden, large increases in NN interval in Holter recordings may be related to the sudden increases in NN interval seen during recovery from short periods of exercise. In 1914, Wenckebach[31] called these sudden lengthenings of NN intervals after exercise *bremsungen,* i.e., braking. In 1923, Kauf[32] called these fluctuations *vagushalt* in subjects recovering from exercise in the supine position. In 1982, Jennett et al[33] reported elegant experiments in 41 healthy male students in whom they explored the mechanism of sudden, large, and periodic changes in heart rate after a short period of exercise. Subjects exercised at 200 W on a bicycle ergometer for one minute to reach a minimum exercise heart rate of $\geq$150 beats/minute, then lay down (supine) to recover. Continuous ECG and respiratory tracings were recorded during recovery. They found braking, defined as a sharp fall in the instantaneous heart rate of >30 beats/minute, in 29 of the 41 subjects (71%) (see Fig. 6). Given the heart rate at which braking occurred, the sudden increases in NN interval were about 200 to 250 milliseconds. Typically breaking began as heart rate fell to about 100 beats/minute, lasted for about one minute, was associated with a decrease in P wave amplitude, and subsided as the preexercise heart rate was approached. There was a constant delay of about three seconds from inspiration to a braking cycle, but *vagushalt* did not necessarily occur after every inspiration. The braking cycles could occur after every second or third inspiration and, in a given subject, the ratio could vary, e.g., 1:1, 2:1, 3:1. Unlike RSA, however, braking was also seen during breath holding. Braking did not occur when subjects recovered from exercise either in the standing position or in the supine position with venous occlusive tourniquets on the thighs.[33] The latter finding suggests that central venous pressure contributes importantly to braking or *vagushalt.*

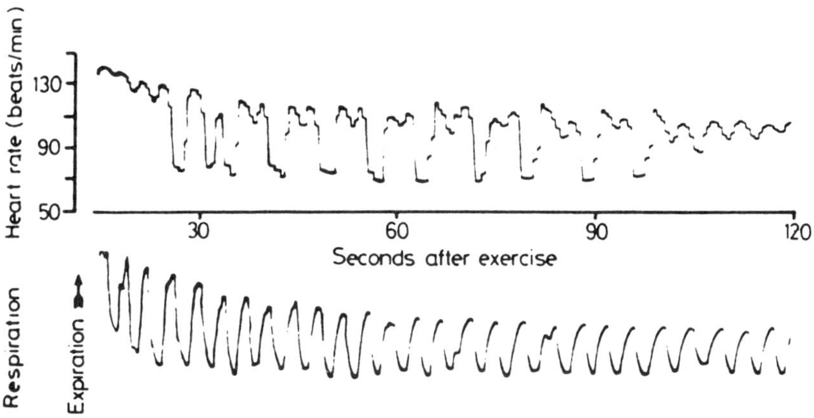

Figure 6. *An example of vagal braking, or vagushalt, in a normal man lying supine after a brief period of vigorous exercise. The upper tracing is the computed instantaneous heart rate and the lower tracing is ventilation (note that inspiration goes down). The first three vagal brakings occur after three consecutive breaths. Thereafter, they occur after every other breath. Vagal braking continues for about 1 min of recovery (from 30 to 90s). Before, during, and after the period of vagal braking, respiratory sinus arrhythmia can be seen in the upper tracing. Reproduced with permission from Jennett S, Lamb JF, Travis P: Sudden large and periodic changes in heart rate in healthy young men after short periods of exercise. Br Med J 285:1154–1156, 1982.*

Measures of Short-Term Variance or Standard Deviation

Early work by psychologists to determine the effect of cognitive tasks on vagal tone often used heart period variability, usually measured as the variance of heart period.[34] For short-term experiments (minutes) when the mean heart period is not changing, the variance or standard deviation can roughly estimate the vagal modulation of sinus rhythm. Smith and associates[35,36] have used the standard deviation of 100 or 255 consecutive normal RR intervals to estimate the vagal modulation of sinus arrhythmia. Standard deviations over such short periods of time are strongly associated with vagal modulation, but also are influenced by other modulating factors, e.g., sympathetic nerve activity. As the period of analysis increases, the fraction of the standard deviation that represents vagal modulation decreases. When the standard deviation of the NN intervals is calculated for a 24-hour period, $<5\%$ of the variance or standard deviation of the NN intervals is due to vagal modulation.[8] We have used the abbreviation SDNN to indicate the standard deviation of NN intervals calculated over a 24-hour period. SDNN over 24 hours reflects modulation of heart period over a wide range of frequencies motivated by many processes other than vagal activity. Even the standard deviation of 512 consecutive NN intervals fails to provide a good index of the parasympathetic withdrawal that occurs during head-up tilt from 0° to 70°, because this measure is influenced as much by the increase in heart period oscillations mediated by sympathetic nerve activity (SNA) as by the decreased oscillations mediated by parasympathetic nervous activity.[37] In order for short-term measures of heart period variance or standard deviation to provide a satisfactory index of vagal tone, the period over which the standard deviation is calculated must be short, e.g., 100 NN intervals or fewer. Also, trends in heart period must be minimal over the interval selected for the calculation. When trends (linear or otherwise) are present in the data, the standard deviation and variance tend to overestimate the variance present in the data (see the section below entitled "Root Mean Square Successive Difference.") When sympathetic activity is changing at the same time as parasympathetic activity, the standard deviation is affected by both sets of changes. A potential weakness in the standard deviation and the variance of NN intervals is that, unlike the other measures of heart period variability, they take no account of the serial nature of the measurements. A time series includes a first measurement, e.g., x_1, a second, x_2, etc. If the measurements are permuted, the standard deviation or variance will remain exactly the same, whereas the values of the other measures of variability, e.g., rMSSD, will almost surely change.

Root Mean Square Successive Difference

The mean square successive differences (MSSD) (δ^2) (also called the successive difference mean square) was developed by von Neumann et al[38,39] in the early 1940s to provide a variance measure that reduces the effects of gradual nonrandom trends in heart period. MSSD is defined as

$$\delta^2 = [\sum_{x=1}^{n-1}(x_{i+1} - x_i)^2]/(n - 1)$$

where i is an index of successive observations, $x_1, x_2, \ldots, x_n$. Unlike SDNN calculated over long periods (e.g., >two minutes), MSSD, NN50, and pNN50 are sensitive to high-frequency variability. MSSD (like NN50 and pNN50) takes the order of observations into account, and thus reduces the effects of linear and other nonrandom trends that spuriously inflate s^2, the sample variance. If variation in NN intervals is essentially random, then $\delta^2/2$ should equal s^2. If there are linear trends in the data, e.g., heart rate is increasing or decreasing, then s^2 can become substantially larger than $\delta^2/2$.

Many years after its properties were described, MSSD or rMSSD began to be used in psychophysiological studies.[40,41] In 1979, Heslegrave et al[42] reported a study that compared MSSD with s^2 for measuring the effects of 20-second periods of cognitive activity on heart period variability. These workers also evaluated whether heart rate or interbeat (i.e., NN) interval was the better scale of measurement. Since cognitive activity reduces vagal tone and, thereby, increases mean heart rate, MSSD was a better measure of heart period variability than s^2. They also found that the NN interval was a more sensitive scale of measurement than heart rate for detecting changing in vagal modulation (the transformation from one of these to the other, being a reciprocal, is highly non-linear). As expected, MSSD decreased substantially during cognitive activity.

rMSSD has been used to measure the decrease in vagal tone during exercise,[43] during treatment with atenolol,[44] and after acute myocardial infarction.[8] rMSSD is a continuous variable and, therefore, has statistical advantages over NN50 or pNN50. The distribution of rMSSD in samples of normal persons or of patients with recent myocardial infarction, however, is so positively skewed that the log transformation is advisable when rMSSD is used for parametric statistics.

Kleiger et al[30] showed that in 14 normal subjects, rMSSD, like pNN50, was remarkably reproducible. The intraclass correlation coefficient was 0.88 and the standard error of the measurement was 7.5. Hence, it is feasible to find differences in vagal tone due to changes in physiological or pharmacological conditions. Bigger et al[8] showed that low values of rMSSD significantly predict death during follow-up after acute myocardial infarction. Like pNN50, adjustment for other risk predictors renders the association between rMSSD and death weak and statistically insignificant.[8]

Correlations Among Measures of Vagal Tone

Ewing et al[45] showed that NN50 was moderately associated ($r = 0.63$) with RSA measured by the difference method during deep breathing. NN50 measured over the course of 24 hours, however, seemed to be more sensitive than short-term measures of respiratory sinus arrhythmia for detecting parasympathetic dysfunction in patients with diabetes mellitus.[45] Bigger et al[8,46] showed that pNN50, rMSSD, and high-frequency power (i.e., power in the 0.15 to 0.40 Hz range) in the 24-hour or five-minute heart period power spectra were strongly correlated with each other ($r \geq 0.89$) when measured about two weeks after myocardial infarction (see Table 2). Kleiger et al[30] showed that these three variables were also strongly correlated in normal young persons.

Table 2.
Correlations Among Measures of Vagal Tone in Normal Subjects and in Patients Studied Two Weeks After Myocardial Infarction

	Normal Subjects (n = 14)			*Postinfarction (n = 715)*		
	Ln HFP	*Ln rMSSD*	*Ln pNN50*	*Ln HFP*	*Ln rMSSD*	*Ln pNN50*
Ln HFP	1.00			1.00		
Ln rMSSD	0.98	1.00		0.92	1.00	
Ln pNN50	0.92	0.96	1.00	0.89	0.93	1.00

HFP: high-frequency power in the 24-hour heart period power spectrum; Ln: natural logarithm; pNN50: proportion of consecutive NN differences >50 msec; rMSSD: root mean square successive difference. Reproduced with permission from Bigger JT Jr, Fleiss JL, Steinman RC, et al: Correlations among time and frequency domain measures of heart period variability two weeks after myocardial infarction. Am J Cardiol 69:891–898, 1992 and from Kleiger RE, Bigger JT Jr, Bosner MS, et al: Stability over time of variables measuring heart rate variability in normal subjects. Am J Cardiol 68:626–630, 1991.

Conclusions

There are a variety of time domain methods for estimating vagal tone in intact humans. These technics range from simple bedside methods requiring <30 seconds to those that provide an average value for vagal tone over a 24-hour period. Thanks to their high correlations, any of these variables can be used to assess vagal tone in health or disease or to evaluate the effect of treatment on vagal modulation of the SA node. Reliable measurements can be made as often as every two minutes or averaged over 24 hours or more; the period depends on the demands of the application. Time domain measurements of vagal tone correlate so strongly with frequency domain measures that they can be used interchangeably. Twenty-four-hour measures of vagal tone are quite stable from day to day. This stability makes it easy to determine changes in vagal tone due to physiological, psychological, pathological, or to drug effects. Measures of vagal tone predict mortality after myocardial infarction and may be subject to experimental and therapeutic manipulation.

References

1. Eckberg DL, Drabinsky M, Braunwald E: Defective cardiac parasympathetic control in patients with heart disease. N Engl J Med 285:877–881, 1971.
2. Wolf M, Varigos G, Hunt D, et al: Sinus arrhythmia in acute myocardial infarction. Med J Aust 2:52–53, 1978.
3. Airaksinen K, Ikaheimo MJ, Linnaluoto MK, et al: Impaired vagal heart rate control in coronary artery disease. Br Heart J 58:592–597, 1988.
4. Ryan C, Hollenberg MM, Harvey DB, et al: Impaired parasympathetic responses in patients after myocardial infarction. Am J Cardiol 37:1013–1018, 1976.
5. La Rovere MT, Specchia G, Mortara A, et al: Baroreflex sensitivity, clinical correlates and cardiovascular mortality among patients with a first myocardial infarction. A prospective study. Circulation 78:816–824, 1988.
6. Schwartz PJ, Vanoli E, Stramba-Badiale M, et al: Autonomic mechanisms and sudden death. New insights from analysis of baroreceptor reflexes in conscious dogs with and without a myocardial infarction. Circulation 78:969–979, 1988.
7. Bigger JT Jr, Fleiss JL, Steinman RC, et al: Frequency domain measures of heart period variability and mortality after myocardial infarction. Circulation 85:164–171, 1992.
8. Bigger JT Jr, Fleiss JL, Steinman RC, et al: Correlations among time and frequency domain measures of heart period variability two weeks after myocardial infarction. Am J Cardiol 69:891–898, 1992.
9. Ludwig C: Beitrage zur Kenntniss des Einflusses der Respirations bewegungen auf den Blutlauf im Aortensysteme. Arch Anat Physiol 13:242–302, 1847.
10. Anrep G, Pascual W, Rossler R: Respiratory variations of the heart rate. I. The reflex mechanism of the respiratory arrhythmia. Proc Soc Lond 119B:191–217, 1936.
11. Anrep G, Pascual W, Rossler R: Respiratory variations of the heart rate. II. The central mechanism of the respiratory arrhythmia and the inter-relations between the central and reflex mechanisms. Proc Soc Lond 119B:218–230, 1936.
12. Katona PG, Poitras JW, Barnett GO, et al: Cardiac vagal efferent activity and heart period in the carotid sinus reflex. Am J Physiol 218:1030–1037, 1970.
13. Katona PG, Jih F: Respiratory sinus arrhythmia: Noninvasive measure of parasympathetic cardiac control. J Appl Physiol 39:801–805, 1975.

14. Wheeler T, Watkins PJ: Cardiac denervation in diabetes. Br Med J 4:584–586, 1969.
15. Hirsch JA, Bishop B: Respiratory sinus arrhythmia in humans: How breathing pattern modulates heart rate. Am J Physiol 241:H620–H629, 1981.
16. Eckberg DL: Human sinus arrhythmia as an index of vagal cardiac outflow. J Appl Physiol 54:961–966, 1983.
17. Fouad FM, Tarazi RC, Ferrario CM, et al: Assessment of parasympathetic control of heart rate by a noninvasive method. Am J Physiol 246:H838–H842, 1984.
18. Sundkvist G, Almer LO, Lilja B: Respiratory influence on heart rate in diabetes mellitus. Br Med J 1:924–925, 1979.
19. Bennett T, Farquhar IK, Hosking DJ, et al: Assessment of methods for estimating autonomic nervous control of the heart in patients with diabetes mellitus. Diabetes 27:1167–1174, 1978.
20. Smith SA: Reduced sinus arrhythmia in diabetic autonomic neuropathy: Diagnostic value of an age-related normal range. Br Med J 285:1599–1601, 1982.
21. Ewing DJ, Clarke BF: Diagnosis and management of diabetic autonomic neuropathy. Br Med J 285:916–918, 1982.
22. Ewing DJ, Martyn CN, Young RJ, et al: The value of cardiovascular autonomic function tests: 10 years experience in diabetes. Diabetes Care 8:491–498, 1985.
23. Ewing DJ, Neilson JMM, Travis P: New method for assessing cardiac parasympathetic activity using 24-hour electrocardiograms. Br Heart J 52:396–402, 1984.
24. Bigger JT Jr, Kleiger RE, Fleiss JL, et al: Components of heart rate variability measured during healing of acute myocardial infarction. Am J Cardiol 61:208–215, 1988.
25. McAreavey D, Neilson JM, Ewing DJ, et al: Cardiac parasympathetic activity during the early hours of acute myocardial infarction. Br Heart J 62:165–170, 1989.
26. Mark AL: The Bezold-Jarisch reflex revisited: Clinical implications of inhibitory reflexes originating in the heart. J Am Coll Cardiol 1:90–102, 1983.
27. Thames MD, Klopfenstein HS, Abboud FM, et al: Preferential distribution of inhibitory cardiac receptors to the inferoposterior wall of the left ventricle activated during coronary occlusion in the dog. Circ Res 43:512–519, 1978.
28. Felder RB, Thames MD. Interaction between cardiac receptors and sinoaortic baroreceptors in the control of efferent cardiac sympathetic nerve activity during myocardial ischemia in dogs. Circ Res 45:728–736, 1979.
29. Zuanetti G, Latini R, Neilson JMM, et al: Heart rate variability in patients with ventricular arrhythmias: Effect of antiarrhythmic drugs. J Am Coll Cardiol 17:604–612, 1991.
30. Kleiger RE, Bigger JT Jr, Bosner MS, et al: Stability over time of variables measuring heart rate variability in normal subjects. Am J Cardiol 68:626–630, 1991.
31. Wenckebach KF: Die unregelmassige Herztatigkeit und ihre Klinische Bedeutung. Leipsiz: 1914.
32. Kauf E: Untersuchungen uber das Verhalten des Herzens nach Muskelarbeit. Wiener archiv fur innere Medizin 5:567–580, 1923.
33. Jennett S, Lamb JF, Travis P: Sudden large and periodic changes in heart rate in healthy young men after short periods of exercise. Br Med J 285:1154–1156, 1982.
34. Porges SW: Heart rate variability and deceleration as indexes of reaction time. J Exp Psychol 92:103–110, 1972.
35. Smith SE, Smith SA: Heart rate variability in healthy subjects measured with a bedside computer-based technique. Clin Sci 61:379–383, 1981.
36. Coker R, Koziell A, Oliver C, et al: Does the sympathetic nervous system influence sinus arrhythmia in man? Evidence from combined autonomic blockade. J Physiol (Lond) 356:459–464, 1984.
37. Vybiral T, Byrg RF, Maddens ME, et al: Effect of passive tilt on sympathetic and parasympathetic components of heart rate variability in normal subjects. Am J Cardiol 63:1117–1120, 1989.

38. von Neumann J, Kent RH, Bellinson HR, et al: The mean square successive difference. Ann Math Stat 12:153–162, 1941.
39. von Neumann J: Distribution of the ratio of the mean square successive difference to the variance. Ann Math Stat 12:367–395, 1941.
40. Liederman PH, Shapiro D: Application of a time series statistic to physiology and psychology. Science 138:141–142, 1962.
41. Varni JG, Clark E, Gidden DB: Analysis of cyclic heart rate variability. Psychophysiology 8:406–413, 1971.
42. Heslegrave RJ, Ogilvie JC, Furedy JJ: Measuring baseline treatment differences in heart rate variability: Variance versus successive difference mean square and beats per minute versus interbeat intervals. Psychophysiology 16:151–157, 1979.
43. Goldsmith R, Bigger JT Jr, Steinman RC, et al: A comparison of 24-hour parasympathetic activity in endurance trained and untrained men. J Am Coll Cardiol 20:552–558, 1992.
44. Cook JR, Bigger JT Jr, Kleiger RE, et al: The effect of atenolol and diltiazem on heart period variability in normal persons. J Am Coll Cardiol 17:480–484, 1991.
45. Ewing DJ, Neilson JMM, Shapiro CM, et al: Twenty four hour heart rate variability: Effects of posture, sleep, and time of day in healthy controls and comparison with bedside tests of autonomic function in diabetic patients. Br Heart J 65:239–244, 1991.
46. Bigger JT Jr, Albrecht P, Steinman RC, et al: Comparison of time- and frequency domain-based measures of cardiac parasympathetic activity in Holter recordings after myocardial infarction. Am J Cardiol 63:536–538, 1989.

CHAPTER 27

Methods for Assessment of Sympatho-Vagal Balance:

Power Spectral Analysis

A. Malliani, M. Pagani, F. Lombardi

The study of rhythmicity furnishes one of the simplest keys to understanding complexity[1] of the relationships between the external environment and life. Indeed, the influence of solar or lunar cycles on biological rhythms was recognized long before the birth of experimental physiology. Conversely, the contemporary framework is that rhythmicity constitutes an inherent property of biological systems.[2] In this chapter, the basic hypothesis that biological rhythms can be markers of functional states, again an ancient thought increasingly reiterated in recent times,[3] is explored in regard to some aspects of the neural regulation of cardiovascular function.

A few premises might be worthwhile. The emerging principles, including rhythmicity, that govern the operation of neural networks have recently been reviewed[2,4] and are outside the scope of this chapter. Suffice it to say that studies on the central pattern generators have evolved from Sherrington's[5] pioneering observations of rhythmic locomotion movements in the chronic spinal dog to the use of invertebrate nervous systems surgically isolated or in vitro neuron cultures. The conclusion was reached that multiple ionic conductance mechanisms can provide a neuron with a capacity for autorhythmic discharge.[2] Circulation and respiration, however, which are strictly related transport functions, are both based on discontinuous events, and oscillations of various orders characterize variables such as arterial pressure and heart period.

Observations on rhythmic fluctuations of systemic arterial pressure probably started in 1733 with Reverend Stephen Hales' experiment,[6] during which oscillations of first and second order were observed, i.e., those related to cardiac cycle and to respiration. As to third order oscillations, i.e., those with a period apparently longer than the respiratory cycle, Koepchen[7] has recently reviewed

From *Vagal Control of the Heart: Experimental Basis and Clinical Implications* edited by MN Levy, PJ Schwartz © 1994, Futura Publishing Co. Inc., Armonk, NY.

their history. According to his conclusions, it is assumed that the waves that were described by Sigmund Mayer,[8] which have a period of about 10 seconds, are the prototype of the third order oscillations of arterial pressure. The period of this type of oscillation however, is highly variable.[9–12]

With regard to the rhythms discernible in the discharge of the autonomic outflow, Adrian and coworkers[13] were the first to record, from sympathetic nerves, efferent impulse activity displaying a dual rhythm in phase with arterial pulse and respiration. Several decades then elapsed before Fernandez de Molina and Perl[14] observed, in spinal cats, increases in sympathetic efferent discharge simultaneous to slow arterial pressure waves. As to the impulse activity of vagal efferent fibers, the existence of cardiac and respiratory rhythms was also reported[15,16] before the description of an additional rhythm in phase with third order arterial pressure oscillations.[17,18]

There has been much debate over the years as to the origin of these neural rhythms. Indeed, these rhythms could depend on either afferent peripheral modulations or on autochthonous oscillating properties of the central nervous system (CNS), or on both mechanisms. Similarly, cardiovascular oscillations could either be due to neural rhythms, or could cause them, or could reflect both influences.[19] In fact, it should be of no surprise if two basic disturbances, such as respiration and vasomotion, shared the same rhythmic code, with the neural mechanisms influenced by and regulating them.

Physiological Background

Neural regulation of circulatory functions is mainly effected through the interplay of the sympathetic and vagal outflows, which are tonically and phasically modulated by the interaction of at least three major factors: the central integration, peripheral inhibitory reflex mechanisms (with negative feedback characteristics), and peripheral excitatory reflex mechanisms (with positive feedback characteristics) (Fig. 1).[20–22] In natural closed loop conditions,[23] simple reflexes are unlikely to exist. In fact, even the bradycardia reflex response to an arterial pressure rise is the result of a composite inhibitory supraspinal reflex mechanism,[23] which may be blunted, however, by the excitatory influence mediated by the cardiovascular sympathetic afferent fibers.[24] In short, the problem is that of reconciling the complexity of neural regulation with a unitary operational scheme that might be the basis for modelling approaches. In our proposal (Fig. 1), this level of uncertainty is inherent to a black box analysis that is simply aimed at assessing the dynamic state of the sympatho-vagal interaction, viewed as a push-pull or reciprocal relationship. In fact, in most physiological conditions, though not in all,[17,18] the activation of either outflow is accompanied by the inhibition of the other.

The core hypothesis of this chapter is that this interaction can be broadly explored in the frequency domain. Data are reviewed that support the assumptions that the second order rhythm of heart period variability, related to respiration and defined as the high-frequency (HF) spectral component, is a marker of vagal modulation; the third order rhythm, present in heart period

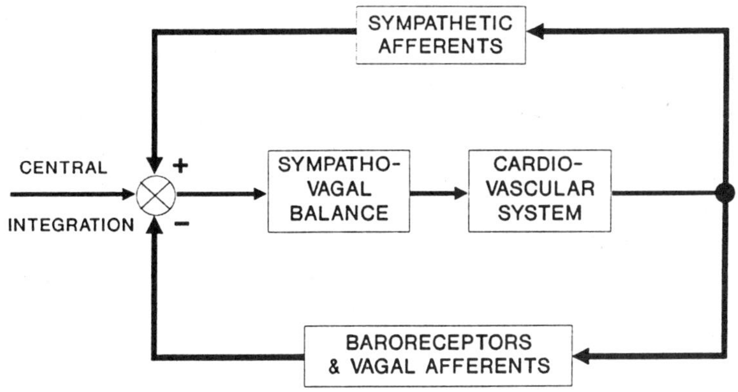

Figure 1. *Schematic representation of the opposite feedback mechanisms that, in addition to central integration, subserve the neural control of the cardiovascular system. Baroreceptive and vagal afferent fibers from the cardiopulmonary region mediate negative feedback mechanisms (exciting the vagal and inhibiting the sympathetic outflow), while positive feedback mechanisms are mediated by sympathetic afferent fibers (exciting the sympathetic and inhibiting the vagal outflow). Reproduced by permission of the American Heart Association, Inc. from Malliani A, Pagani M, Lombardi F: Cardiovascular neural regulation explored in the frequency domain. Circulation 84:482–492, 1991.*

and arterial pressure variabilities and defined as the low-frequency (LF) component, is a marker of sympathetic modulation; and a reciprocal relation exists between these two rhythms, and it is similar to the relation characterizing the sympatho-vagal balance.

Methodology

In recent years, even quite simple analyses of the variability phenomena, such as those offered by the use of standard deviation, frequency histograms, or scattergrams of discrete series of events, have provided important information on pathophysiological processes like myocardial infarction[25] and diabetic neuropathy.[26] In this context, however, this chapter discusses the application of spectral techniques that can specifically assess the dynamics of any given variability by quantifying any rhythmicity hidden in the signal.

Sayers and his coworkers,[27,28] employing the algorithm of Fast Fourier Transform (FFT), first reported the existence of three major components in human RR variability that occurred at frequencies around 0.25, 0.10, and 0.03 Hz; i.e., a component related to respiration (0.25 Hz) and two others at lower frequencies. The FFT algorithm is still widely used and has provided valuable results.

We shall, however, briefly describe a partially different methodology, which is based on autoregressive algorithms and which is used in our[29–32] and other laboratories.[33–35] After appropriate acquisition of the electrocardiogram, the individual R waves are sequentially recognized. The series of consecutive RR intervals constitutes the interval tachogram. An important feature of autoregressive algorithms is that a reliable estimate of spectral parameters can be obtained from data series as short as 200 intervals. Additionally, the computer algorithm[30,31] automatically calculates the autoregressive coefficients necessary to define the model of the signal generation mechanism and, hence, the power spectral density estimate. The power and center frequency of every spectral component is presented in absolute units as well as in normalized units (nu) (Fig. 2).

Nu are obtained by dividing any given spectral component by the total variance cleared of the power of the component near 0 Hz (component 1 in the left upper panel of Fig. 2), and this ratio is then multiplied by 100.[11,12,30] Recent development of the methodology involves the analysis of recordings over a 24-hour period.[11,32]

Spectral analysis, in principle, can be applied to any variability phenomenon. For instance, a similar procedure can be used to compute the spectrum of systolic arterial pressure (SAP) (Fig. 2).[11,30,32,36,37] Further computations can be performed on the data in a multivariate form, such as cross-spectral and coherence analysis, that can provide quantitative information on the statistical link between the two signals at any given frequency and on their phase relationships (Fig. 2).[30,36–40]

Spectral analysis requires, per se, stationary conditions which, paradoxically, are unknown to biology. Thus, a theoretical and practical compromise has to be found between the length of a series of events and the confidence level of stationarity.[41] Short segments of data are more likely to be stationary. Thus, methods of spectral estimation capable of operating efficiently even on short series of data are preferable. The very slow oscillations that are considered the D.C. component can only be properly assessed with this technique with much longer series of data[42] or with different algorithms.[43,44] This low part of the spectrum, however, may contain information on thermoregulation.[28,45] Experiments have shown that very low-frequency thermal stimuli produce synchronous peaks in digital flow. This hypothesis, however, disregards the question of whether the primary mechanism involved is vasomotion or thermoregulation.[45]

In resting conditions, when noise and components near 0 Hz are minimal, the meaningful portion of the signal can be greater than 50% in man and 90% in conscious dogs,[12] while it can be as low as 15% in dynamic conditions.[11]

Human Physiological Studies

Total Power

RR interval variability decreases as age increases[30,32,46–49] and has been interpreted as a selective[25,26] index of cardiac parasympathetic tone. This interpretation requires a few comments, however, that are essential in clarifying the usefulness of spectral analysis.

It is self-evident that total power, or its measures in the time domain (i.e.,

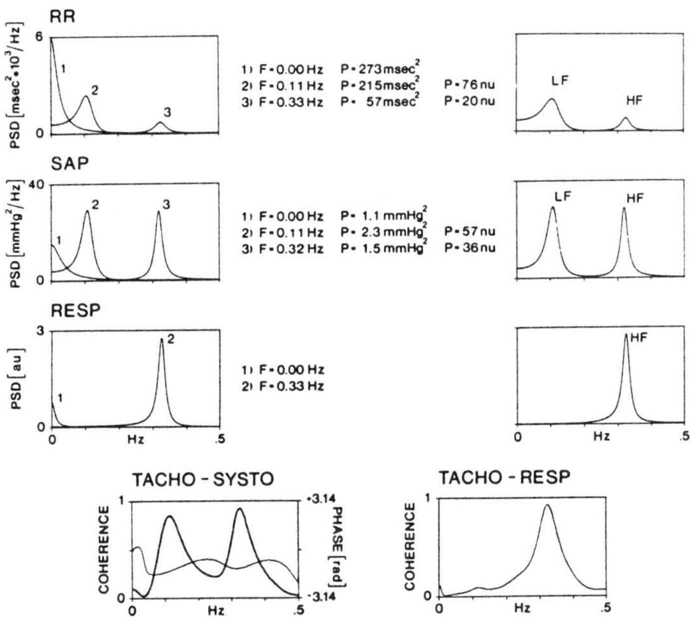

Figure 2. *Spectral analysis of RR and systolic arterial pressure (SAP) variabilities and of respiratory activity (Resp) in a healthy human subject, at rest. The left panels depict the separate components detected by the computer algorithm in the three variability series. The right panels represent the autospectra, plotted without using the coefficients of the component (1), centered at 0.00 Hz. Notice the presence of two major (LF and HF) components in the case of RR and SAP variability spectra and of only a major HF component in the case of respiration. For each autospectrum, in the case of both RR and SAP variabilities, the computer provides the center frequency (in Hz) and associated power (P), both in absolute (i.e., respectively msec² or mm Hg²) and normalized units (nu) for all components detected. In the case of respiration, only the center frequency of the major component is considered. In the bottom panels, the coherence function (thick tracing) is presented between the RR and SAP variabilities (tacho-systo) and between RR variability and respiration (tacho-resp), while the phase function (thin tracing) is presented only in the case of the tachogram-systogram relationship. In the case of the tachogram-systogram relationship, notice the high values (approaching 1) of the coherence function in correspondence of both LF and HF components, and only in correspondence of the HF component in the case of the tachogram-respiration relationship.*

variance or standard deviation), includes both rhythmic and nonrhythmic components to which most, if not all, of the D.C. component also pertains. The main reason for attributing the significance of a pure vagal marker to variance is probably due to the fact that variance usually increases with bradycardia and decreases with tachycardia. This phenomenon, however, affects not only total power but, in general, the absolute power of all spectral components. Also, it probably represents a simple consequence of the fact that the absolute variability of the cardiac cycle is larger around 60 to 70 beats/minute than around 140 beats/minute. In other words, variance does not reflect the property that only vagal activity induces fluctuations in heart period, but it probably depends upon the oscillations that are present when both vagal and sympathetic influences are active. On the contrary, variance is obviously reduced when the functional change is close to saturation and is under the almost exclusive influence of sympathetic drive, as in the case of marked tachycardia. Consequently, a drastic reduction of variance accompanying various pathophysiological states cannot always be interpreted as a sign of a reduced parasympathetic and, simultaneously, increased sympathetic modulation. Indeed, an abatement of variance can also depend on the reduced responsiveness of the target function (such as heart period) or on the viability of the neural pathways.

As an experimental proof, it has been found that during passive tilt, a maneuver that excites the sympathetic activity but in which tachycardia is not marked, total variance is not a sensitive marker of vagal withdrawal.[30,50–52] Thus, increases in variance are also described during passive tilt.[49]

Spectral Components

In the resting normal subject, power spectral analysis reveals two main rhythmic oscillations[11,29–37,50,51,53] in heart period and in arterial pressure (Fig. 2). The LF component has a center frequency usually around 0.1 Hz (0.11 Hz in the case of Fig. 2), while the HF component, synchronous with respiration, occurs at about 0.25 Hz (0.33 Hz in Fig. 2). Cross-spectral analysis[30,36,37,39,40] of RR interval and SAP variabilities indicates (see Fig. 2) that a high degree of coherence (approaching 1) exists between the fluctuations of these two variables only in correspondence to the LF and HF components. Similarly, a high coherence is found between the HF component of RR or SAP variability and the main component in the spectrum of respiratory movements (Fig. 2). Vice versa, with this length of time series, the coherence function between RR and SAP variability is virtually nil, near 0 Hz. The LF component and the corresponding Mayer waves do not have a fixed period and their center frequency can vary considerably.[11] Therefore, dividing the lower part of the spectrum into two preselected bands with a cut-off frequency of 0.07 to 0.09 Hz[54,55] appears now totally unjustified.

The power of the LF component usually prevails over that of the HF component in the RR variability, with a LF/HF ratio of more than 1.[30,32] With ageing, in spite of a progressive reduction in variance, this ratio is preserved when measured with autoregressive algorithms.[30] When Fourier analysis was used,[49] however, a greater attenuation of the HF component occured in elderly subjects.

Increases in Sympathetic Activity and RR Variability

Passive tilt or, more simply, standing up increases sympathetic activity and thus shifts the sympatho-vagal balance. According to the scheme of Figure 1, the new equilibrium should mainly be due to a decreased central restraint by negative feedback mechanisms, although some variation in central command and an interplay with excitatory reflexes elicited by the redistribution of blood cannot be dismissed.[20,21,56] Such a change in the sympatho-vagal balance is accompanied by an increase in the LF component and a decrease in the HF component of RR variability (Fig. 3).[29,30,32,50,51,57–60] In the presence of a simultaneous reduction of variance, the use of nu[32] facilitates the appreciation of the new state. The LF/HF ratio is greatly enhanced, up to values of about 20 in young subjects.[30] The increase in the LF component and the reciprocal decrease in the HF component of RR variability during tilt may[30,48] or may not[49] be spared by ageing.

Mental stress, as induced by arithmetic calculation, may be used in human experiments to enhance sympathetic tone. In this case, a modified central command should represent the fundamental mechanism that alters sympatho-vagal balance. The total power is reduced,[61] but the LF component is increased and the HF component is decreased (Fig. 3).[62,63]

Finally, physical exercise is a crucial biological condition that influences the sympatho-vagal balance. Yet, this condition is associated with various factors, such as enhanced respiratory activity, decreased variance, and increased nonstationarity, that might complicate the analysis. Indeed, while Pagani et al[36] have described an increase in the LF component of RR variability with mild levels of exercise, this phenomenon has been refuted by Arai et al.[64] In general, however, when a sympathetic activation is accompanied by an abatement of RR variance, as occurs during physical exercise[65] or after

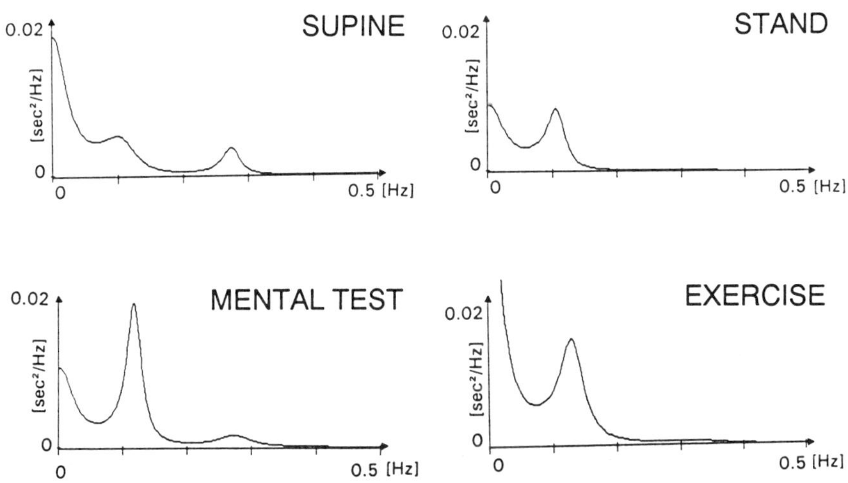

Figure 3. *Example of the spectral analysis of RR variability in a young normal subject during supine rest (supine, top left panel), during active orthostatism (stand, top right panel), during mental arithmetic test (mental test, bottom left panel), and during a mild level of bicycle exercise (exercise, bottom right panel). The mental arithmetic test consisted of subtracting a two-digit number (usually 17) from a four-digit number (usually 2021) as fast as possible, for about five minutes. The bicycle exercise consisted of a single bout of 75 W for about five minutes. Note the presence, during supine rest, of two similar components, respectively, at low and high frequency. On the contrary, in the other experimental conditions in which all are accompanied by sympathetic activation, the LF component prevailed. From Lucini et al, unpublished material.*

atropine administration,[12] it is crucial to determine where the residual power is distributed. The balance would still be reflected by the relationship between the two components, evaluated in nu or by the LF/HF ratio.[66]

Increases in Vagal Activity and RR Variability

The relationship between respiration and sinus arrhythmia is nonlinear.[67] Controlled respiration at frequencies within the resting physiological range,[67] however, is a convenient tool for enhancing the vagal modulation of heart rate.[30,57] In concrete terms, the power of the HF component predominates during metronome breathing (Fig. 4).[30,57] Under these conditions, the increase in the LF component observed with tilt is blunted in respect to that which is when it is obtained during spontaneous respiration.[30] If the frequency of controlled respiration is decreased enough to approach the third order rhythm, the two components merge into a single, more powerful oscillation.[67] The numerous studies that have been performed under controlled respiration in a

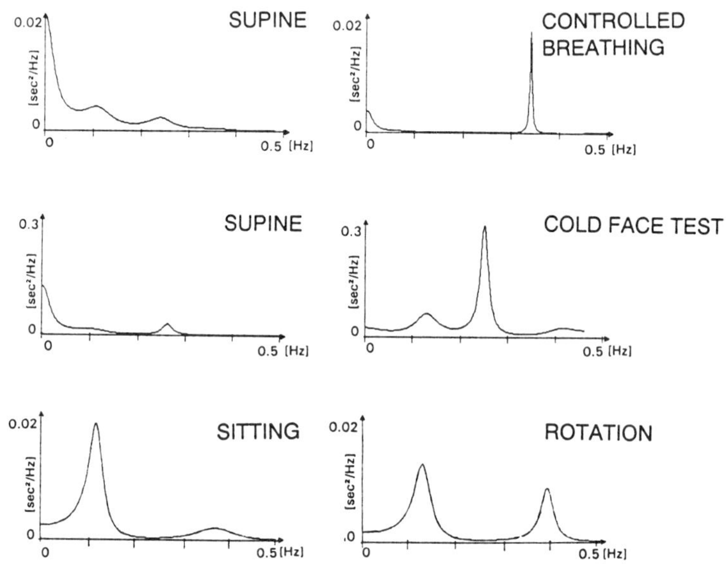

Figure 4. *Examples of the spectral analysis of RR variability in three different subjects, undergoing different experimental maneuvers, attended by increases in indices of vagal activity. Controlled breathing, at 20 cycles per min, was performed by asking the subjects to breathe following a metronome, and was not accompanied by significant changes in tidal volume or in blood gases. The cold face test was obtained by applying to both sides of the faces an ice pack, which contained a cold chemical mixture calibrated at 4°C. The rotation test was obtained by having the subjects sit on a motor-driven chair, which slowly rotated back and forth for about 200°. In this latter case, note the prevailing LF component during the control sitting recording, as already reported,[63] and the smaller increase in the HF component during the rotation, as compared to the other vagal stimuli, that were performed in the supine position. From Pizzinelli et al, unpublished material.*

broad range of 0.20 to 0.30 Hz are characterized, however, by a baseline sympatho-vagal balance that is likely to be shifted in favor of the latter component. In these conditions, which might approximate the near saturation of the system, the HF component is more likely to decrease than to increase.[68] Additional maneuvers that can be carried out in order to shift the sympatho-vagal balance in favor of the latter component are represented by cold stimulation of the face or by a mild rotational stimulus (Fig. 4). In both cases, the HF component increases.

Pharmacological Blockades and RR Variability

Selman et al[69] showed that atropine administration practically abolished the respiratory component of RR variability. This finding was corroborated by the study of Pomeranz et al,[57] who also noticed that I.V. administration of atropine reduced the absolute power of the LF component by 85% in supine subjects and reduced it by 72% when the subjects stood. Conversely, I.V. administration of propranolol, while leaving the LF and HF components unchanged in supine subjects, reduced the LF component by 73% in the standing subjects. Pomeranz et al[57] concluded that HF was mediated solely by the parasympathetic system in supine subjects and by the sympathetic system during standing.

The following considerations, however, suggested that these conclusions were unwarranted. The subjects were under controlled respiration and, therefore, in a condition of marked vagal predominance as suggested by recalculating the data.[57] Thus, the effects of atropine on the LF component were not assessed during spontaneous breathing. In fact, it is quite likely that the remaining power after atropine and under spontaneous breathing would all be distributed in the low-frequency region, similar to what has been observed in the conscious dog.[12] In order to assess this new equilibrium, however, the use of nu or of the LF/HF ratio is essential.[12] Finally, the study was performed on only eight subjects in whom tidal volume, pO_2, and pCO_2 were not measured to ensure the maintenance of comparable conditions.[30] These criticisms were prompted by the attention that this study has received concerning the interpretation of the LF component of RR variability.

The effects of β-adrenergic (β-AR) receptor blockade have also been variously interpreted. Pagani et al[30] observed that, although acute I.V. administration of propranolol blunted only the LF component increase induced by tilt, as described also by Pomeranz et al,[57] chronic oral administration significantly reduced the LF component, in subjects either at rest or during tilt (Fig. 5). In addition, β blockade was often accompanied by an increase in total power, and, thus, it could raise the absolute values of any single component. Therefore, the state of the sympatho-vagal balance, which is usually shifted toward vagal predominance, should be evaluated by using nu or the LF/HF ratio. In this regard, Cook et al[70] evaluated the absolute power of a LF component. It was measured with the FFT algorithm and, therefore, it only partly corresponded to the LF component measured with autoregressive algorithms. They

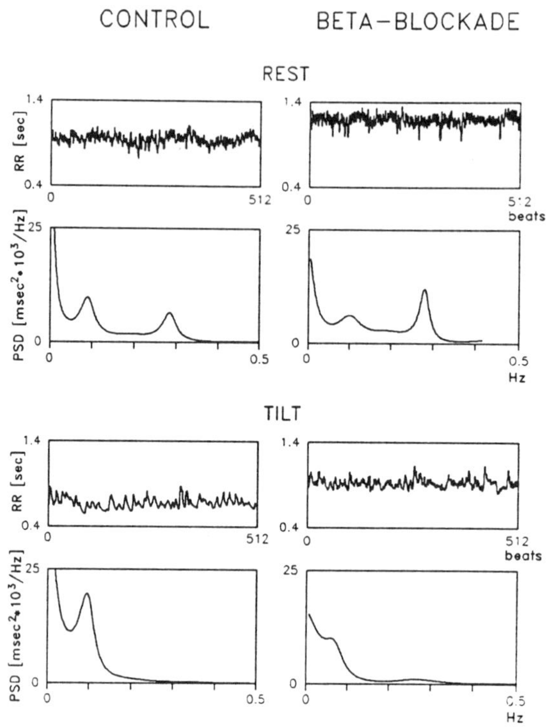

Figure 5. *Example of the effects of chronic β-AR receptor blockade (propranolol, [INDERAL, ICI] 0.6 mg/kg po per six days) on RR interval variability in a young healthy subject, examined before and during β-blockade both at rest and during passive tilt. Note the increase in average RR interval length both at rest and during tilt. The effects of β-blockade on the changing balance between sympathetic and vagal activities controlling the SA node are more easily described by considering the changes in the relative powers of both LF and HF components than variance alone. Accordingly, at rest, the reduced sympathetic activity and attendant relative increase in vagal control were paralleled by smaller LF and greater HF components. During tilt, a smaller increase in the LF component and reduction in the HF component indicated the reduced responsiveness to sympathetic activation.*

arrived at the conclusion, unjustified in our opinion, that LF is a marker of parasympathetic activity, because its absolute value increased over the 24 hours after β blockade.

A better evaluation of this point, however, may be derived from approaches other than pharmacological blockade. In particular, note that, in tetraplegic patients, the LF component was absent in the study by Inoue et al[35] and absent in about 50% of patients in our own current work, and yet the vagal modulation of heart rate is unimpaired in tetraplegic patients. Therefore, the interruption of the spinal pathways that connect supraspinal centers with the spinal sympathetic outflow may impede the transmission of the LF oscillation; therefore, it is likely to normally take place in brain structures. In addition, patients with idiopathic orthostatic hypotension (vide infra) have practically no LF component in their RR variability.

In short, the LF component seems to represent a reliable marker of the sympathetic contribution to the sympatho-vagal balance.

RR and Systolic Arterial Pressure Variability

Continuous recording of arterial pressure provides the opportunity of measuring those pressure waves that appear as a main expression of the third order rhythm and of testing the hypothesis that increases in sympathetic activity enhance this rhythm.[19,71] In resting subjects, recordings adequate for spectral analysis can be obtained both with noninvasive, indirect measurements[72,73] and with traditional fluid-filled, intra-arterial catheters.[30,40]

Whereas, the HF component of SAP variability is largely influenced by the mechanical effects of respiration,[11,12,74] its LF component appears to be the elective index for the third order rhythm. The LF component increases during tilt,[30,75] mental stress,[62] and physical exercise.[36,75]

The analysis of arterial pressure variability during physical exercise seems particularly suited to demonstrate an increased sympathetic activity, because its total variance and LF component remain elevated, at least during mild levels of activity.[11,36,75]

Continuous 24-Hour Recording of RR and Systolic Arterial Pressure Variability

In dynamic conditions, the direct recording of arterial pressure with a fluid-filled catheter-manometer system cannot avoid motion artifacts and an unpredictable deterioration of waveforms.[76] To overcome these problems, a high-fidelity recording technique has been developed[77] using microminiature tip transducers (Millar, Houston, Texas) and appropriately modified Holter recorders (Remco, Milan, Italy).

Since the initial observations,[78] a clear circadian oscillation characterizes the sympatho-vagal balance.[36] In a recent study,[11] the LF component of SAP variability increased abruptly upon waking, while the subjects were still lying in bed. The LF component remained elevated during the day, especially during physical exercise, and then diminished markedly during the night. A similar circadian pattern in which LF and HF components of RR variability underwent reciprocal changes over 24 hours could also be assessed with electrocardiographic Holter (Remco, Milan, Italy) monitoring (Fig. 6).[11] This circadian pattern strongly favors the hypothesis that the LF component is a marker of sympathetic modulation and that the HF component is a marker of vagal modulation of heart rate variability. Such a circadian pattern is obviously concealed when a 24-hour recording is compressed into a single spectrum, as proposed by several studies.[70,79] As to the clinical relevance of this circadian rhythmicity, a recent investigation has clearly demonstrated the occurrence of several types of acute cardiovascular events in the early morning hours.[80]

The importance of appropriate recording techniques and adequate algo-

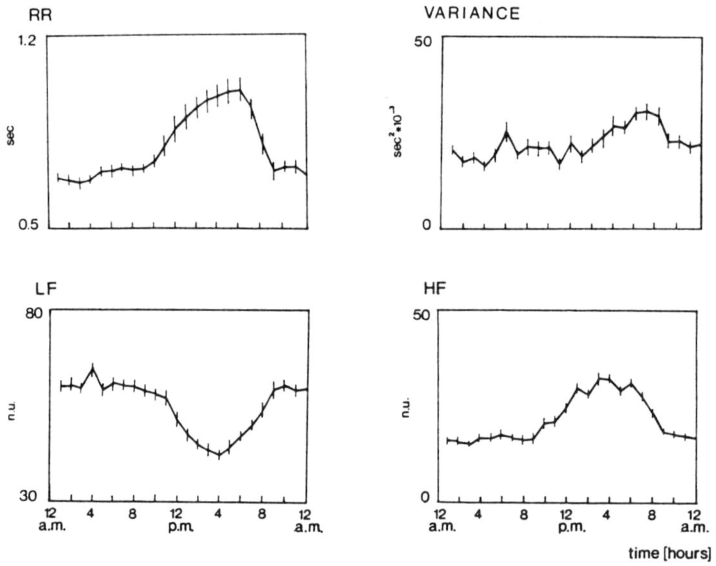

Figure 6. *Plots of average hourly values of RR interval (RR) of its variance (in absolute units) (variance), and of LF and HF components (LF and HF) (in nu) during 24 hours in a group of nonhospitalized subjects free to move. Reproduced by permission of the American Heart Association, Inc. from Furlan R, Guzzetti S, Crivellaro W, et al: Continuous 24-hour assessment of the neural regulation of systemic arterial pressure and R-R variabilities in ambulant subjects. Circulation 81:537–547, 1990.*

rithms has again been proposed by the description[55] of a third frequency component in SAP variability in the range of 0.025 to 0.07 Hz. Arterial pressure was recorded[81] with fluid-filled catheters and analyzed on short segments of 256 beats. Under such conditions, the drift of the recording system and the noise of the dynamic state could contribute particularly to the energy content of that low region of the spectrum that, moreover, could also include part of the LF component during the transient decreases of its center frequency.[11]

Animal Studies

A dominant role of the vagi in determining the HF component of RR variability was inferred from experiments in acute decerebrate cats[82] and in conscious dogs.[12,83,84] Accordingly, the power of the HF component of RR variability has been used to assess vagal control of heart rate in conditions such as dynamic exercise[85] and in species such as fetal sheep.[86]

Additionally, in experiments on conscious dogs, Akselrod et al[83] addressed the problem of oscillations with a frequency lower than respiration; namely, two bands with frequencies that centered at about 0.04 and 0.12 Hz. The former component was linked to the renin-angiotensin system, and the latter component was attributed to baroreflex mechanisms[83] but, being poorly detectable, was disregarded in subsequent studies.[84,87]

Recently, Rimoldi et al[12] reported that, in resting conscious dogs, a small LF component was always present in SAP variability, but in only 50% of the cases in RR variability. Whenever the sympathetic system was excited, however, (as during baroreceptor unloading with nitroglycerin infusion, transient coronary artery occlusion, or physical exercise), the LF component increased significantly. The mechanisms for this excitation were probably different. In the case of a nonhypotensive episode of myocardial ischemia, an excitatory sympathetic reflex from the heart[20,21] was likely to be the main factor. An increased central command, together with a peripheral reinforcement, however, may have been paramount during physical exercise.[88] Thus, the LF component may not simply reflect a baroreflex compensatory response[89] but, rather, it may be an unspecific marker of sympathetic excitation, whatever its mechanism might be.

Attempts to increase the vagal predominance with phenylephrine infusion in conscious dogs[90] markedly augment RR and SAP variance, but induce only minor changes in the spectral profile.[12] Conversely, during muscarinic receptor (mAChR) blockade, which drastically reduces the total RR variance, the remaining power during baroreceptor unloading is all concentrated in the LF region. This emphasizes the importance of using nu or the LF/HF ratio to assess the actual sympatho-vagal balance. After chronic bilateral stellectomy to produce a sympathetic denervation of the heart, however, baroreceptor unloading still increased the LF component of SAP variability, even though its increase in RR variability was prevented.[12,30] Hence, the HF component appeared to be mediated mainly by vagal mechanisms, while the sympathetic outflow appeared to govern the LF component. In addition, the importance of neural mechanisms in mediating the LF and HF components of RR variability and the LF component of SAP variability was proven[12] by their disappearance during ganglionic transmission blockade with trimethaphan.

The conceptual approach based on this type of subtractive logic is potentially misleading, however, not only because vagotomy,[82] stellectomy,[12,30] pharmacological blockades,[12,30,57,82–84] and spinal transection[35] are all likely to alter the basal conditions profoundly, but mainly because it might suggest that a rhythm should coincide with a given neural apparatus to convey a functional meaning. In fact, the opposite is true. Both the LF and HF components can be directly and simultaneously recorded from the vagal and sympathetic outflows[32,91] (see the section below entitled "General Conclusions").

Modelling Approaches

When the circulation is modelled as a closed-loop coupling between heart period and arterial pressure, the transfer function between SAP and RR variabilities describes the neural links between these two signals, and the simultaneous mechanical coupling between RR and SAP is also considered.[84] All perturbations, such as respiration, that are not explicitly accounted for by this model are labelled as noise external to the loop. The closed loop can be experimentally opened by nullifying one variable, e.g., RR variability by way of ventricular pacing.[84]

By making the simple assumption that the direct influence of respiration (i.e., noise) on RR variability is negligible, an index (α) can be computed that quantifies the overall gain of the relationship between heart period and arterial pressure.[39,73,92] The numerical value of this index equals the square root of the ratios of the spectral components of RR and SAP variabilities for both the LF and HF components.[36,40,93] This approach, which requires neither preselection of data[94] nor injections of pressor drugs, has furnished results in man comparable[36] to those obtained with the phenylephrine method.[95] This approach, however, also enables the continuous evaluation of the minute-to-minute and circadian changes that characterize the gain of the complex baroreflex mechanisms.[36]

More elaborate models and algorithms have recently been proposed in order to consider respiration together with the RR and SAP variabilities.[74] This approach, by quantifying separately the effects of respiration on RR and SAP variabilities, yields the index (α) cleared of respiratory influences, and it also quantifies the effects of changes in SAP over successive SAP values.

In short, these black box approaches seem capable of evaluating the regulatory neural functions and the regulated cardiovascular variables as a whole in relation to their various functional states. The physiological mechanisms that attend these functions need not be oversimplified. Vice versa, other modelling attempts prefer to focus on a simple baroreflex in order to explain Mayer waves. Such attempts may conclude that a central oscillator is not needed.[96]

Assessment of Sympatho-Vagal Interaction in Various Pathological Conditions

In view of the inherent noninvasiveness of the methodology, spectral analysis of cardiovascular variabilities represents a potentially useful tool to explore the role played by neural regulatory mechanisms in various pathophysiological conditions.

Essential Arterial Hypertension

An appealing hypothesis is that essential hypertension, at least in its early stages, is largely based on increased sympathetic activity.[22,97] In a study[58] comparing RR variability in hypertensive patients with that in normotensive, age-matched controls, it was found that, under resting conditions, the LF component was greater (LF, 68 ± 3 versus 54 ± 3 nu) and the HF component was less (HF, 24 ± 3 versus 33 ± 2 nu) in hypertensive patients. These data suggest an enhanced sympathetic and a reduced vagal activity. In hypertensive patients, passive tilt produced smaller increases in the LF component (LF, 6.3 ± 3 versus 26 ± 3 nu) and decreases in the HF component (HF, -7.5 ± 2 versus -21.5 ± 2 nu) than in normotensive controls. Furthermore, the values of the LF component at rest and the altered effects of tilt on the LF and HF components correlated significantly with the degree of hypertension; this correlation suggests a continuum distribution.[98]

When RR variability was studied throughout the 24-hour period with the use of Holter (Remco, Milan, Italy) recordings, patients with essential hypertension were characterized by the loss of the circadian rhythmicity of the LF component, whereas a small nocturnal increase in the HF component was still detectable.[99] These data, although difficult to interpret, suggest that in hypertensive patients, an increased sympathetic drive under basal conditions might be associated with a reduced circadian oscillation of neural regulatory mechanisms, as assessed by spectral analysis.

In an invasive study[36] in normotensive and hypertensive subjects undergoing 24-hour continuous recording of electrocardiogram and arterial pressure measured with a high-fidelity technique, the overall gain of the baroreceptive mechanisms was evaluated with index (α) (see the section entitled "Modelling Approaches"). This index underwent a clear circadian variation, being smaller during the day, and it was decreased at rest in the hypertensive group, which confirms that neural buffering mechanisms may be attenuated in essential hypertension.

Myocardial Infarction

Since pioneering observations of Pantridge's group,[100] it has been commonly accepted that the hyperacute phase of myocardial infarction can be accompanied by signs of sympathetic overactivity, particularly in the case of anterior localization, or by signs of vagal predominance, particularly in the case of inferior myocardial infarction.

In on-going studies, we are addressing this problem with spectral analysis of RR variability. We find that, in patients examined within three hours from the onset of symptoms, the LF component is clearly predominant both in cases of anterior and posterior localization. Thus, the vagal hyperactivity, which has been reported in the case of hyperacute inferior wall myocardial infarction, might be short-lasting and sympathetic predominance is rapidly substituted.

We studied patients two weeks, six months, and 12 months after the acute episode to address the progressive changes in the neural regulatory mechanisms that occur during convalescence after myocardial infarction.[50] In comparison to control subjects, patients at two weeks after myocardial infarction exhibited a significant increase in the LF component and a diminished HF component. Furthermore, increases of the LF component induced by tilt[50] or psychological stress[101] were blunted. At six and 12 months, the LF component progressively decreased and the HF component increased, which suggested a normalization of sympatho-vagal interaction. More recently, the sympathetic predominance observed two weeks after myocardial infarction was studied during a 24-hour period in patients one month after the acute event.[102] We found that the normal circadian rhythm was markedly blunted. Moreover, in these same patients, physical training significantly diminished the LF component, and the LF/HF ratio, and the increase was restored during tilt.[103]

Congestive Heart Failure

Congestive heart failure, which is characterized by a reduced RR variance, has been generally considered a condition in which vagal modulation of heart period is greatly reduced. We propose that excitatory sympathetic reflexes might play a crucial role.[104]

In an on-going study in patients with congestive heart failure of moderate degree (New York Heart Association [NYHA] Class 2–3), we observed a significant increase in the LF component.[32] This finding suggests the presence of sympathetic hyperactivity. Vice versa, in NYHA Class 4 patients, there was a further reduction in RR variance while, in the autospectrum, no LF component was detectable, and only a predominant HF (respiration-related) component was evident. These preliminary results suggest that a persistent sympathetic activation is more easily detectable in the less advanced phase of the disease, when the heart maintains its responsiveness to adrenergic stimulation.

Diabetic Neuropathy

Functional tests based on reflex cardiovascular responses are commonly used to evaluate the presence of initial alterations of neural mechanisms controlling cardiovascular function before the appearance of overt clinical signs of neuropathy.[105]

Studies of RR variability have shown that diabetic patients have a reduced variance.[26,54,106] Moreover, we observed that, in patients without clinical signs of visceral neuropathy, the spectral profile was normal at rest.[106] Conversely, during sympathetic activation induced by tilt, the increase in the LF component and in the LF/HF ratio and the decrease in HF component were significantly smaller than observed in control subjects. These findings indicate that diabetic neuropathy is characterized by both sympathetic and parasympathetic alterations.

Cardiac Transplantation

The condition after human heart transplantation represents a clinical model of the denervated heart that has prompted various studies with spectral analysis.[107–109] In general, the total RR variance was reduced. Although in some studies[107,109] no discrete HF or LF components were consistently found in the RR variability, Bernardi et al[108] described a small HF component that appeared to be independent of neural mechanisms. Furthermore, in one patient studied by Fallen et al[107] three years after transplantation, both LF and HF components were present. The latter was increased by synchronous respiration and was abolished by atropine. The authors concluded that spectral analysis might establish the state of reinnervation of the transplanted heart in humans. Finally, Sands et al[109] reported an increased variance in patients developing an allograft rejection. Their finding, however, has been challenged by others.[107,110]

Idiopathic Orthostatic Hypotension

Finally, in idiopathic orthostatic hypotension, catecholamine depletion at the neural endings produces a condition similar to sympathetic denervation. In five out of six such patients (Furlan et al, work in progress) who presented with very low levels of circulating catecholamines, no LF component was detectable in the RR or systolic arterial pressure variabilities. During 45° head-up tilt, the SAP was, as expected, markedly reduced. In two patients, a small LF component appeared in systolic arterial pressure variability. No LF component, however, appeared in RR variability.

Thus, patients with idiopathic orthostatic hypotension, both at rest and during tilt, are characterized by a disappearance of spectral indices of sympathetic modulation of heart period and vasomotion. These results further confirm the importance of altered sympathetic neural regulatory mechanisms in this clinical condition.

General Conclusions

Spectral analysis of the variability of cardiovascular responses and, in particular, of heart period, offers a new opportunity to examine the complexities of neural regulation, and it does not artificially isolate the influence of either autonomic outflow. Rhythmicity is a flexible and dynamic property of neural networks. Any given rhythm, like electroencephalographic synchronization or desynchronization, need not be restricted to one specific structure or pathway in order to carry a functional significance. Hence, we believe that rhythms and their neural components always interact, just like flexor and extensor tones or excitatory and inhibitory cardiovascular reflexes. Accordingly, to consider vagal and sympathetic modulations of cardiovascular function separately might be misleading. In concrete terms, in humans and experimental animals, functional states likely to be accompanied by an increased sympathetic activity are characterized by a shift in the LF/HF balance in favor of LF components; the opposite occurs during presumed increases in vagal activity. In this respect, the absolute values of the LF or HF components are unlikely to provide the information that instead can be derived from their ratio or from their appraisal in nu. To illustrate, no isolated information either on flexor or extensor tone can predict the position of a joint, as the same position can be sustained by different levels of absolute tone in the antagonistic muscles. As we have recently concluded,[32] the exploration in the frequency domain, although based on indirect markers, might disclose a unitary view of cardiovascular neural regulation that is hard to reach through the assemblage of more specific but fragmented pieces of information.

References

1. Blois MS: Medicine and the nature of vertical reasoning. N Engl J Med 318:847–851, 1988.
2. Lydic R: Central pattern-generating neurons and the search for general principles. FASEB J 3:2457–2468, 1989.
3. Koepchen HP: Respiratory and cardiovascular "centres": Functional entirety or separate structures? In ME Schlafke, HP Koepchen, WR See (eds): Central Neurone Environment and the Control of Breathing and Circulation. Berlin, Springer-Verlag, 1983, pp. 221–237.
4. Getting PA: Emerging principles governing the operation of neural networks. Ann Rev Neurosci 12:185–204, 1989.
5. Sherrington CS: Ferrier Lecture. Some functional problems attaching convergence. Proc R Soc (London) Ser. B 105B:332–362, 1929.
6. Hales S: Statistical Essays: Containing Haemastaticks. London, Innys, Manby and Woodward, 1733, Vol II.
7. Koepchen HP: History of studies and concepts of blood pressure waves. In K Miyakawa, HP Koepchen, C Polosa (eds): Mechanism of Blood Pressure Waves. Tokyo, Japanese Science Society Press, Berlin, Springer Verlag, 1984, pp. 3–23.
8. Mayer S: Studien zur Physiologie des Herzens und der Blutgefasse: 5. Abhandlung: Uber spontane Blutdruckschwankungen. Sber. Akad. Wiss., 3. Abteilung 74:281–307, 1876.
9. Monos E, Szucs B: Effect of changes in mean arterial pressure on the structure of short-term blood pressure waves. Automedica 2:149–160, 1978.
10. Penaz J: Mayer waves: History and methodology. Automedica 2:135–141, 1978.
11. Furlan R, Guzzetti S, Crivellaro W, et al: Continuous 24-hour assessment of the neural regulation of systemic arterial pressure and R-R variabilities in ambulant subjects. Circulation 81:537–547, 1990.
12. Rimoldi O, Pierini S, Ferrari A, et al: Analysis of short-term oscillations of R-R and arterial pressure in conscious dogs. Am J Physiol 258:H967–H976, 1990.
13. Adrian ED, Bronk DW, Phillips G: Discharges in mammalian sympathetic nerves. J Physiol (Lond) 74:115–133, 1932.
14. Fernandez de Molina A, Perl ER: Sympathetic activity and the systemic circulation in the spinal cat. J Physiol (Lond) 181:82–102, 1965.
15. Jewett DL: Acitivity of single efferent fibres in the cervical vagus nerve of the dog, with special reference to possible cardio-inhibitory fibres. J Physiol (Lond) 175:321–357, 1964.
16. Kunze DL: Reflex discharge patterns of cardiac vagal efferent fibres. J Physiol (Lond) 222:1–15, 1975.
17. Kollai M, Koizumi K: Cardiovascular reflexes and interrelationships between sympathetic and parasympathetic activity. J Autonom Nerv Syst 4:135–148, 1981.
18. Koizumi K, Terui N, Kollai M: Relationships between vagal and sympathetic activities in rhythmic fluctuations. In K Miyakawa, HP Koepchen, C Polosa (eds): Mechanisms of Blood Pressure Waves. Tokyo/Berlin, Japan Science Society Press/Springer Verlag, 1984, pp. 43–56.
19. Miyakawa K, Koepchen HP, Polosa CL: Mechanisms of Blood Pressure Waves. Tokyo/Berlin, Japanese Science Society Press/Springer Verlag, 1984, pp. 43–56.
20. Malliani A: Cardiovascular sympathetic afferent fibers. Rev Physiol Biochem Pharmacol 94:11–74, 1982.
21. Bishop VS, Malliani A, Thorén P: Cardiac mechanoreceptors. In JT Shepherd, FM Abboud, SR Geiger (eds): Handbook of Physiology. Section 2: The Cardiovascular System, Vol. 3: Peripheral Circulation and Organ Blood Flow. Bethesada, MD, American Physiological Society, 1983, pp. 497–555.
22. Malliani A, Pagani M, Lombardi F: Positive feedback reflexes. In A Zanchetti, RC

Tarazi (eds): Handbook of Hypertension. Vol. 8: Pathophysiology of Hypertension. Amsterdam, Elsevier Science Publishing B.V., 1986, pp. 69–81.
23. Sagawa K: Baroreflex control of systemic arterial pressure and vascular bed. In JT Shepherd, FM Abboud, SR Geiger (eds): Handbook of Physiology. Section 2: The Cardiovascular System, Vol. 3: Peripheral Circulation and Organ Blood Flow. Bethesda, MD, American Physiological Society 1983, pp. 453–496.
24. Gnecchi Ruscone T, Lombardi F, Malfatto G, et al: Attenuation of baroreceptive mechanisms by cardiovascular sympathetic afferent fibers. Am J Physiol 253:H787–H791, 1987.
25. Kleiger RE, Miller JP, Bigger JT, et al: Decreased heart rate variability and its association with increased mortality after acute myocardial infarction. Am J Cardiol 59:256–262, 1987.
26. Ewing DJ, Neilson JMM, Travis P: New method for assessing cardiac parasympathetic activity using 24-hour electrocardiograms. Br Heart J 52:396–402, 1984.
27. Hyndman BW, Kitney RI, Sayers BM: Spontaneous rhythms in physiological control systems. Nature 233:339–341, 1971.
28. Sayers BM: Analysis of heart rate variability. Ergonomics 16:17–32, 1973.
29. Brovelli M, Baselli G, Cerutti S, et al: Computerized analysis for an experimental validation of neurophysiological models of heart rate control. In Computers in Cardiology. Silver Spring, MD, IEEE Computer Society Press, 1983, pp. 205–208.
30. Pagani M, Lombardi F, Guzzetti S, et al: Power spectral analysis of heart rate and arterial pressure variabilities as a marker of sympatho-vagal interaction in man and conscious dog. Circ Res 59:178–193, 1986.
31. Baselli G, Cerutti S, Civardi S, et al: Heart rate variability signal processing: A quantitative approach as an aid to diagnosis in cardiovascular pathologies. Int J BioMed Computing 20:51–70, 1987.
32. Malliani A, Pagani M, Lombardi F, et al: Cardiovascular neural regulation explored in the frequency domain. Circulation 84:482–492, 1991.
33. Fallen EL, Kamath MV, Ghista DN: Power spectrum of heart rate variability: A non-invasive test of integrated neurocardiac function. Clin Invest Med II:331–340, 1988.
34. Hayano J, Sakakibara Y, Yamada M, et al: Decreased magnitude of heart rate spectral components in coronary artery disease. Circulation 81:1217–1224, 1990.
35. Inoue K, Miyake S, Kumashiro M, et al: Power spectral analysis of heart rate variability in traumatic quadriplegic humans. Am J Physiol 258:H1722–H1726, 1990.
36. Pagani M, Somers V, Furlan R, et al: Changes in autonomic regulation induced by physical training in mild hypertension. Hypertension 12:600–610, 1988.
37. Baselli G, Cerutti S, Civardi S, et al: Spectral and cross-spectral analysis of heart rate and arterial blood pressure variability signals. Comput Biomed Res 19:520–534, 1986.
38. Zwiener U: Physiological interpretation of autospectra, coherence and phase spectra of blood pressure, heart rate, and respiration waves in man. Automedica 2:161–169, 1978.
39. DeBoer RW, Karemaker JM, van Montfrans GA: Determination of baroreflex sensitivity by spectral analysis of spontaneous blood-pressure and heart-rate fluctuations in man. In B Lown, A Malliani, M Prosdocimi (eds): Neural Mechanisms and Cardiovascular Disease. Padova, Liviana Press, 1987, pp. 303–315.
40. Robbe HWJ, Mulder LJM, Ruddel H, et al: Assessment of baroreceptor reflex sensitivity by means of spectral analysis. Hypertension 10:538–543, 1987.
41. Jenkins GM, Watts KG: Spectral analysis and its applications. San Francisco, Holden-Day Inc, 1968.
42. Shimada SG, Marsh DJ: Oscillations in mean arterial blood pressure in conscious dogs. Circ Res 44:692–700, 1979.
43. Kobayashi M, Musha T: 1/f Fluctuations of heartbeat period. IEEE Trans Biomed Eng 29:456–457, 1982.

44. Saul JP, Albrecht P, Berger RD, et al: Analysis of long-term heart rate variability: Methods, 1/f scaling and implications. In Computers in Cardiology. Silver Springs, MD, IEEE Computer Society Press, 1988, pp. 419–422.
45. Kitney RI: An analysis of the nonlinear behaviour of the human thermal vasomotor control system. J Theor Bio 52:231–248, 1975.
46. Waddington JL, MacCulloch MJ, Sambrooks JE: Resting heartrate variability in man declines with age. Experientia 35:1197–1198, 1979.
47. Smith SE, Smith SA: Heart rate variability in healthy subjects measured with a bedside computer-based technique. Clin Sci 61:379–383, 1981.
48. Simpson DM, Wicks R: Spectral analysis of heart rate indicates reduced baroreceptor-related heart rate variability in elderly persons. J Gerontology 43:M21–M24, 1988.
49. Lipsitz LA, Mietus J, Moody GB, et al: Spectral characteristics of heart rate variability before and during postural tilt. Circulation 81:1803–1810, 1990.
50. Lombardi F, Sandrone G, Pernpruner S, et al: Heart rate variability as an index of sympathovagal interaction after acute myocardial infarction. Am J Cardiol 60:1239–1245, 1987.
51. Pagani M, Malfatto G, Pierini S, et al: Spectral analysis of heart rate variability in the assessment of autonomic diabetic neuropathy. J Autonom Nerv Syst 23:143–153, 1988.
52. Vybiral T, Bryg RJ, Maddens ME, et al: Effect of passive tilt on sympathetic and parasympathetic components of heart rate variability in normal subjects. Am J Cardiol 63:1117–1120, 1989.
53. DeBoer RW, Karemaker JM, Strackee J: Comparing spectra of a series of point events particularly for heart rate variability data. IEEE Trans Biomed Eng 31:384–387, 1984.
54. Lishner M, Akselrod S, Avi VM, et al: Spectral analysis of heart rate fluctuations. A noninvasive, sensitive method for the early diagnosis of autonomic neuropathy in diabetes mellitus. J Autonom Nerv Syst 19:119–125, 1987.
55. Di Rienzo M, Castiglioni P, Mancia G, et al: 24 hour sequential spectral analysis of arterial blood pressure and pulse interval in free-moving subjects. IEEE Trans Biomed Eng 36:1066–1075, 1989.
56. Kostreva DR, Castaner A, Kampine JP: Reflex effects of hepatic baroreceptors on renal and cardiac sympathetic nerve activity. Am J Physiol 238:R390–R394, 1980.
57. Pomeranz B, Macaulay RJB, Caudill MA, et al: Assessment of autonomic function in humans by heart rate spectral analysis. Am J Physiol 248:H151–H153, 1985.
58. Guzzetti S, Piccaluga E, Casati R, et al: Sympathetic predominance in essential hypertension: A study employing spectral analysis of heart rate variability. J Hypertens 6:711–717, 1988.
59. Lindquist A, Jalonen J, Parviainen P, et al: Effect of posture on spontaneous and thermally stimulated cardiovascular oscillations. Cardiovas Res 24:373–380, 1990.
60. Bekheit S, Tangella M, El-Sakr A, et al: Use of heart rate spectral analysis to study the effects of calcium channel blockers on sympathetic activity after myocardial infarction. Am Heart J 119:79–85, 1990.
61. Hyndman BW, Gregory JR: Spectral analysis of sinus arrhythmia during mental loading. Ergonomics 18:255–270, 1975.
62. Pagani M, Furlan R, Pizzinelli P, et al: Spectral analysis of R-R and arterial pressure variabilities to assess sympatho-vagal interaction during mental stress in humans. J Hypertens 7(suppl 6):S14–S15, 1989.
63. Pagani M, Rimoldi O, Pizzinelli P, et al: Assessment of the neural control of the circulation during psychological stress. J Autonom Nerv Syst 35:33–42, 1991.
64. Arai Y, Saul JP, Albrecht P, et al: Modulation of cardiac autonomic activity during and immediately after exercise. Am J Physiol 256:H132–H141, 1989.
65. Rimoldi O, Furlan R, Pagani MR, et al: Analysis of neural mechanisms accompanying different intensities of dynamic exercise. Chest 101 (suppl 5):2265–2305, 1992.
66. Yamamoto Y, Hughson RL, Peterson JC: Autonomic control of heart rate during

exercise studied by heart rate variability spectral analysis. J Appl Physiol 71:1136–1142, 1991.
67. Kitney R, Linkens D, Selman A, et al: The interaction between heart rate and respiration: Part II–nonlinear analysis based on computer modelling. Automedica 4:141–153, 1982.
68. Saul JP, Rea RF, Eckberg DL, et al: Heart rate and muscle sympathetic nerve variability during reflex changes of autonomic activity. Am J Physiol 258:H713–H721, 1990.
69. Selman A, McDonald A, Kitney R, et al: The interaction between heart rate and respiration: Part I–experimental studies in man. Automedica 4:131–139, 1982.
70. Cook JR, Bigger JT, Kleiger RE, et al: Effect of atenolol and diltiazem on heart period variability in normal persons. J Am Coll Cardiol 17:480–484, 1991.
71. Preiss G, Polosa C: Patterns of sympathetic neuron activity associated with Mayer waves. Am J Physiol 226:724–730, 1974.
72. Wesseling KH, Dewit B, Settels JJM, et al: On the indirect registration of blood pressure after Penaz. Fukt Biol Med 1:245–250, 1982.
73. DeBoer RW: Beat-to-beat blood-pressure fluctuations and heart-rate variability in man: Physiological relationships, analysis techniques and a simple model. Amsterdam, University of Amsterdam, 1985. Thesis.
74. Baselli G, Cerutti S, Civardi S, et al: Cardiovascular variability signals: Towards the identification of a closed-loop model of the neural control mechanisms. IEEE Trans Biomed Eng 35:1033–1046, 1988.
75. Furlan R, Dell'Orto S, Crivellaro W, et al: Effects of tilt and treadmill exercise on short-term variability in systolic arterial pressure in hypertensive men. J Hypertens 5 (suppl. 5):S423–S425, 1987.
76. Millar-Craig M: Techniques for intra arterial recording. In D Magometschnigg, G Hitzenberger (eds): Blood Pressure Variability. Vienna, Uhlen Verlaggesellschaft, 1983, pp. 15–22.
77. Pagani M, Furlan R, Dell'Orto S, et al: Continuous recording of direct high fidelity arterial pressure and electrocardiogram in ambulant patients. Cardiovasc Res 20:384–388, 1986.
78. Pagani M, Furlan R, Dell'Orto S, et al: Simultaneous analysis of beat by beat systemic arterial pressure and heart rate variabilities in ambulatory patients. J Hypertens 3 (suppl. 3):S83–S85, 1985.
79. Bigger JT, Fleiss JL, Rolnitzky LM, et al: Time course of recovery of heart period variability after myocardial infarction. J Am Coll Cardiol 18:1643–1649, 1991.
80. Muller JE, Toffler GH, Stone PH: Circadian variation and triggers of onset of acute cardiovascular disease. Circulation 79:733–743, 1989.
81. Parati G, Castiglioni P, Di Rienzo M, et al: Sequential spectral analysis of 24-hour blood pressure and pulse interval in humans. Hypertension 16:414–421, 1990.
82. Chess GF, Tam RMK, Calaresu FR: Influence of cardiac neural inputs on rhythmic variations of heart period in the cat. Am J Physiol 228:775–780, 1975.
83. Akselrod S, Gordon D, Ubel FA, et al: Power spectrum analysis of heart rate fluctuations: A quantitative probe of beat-to-beat cardiovascular control. Science 213:220–222, 1981.
84. Akselrod S, Gordon D, Madwed JB, et al: Hemodynamic regulation: Investigation by spectral analysis. Am J Physiol 249:H867–H875, 1985.
85. Billman GE, Dujardin JP: Dynamic changes in cardiac vagal tone as measured by time-series analysis. Am J Physiol 258:H896–H902, 1990.
86. Donchin Y, Caton D, Porges SW: Spectral analysis of fetal heart rate in sheep: The occurrence of respiratory arrhythmia. Am J Obstet Gynecol 148:1130–1135, 1984.
87. Brown DR, Randall DC, Knapp CF, et al: Stability of the heart rate power spectrum over time in conscious dogs. FASEB J 3:1644–1650, 1989.
88. Rimoldi O, Pagani M, Pagani MR, et al: Sympathetic activation during treadmill exercise in the conscious dog: Assessment with spectral analysis of heart period and systolic pressure variabilities. J Autonom Nerv Syst 30 (suppl):S129–S132, 1990.

89. Appel ML, Berger RD, Saul JP, et al: Beat to beat variability in cardiovascular variables: Noise or music? J Am Coll Cardiol 14:1139–1148, 1989.
90. Haddad GG, Jeng HJ, Lee SH, et al: Rhythmic variations in R-R interval during sleep and wakefulness in puppies and dogs. Am J Physiol 247:H67–H73, 1984.
91. Lombardi F, Montano N, Finocchiaro ML, et al: Spectral analysis of sympathetic discharge in decerebrate cats. J Auton Nerv Syst 30 (suppl):S97–S99, 1990.
92. DeBoer RW, Karemaker JM, Strackee J: Hemodynamic fluctuations and baroreflex sensitivity in humans: A beat-to-beat model. Am J Physiol 253:H680–H689, 1987.
93. Cerutti S, Baselli G, Civardi S, et al: Spectral analysis of heart rate and arterial blood pressure variability signals for physiological and clinical purposes. In Computers in Cardiology. Silver Spring, MD, IEEE Computer Society Press, 1987, pp. 435–438.
94. Bertinieri G, Di Rienzo M, Cavallazzi A, et al: A new approach to analysis of the arterial baroreflex. J Hypertens 3 (suppl. 3):s79–s81, 1985.
95. Smyth HS, Sleight P, Pickering GW: A quantitative method of assessing baroreflex sensitivity. Circ Res 24:109–121, 1969.
96. Madwed JB, Albrecht P, Mark RG, et al: Low-frequency oscillations in arterial pressure and heart rate: A simple computer model. Am J Physiol 256:H1573–H1579, 1989.
97. Goldstein DS: Plasma catecholamines and essential hypertension. Hypertension 5:86–89, 1983.
98. Pickering G: The Nature of Essential Hypertension. London, J&A Churchill Ltd, 1961.
99. Guzzetti S, Dassi S, Pecis M, et al: Altered pattern of circadian neural control of heart period in mild hypertension. J Hypertens 9:831–838, 1991.
100. Webb SW, Adgey AA, Pantridge JF: Autonomic disturbance at onset of acute myocardial infarction. Br Med 3:89–92, 1972.
101. Lombardi F, Sandrone G, Mortara A, et al: Circadian variation of spectral indices of heart rate variability after myocardial infarction. Am Heart J 123:1521–1529, 1992.
102. Pagani M, Mazzuero G, Ferrari A, et al: Sympathovagal interaction during mental stress: A study employing spectral analysis of heart rate variability in healthy controls and in patients with a prior myocardial infarction. Circulation (suppl. II):II–43–II–51, 1991.
103. La Rovere MT, Mortara A, Sandrone G, et al: Autonomic nervous system adaptations to short-term exercise training. Chest 101 (suppl):2995–3035, 1992.
104. Malliani A, Pagani M: The role of the sympathetic nervous system in congestive heart failure. Eur Heart J 4 (suppl A):49–54, 1983.
105. Ewing DJ, Martyn CN, Young RJ, et al: The value of cardiovascular autonomic function tests: 10 years experience in diabetes. Diabetes Care 8:491–498, 1985.
106. Pagani M, Malfatto G, Pierini S, et al: Spectral analysis of heart rate variability in the assessment of autonomic diabetic neuropathy. J Autonom Nerv Syst 23:143–153, 1988.
107. Fallen EL, Kamath MV, Ghista DN, et al: Spectral analysis of heart rate variability following human heart transplantation: Evidence for functional reinnervation. J Autonom Nerv Syst 23:199–206, 1988.
108. Bernardi L, Keller F, Sanders M, et al: Respiratory sinus arrhythmia in the denervated human heart. J Appl Physiol 67:1447–1455, 1989.
109. Sands KEF, Appel ML, Lilly LS, et al: Power spectrum analysis of heart rate variability in human cardiac transplant recipients. Circulation 79:76–82, 1989.
110. Zbilut JP, Lawless CE: Power spectrum analysis of heart rate variability in human cardiac transplant recipients. Circulation 80:1498, 1989.

CHAPTER 28

Methods for Assessment of Vagal Reflexes

E. Vanoli, M.T. La Rovere, A. Mortara, P.J. Schwartz

The evidence linking the autonomic nervous system, cardiovascular mortality, and sudden death, particularly after myocardial infarction,[1–3] has increased the interest for methods and tests available to assess tonic and reflex autonomic activity. Recent experimental and clinical observations (see Ch. 34) have highlighted the prognostic value of the analysis of reflex cardiac vagal activity as estimated by determining the heart rate decrease secondary to a blood pressure rise, i.e. baroreflex sensitivity.

Several methods have been described to alter human arterial baroreceptive activity.[4–6] They include bolus injection or infusion of vasoactive drugs, the Valsalva maneuver, and mechanical alteration of transmural carotid sinus pressure by means of the neck chamber. Each of these methods suffers from some technical or theoretical limitations and, overall, they allow only indirect assessment of the neural vagal outflow to the heart. Among the different methods, the use of bolus injections of phenylephrine is the one that has been more extensively described in the experimental setting and that has also been used in a large number of patients with different cardiovascular diseases. Specifically, this test has been used in studies aimed to evaluate the link between cardiac reflexes and risk for cardiac mortality and sudden death after myocardial infarction. Since the main objective of this chapter concerns the discussion of methods useful to assess risk profile in coronary artery disease patients, we will focus mainly on the technical and theoretical aspects of the analysis of baroreflex sensitivity as calculated from the reflex response to blood pressure rise induced by bolus injection of phenylephrine. A brief review of the other methods used to induce vagal activation, more largely discussed in Ch. 25, is also presented.

From *Vagal Control of the Heart: Experimental Basis and Clinical Implications* edited by MN Levy, PJ Schwartz © 1994, Futura Publishing Co. Inc., Armonk, NY.

Direct Neural Recording Versus the Use of "Markers" of Autonomic Activity

Between the options of directly monitoring neural activity directed to the heart and of drawing inferences from indirect markers, it is obvious that the preference would go to the first approach. Major technical problems, however, still exist that severely limit the first possibility. Furthermore, the situation is profoundly different for sympathetic and for vagal activity. After the first description in 1968 by Hagbarth and Vallbo,[7] several investigators have used the direct measurement of tonic and reflex sympathetic postganglionic activity from human peroneal and brachial nerves under different conditions.[8–12] The method is based on the insertion of a tungsten microelectrode that records bursts of neural activity directed to skeletal muscle and skin blood vessels. Data obtained by this technique seem to allow, in general, a good estimate of the efferent sympathetic activity. For instance, a close positive relationship between the number of bursts of muscle sympathetic activity recorded by microneurography and plasma noradrenaline has been described in normal subjects[10] and hypertensive[10,11] and congestive heart failure patients.[12] Whether sympathetic activity to muscle and skin is truly representative of the outflow to the heart, however, remains an open question.[13] When major and widespread reflexes, such as baroreceptive reflexes, are elicited, there is no question that activation or inhibition of sympathetic activity will occur and will be recorded at different levels.

The situation, however, is more complex and very different for selective activation of sympathetic reflexes, such as with acute myocardial ischemia.[14,15] This problem is enhanced by the high degree of specificity of the sympathetic outflow directed to the heart (Fig. 1).[16] Another very serious, and often underestimated limitation of this technique, is that it is unavoidably based on whole nerve recording (but the same criticism would apply to recordings from large multifiber preparations). This may be quite misleading, because the neural activity is quantified not by direct count of individual action potentials (spikes), but by counting whatever exceeds a selected voltage and passes though a window discriminator. This method has been criticized by two careful quantitative analyses.[17,18] Andresen and Yang[18] have concluded that "interactions among spike trains. . . . lead to serious underestimation of activity levels" and that "interpretation of results of multifiber or whole nerve recording whether analyzed with integrative, time-averaging, or spike counting techniques needs to be viewed with caution" (p. R997).

These considerations represent a significant limitation for the use of this technique to study cardiac autonomic reflexes related to ischemic heart disease. This limitation may be less relevant, however, for studies related to hypertension, where the peripheral outflow is quite important and where the peripheral component of baroreceptive reflexes is a major target for studies and interventions.

This type of problem does not exist with cardiac vagal activity, because, only indirect approaches can be used for this component of autonomic activity.

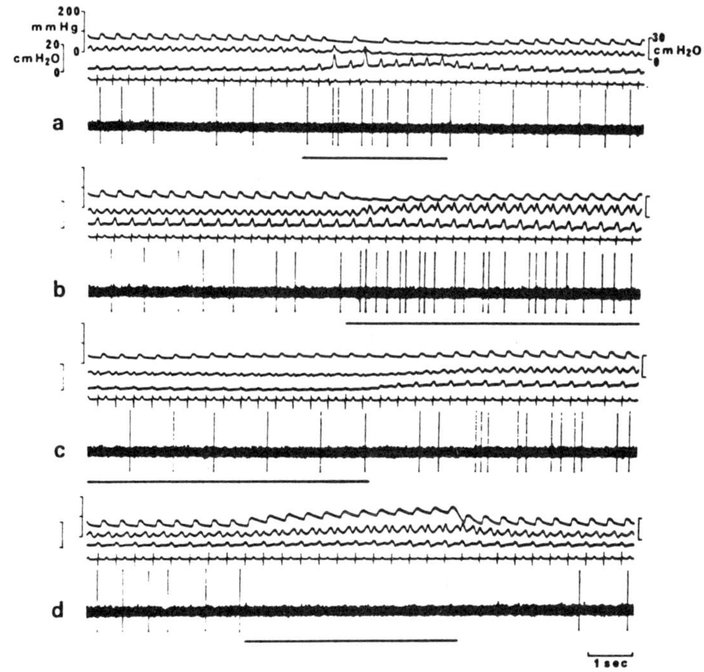

Figure 1. *Anesthetized cat, with spinal section at C1, bilateral vagotomy, and bilateral carotid sinus denervation. Increases or decreases in the discharge of the same sympathetic preganglionic neuron obtained with different stimuli. Tracings represent, from top to bottom, carotid arterial blood pressure, left atrial pressure, right atrial pressure, ECG, and nervous recording from a single efferent sympathetic fiber isolated from the left white ramus communicans T3, the most important sympathetic outflow to the heart. a: Stenosis of the pulmonary artery by a snare; b: Obstruction of the left ventricular outflow by inflating a balloon in the root of the aorta; c: Release of a transient occlusion of the inferior vena cava; and d: Obstruction of the midthoracic aorta by a snare. The first three maneuvers activate cardiac receptors and elicit a reflex increase in sympathetic efferent activity, while the latter also activates aortic receptors and induces an inhibition of the sympathetic outflow. Reproduced with permission from Pagani M, Schwartz PJ, Banks R, et al: Reflex responses of sympathetic preganglionic neurones initiated by different cardiovascular receptors in spinal animals. Brain Res 68:220, 1974.*

The direct relation between stimulation of the baroreceptors and vagal outflow to the heart, however, has been clearly documented by direct recording from cardiac efferent vagal fibers during blood pressure changes. Figure 2 illustrates the reflex vagal responses to different levels of arterial blood pressure. In the three panels, the upper trace shows the electrocardiogram and the lower trace shows the recording of neural activity from a single unit isolated from the central cut end of the cardiac branch of the right vagus, a branch largely directed to the sinoatrial (SA) node.[19] It is evident that the firing of this cardiac vagal fiber is synchronous with the heartbeat and that higher levels of blood pressure are associated with a progressive increase in the number of action potentials per cardiac cycle. Thus, changes in SA node activity (expressed as sinus heart rate) can be taken as representing concordant variations in vagal efferent activity.

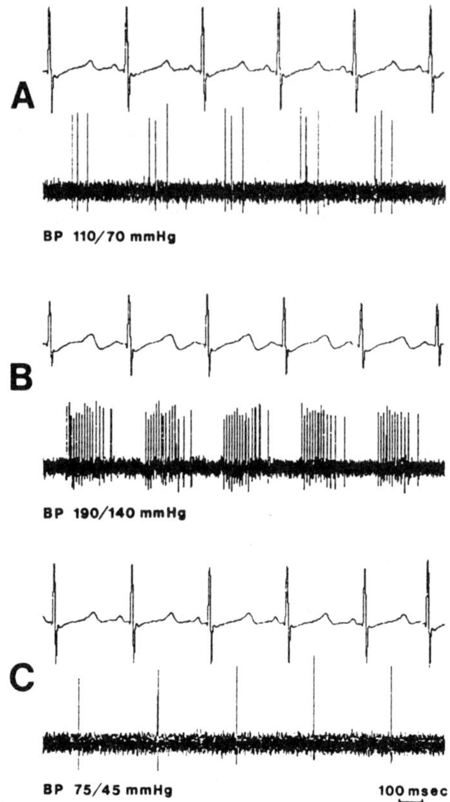

Figure 2. *Activity of a single cardiac vagal efferent fiber at three different levels of arterial blood pressure. In each panel, the upper trace shows the electrocardiogram and the lower trace shows the electroneurogram. A: At the resting level of blood pressure, a pulse-synchronous activity, with three impulses in each burst, was present. B: When blood pressure was raised by phenylephrine, the activity of the fiber increased markedly. The activity was still synchronous with the cardiac cycle, it started 60 msec earlier, and each burst showed many more impulses. C: When blood pressure was reduced by bleeding, the activity of the fiber decreased. The activity was still synchronous with the cardiac cycle, but only one impulse per cycle was present. Changes in vagal activity do not modify heart rate because the nerve is cut in order to allow the recording from the central cut end of the nerve. Reproduced by permission of the American Heart Association, Inc. from Cerati D, Schwartz PJ: Single cardiac vagal fiber activity, acute myocardial ischemia, and risk for sudden death. Circ Res 69:1392, 1991.*

Under conditions other than myocardial ischemia, vagal efferent firing is, of course, greatly influenced by the activity in the carotid sinus nerve. When this afferent activity increases it has, via vagal activation, a profound effect on the RR interval, as has been documented in experimental preparations[20] and in hypertensive[21] or in anginal[22] patients. In a study by Eckberg et al,[23] the electrical stimulation of the carotid sinus nerve, performed in unsedated subjects by means of a chronically implanted device, produced a mean RR interval lengthening of 269 milliseconds. Additional important information provided by the same investigation was that, with the patients relaxed and in supine positions, the effects of carotid sinus nerve stimulation were not influenced by propranolol in seven out of the eight patients studied.

The existence of a linear relation between frequency of electrical vagal stimulation and RR interval lengthening was initially described by Levy and Zieske[24] in anesthetized preparations. These observations have been extended recently by studying the effect of vagal stimulation in conscious dogs at rest and during exercise.[25] In these conditions, the relation between vagal activity and heart rate, described initially by Levy and Zieske,[24] was documented in the recent study[25] in absence of the confounding effects of anesthesia and at different levels of sympathetic activity produced by exercise.

Particularly relevant to the pattern of firing of vagal fibers during baroceptive reflexes is the study performed by Levy et al in 1972.[26] In these experiments, the authors documented a linear increase in PP intervals with the progressive increase in numbers of impulses delivered in a single burst of electrical vagal stimulation with a fixed delay from the cardiac beat.[26] This observation has been recently reappraised in conscious dogs in our laboratory. We have developed a system capable of delivering bursts of electrical stimuli, synchronous with the cardiac beat, to the right vagus while the dogs are either resting on the laboratory table or are exercising on a treadmill. By this means, we studied the effect of progressive increase in vagal activity to the heart. The pattern mimicked the spontaneous physiological firing as it occurs during a baroreceptive reflex at rest or during an exercise-induced increase in sympathetic activity. Figure 3 illustrates an example obtained during exercise. As the number of impulses in bursts of vagal stimulation increases, the RR interval prolongs.

Vagal activity is, of course, not the sole determinant of SA node activity, and this always has to be kept in mind to avoid the risk of excessive simplifications. Experimental[27–29] and clinical[30,31] observations document the role of sympathetic activity in modulating reflex RR interval lengthening during a blood pressure rise (see also Ch. 25). This modulating effect has special importance for the conditions under which the various tests, to be discussed below, are executed. With these limitations in mind, the evidence of a linear relation between efferent vagal activity and heart rate slowing supports the use of heart rate at rest and during mild perturbations of the autonomic nervous system activity as a reliable marker of cardiac vagal activity.

Techniques

The Valsalva Maneuver

The Valsalva maneuver is a time-honored procedure that is still used in testing autonomic function,[4,5] largely because of its apparent simplicity. Autonomic reflexes are produced by a transient increase of intrathoracic and intraabdominal pressures provoked by straining. Straining is initiated after a

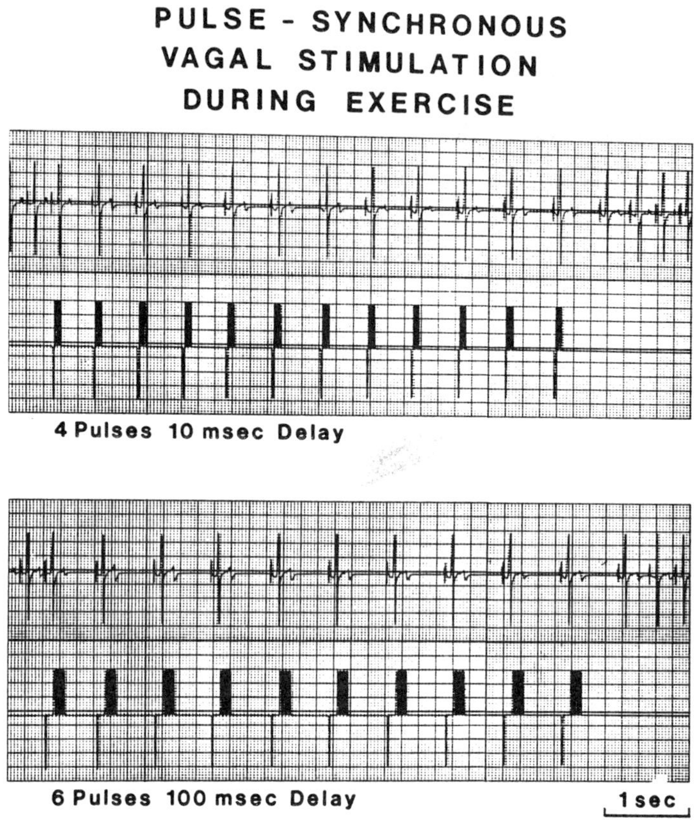

Figure 3. *Two examples of pulse-synchronous stimulation of the right cervical vagus during exercise in a dog. The upper trace shows a transthoracic electrocardiogram and the lower trace shows the output of the stimulator. In the lower trace, the negative deflection represents the activation of the sensing system of the stimulator by the P wave, the positive deflections the number of pulses delivered in each burst. By increasing the number of pulses and the delay from the atrial activation, a greater reduction in heart rate is obtained.*

maximal or full inspiration. Hamilton et al[32] proposed that the response to the maneuver occurs in four phases. One, a rapid transient rise in blood pressure is associated with a heart rate reduction immediately after the onset of straining. This initial response is likely to be due to the compressive effect on the aorta of the increased intrathoracic pressure and to the increase in stroke volume. Two, the continuation of straining impedes venous return and leads to a reduced stroke volume and cardiac output. As a consequence, blood pressure transiently falls and then recovers, and heart rate increases. Three, at the release of straining, venous inflow and stroke volume return toward normal, and blood pressure rises because of the reflex vasoconstriction.

Phase 1 of the maneuver has been used mainly to assess vagal reflexes. Indeed, in phase 4 of the maneuver, the blood pressure rise depends mainly upon neural mechanisms that can also influence the reflex heart rate response, but in phase 1, this occurrence is due primarily to mechanical effects.

The simplicity of the Valsalva maneuver has been described as "illusory."[5] It is a complex test that involves several types of receptors (baroreceptors, cardiopulmonary receptors, and chemoreceptors). The main limitation for the widespread use of this maneuver is the problem of individual and interindividual reproducibility, particularly when normal subjects and patients with cardiac diseases are compared.[33–36] The blood pressure response during phase 2 is different in normal subjects than in patients with congestive heart failure (CHF).[35] The overall response is obviously affected by the intensity and duration of the strain, and this requires monitoring of intraoral pressure and the maintenance of a constant pressure.[36] The patient is obviously aware of the stimulus.

The Valsalva maneuver has been used to test autonomic reflexes in two studies of postmyocardial infarction patients.[33,37] In the first study,[33] the pressor responses during the different phases of the Valsalva maneuver were examined in 22 patients with a recent myocardial infarction. The main finding was that the blood pressure rise occurring in phase 4 was significantly less than that in normal subjects. This finding was proposed as evidence for autonomic imbalance occurring after a myocardial infarction. In the second study,[37] patients with a one-year-old myocardial infarction had less reflex tachycardia than did control subjects during the blood pressure decrease in phase 2 of the Valsalva maneuver. The small size of the two populations under study precluded any inference about the prognostic value of the Valsalva maneuver.

The Neck Chamber

The variable pressure neck chamber is another valuable means to study baroreflexes. Among the different types, the Eckberg model[38] is the one that has been mostly used. This chamber consists of a malleable lead collar that encompasses the anterior and lateral aspects of the neck. The chamber can be used to activate or deactivate the receptors by altering transmural pressure in the receptor area of the carotid arteries. The stimulus is produced by a measurable increase or decrease of the pressure in the collar. Eckberg found the data obtained by the neck chamber to be highly reproducible,[39] but a greater degree of variability has been reported by Mancia et al.[40] Overall, this method presents several advantages:

1. it allows selective stimulation of the carotid baroreceptors over a large range of their activity;
2. the stimuli can be delivered rapidly to assess fast reflex responses, such as those for heart rate; and
3. it allows analysis of reflex control of both heart rate and peripheral resistance.

Even this method, however, has some drawbacks. The technique is complex to use and the patients, aware of the stimulus, may have some emotional reactions. Furthermore, the selectivity of the stimulus at the level of the carotid receptors itself represents a potential problem. In fact, the reflex pressor changes induced by the stimulus activates aortic baroreceptors that, in turn, oppose the effects of carotid receptor stimulation. This occurrence creates a complex interaction of different receptors on the reflex heart rate response.[4]

Vasoactive Drugs

In the 1960s, the reflex heart rate responses to blood pressure changes induced by vasoactive drugs have been proposed to test autonomic function. Two groups described two different methodologies to study and quantify the reflex bradycardia during the blood pressure rise. Korner et al[41] proposed the use of infusion of phenylephrine to study the relation between different levels of blood pressure and heart rate in steady state condition, while Smyth and the Oxford group[42] used a rapid (in a few seconds) bolus injection of phenylephrine, usually 100 to 200 μg.

Whether blood pressure rises slowly during an infusion or more rapidly after a bolus injection, the main feature common to these two methods is that values of blood pressure can be plotted versus RR intervals and a regression analysis is performed. The relation is linear between the two variables over a limited pressure range, and the slope of the regression line allows a quantification of the sensitivity of the reflex. The measurement of baroreflex sensitivity is then expressed in milliseconds of RR interval lengthening (or shortening) per one mm Hg of blood pressure change. Figure 4 illustrates two extreme patterns of response that can be observed with the phenylephrine bolus injection. A steep slope of the regression line (Fig. 5) indicates strong vagal reflexes and weak sympathetic reflexes. Conversely, a relatively flat slope (Fig. 6) indicates weak vagal reflexes, probably accompanied by strong sympathetic reflexes, a condition that denotes sympathetic dominance. In general, these slopes provide reasonable information about autonomic balance.

A theoretical limitation of this mathematical approach is that the relation between baroreceptor stimulation and SA node response is, once the entire range of the reflex is considered, sigmoidal rather than linear.[43] In most subjects, however, the 20 to 30 mm Hg pressure rise induced by the drug injection is well below the saturation levels of the reflex and, thus, it explores its linear part. A similar relation has also been described for the reflex tachycardia that follows the administration of a vasodilator drug. Nevertheless, because the vagal component of the reflex appears to carry the more meaningful information concerning cardiovascular patients, the attention of most investigators has focused on vasopressor interventions.

Among the two methods involving a blood pressure rise, the one described by the Oxford group,[42] has been more frequently used, because it has some advantages over the infusion technique. The bolus injection measures the reflex response beat by beat, and not as an average over several beats; it does not involve the problem of receptor adaptation[44]; and the test can be repeated several times in a relatively brief session. The last point is important, as the length of the protocol and the consequent emotional response of the patient can affect the reproducibility of the measurement.

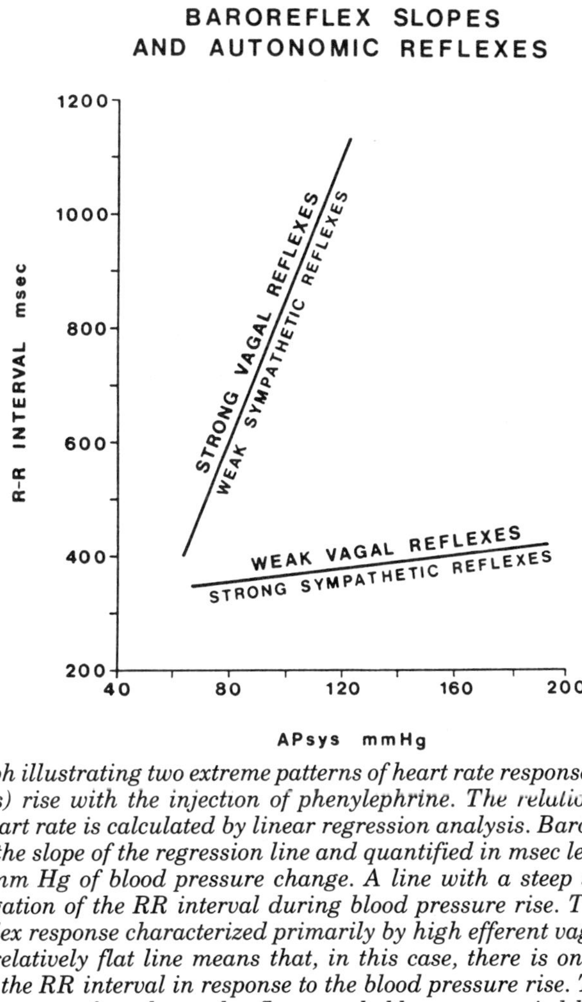

Figure 4. *Graph illustrating two extreme patterns of heart rate response to systolic blood pressure (APsys) rise with the injection of phenylephrine. The relation between blood pressure and heart rate is calculated by linear regression analysis. Baroreflex sensitivity is expressed by the slope of the regression line and quantified in msec lengthening of RR interval per 1 mm Hg of blood pressure change. A line with a steep slope indicates a marked prolongation of the RR interval during blood pressure rise. This prolongation represents a reflex response characterized primarily by high efferent vagal activity to the SA node. The relatively flat line means that, in this case, there is only a very modest prolongation of the RR interval in response to the blood pressure rise. The prolongation indicates the presence of weak vagal reflexes probably accompanied by strong sympathetic reflexes. Reproduced with permission from Schwartz PJ, Stone HL: The analysis and modulation of autonomic reflexes in the prediction and prevention of sudden death. In DP Zipes, J Jalife (eds): Cardiac Electrophysiology and Arrhythmias. Orlando, FL, Grune & Stratton, 1985, p. 172.*

The vasoactive drug technique has the following major advantages:

1. the heart rate response is neurally mediated;
2. the technique is easy to perform and the subject is unaware of the stimulus; and
3. the stimulus acts in the same direction on all receptors.

One potentially important source of interference, however, has to be remembered: any type of stress, by activating sympathetic activity and there-

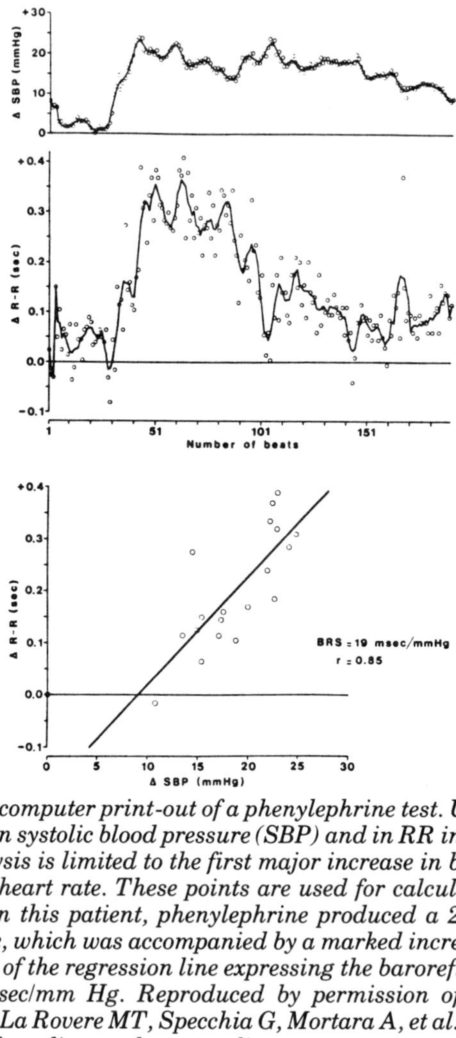

Figure 5. *Retouched computer print-out of a phenylephrine test. Upper and mid-panels: Beat-to-beat changes in systolic blood pressure (SBP) and in RR intervals compared with baseline values. Analysis is limited to the first major increase in blood pressure with the attendant changes in heart rate. These points are used for calculation of the regression line (bottom panel). In this patient, phenylephrine produced a 25 mm Hg increase in systolic blood pressure, which was accompanied by a marked increase of the RR interval. Accordingly, the slope of the regression line expressing the baroreflex sensitivity (BRS) is rather high = 19 msec/mm Hg. Reproduced by permission of the American Heart Association, Inc. from La Rovere MT, Specchia G, Mortara A, et al: Baroreflex sensitivity, clinical correlates and cardiovascular mortality among patients with a first myocardial infarction. A prospective study. Circulation 78:817, 1988.*

by augmenting the release of norepinephrine (NE), reduces the effect of vagal activation. This occurrence produces smaller values of baroreflex sensitivity.[45]

The bolus injection of phenylephrine has been proposed by our group[46] to study the prognostic value of the analysis of vagal reflexes in patients with a recent myocardial infarction. It has also been used by other groups with similar results.[47] The advantages and problems of this technique in coronary artery disease patients is discussed below.

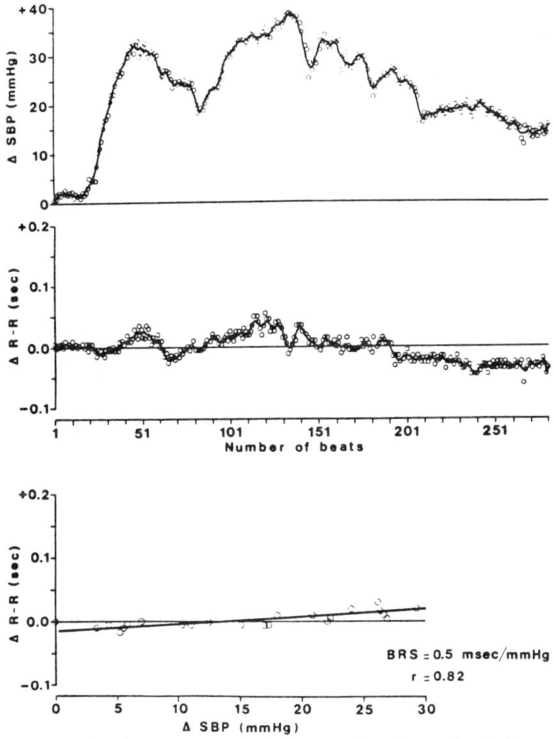

Figure 6. *Similar retouched computer print-out of a phenylephrine test, as in Figure 5. Heart rate in this patient did not change despite a clear-cut increase in systolic blood pressure (SBP). Accordingly, baroreflex sensitivity (BRS) is extremely depressed = 0.5 msec/mm Hg (bottom panel). Reproduced by permission of the American Heart Association, Inc. from La Rovere MT, Specchia G, Mortara A, et al: Baroreflex sensitivity, clinical correlates and cardiovascular mortality among patients with a first myocardial infarction. A prospective study. Circulation 78:818, 1988.*

Baroreflex Sensitivity in Patients with Myocardial Infarction

In this section, several practical aspects related to the determination and analysis of baroreflex sensitivity are examined. They include a thorough description of the actual methodology, and a discussion of the clinical factors that are either associated with or that may modify baroreflex sensitivity.

Methods

The technique for the execution of the test has been extensively described.[42,46] To define the reflex heart rate change accurately during the blood pressure rise, it is important to avoid the influence of any factor that might affect it, such as environmental noise, temperature, and the effects of digestion. The study should be carried out with the patient fasting, resting, and feeling comfortable with the environment and personnel. One electrocardiographic lead and systolic blood pressure are continuously recorded throughout the test. Once blood pressure is stable, phenylephrine is injected at a dose that increases the systolic blood pressure by at least 15 mm Hg and by no more than 40 mm Hg. At variance with the initial description of the method, phenylephrine is administered slowly (in 30 seconds) in post-myocardial infarction patients. As a consequence, a slightly higher dose is used; 3 to 4 μg/kg are usually sufficient. In patients with a depressed cardiac function, however, a greater dose may be needed. Baroreflex sensitivity is then expressed by the slope of the regression line correlating RR intervals and blood pressure during the response to the vasoactive drug.

Three different studies in patients with a prior myocardial infarction, without overt cardiac failure, have provided information about the values of baroreflex sensitivity that can be expected in a patient with a recent myocardial infarction.[46–48] In these studies, mean baroreflex sensitivity was approximately 7 to 8 milliseconds/mm Hg, with a standard deviation of 4 to 5 milliseconds/mm Hg (see also Ch. 30). To better interpret this information, a comparison with a group of age- and sex-matched control subjects was performed.[48] Mean baroreflex sensitivity of the control group was 12.3 ± 2.9 milliseconds/mm Hg. The analysis of individual data provided additional insights; indeed, 15 out of 32 (47%) patients had baroreflex slopes lower than 7 milliseconds/mm Hg, whereas this finding was never observed in control subjects (Fig. 7). This information is relevant to the effects that myocardial infarction has on baroreflex sensitivity.

The main limitation of this issue in clinical studies is the necessity of drawing conclusions from cross-sectional group comparisons. To overcome this clinical limitation, we evaluated the effect of a myocardial infarction on baroreflex sensitivity in a large, prospective experimental study.[49] We first compared the baroreflex sensitivity of 85 conscious dogs with normal hearts to that of 192 conscious dogs with a one-month-old myocardial infarction. This study is similar to the procedure in clinical studies. We found that baroreflex sensitivity was significantly lower in the infarcted group (12.9 ± 7.6 milliseconds versus 19.7 ± 7.9 mm Hg, $p<0.001$). We then performed an internal control study by comparing baroreflex sensitivity before and 30 days after myocardial infarction in 55 dogs. This is what clinical studies cannot do. In 40 of these 55 (73%) dogs, baroreflex sensitivity decreased after myocardial infarction (change $\geq$3 milliseconds/mm Hg), but it did not change in 11 (20%) dogs and it increased in 4 dogs (Fig. 8). This study definitively documented that myocardial infarction decreases baroreflex sensitivity in approximately 70% of individuals. The fact that almost 30% of the dogs had either no change or an increase in baroreflex sensitivity calls for great caution in the interpretation of clinical findings obtained in small clinical studies based on group comparison.[50]

A practical issue that was viewed as a potential limit for the wide use of baroreflex sensitivity testing concerns the measurement of arterial blood pressure. To date, arterial blood pressure has been mostly measured from a

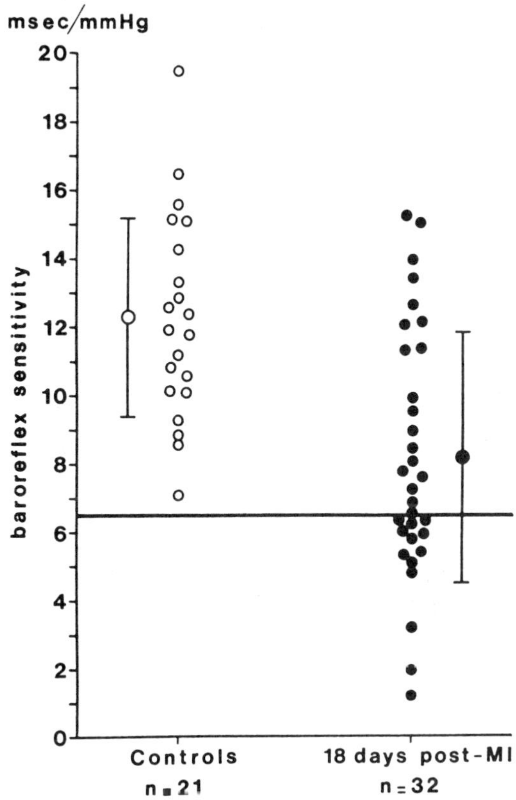

Figure 7. *Plot showing individual values of baroreflex sensitivity among 32 patients, studied 18 days after myocardial infarction (post-MI), and 21 age- and sex-matched control subjects. The horizontal line at 6.5 msec/mm Hg represents two standard deviations below the mean value for the control subjects. The mean values ±1 SD are also indicated. From Schwartz PJ, Zaza A, Pala M, et al: Baroreflex sensitivity and its evolution during the first year after a myocardial infarction. Reprinted with permission from the American College of Cardiology (Journal of the American College of Cardiology, 1988, 12:632).*

teflon cannula (22 G)[51] or from a miniature catheter tip transducer[52] positioned in the radial or brachial artery. The invasive approach has been used both for short-term tests and for 24-hour blood pressure monitoring in man.[51,52] In the early 1970s, however, Ian Penaz[53] described a new technique for noninvasive recording of blood pressure. The device that was subsequently developed from this initial report was called FINAPRES (FINger Arterial PRESsure).[54] The FINAPRES operates through a small finger cuff equipped with an infrared digital photoplethysmograph to measure the arterial blood volume under the cuff. The accuracy of blood pressure measurement of FINAPRES has been documented recently in a small group of hypertensive patients during a 24-hour monitoring period and also during vasoactive interventions that produce brief changes in blood pressure.[55]

Given the importance of the availability of a noninvasive method to

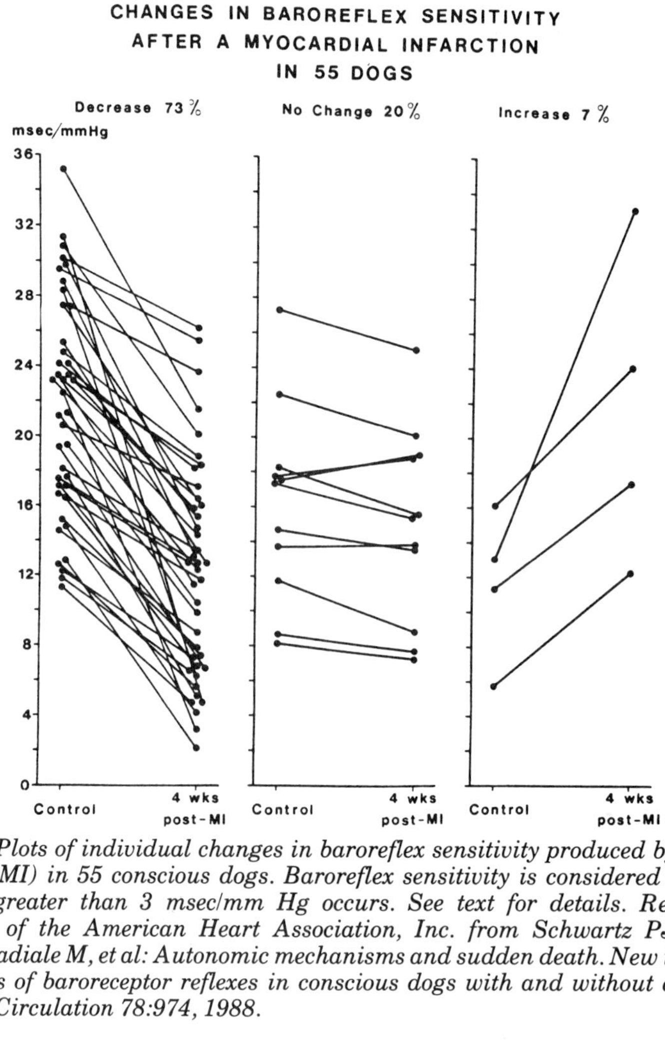

Figure 8. *Plots of individual changes in baroreflex sensitivity produced by myocardial infarction (MI) in 55 conscious dogs. Baroreflex sensitivity is considered changed if a difference greater than 3 msec/mm Hg occurs. See text for details. Reproduced by permission of the American Heart Association, Inc. from Schwartz PJ, Vanoli E, Stramba-Badiale M, et al: Autonomic mechanisms and sudden death. New insights from the analysis of baroreceptor reflexes in conscious dogs with and without a myocardial infarction. Circulation 78:974, 1988.*

measure blood pressure beat by beat, a validation of FINAPRES over a large number of patients was needed. An ongoing, international follow-up study (described in detail in Ch. 30) is currently evaluating the prognostic values of the analysis of baroreflex sensitivity and of heart rate variability in the identification of post-myocardial infarction patients at higher risk for cardiac mortality and sudden death. This study (ATRAMI, acronym for Autonomic Tone and Reflexes After Myocardial Infarction) is also assessing the accuracy of FINAPRES in a large population. So far, the phenylephrine test, which includes both the invasive and noninvasive measurement of blood pressure, has been performed in more than 500 patients with recent myocardial infarctions. An initial linear regression analysis of 246 baroreflex sensitivity tests was performed using blood pressure values from the two approaches. Figure 9 shows the strong correlation (correlation coefficient “r” = 0.94) between the invasive and noninvasive measurements.

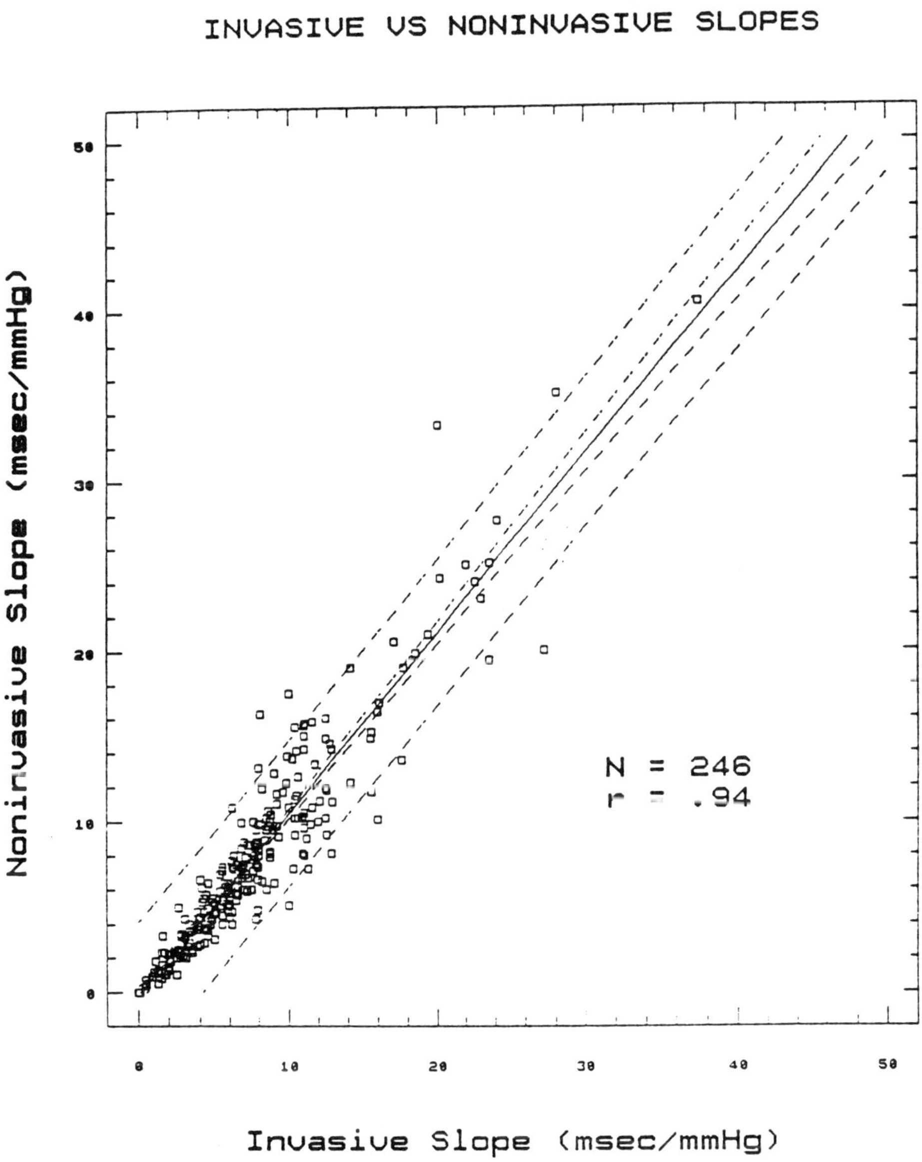

Figure 9. *Plot of the linear regression analysis of 246 baroreflex sensitivity values obtained in the same patients by measuring blood pressure by the invasive procedure (teflon cannula in the brachial artery) and by the noninvasive procedure (FINAPRES). The correlation coefficient between the baroreflex sensitivities obtained with the two methods = 0.94.*

Figure 10 describes in detail the relation between the two methods in 142 tests with values lower than 10 milliseconds/mm Hg. In this figure, the analysis focuses on the area of slopes lower than 3 milliseconds/mm Hg. This area is associated with a greater risk for cardiac mortality and sudden death in the first year after a myocardial infarction.[46] The main information is that in the area of slopes lower than 3 milliseconds/mm Hg with the invasive method,

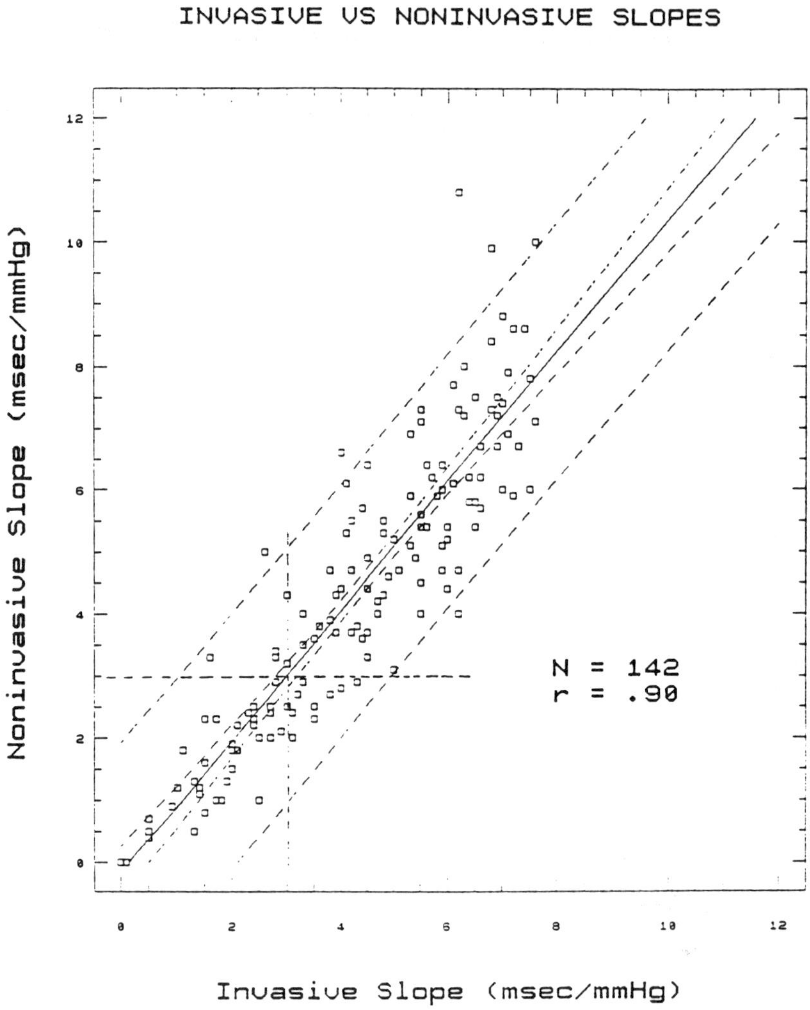

Figure 10. *Magnification of the data shown in Figure 9 that describes in detail the comparisons between baroreflex sensitivity values lower than 12 msec/mm Hg obtained by the invasive and noninvasive measurement of blood pressure. The area within the two dotted lines includes values (lower than 3 msec/mm Hg) associated in previous studies with a significant increase in risk for cardiac mortality and sudden death after myocardial infarction. In only 6 out of 41 values <3 msec/mm Hg, the slope calculated from blood pressure recorded by FINAPRES exceeded the value obtained with the invasive procedure. In 4 of these 6 cases, the values obtained by FINAPRES were higher than those obtained by the invasive procedure by <1 msec/mm Hg.*

only six patients exceeded the area that denotes high risk when the noninvasive method is used. In four of these six cases the excess in the calculation obtained from data collected by FINAPRES was <1 mm Hg. This finding suggests that, by using the noninvasive approach, there is only a modest loss of accuracy in the identification of high-risk patients. Thus, this initial analysis indicates that FINAPRES may represent a dependable device to more easily evaluate cardiac reflexes in large populations.

Test Execution and Reproducibility

A potential problem in the execution of the test concerns the presence of a systematic trend or of a drift caused by the carry-over effect of the drug in successive determinations. To assess this problem and to quantify any potential effect of repeated injections of phenylephrine on baroreceptor responses, three series of consecutive bolus injections in 150 patients with a previous myocardial infarction were analyzed. The injections, given at least 10 minutes apart, were repeated until the blood pressure and heart rate had returned to their control values. Among the entire series of injections, the three slopes obtained with a similar dose of the drug and with the highest correlation coefficient were then selected and analyzed for each patient. To test the hypothesis of a systematic error among the sequence of the three tests, an analysis of variance for repeated measurements was performed. The means and the standard deviations did not differ from each other (8.1 ± 5.9, 8.3 ± 6.3, and 8.1 ± 6.1 milliseconds/mm Hg respectively; $F = 0.1$, $p = 0.9$). These data suggest that, provided that all methodological rules are fulfilled, the drug had no effect on consecutive determinations of baroreflex sensitivity.

The usefulness of a test for risk stratification in large populations depends also on the reproducibility of the results (from a quantitative point of view) when data are collected and analyzed by investigators with different degrees of experience. ATRAMI (see above and Ch. 30) is also addressing this issue, as it is currently enrolling patients in over 25 centers in Europe, the United States, and Japan. As a consequence, not all the investigators can be expected to have the same expertise of those involved in the initial studies.[46,47] An internal double-blind control between one experienced investigator at the ATRAMI coordinating center and one of the enrolling centers provided an initial answer to this issue. Figure 11 describes the relation between the analyses performed at the two sites on the same set of data collected by the enrolling center. Two points deserve a specific comment. First, the significant correlation ($r = 0.93$) between the two calculations documents that data analysis of baroreflex sensitivity is highly reproducible among different investigators. Second, the distribution of the data observed at this enrolling center closely resembles that obtained in the initial study.[46] This finding coincides with the similarity already noted[1] between the two studies by La Rovere et al[46] and by Farrell et al.[47]

Calculation of Baroreflex Sensitivity

In the initial description of the technique in 1969,[42] the authors explored the role of respiration during the reflex response to blood pressure rise and proposed that only beats occurring during expiration should be used. A subsequent analysis by the same authors indicated that respiration has only a modest effect on the calculation of the index,[56] especially when one deals with slopes lower than 15 milliseconds/mm Hg. This information is relevant to the issue of measuring baroreflex sensitivity in post-myocardial infarction patients, in whom only a minority are likely to be at high risk for cardiovascular mortality and sudden death and have indices higher than 15 milliseconds/mm Hg.

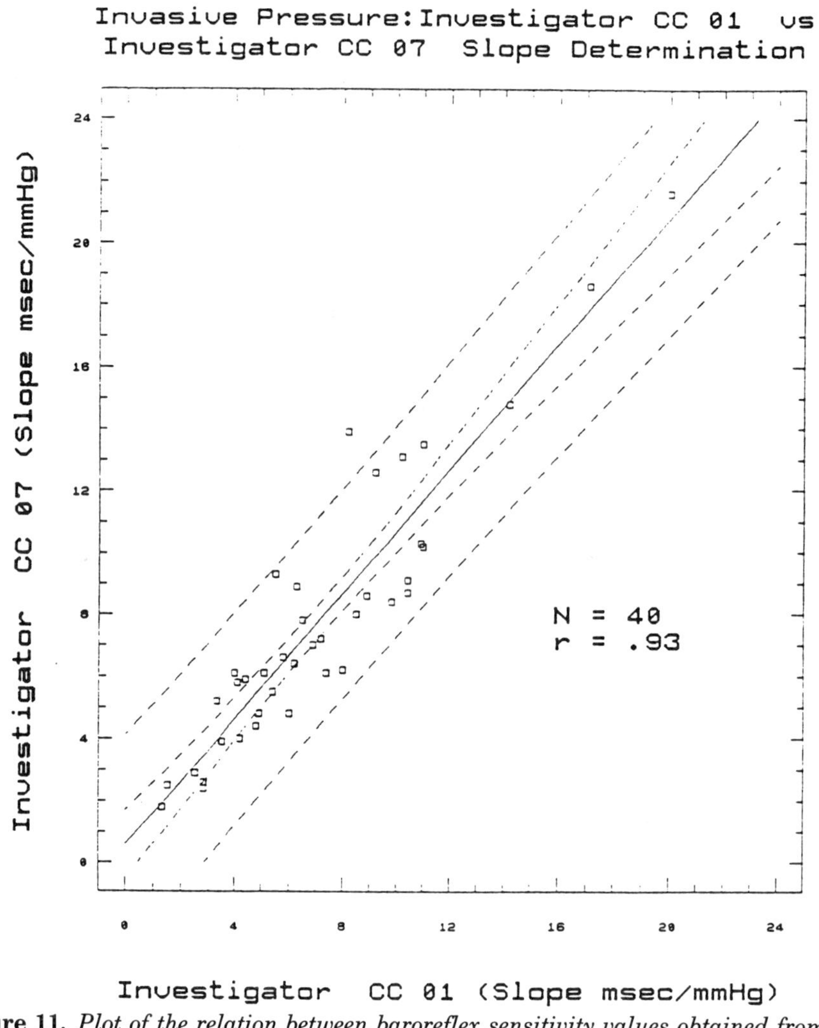

Figure 11. *Plot of the relation between baroreflex sensitivity values obtained from the same set of data but calculated by two different investigators. CC 01 is the code of the coordinating center of ATRAMI (see text for details). CC 07 is one of the enrolling centers of ATRAMI. The high correlation between the two calculations documents the high reproducibility of baroreflex sensitivity calculation even when made by investigators with very different experience with the method.*

Another issue in the analysis concerns the selection of starting points for the calculation and the best coupling between blood pressure values and RR intervals. In our experience, the best approach is to collect data starting from the first noticeable pressure change and to continue until blood pressure reaches its peak. The best coupling between blood pressure and RR interval for the analysis largely depends upon the initial values of RR interval. The conduction time of the reflex is, in humans, around 800 milliseconds. This value means that for RR longer than 800 milliseconds the reflex vagal activation is potentially able to influence the occurrence of the QRS that immediately follows the one that generated the pressor event. As a consequence, for heart rates lower than 75 beats/minute, the pulse interval should be correlated with the immediately preceding pulse pressure. Software available for automatic calculation of baroreflex sensitivity allows the best choice by providing simultaneous calculation of slopes from the same data with eight different shifts between blood pressure and RR intervals. Such software includes the one developed by the bioengineering staff supporting ATRAMI.

Baroreflex Sensitivity and Test-Related Variables

The issue of the possible relation between baroreflex sensitivity and several variables related to the execution of the test was addressed by La Rovere et al.[46] In 78 post-myocardial infarction patients, baroreflex sensitivity was not correlated significantly with heart rate ($p = 0.08$), basal systolic blood pressure ($p = 0.08$), dosage of phenylephrine ($p = 0.3$), or the attendant increase in blood pressure after the injection ($p = 0.13$) (Fig. 12). The lack of correlation between baroreflex sensitivity and basal blood pressure and heart rate disagreed somewhat with previous findings in noninfarcted individuals.[57] This finding may reflect a consequence of the autonomic derangements occurring after myocardial infarction and influencing the normal relation between blood pressure and heart rate.

Baroreflex Sensitivity and Clinical Correlates

The inverse relation between age and baroreflex sensitivity is well known[56,58] and it has been also documented in patients with coronary artery disease.[46,47] Several pathological conditions such as diabetes and heart failure, may also influence baroreflex sensitivity (see Ch. 25). As far as patients with a recent myocardial infarction are concerned, the relation between baroreflex sensitivity and several clinical aspects of coronary artery disease has been investigated. Specifically, patients with three vessel diseases have a baroreflex sensitivity significantly lower than patients with one vessel disease (4.8 ± 2.7 versus 7.1 ± 3.1 milliseconds/mm Hg). This finding could be the consequence of a greater afferent discharge from sympathetic mechanoreceptors[15] located in the hypoperfused areas.[29]

The site of the infarction was also expected to influence baroreflex sensitivity on the basis of the described prevalence of sensory endings connected to vagal afferent fibers in the inferoposterior wall[59] and to sympathetic afferent fibers in the anterior wall of the left ventricle. The information obtained in the three studies[46–48] is not unequivocal. La Rovere et al[46] found that patients with an inferior myocardial infarction had a baroreflex sensitivity lower than patients with an anterior myocardial infarction: 6.1 ± 3.3 versus 8.9 ± 5.8 milliseconds/mm Hg ($p = 0.03$). A potential explanation of this finding involves the possibility of a greater destruction of vagal sensory endings, secondary to the necrosis of the inferior portion of the left ventricle. In the other two studies,[47,48] however, such a difference was not observed. Thus, larger populations may be needed to address the issue of infarct site.

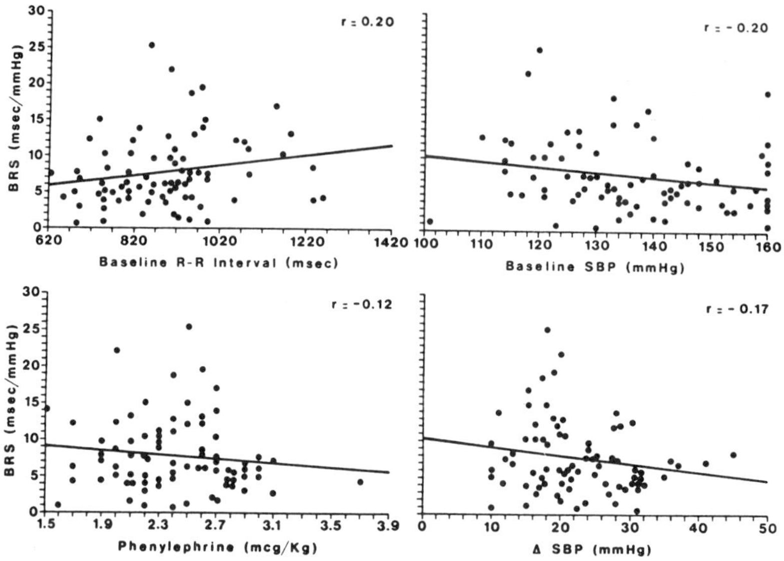

Figure 12. *Plots of the correlation between baroreflex sensitivity (BRS) and some important test-related variables: baseline RR interval (top left panel); baseline systolic blood pressure (SBP) (top right panel); dose of phenylephrine (bottom left panel); and phenylephrine-induced changes in SBP (ΔSBP) (bottom right panel). These data are calculated from the first injection of phenylephrine and indicate lack of correlation between baroreflex sensitivity and these test-related variables. Reproduced by permission of the American Heart Association, Inc. from La Rovere MT, Specchia G, Mortara A, et al: Baroreflex sensitivity, clinical correlates and cardiovascular mortality among patients with a first myocardial infarction. A prospective study. Circulation 78:819, 1988.*

Given the fact that patients with CHF have a depressed baroreflex sensitivity,[60] a significant correlation with markers of left ventricular function might have been expected. In post-myocardial infarction patients, however, baroreflex sensitivity was not at all correlated with left ventricular ejection fraction (Fig. 13), pulmonary wedge pressure at peak exercise (Fig. 14), or several quantitative measures of systolic function (Figs. 15 and 16).[61] The lack of correlation between baroreflex sensitivity and left ventricular ejection fraction has already been confirmed by Farrell et al.[47]

Another important issue that must be considered when dealing with cardiovascular reflexes in patients with prior myocardial infarctions concerns the possible interference of concomitant drug therapy. Of particular relevance here are the effects of β-adrenergic receptor blockers. Baroreflex sensitivity increased after administration of β blockers in several,[62–66] but not all,[67,68] studies in normal subjects[62–64] and in hypertensive patients.[65,67,68] This issue, however, has not yet been addressed in post-myocardial infarction patients, in whom β-adrenergic blockade is often used and it still remains the only intervention with a demonstrated ability to improve prognosis.[69] In an ongoing study,[70] the effect of chronic therapy with β-blocking agents on baroreflex sensitivity has been evaluated in 20 post-myocardial infarction patients. One month after the infarction, baroreflex sensitivity was tested before and after one week of oral therapy

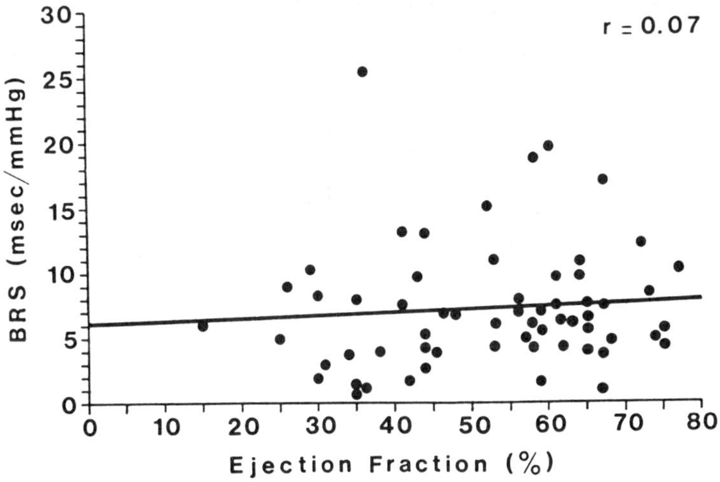

Figure 13. *Plot of relation between baroreflex sensitivity (BRS) and left ventricular ejection fraction at rest. Reproduced by permission of the American Heart Association, Inc. from La Rovere MT, Specchia G, Mortara A, et al: Baroreflex sensitivity, clinical correlates and cardiovascular mortality among patients with a first myocardial infarction. A prospective study. Circulation 78:818, 1988.*

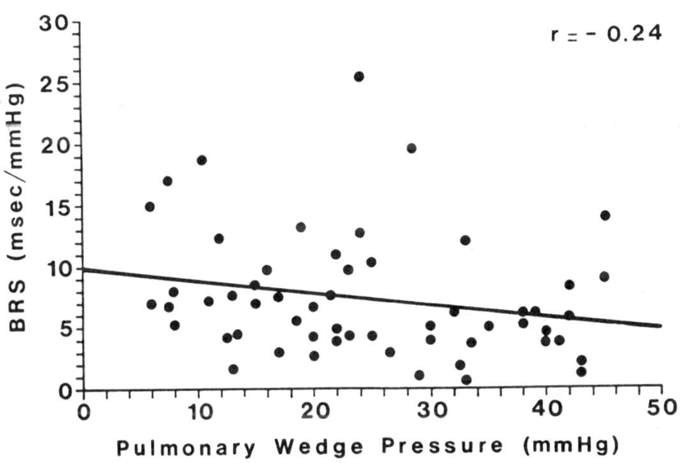

Figure 14. *Plot of relation between baroreflex sensitivity (BRS) and mean pulmonary wedge pressure at peak exercise. Reproduced by permission of the American Heart Association, Inc. from La Rovere MT, Specchia G, Mortara A, et al: Baroreflex sensitivity, clinical correlates and cardiovascular mortality among patients with a first myocardial infarction. A prospective study. Circulation 78:822, 1988.*

with atenolol or metoprolol. Baroreflex sensitivity did not change in 10 patients treated with placebo, whereas it increased by at least 2 milliseconds/mm Hg in 40% of the patients treated with β-blocking agents. These data should, however, be considered with caution, because the baroreflex sensitivity of the patients studied was not particularly low. This pilot study may suggest that β-blockade

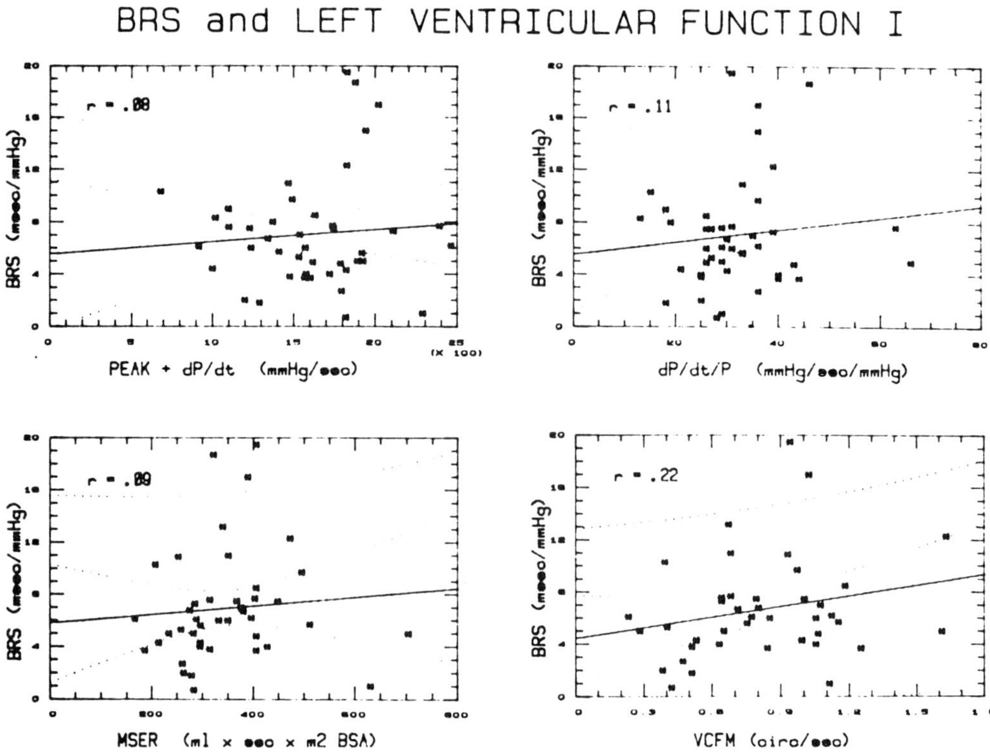

Figure 15. *Plot of the relation between baroreflex sensitivity (BRS) and measures of left ventricular function. No correlation exists between baroreflex sensitivity and peak dP/dt, dP/dt/P, mean systolic ejection rate (MSER), and mean ventricular circumferential fraction (VCFM).*

improves baroreflex sensitivity modestly and in less than half of the post-myocardial infarction patients. An unproven, but tenable, implication is that administration of β-blockers might not significantly alter the potential of baroreflex sensitivity to identify high-risk patients.

Side Effects

The possible occurrence of side effects while using an intervention that increases blood pressure in patients with a recent myocardial infarction has to be considered. The recovery time between each injection is an aspect of particular importance. In patients with left ventricular dysfunction, the vasoconstrictor effect of phenylephrine might influence hemodynamics negatively. This issue was addressed in patients with different degrees of hemodynamic impairment and in whom mean pulmonary artery and capillary pressures were monitored during phenylephrine injections. In all patients, phenylephrine slightly increased both pressures. In patients with left ventricular dysfunction, this increase persisted for a few minutes after the systolic blood pressure had returned to control values. Within 15 minutes of the injection, however, all

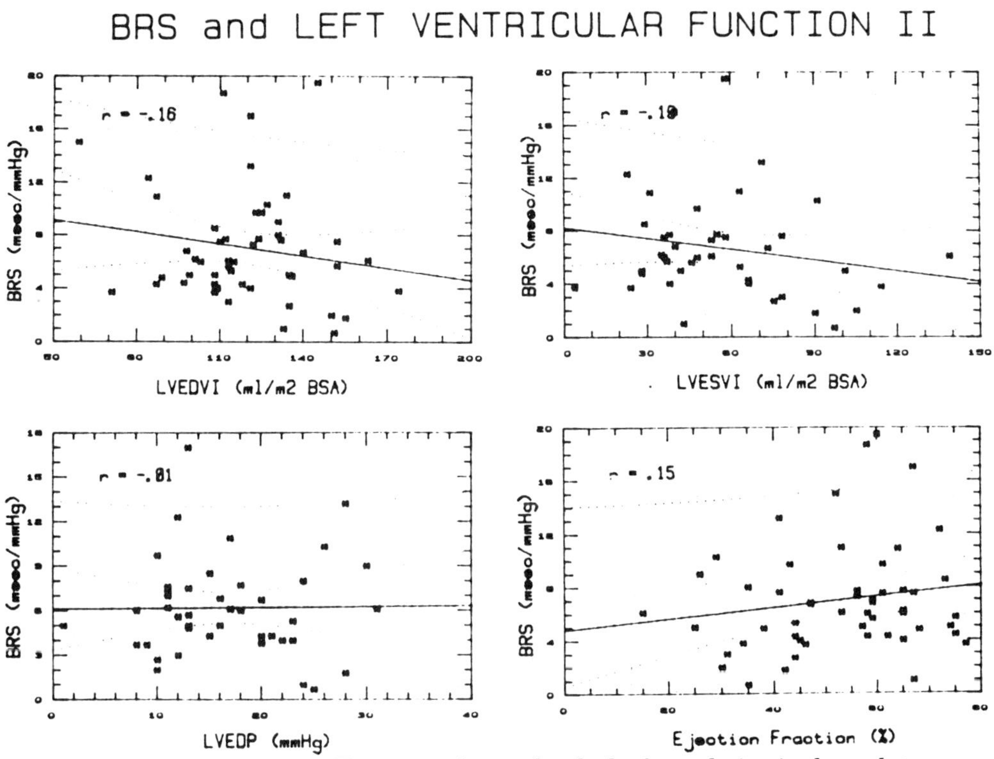

Figure 16. *Same plot as in Figure 15. A complete lack of correlation is shown between baroreflex sensitivity (BRS) and left ventricular end diastolic volume index (LVEDVI), left ventricular and systolic volume index (LVESVI), left ventricular end diastolic pressure (LVEDP), and left ventricular ejection fraction.*

patients had returned to the control situation. Among almost 1800 phenylephrine injections performed in approximately 400 patients with a previous myocardial infarction and, in some cases, with CHF, no major side effects were reported. The only complaints reported, and in a quite limited number of cases (<1%), were headache and a rash of short duration.

Conclusions

Baroreflex sensitivity is a useful tool for the study of vagal reflexes, and it can be safely determined even in patients with a recent myocardial infarction. It provides a reliable quantitative assessment of autonomic balance, even though it explores the vagal more than the sympathetic component.

References

1. Schwartz PJ, La Rovere MT, Vanoli E: Autonomic nervous system and sudden cardiac death. Experimental basis and clinical observations for post-myocardial infarction risk stratification. Circulation 85(suppl I):I-77, 1992.

2. Corr PB, Yamada KA, Witkowski FX: Mechanisms controlling cardiac autonomic function and their relation to arrhythmogenesis. In HA Fozzard, E Haber, RB Jennings, et al (eds): The Heart and Cardiovascular System. New York, NY, Raven Press, 1986, p. 1343.
3. Schwartz PJ, Priori SG: Sympathetic nervous system and cardiac arrhythmias. In DP Zipes, J Jalife (eds): Cardiac Electrophysiology. From Cell to Bedside. Philadelphia, PA, WB Saunders Co, 1990, p. 330.
4. Mancia G, Mark AL: Arterial baroreflexes in humans. In Handbook of Physiology. Section 3: The Cardiovascular System. Bethesda, MD, American Physiological Society, 1983, p. 755.
5. Eckberg DL: Parasympathetic cardiovascular control in human disease: A critical review of methods and results. Am J Physiol 239:H581, 1980.
6. Goldstein DS, Horwitz D, Keiser HR: Comparison of techniques for measuring baroreflex sensitivity in man. Circulation 66:432, 1982.
7. Hagbarth KE, Vallbo AB: Pulse and respiratory grouping of sympathetic impulses in human muscle nerves. Acta Physiol Scand 74:96, 1968.
8. Vallbo AB, Hagbarth KE, Torebjork HE, et al: Somatosensory, proprioceptive, and sympathetic activity in human peripheral nerves. Physiol Rev 59:919, 1979.
9. Anderson EA, Balon TW, Hoffman RP, et al: Insulin increases sympathetic activity but not blood pressure in borderline hypertensive humans. Hypertension 19:621, 1992.
10. Morlin C, Wallin BG, Erikson BM: Muscle sympathetic activity and plasma noradrenaline in normotensive and hypertensive man. Acta Physiol Scand 119:117, 1983.
11. Yamada Y, Miyajima E, Tochikubo O, et al: Age-related changes in muscle sympathetic nerve activity in essential hypertension. Hypertension 13:870, 1989.
12. Leimbach WN, Wallin GB, Victor RG, et al: Direct evidence from intraneural recordings for increased central sympathetic outflow in patients with heart failure. Circulation 73:913, 1986.
13. Mancia G, Grassi G: Assessment of sympathetic cardiovascular influences in man: Haemodynamic and humoral markers versus microneurography. Clin Autom Res 1:245, 1991.
14. Malliani A, Schwartz PJ, Zanchetti A: A sympathetic reflex elicited by experimental coronary artery occlusion. Am J Physiol 217:703, 1969.
15. Malliani A, Recordati G, Schwartz PJ: Nervous activity of afferent cardiac sympathetic fibers with atrial and ventricular endings. J Physiol (Lond) 229:457, 1973.
16. Pagani M, Schwartz PJ, Banks R, et al: Reflex responses of sympathetic preganglionic neurones initiated by different cardiovascular receptors in spinal animals. Brain Res 68:215, 1974.
17. Hopp FA, Seagard JL, Kampine JP: Comparison of four methods of averaging nerve activity. Am J Physiol 251:R700, 1986.
18. Andresen MD, Yang M: Interaction among unitary spikes trains: Implications for whole nerve measurements. Am J Physiol 256:R997, 1989.
19. Kunze DL: Reflex discharge patterns of cardiac vagal efferent fibers. J Physiol (Lond) 222:1, 1972.
20. Vatner SF, Franklin D, Van Citters RL, et al: Effects of carotid sinus nerve stimulation on blood flow distribution in conscious dogs at rest and during exercise. Circ Res 27:495, 1970.
21. Brest AN, Wiener L, Bachrach B: Bilateral carotid sinus nerve stimulation in the treatment of hypertension. Am J Cardiol 29:821, 1972.
22. Braunwald E, Epstein SE, Glick G, et al: Relief of angina pectoris by electrical stimulation of the carotid sinus nerves. N Engl J Med 277:1278, 1967.
23. Eckberg DL, Fletcher GF, Braunwald E: Mechanism of prolongation of the RR interval with electrical stimulation of the carotid sinus nerves in man. Circ Res 30:131, 1972.
24. Levy MN, Zieske H: Autonomic control of cardiac pace-maker activity and atrioventricular transmission. J Appl Physiol 27:465, 1969.

25. Stramba-Badiale M, Vanoli E, De Ferrari GM, et al: Sympathetic-parasympathetic interaction and accentuated antagonism in conscious dogs. Am J Physiol 260:H335, 1991.
26. Levy MN, Iano T, Zieske H: Effects of repetitive bursts of vagal activity on heart rate. Circ Res 30:286, 1972.
27. Schwartz PJ, Pagani M, Lombardi F, et al: A cardio-cardiac sympatho-vagal reflex in the cat. Circ Res 32:215, 1973.
28. Gnecchi-Rusconi T, Lombardi F, Malfatto G, et al: Attenuation of baroceptive mechanisms by cardiovascular sympathetic afferent fibers. Am J Physiol 253:H787, 1987.
29. Cerati D, Schwartz PJ: Single cardiac vagal fiber activity, acute myocardial ischemia, and risk for sudden death. Circ Res 69:1389, 1991.
30. Bristow JD, Brown EB Jr, Cunningham DJC, et al: The effect of bicycling on the baroreflex regulation of pulse interval. Circ Res 28:582, 1971.
31. Goldstein DS: Arterial baroreflex sensitivity, plasma catecholamines, and pressor responsiveness in essential hypertension. Circulation 68:234, 1983.
32. Hamilton WF, Woodbury RA, Harper HT Jr: Physiologic relationships between intrathoracic, intraspinal and arterial pressures. JAMA 107:853, 1936.
33. Bennett T, Wilcox RG, Hampton JR: Cardiovascular reflexes in patients after myocardial infarction. Effect of long-term treatment with beta-adrenoceptor antagonists. Br Heart J 44:265, 1980.
34. Korner PI, Tonkin AM, Uther JB: Valsalva constrictor and heart rate reflexes in subjects with essential hypertension and with normal blood pressure. Clin Exp Pharmacol Physiol 6:97, 1979.
35. Parisi AF, Harrington JJ, Askenazi J, et al: Echocardiographic evaluation of the Valsalva maneuver in healthy subjects and patients with and without heart failure. Circulation 54:921, 1976.
36. Robertson D, Stevens RM, Friesinger GC, et al: The effect of the Valsalva maneuver on echocardiographic dimension in man. Circulation 55:596, 1977.
37. Kirby BJ: Circulatory reflexes in myocardial infarction. Br Heart J 39:168, 1977.
38. Eckberg DL, Cavanaugh MS, Mark AL, et al: A simplified neck suction device for activation of carotid baroreceptors. J Lab Clin Med 85:167, 1975.
39. Eckberg DL: Adaptation of the human carotid baroreceptor cardiac reflex. J Physiol (Lond) 269:579, 1977.
40. Mancia A, Ferrari A, Gregorini L, et al: Circulatory reflexes from carotid and extracarotid baroreceptor areas in man. Circ Res 41:309, 1977.
41. Korner PI, West MJ, Shaw J, et al: Steady-state properties of the baroreceptors-heart rate reflex in essential hypertension in man. Clin Exp Pharmacol Physiol 1:65, 1974.
42. Smyth HS, Sleight P, Pickering GW: Reflex regulation of arterial pressure during sleep in man: A quantitative method of assessing baroreflex sensitivity. Circ Res 24:109, 1969.
43. Downing SE: Baroreceptor regulation of the heart. In Handbook of Physiology. Section 3: The Cardiovascular System. Bethesda, MD, American Physiological Society, 1983, p. 621.
44. Brown AM: Receptors under pressure. An update on baroreceptors. Circ Res 46:1, 1980.
45. Sleight P, Fox P, Lopez R, et al: The effect of mental arithmetic on blood pressure variability and baroreflex sensitivity in man. Coeur et Medecine Interne 17:23, 1978.
46. La Rovere MT, Specchia G, Mortara A, et al: Baroreflex sensitivity, clinical correlates and cardiovascular mortality among patients with a first myocardial infarction. A prospective study. Circulation 78:816, 1988.
47. Farrell TG, Odemuyiwa O, Bashir Y, et al: Prognostic value of baroreflex sensitivity testing after acute myocardial infarction. Br Heart J 67:129, 1992.
48. Schwartz PJ, Zaza A, Pala M, et al: Baroreflex sensitivity and its evolution during the first year after a myocardial infarction. J Am Coll Cardiol 12:629, 1988.
49. Schwartz PJ, Vanoli E, Stramba-Badiale M, et al: Autonomic mechanisms and

sudden death. New insights from the analysis of baroreceptor reflexes in conscious dogs with and without a myocardial infarction. Circulation 78:969, 1988.
50. Osculati G, Grassi G, Giannattasio C, et al: Early alterations of the baroreceptor control of heart rate in patients with acute myocardial infarction. Circulation 81:939, 1990.
51. Parati G, Di Rienzo M, Bertinieri G, et al: Evaluation of the baroreceptor-heart rate reflex by 24-hour intra-arterial blood pressure monitoring in humans. Hypertension 12:214, 1988.
52. Furlan R, Guzzetti S, Crivellaro W, et al: Continuous 24-hour assessment of the neural regulation of systemic arterial pressure and RR variabilities in ambulant subjects. Circulation 81:537, 1990.
53. Penaz I: Photoelectric measurement of blood pressure, volume and flow in the finger. Digest of the International Conference on Medicine and Biological Engineering. Dresden, Conference Committee of the 10th International Conference on Medicine and Biological Engineering, 1973, p. 104.
54. Wesseling KH, De Wit B, Settels JJ, et al: On the indirect registration of finger blood pressure after Penaz. Funkt Biol Med 1:245, 1982.
55. Parati G, Casadei R, Groppelli A, et al: Comparison of finger and intra-arterial blood pressure monitoring at rest and during laboratory testing. Hypertension 13:647, 1989.
56. Gribbin B, Pickering TG, Sleight P, et al: Effect of age and high blood pressure on baroreflex sensitivity in man. Circ Res 29:424, 1971.
57. Eckberg DL: Baroreflex inhibition of the human sinus node: Importance of stimulus intensity, duration and rate of pressure change. J Physiol (Lond) 269:561, 1977.
58. Karemaker JM, Wieling W, Dunning AJ: Aging and the baroreflex. In A Amery, J Staessen (eds): Handbook of Hypertension. North Holland, Elsevier Science Publishers BV, 1989, Vol. 12, p. 24.
59. Thames MD, Klopfenstein HS, Abboud FM, et al: Preferential distribution of inhibitory cardiac receptors with vagal afferents to the inferoposterior wall of the left ventricle activated during coronary occlusion in the dog. Circ Res 43:512, 1978.
60. Eckberg DL, Drabinsky M, Braunwald E: Defective cardiac parasympathetic control in patients with heart disease. N Engl J Med 285:877, 1971.
61. La Rovere MT, Mortara A, Ghio S, et al: Baroreflex sensitivity and left ventricular function in post-myocardial infarction patients. Circulation 76(suppl 4):59, 1987.
62. Pickering TG, Gribbin B, Strange-Petersen E, et al: Effects of autonomic blockade on the baroreflex in man at rest and during exercise. Circ Res 30:177, 1972.
63. Eckberg DL, Abboud FM, Mark AL: Modulation of carotid baroreflex responsiveness in man: Effects of posture and propranolol. J Appl Physiol 413:383, 1976.
64. Takeshita A, Mark AL, Eckberg DL, et al: Effect of central venous pressure on arterial baroreflex control of heart rate. Am J Physiol 236:H42, 1979.
65. Takeshita A, Tanaka S, Nakamura M: Effects of propranolol on baroreflex sensitivity in borderline hypertension. Cardiovasc Res 12:148, 1978.
66. Billman GE, Schwartz PJ, Stone HL: Baroreceptor reflexes and cardiac beta receptor blockade: Prediction and protection from sudden death. Circulation 66(suppl II):II-35, 1982.
67. Simon G, Kiowski W, Julius S: Effect of beta-adrenoceptor antagonists on baroreceptor reflex sensitivity in hypertension. Clin Pharmacol Ther 22:296, 1977.
68. Parati G, Pomidossi G, Grassi C: Mechanisms of antihypertensive action of beta-adrenergic blocking drugs: Evidence against potentiation of baroreflexes. Eur Heart J 4(suppl D):19, 1983.
69. Yusuf S, Wittes J, Friedman L: Overview of results of randomized clinical trials in heart disease. JAMA 260:2088, 1988.
70. La Rovere MT, Mortara A, Capomolla S, et al: Autonomic reflexes and beta-blockade in post-MI patients. Eur Heart 11(abs suppl):267, 1990.

CHAPTER 29

Markers of Vagal Activity and the Prediction of Cardiac Death After Myocardial Infarction

J.T. Bigger, Jr., P.J. Schwartz

For several years, the interest in the relationship between the autonomic nervous system and cardiac arrhythmias has focused primarily on the electrophysiological mechanisms involved,[1–4] and on the evidence that ventricular fibrillation could be enhanced by sympathetic[5–7] and antagonized by vagal activity.[8–10] The clinical implications of these concepts were applied only to therapy. Examples are the widespread use of β-blockers after myocardial infarction[11] and the use of left cardiac sympathetic denervation for selected populations at high risk for sudden death.[12,13]

A major change occurred as a consequence of the first experimental[14] observations that suggested that analysis of autonomic tone and reflexes might have prognostic value in identifying individuals who were postmyocardial infarction and who were at higher risk for subsequent cardiac death. These initial observations have been followed by several larger studies that have confirmed and reinforced this concept.

In this chapter, those studies that were critical in the development of the concept that the analysis of vagal tone and reflexes carries important prognostic information that contributes, together with the traditional risk factors, to a more accurate identification of the patients at high risk for cardiac death are reviewed. We then examine the data available on normal individuals who have not yet suffered a myocardial infarction. The chapter then concludes by discussing a large prospective study specifically designed to provide the definitive information about the prognostic value of measures of vagal tone (such as the various indices of heart rate variability) and of vagal reflexes (such as baroreflex sensitivity [BRS]).

From *Vagal Control of the Heart: Experimental Basis and Clinical Implications* edited by MN Levy, PJ Schwartz

Heart Rate Variability

Clinical Studies

In 1978, Wolf et al[15] first reported an association between heart period (RR) variability and mortality in patients with acute myocardial infarction. They recorded the ECG for 60 seconds in 176 patients when they were admitted to the Royal Melbourne Hospital coronary care unit. Heart period variability was estimated as the variance of 30 consecutive RR intervals from the 60-second strip. A variance for such a short time measures primarily respiratory sinus arrhythmia (RSA); i.e., the vagal modulation of RR intervals. The investigators arbitrarily chose a variance value of 1,000 milliseconds (SD 31.6 milliseconds), which separated their group into 103 patients (59%) with sinus arrhythmia and 73 patients (42%) without sinus arrhythmia. They found that patients in the lower category (RR variance $<$1,000 milliseconds^2) were more likely to have anterior myocardial infarction, a Norris index $\geq$10, low values for average RR interval, and later admission to a hospital.

Patients were discharged 9 to 14 days after admission. The hospital mortality of patients with an RR variance $<$1,000 milliseconds^2 was 15.5%, compared to 4.1% for patients with an RR variance $\geq$1,000 milliseconds^2. The relative risk was 3.8. After adjusting for heart rate or location of the infarct, a low RR variance was still significantly associated with higher mortality rates.

The study by Wolf et al[15] showed that heart period variance, measured over a period less than 30 seconds, predicted mortality over the next 9 to 14 days. The study included only a small number of deaths so that the strength of the association was not estimated precisely. Also, no account was taken of left ventricular function, ventricular arrhythmias, or myocardial ischemia as covariates. Hence, the independent predictive value of heart period variability was not established. Nevertheless, this study was an important milestone in calling attention to the possible prognostic significance of measures of heart period variability in coronary heart disease. Of special relevance here, Wolf et al[15] mentioned vagal activity only in association with the faster heart rate of the patients with reduced sinus arrhythmia. They did not relate this finding to a potential causal relationship between reduced vagal activity and increased mortality.

Myers et al[16] compared power spectra of heart period variability measured in 24-hour ECG recordings in three groups of six patients each, as follows: normal subjects; patients with cardiac disease and unsustained ventricular arrhythmias, but who did not have ventricular tachycardia induced by programmed ventricular stimulation; and patients who had been resuscitated from ventricular fibrillation. Digitized 24-hour ECG recordings were divided into two-minute, nonoverlapping segments, sampled, and submitted to a Fast Fourier Transform (FFT) algorithm. The following frequency bands from the heart period spectra were evaluated for their prognostic significance: 0.0167 to 0.05 Hz, 0.05 to 0.15 Hz, 0.15 to 0.35 Hz, and 0.35 to 0.50 Hz. Also, a number of time domain measures of heart period variability were calculated. Myers et al[16] found that the 0.35 to 0.50 Hz band provided the best separation among the three groups. Inspection of the data yielded a cutoff point that gave 100% sensitivity and 100% specificity for separating the malignant arrhythmia group from the normal subjects and the patients with potentially malignant ventricular arrhythmias. The 0.15 to 0.35 Hz band also provided good separation among the groups. Both of these bands reflect RSA. The only time domain variable that separated the three groups well was the average number per hour of consecutive RR intervals that differed by 50 seconds or more (NN50).

These findings indicated which measures of vagal activity best separated the three groups under investigation. The study of Myers et al[16] stimulated interest in the use of 24-hour recording of ECG data to compute the average power spectral values over the course of a day. The relationship between heart period variability and mortality was not explored. Instead, patients resuscitated from ventricular fibrillation were used as a surrogate for sudden cardiac death. The association between high-frequency (HF) power spectral components and the surrogate endpoint (ventricular fibrillation) has not been confirmed in studies where death was the endpoint, possibly because the mechanisms for ventricular fibrillation are so heterogeneous. Also, patients with nonfatal ventricular fibrillation may not be representative of all patients who develop ventricular fibrillation, i.e., those who live are different from those who die.

Martin et al[17] compared two measures of heart period variability in three patients who died suddenly during a 24-hour ECG recording with those measured in 20 normal volunteers. The three patients all had coronary heart disease and prior myocardial infarction; two patients had congestive heart failure (CHF); and both had intraventricular conduction defects and prolonged QT_c in their 12-lead ECG. The 20 normal volunteers were not characterized for age and gender. All three patients died as a result of ventricular tachycardia that degenerated into ventricular fibrillation.

Two time domain measures of heart period variability were calculated from the beginning of the Holter recording to the time of ventricular fibrillation: SDNN index (the average of the five-minute standard deviations of NN intervals) and SDANN (the standard deviation of the five-minute average NN intervals). In the three patients who died during the Holter recording, the SDNN index (a measure of very low-frequency [VLF] and low-frequency [LF] variation) and the SDANN index (a measure of ultra low-frequency [ULF] variation) differed markedly from the respective indices in the 20 normal subjects. The changes in heart period variability as the time of death approached were not reported. Ventricular arrhythmias increased in frequency and complexity in the hour before death.

The contrast between the patients who died suddenly with ventricular fibrillation and the normal subjects (who probably were younger) is not very interesting, because the heart period variability is expected to be much less in a group of older patients who had previous myocardial infarction and CHF than in young normal volunteers. The study does not address the following important questions. Can heart period variability measurements identify heart failure patients who are at highest risk of all-cause mortality or sudden cardiac death? Do heart period variability measurements predict sudden cardiac death better than other modes of death, e.g., heart failure deaths? Can heart period variability measured long before death predict death?

Kleiger et al[18,19] reported a strong association between the standard deviation of the normal RR intervals (SDNN) and all-cause mortality after myocardial infarction. Of the 867 patients enrolled in a natural history study of myocardial infarction (The Multicenter Post Myocardial Infarction Program [MPIP]), 820 had Holter recordings performed 11 ± 3 days after infarction. Twelve patients had atrial fibrillation, implanted pacemakers, or technical problems; thus, 808 patients were suitable for calculation of heart period variability. SDNN <50 milliseconds was found in 15.5% of the patients, and this subgroup had a mortality rate of 34.4%, compared to a 12.3% mortality rate for patients with SDNN ≥50 milliseconds; the relative risk was 2.8 (see Fig. 1). SDNN correlated weakly but significantly with age, heart rate, and measures of left ventricular function, but it did not correlate with ventricular arrhythmias. Of all the Holter variables, SDNN had the strongest association with all-cause mortality. After other risk predictors (age, New York Heart Association [NYHA] functional class, rales in coronary care unit, left ventricular ejection fraction, and ventricular arrhythmias) were adjusted statistically, SDNN was still significantly associated with all-cause mortality over the next

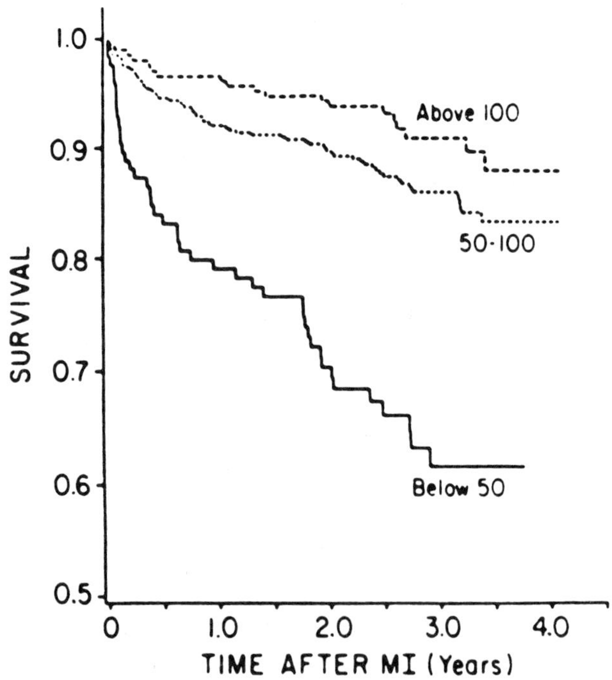

Figure 1. *Survival after myocardial infarction for patients grouped according to the SDNN computed over a 24-hour period <50, 50 to 100, and >100. Reproduced with permission from Kleiger RE, Miller JP, Bigger JT Jr, et al: Decreased heart rate variability and its association with increased mortality after acute myocardial infarction. Am J Cardiol 59:256, 1987.*

four years. This result is definitive, because of the large group (808) of representative patients and the 127 deaths that occurred during the follow-up. SDNN measures both the slow and the fast oscillations in the RR interval, and it does not, therefore, provide specific information on the vagal or sympathetic modulation of the RR intervals. Its independence from left ventricular function and ventricular arrhythmias, however, does suggest that it provides information about a different lethal force, probably involving the autonomic nervous system.

To understand the contribution of autonomic nervous activity to the prediction of all-cause and cause-specific (cardiac and arrhythmic) death, Bigger et al[20] reanalyzed 24-hour ECG recordings from 715 patients who participated in the MPIP. Digitized 24-hour ECGs were analyzed to compute the power spectra for the entire 24-hour period, and power in four frequency bands was calculated:

1. <0.0033 Hz, ULF power;
2. 0.0033 to <0.04 Hz, VLF power;
3. 0.04 to 0.15 Hz, LF power; and
4. 0.15 to 0.40 Hz, HF power.

In addition, total power (≤0.40 Hz) and the ratio of low to high frequency power (LF/HF ratio) power were calculated.

Each measure of heart period variability had a significant and at least moderately strong univariate association with the following mortality endpoints: all-cause mortality, cardiac failure death, and arrhythmic death (see Fig. 2). The estimates of mortality rates were precise because there were 119 deaths in the 715 patient study group; 88 of these were classified as cardiac failure and 68 were classified as arrhythmic. After adjustment for important covariates (age, NYHA functional class, rales in the CCU phase of acute myocardial infarction, left ventricular ejection fraction, and ventricular arrhythmias) in a Cox regression model, ultra low and LF power were still strongly and significantly associated with death. LF and HF power were not strongly associated with death after adjusting for these covariates. Very LF power was more strongly associated with arrhythmic death than with all-cause mortality or cardiac failure death, before and after adjustment with covariates. Combining measures of heart period variability with left ventricular ejection fraction or ventricular arrhythmias identified small subgroups of postinfarction patients with a 2.5-year mortality rate greater than 50% (Fig. 3). This study suggested that slow cyclic variability was a stronger predictor than was the HF variability that reflects vagal tone. The physiological mechanism for ULF modulation of RR intervals is not known.

Bigger et al[21] explored the correlations between the most commonly used time domain and frequency domain measures of heart period variability. The definitions of these variables are given in Table 1. They used an MPIP data set of 715 patients for this analysis. Two bands in the heart period power spectrum have well-known physiological significance: the LF power and the HF power bands together comprise <10% of the 24-hour heart period variance (Fig. 4). Therefore, selective changes in these two bands could be missed by global

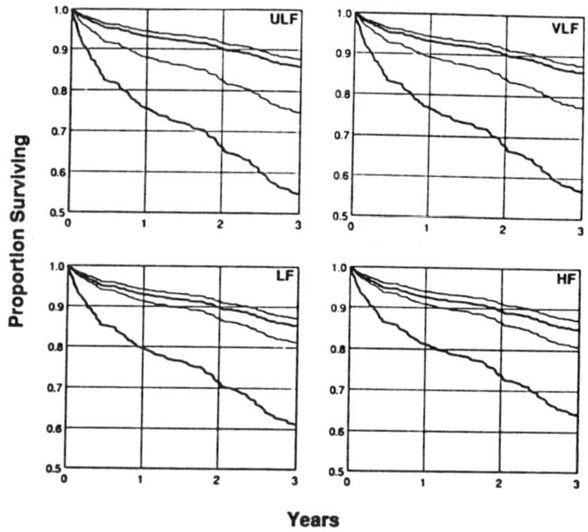

Figure 2. *Survival curves for 673 postinfarction patients in the high or low category for the four mutually exclusive frequency domain measures of heart period variability: ultra low frequency (ULF), very low frequency (VLF), low frequency (LF), and high frequency (HF) power, using all-cause mortality as the endpoint. Thick lines represent unadjusted heart period variability data and thin lines represent data adjusted for the five covariates: age, New York Heart Association (NYHA) functional class, rales in the coronary care unit, radionuclide ejection fraction, and the frequency of ventricular premature complexes. In each panel, the upper two curves represent patients in the high category and the lower two curves represent patients in the low category. Reproduced by permission of the American Heart Association, Inc. from Bigger JT Jr, Fleiss JL, Steinman RC, et al: Frequency domain measures of heart period variability and mortality after myocardial infarction. Circulation 85:164, 1992.*

measures, such as total power or SDNN. Each of the four bands in the heart period power spectrum had one or two corresponding variables in the time domain that correlated with it so strongly ($r \geq 0.90$) that the variables were essentially equivalent (Table 2).

There were three natural clusters among the time and frequency domain variables:

1. SDNN, SDANN index, total power, and ULF power;
2. VLF power, LF power, and SDNN index; and
3. HF power, root of mean square successive difference (r-MSSD), and proportion of differences in normal RR intervals >50 milliseconds (pNN50).

The correlations between measures of heart period variability and other risk predictors previously identified in this data set were weak, from −0.40 to 0.34.[22,23] All of the time domain measures of heart period variability were significantly associated with all-cause mortality, but the SDANN index and the SDNN index had the strongest univariate associations with death. After other risk predictors were adjusted, only SDNN, SDANN index, and SDNN index were significantly associated with all-cause mortality. These findings

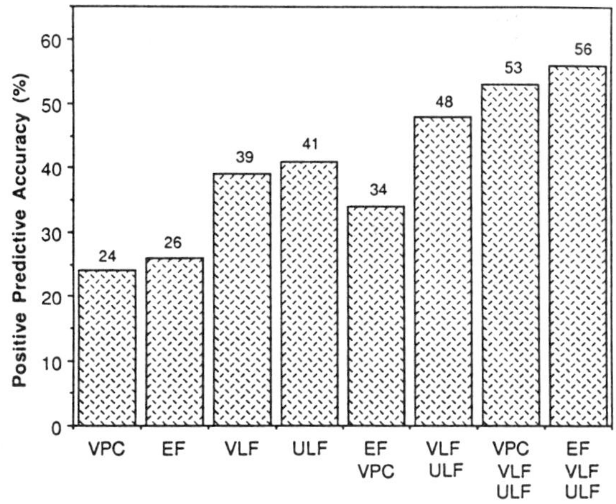

Figure 3. *Sensitivity, specificity, and positive predictive accuracy using measures of heart period variability alone or combined with other risk predictors. Note that measures of RR variability have a higher positive predictive accuracy than left ventricular ejection fraction (EF) and frequent ventricular premature complexes (VPC) in a 24-hour ECG recording. Also, combination of RR variability measures with either left ventricular ejection fraction or ventricular premature complexes yielded positive predictive accuracies greater than 50%. Reproduced by permission of the American Heart Association, Inc. from Bigger JT Jr, Fleiss JL, Steinman RC, et al: Frequency domain measures of heart period variability and mortality after myocardial infarction. Circulation 85:164, 1992.*

are similar to those for the corresponding frequency domain variables in this same data set.[20]

Odemuyiwa et al[24] studied 385 survivors of myocardial infarction to compare the sensitivity and specificity of left ventricular ejection fraction and a heart rate variability index. This index was a time domain measure derived from the frequency distribution of normal RR intervals in a 24-hour ECG recording (the baseline width of triangular interpolation). This measure is dominated by ULF information. The ambulatory ECG was recorded about seven days after myocardial infarction. The endpoints evaluated were all-cause mortality (n = 44), arrhythmic events (sudden death or symptomatic, sustained ventricular tachycardia) (n = 26), and sudden death (n = 14). For all-cause mortality, heart rate variability index and left ventricular ejection fraction had similar sensitivity and specificity (75% and 50%, respectively). For arrhythmic events, a heart rate variability index of ≤30 units had a sensitivity of 75% and a specificity of 76%, whereas a left ventricular ejection fraction ≤0.40 had a sensitivity of 42% and a specificity of 75%. For sudden death, when sensitivity was set at 75%, heart rate variability index had a specificity of 75% compared to a specificity of 47% for left ventricular ejection fraction. The authors concluded that, although the left ventricular ejection fraction and the heart rate variability index had similar sensitivity and specificity for all-cause mortality, the heart rate variability index was a better predictor of sudden death or arrhythmic events. These findings suggest that heart period variability predicts arrhythmic events better than it does nonarrhythmic events.

Farrell et al[25] studied 416 survivors of myocardial infarction to investigate

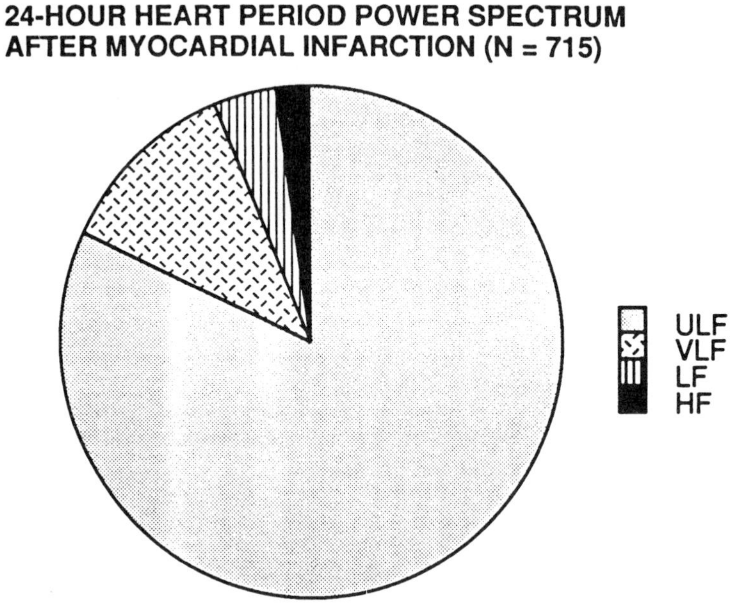

Figure 4. *The fraction of the total power in the 24-hour heart period power spectrum that is in the four mutually exclusive frequency domain measures of heart period variability: ultra low frequency (ULF), very low frequency (VLF), low frequency (LF), and high frequency (HF) power. Reproduced with permission from Bigger JT Jr, Fleiss JL, Steinman RC, et al: Correlations among time and frequency domain measures of heart period variability two weeks after acute myocardial infarction. Am J Cardiol 69:891–898, 1992.*

the prognostic value of heart period variability in combination with ventricular arrhythmias found in a Holter recording of a positive signal-averaged ECG. They hypothesized that the combination of abnormal autonomic tone and an arrhythmogenic substrate would be an excellent predictor of arrhythmic events.[25] Their results apply to current practice, because their sample was collected after thrombolysis was in routine use. Forty-eight percent of these patients received thrombolytic therapy and 24% had coronary artery bypass graft surgery or percutaneous transluminal coronary angioplasty. The Holter and signal-averaged ECG were done five to seven days after infarction. The heart rate variability index (measure of ULF RR variability) was <20 milliseconds in 113 (27%) of the 416 patients. The ventricular premature complex frequency >10/hour was found in 84 (20%) patients and repetitive ventricular premature complexes were found in 86 (21%). Also, 110 (26%) of the patients had a left ventricular ejection fraction less than 0.40 and 210 (50%) had a positive exercise test. A low value of heart rate variability index was significantly associated with average normal RR (NN) interval, age, left ventricular ejection fraction, and a positive signal-averaged ECG. The strongest association was with average NN interval ($r = 0.56$). The signal-averaged ECG was abnormal in 89 (21%) of the 416 patients. A positive signal-averaged ECG was associated significantly with age >65 years, ventricular ectopy, and low values of heart period variability (odds ratio = 3.0, $p<0.001$), but not with left

Table 1.
Definitions for Time and Frequency Domain Measures of Heart Period Variability

Variable	*Domain*	*Units*	*Definition*
Night-day Difference	Time	msec	Difference between the avarage of all the normal RR intervals at night (24:00 to 5:00) and the average of all the normal RR intervals during the day (07:30 to 21:30).
SDNN	Time	msec	Standard deviation of all normal RR intervals in the entire 24-hour ECG recording.
SDANN Index	Time	msec	Standard deviation of the average normal RR intervals for all five-minute segments of a 24-hour ECG recording (each average is weighted by the fraction of the five minutes that has normal RR intervals).
SDNN Index	Time	msec	Mean of the standard deviations of all normal RR intervals for all five-minute segments of a 24-hour ECG recording.
r-MSSD	Time	msec	Root mean square successive difference, the square root of the mean of the squared differences between adjacent normal RR intervals over the entire 24-hour ECG recording.
pNN50	Time	percent	Percent of differences between adjacent normal RR intervals that are greater than 50 msec computed over the entire 24-hour ECG recording.
Total Power	Frequency	ms^2	The energy in the heart period power spectrum up to 0.40 Hz.
Ultra Low-frequency (ULF) Power	Frequency	$msec^2$	The energy in the heart period power spectrum up to 0.0033 Hz.
Very Low-frequency (VLF) Power	Frequency	$msec^2$	The energy in the heart period power spectrum between 0.0033 and 0.04 Hz.
Low-frequency (LF) Power	Frequency	$msec^2$	The energy in the heart period power spectrum between 0.04 and 0.15 Hz.
High-frequency (HF) Power	Frequency	$msec^2$	The energy in the heart period power spectrum between 0.15 and 0.40 Hz.
LF/HF Ratio	Frequency	none	The ratio of low to high frequency power.

Reproduced with permission from Bigger JT Jr, Fleiss JL, Steinman RC, et al: Correlations among time and frequency domain measures of heart period variability two weeks after acute myocardial infarction. Am J Cardiol 69:891–898, 1992.

ventricular ejection fraction, positive exercise test, or site of myocardial infarction.

During a mean follow-up of 612 days, there were 24 arrhythmic events, 47 cardiac deaths, and 40 nonfatal myocardial infarctions. The best univariate predictors of cardiac death were heart rate variability index (relative risk = 7 [95% confidence interval (CI) 4-12]) and Killip class ≥2 (relative risk = 6 [95% CI 3-10]). Left ventricular ejection fraction, positive exercise test, and ventricular arrhythmias in the Holter recording all were substantially weaker predictors of cardiac death. A step-up Cox regression analysis identified the best multivariate (independent) predictors of cardiac mortality: heart rate variability index <20 units, Killip class ≥2, and repetitive ventricular premature complexes.

The best univariate predictor of arrhythmic events (arrhythmic deaths [Cardiac Arrhythmia Pilot Study definition]) was heart rate variability index (relative risk = 32 [95% CI 8-138]), followed by signal-averaged ECG (relative risk = 7 [95% CI 3-15]), and frequent or repetitive ventricular premature complexes in the Holter recording (relative risk = 5 [95% CI 2-11]). Left ventricular ejection fraction and Killip class were weaker predictors of arrhythmic events. In a Cox regression analysis, the best combination of predictors for arrhythmic events was: heart rate variability index <20 units, a positive signal-averaged ECG, and repetitive ventricular premature complexes. After these three variables were entered in the model, heart rate, left ventricular ejection fraction, and positive exercise test did not significantly improve the prediction of arrhythmic events. Heart rate variability index did not predict nonfatal myocardial infarction. Combining heart rate variability index, a positive signal-averaged ECG, and repetitive ventricular premature complexes yielded a positive predictive accuracy of 58% and a negative predictive accuracy of 95%.

These results again suggest that the heart rate variability index has some specificity for predicting arrhythmic events; i.e., it predicts arrhythmic events better than cardiac death or nonfatal reinfarction. Even though the heart rate variability index is significantly associated with a positive signal-averaged ECG, these two risk predictors each have a substantial predictive power that is independent of the other. The prediction of arrhythmic events by a heart rate variability index also seems independent of left ventricular ejection fraction values and positive exercise tests.

Recently, Counihan et al studied the predictive accuracy of heart period variability measurements in a sample of patients with hypertrophic cardiomyopathy (personal communication). They recorded the 24-hour ECG in a group of 104 patients. Ten had cardiac arrest due to ventricular fibrillation or sudden death during the follow-up. Five time domain measures (SDNN, SDANN, SDNN index, mean square successive difference [MSSD], and pNN50) and two frequency domain measures (LF and HF power in the heart period power spectrum) were calculated. The patients with low values for heart period variability revealed no tendency toward higher mortality. This study raises the question about whether measures of heart period variability predict all-cause mortality or arrhythmic death in all patient groups or only in some (e.g., the postmyocardial infarction group). The design of this study, especially the time of follow-up, however, is not clear and, hence, the relationship could be obscure.

Studies in additional patient groups are needed to determine how general is the predictive capability of heart period variability.

Experimental Studies

The experimental studies on heart rate variability and risk for sudden death followed, and did not precede, the clinical investigations. The opposite chronology applies to BRS, as described in the following section.

Hull et al[26] examined the prognostic value of heart rate variability, measured in a 30-minute period in a canine animal model, that is extensively described in Ch. 34. These investigators needed this model to predict the outcome (ventricular fibrillation or survival) during a brief ischemic episode in conscious dogs with a one-month-old myocardial infarction. Their study was performed in 50 dogs, of which 25 had developed ventricular fibrillation (susceptible) and 25 had survived (resistant). Heart period variability, just a few days prior to exposing the animals to the exercise and ischemia test, was significantly lower among the susceptible dogs than among the resistant ones (106 ± 9 versus 209 ± 13 milliseconds, $p<0.001$). As shown in Figure 5, this difference was independent of the difference in heart rate. The results remained unchanged when they used the coefficient of variance, which corrects for heart rate.

These experimental data confirm in dogs what Kleiger et al[19] had already demonstrated in man. The agreement between the two studies underlines the clinical applicability (or vice versa) of this canine model for sudden death. This notion is particularly important for those studies that do not yet have a clinical counterpart. The study by Hull et al[26] also provides a new and important piece of information that, however, is discussed later in the chapter because it concerns the problem of the predictive value in absence of a myocardial infarction.

Baroreflex Sensitivity

In 1982, we[14] published the first study suggesting that depressed BRS was closely associated with an increased risk for ventricular fibrillation in conscious dogs with a healed myocardial infarction. The definitive demonstration of this relationship was provided in 1988 by Schwartz et al[27] in an unusually large ($n = 192$) experimental study of a canine model for sudden death, generally regarded as highly relevant to clinical reality.[28] These results paved the way for the clinical studies that followed shortly afterwards, and contributed significantly to the development of the concept that depressed vagal activity may often be the harbinger of cardiac mortality. The experimental basis is reviewed first, followed by a discussion of the clinical studies.

Experimental Studies

The potential clinical extrapolation of an experimental study depends largely on the characteristics of the animal preparation in which the study is

Table 2.
Correlations Among Measures of Heart Period Variability (n = 715)

	Night-Day Difference	*SDNN*	*Ln Total Power*	*Ln ULF Power*	*SDANN Index*	*Ln VLF Power*	*SDNN Index*	*Ln LF Power*	*Ln r-MSSD*	*Ln pNN50*	*Ln HF Power*	*Ln LF/HF Power*
Night-day Difference	1.00											
SDNN	0.71	1.00										
Ln Total Power	0.68	0.96	1.00									
Ln ULF Power	0.71	0.95	0.99	1.00								
SDANN Index	0.75	0.98	0.94	0.96	1.00							
Ln VLF Power	0.43	0.78	0.82	0.75	0.68	1.00						
SDNN Index	0.44	0.82	0.79	0.71	0.70	0.90	1.00					
Ln LF Power	0.42	0.72	0.75	0.67	0.61	0.91	0.89	1.00				
Ln r-MSSD	0.28	0.62	0.58	0.52	0.51	0.60	0.78	0.65	1.00			
Ln pNN50	0.27	0.57	0.56	0.50	0.49	0.59	0.71	0.64	0.93	1.00		
Ln HF Power	0.35	0.67	0.66	0.59	0.57	0.70	0.82	0.77	0.92	0.89	1.00	
Ln LF/HF Power	0.17	0.20	0.26	0.23	0.17	0.45	0.25	0.49	−0.25	−0.22	−0.18	1.00

Ln = natural logarithm. Abbreviations defined in Table 1. Reproduced with permission from Bigger JT Jr, Fleiss JL, Steinman RC, et al: Correlations among time and frequency domain measures of heart period variability two weeks after acute myocardial infarction. Am J Cardiol 69:891–898, 1992.

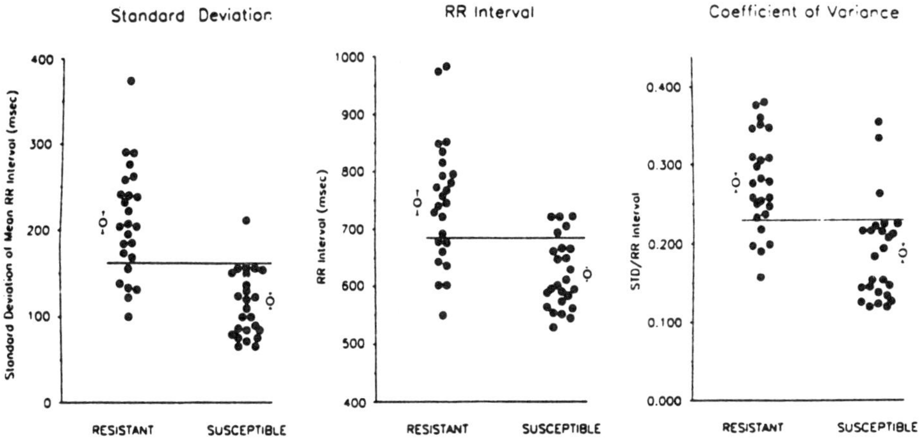

Figure 5. *Scattergrams of the standard deviation (STD) of the mean RR intervals (left), RR interval (middle), and coefficient of variance (right) in 25 dogs resistant (left aspect of the diagrams) and 25 dogs susceptible (right aspect of the diagrams) to sudden death one month after myocardial infarction. Group mean values (±SEM) (O) are displayed adjacent to the scatter data. Discriminator is placed at the midpoint of group mean values; p<0.05. Reproduced with permission from Hull SS, Evans AR, Vanoli E, et al: Heart rate variability before and after myocardial infarction in conscious dogs at high and low risk of sudden death. J Am Coll Cardiol 16:978, 1990.*

performed. This process makes necessary a brief recapitulation of the animal model used for these studies. More details can be found in Ch. 29.

Three elements involved often in the genesis of malignant arrhythmias in man are present in this experimental model: one, a healed myocardial infarction that acts as a substrate; two, a transient episode of acute myocardial ischemia; and three, a physiologically-elevated sympathetic activity that acts as a trigger. In short, one month after an anterior wall myocardial infarction, chronically instrumented dogs perform a submaximal exercise stress test. Whenever heart rate reaches approximately 220 beats/minute, a two-minute occlusion of the circumflex coronary artery is performed by means of an occluder previously positioned around the vessel. After one minute, exercise ends, but the occlusion continues for one additional minute. This exercise and ischemia test produces ventricular fibrillation in more than 50% of the animals. Whenever this occurs, the dogs are immediately defibrillated through steel paddles ligated to their chest prior to the test. An important feature of the model is the very high reproducibility of the outcome, fibrillation in susceptible or survival in resistant animals, in subsequent tests.

After the observation that survival was often associated with vagally-mediated reflex reductions in heart rate during myocardial ischemia, it became logical to evaluate vagal reflexes prior to exposing the dogs to the exercise and ischemia test. The methodology used has been described in detail in the original study[28] and in Ch. 29.

The finding most specifically relevant to the question of early recognition of individuals at high risk for sudden death was that BRS was significantly lower in susceptible than in resistant dogs. After the first report in a small size study,[14] the definitive results appeared in 1988[27] and were based on a very large population of conscious and infarcted dogs (n = 192). As illustrated in Figures 6 and 7, which show the group and individual data, BRS was 17.7 ± 6.0 milliseconds/mm Hg in the resistant dogs and only 9.1 ± 6.5 milliseconds/mm Hg in the susceptible group ($p<0.001$). This finding indicates that the capability of reflexly increasing vagal activity, as expressed by BRS, was significantly lower in those animals that were at higher risk of developing ventricular fibrillation. This study also allowed a calculation of the risk of developing ventricular fibrillation from a given value of BRS, as shown in Table 3. Sensitivity was 58%, and both specificity and predictive value exceeded 90%.

The strong correlation between BRS assessed in resting conditions and survival during the exercise and ischemia test suggests that the magnitude of the neural response to a blood pressure increase may be predictive of the neural response to acute myocardial ischemia. This concept is supported by the observation that the resistant dogs were those that could respond to acute

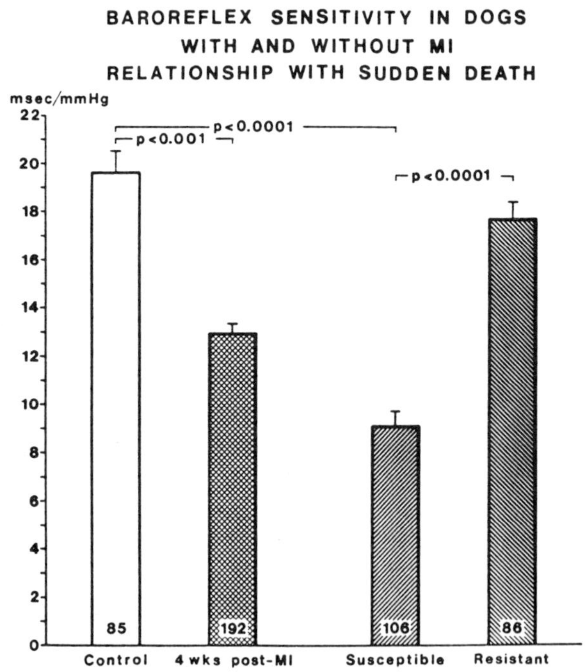

Figure 6. *Bar graph of BRS of 85 control dogs and 192 dogs postmyocardial infarction. Former are without myocardial infarction, whereas the latter are tested four weeks after the production of an anterior myocardial infarction. Among the animals with myocardial infarction, 106 were susceptible and 86 were resistant to ventricular fibrillation during the exercise and ischemia test. Their baroreflex sensitivities are shown in the third and fourth columns. Reproduced by permission of the American Heart Association, Inc. from Schwartz PJ, Vanoli E, Stramba-Badiale M, et al: Autonomic mechanisms and sudden death. New insight from the analysis of baroreceptor reflexes in conscious dogs with and without a myocardial infarction. Circulation 78:969, 1988.*

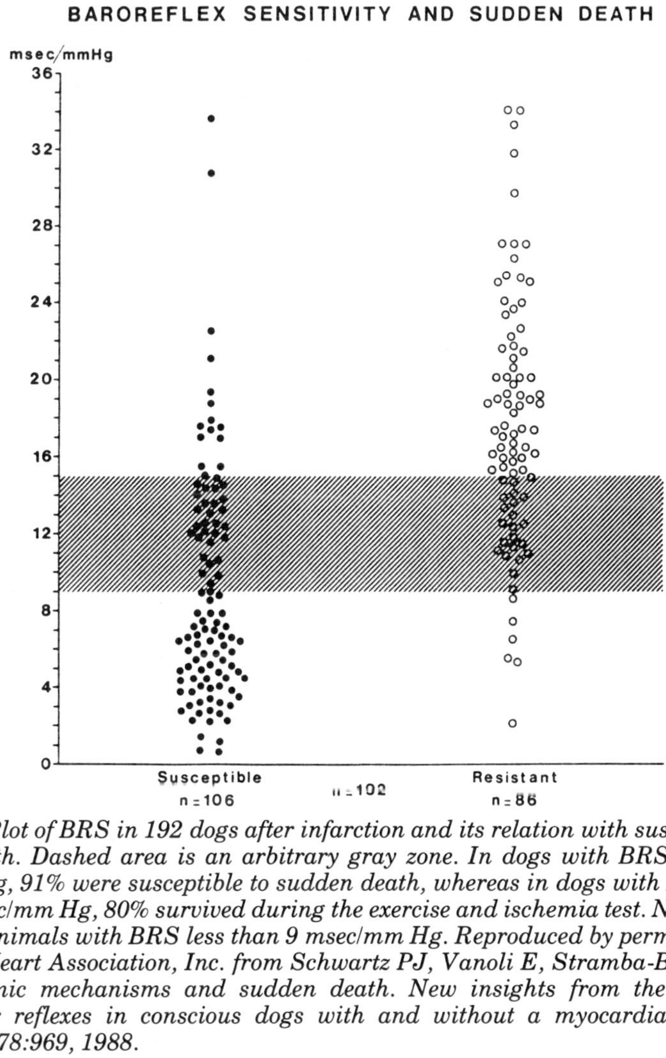

Figure 7. *Plot of BRS in 192 dogs after infarction and its relation with susceptibility to sudden death. Dashed area is an arbitrary gray zone. In dogs with BRS less than 9 msec/mm Hg, 91% were susceptible to sudden death, whereas in dogs with BRS greater than 15 msec/mm Hg, 80% survived during the exercise and ischemia test. Note the large number of animals with BRS less than 9 msec/mm Hg. Reproduced by permission of the American Heart Association, Inc. from Schwartz PJ, Vanoli E, Stramba-Badiale M, et al: Autonomic mechanisms and sudden death. New insights from the analysis of baroreceptor reflexes in conscious dogs with and without a myocardial infarction. Circulation 78:969, 1988.*

myocardial ischemia with vagally-mediated reductions in heart rate. This concept fits well also with the finding that the cats surviving a one-hour coronary artery occlusion were those who evinced greater increases in the firing rate of single cardiac vagal fibers in response to a blood pressure rise and during the first few minutes of myocardial ischemia.[29]

The study by Schwartz et al[27+] definitively demonstrated that a depressed BRS can accurately identify those animals at very high risk for sudden cardiac death. It also represented the first example of the use of autonomic responses to provide prognostic information. The clinical implications of these results were immediately evident and led to the design of the first clinical study to test the applicability to man of the striking observations made in conscious dogs with a healed myocardial infarction.

Table 3.
Baroreflex Sensitivity and Sudden Death in Dogs After Myocardial Infarction

Baroreflex Sensitivity (msec/ mm Hg)	*Sudden Death (n)*	*Percentage*
> 20	4/32	12
> 15	15/73	20
9 to 15	28/51	55
< 9	62/68	91
< 4	23/24	96

n = 192 dogs

Clinical Studies

On the basis of the experimental studies just described, a prospective clinical study was designed in order to test the hypothesis that BRS might be correlated with cardiac mortality in patients. In this first study, La Rovere et al[30] evaluated BRS in 78 patients with a one-month-old myocardial infarction. The correlations between BRS and several clinical variables is described in Ch. 28. Only the data with prognostic implications are presented here.

This study was performed in a cardiac rehabilitation center and the entry criteria were such to favor the enrollment of patients at relatively low risk. All patients had survived their first myocardial infarction by 30 days, they were below age 65, and they were all able to perform a maximal exercise stress test in pharmacological washout, i.e., after all drugs had been withheld for at least five half-lives. These entry criteria were chosen correctly because the two-year mortality rate for the entire group was indeed only 9%.

During this average follow-up of two years, seven patients died and four of them died suddenly. When their BRS was compared to that of the 71 survivors (Fig. 8), it became evident that their BRS was markedly lower (2.4 ± 1.5 versus 8.2 ± 4.8 milliseconds/mm Hg, $p = 0.004$). When mortality was correlated with the presence or absence of a markedly depressed BRS ($\leq$3.0 milliseconds/mm Hg, i.e., one standard deviation below the mean for the entire group), a striking difference became evident, as illustrated in Table 4. Indeed, the risk of dying was 17 times greater for those patients who one month after a myocardial infarction had a depressed BRS. These calculations had to be accepted with caution because of the small number of patients ($n = 10$) with depressed BRS. On the other hand, the difference in mortality was sufficiently large to have meaningful implications.

Another important aspect of this study was that it documented that BRS is not correlated with left ventricular ejection fraction ($r = 0.07$) and, moreover, that a depressed BRS did not merely identify the patients with poor left ventricular function. Figure 9 shows the relationship between BRS, left ventricular ejection fraction, and mortality. It is clear that, within the group of

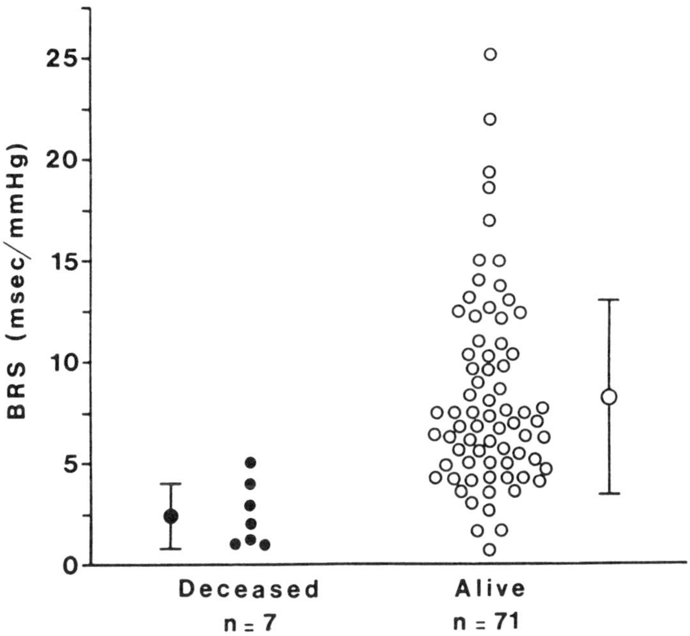

Figure 8. *Plot of relation between BRS and cardiovascular mortality. Besides the clear difference in BRS (p = 0.004) between the deceased patients and the survivors, it is worthy of note that while all deceased patients had a reduced BRS, four of them were in the extreme lower end of the distribution of BRS for the entire population. Modified by permission of the American Heart Association, Inc. from La Rovere MT, Specchia G, Mortara A, et al: Baroreflex sensitivity, clinical correlates and cardiovascular mortality among patients with a first myocardial infarction: A prospective study. Circulation 78:816, 1988.*

Table 4.
Baroreflex Sensitivity and Mortality

	n	*Mortality %*
Whole Population	7/78	9.0%
BRS > 3.0 msec/mm Hg	2/68	3.0%
BRS ≤ 3.0 msec/mm Hg	5/10	50.0%

BRS: baroreflex sensitivity

patients with reduced left ventricular ejection fraction, the risk of dying was increased when the BRS was depressed. This finding implies that a depressed pump function remains an important substrate on which an autonomic imbalance (characterized by reduced vagal activity and increased sympathetic activity) can trigger lethal arrhythmias.

This prospective clinical study has, for the first time, suggested that the analysis of BRS in patients after myocardial infarction may help identify individuals at high risk for subsequent mortality.

With a few exceptions, whenever a new concept is based on a study of a

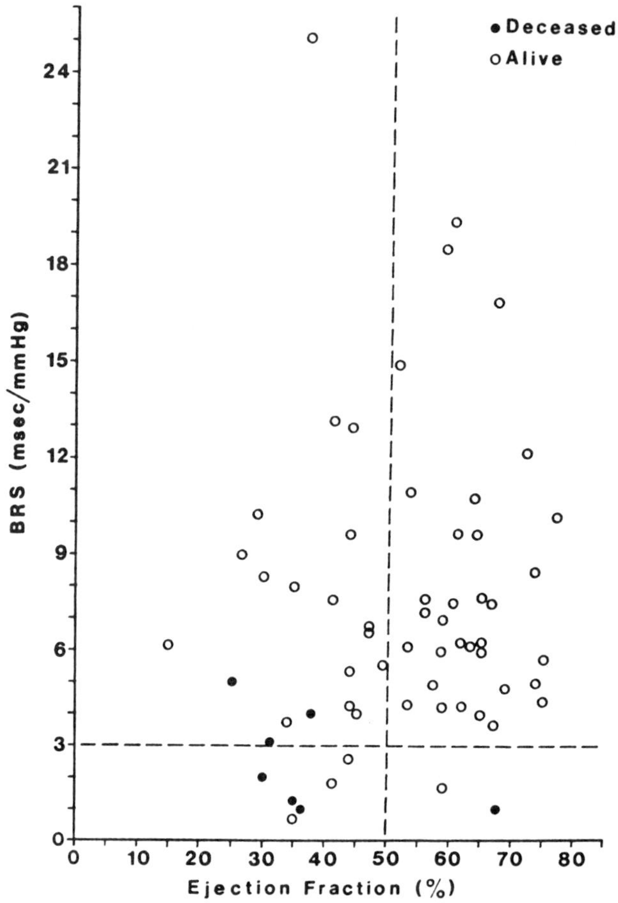

Figure 9. *Plot of relation between BRS, left ventricular ejection fraction, and cardiovascular mortality. Broken lines indicate the arbitrary limits for reduced ejection fraction (<50%) and for markedly reduced BRS (<3 msec/mm Hg). It is evident that, among patients with depressed left ventricular function, the prediction of mortality is enhanced by the analysis of BRS. Reproduced by permission of the American Heart Association, Inc. from La Rovere MT, Specchia G, Mortara A, et al: Baroreflex sensitivity, clinical correlates and cardiovascular mortality among patients with a first myocardial infarction: A prospective study. Circulation 78:816, 1988.*

small population, the conclusions are somewhat shaky. It then becomes very important to wait for additional studies. Therefore, the recent studies by Farrell et al[31,32] are very important. These investigators used the same methodology and the same cutoff points described by La Rovere et al.[30] These similarities allow a meaningful comparison between the studies and will facilitate a meta-analysis in the future, if necessary.

In the first study, Farrell et al[31] measured BRS and heart rate variability in 68 patients who had suffered a myocardial infarction 7 to 10 days earlier. They also assessed the presence of late potentials and used programmed ventricular stimulation to evaluate the inducibility of sustained monomorphic ventricular tachycardia. Note that the correlations between BRS and age and between BRS and left ventricular ejection fraction were strikingly similar in the Italian and the British study. BRS was the most significant predictor of inducibility by the electrophysiological test. During follow-up, there were five major arrhythmic events (ventricular tachycardia, with or without sudden death). The events were all correctly identified by depressed BRS and by inducibility by electrical testing. When Farrell et al[31] compared the BRS of their patients with and without major cardiac events, they found that, as in the study by La Rovere et al,[30] the patients destined to develop life-threatening arrhythmias had BRS values that were markedly lower (0.9 ± 0.8 versus 7.4 ± 4.6 milliseconds/mm Hg, $p = 0.002$). Farrell et al[31] concluded that their study "... confirms that depressed BRS identifies a subgroup at high risk for arrhythmic events following myocardial infarction" (p. 9).

In the second report, Farrell et al[32] extended their study population to include 122 patients with a one-year follow-up. During this period, there were 13 deaths and 10 documented life-threatening events (five sudden deaths and five sustained ventricular tachycardias requiring hospital admission). For these patients, they calculated the risk associated with depressed BRS, depressed heart rate variability, and depressed left ventricular function.

They confirmed in this larger group that the BRS of the patients developing major arrhythmic events was markedly lower than that of the remaining patients (1.73 ± 1.49 versus 7.83 ± 4.5 milliseconds/mm Hg, $p = 0.0001$). Their most important finding, however, was derived from the calculation of the relative risk for arrhythmic events, based on a comparison of the three major prognostic variables under study. They found that depressed BRS carried the highest relative risk (relative risk = 23 [95% CI 7.7–69.2]). It was superior to both depressed left ventricular function (relative risk = 10.4 [95% CI 3.3–32.6]) and reduced heart rate variability (relative risk = 10.1 [95% CI 5.6–18.1]). Even if this study is too small to allow valid conclusions about relative prognostic power, one must note that BRS appears as the most powerful predictor of arrhythmic death in patients with ischemic heart disease. Another important contribution of this study is the suggestion (Fig. 10) that a depressed BRS is particularly effective in identifying patients at risk for major arrhythmic events and for sudden death. It is less effective when the risk is related to cardiac deaths in general.

We would also like to draw another important implication from this study. Farrell et al[33] found that depressed heart rate variability was almost equally effective in identifying patients at risk either for cardiac death in general or for sudden death. By contrast, a depressed BRS appeared to be a good predictor only for sudden deaths. If confirmed in a larger study, this finding may indicate that, by analyzing both BRS and heart rate variability, one may derive specific information about the type of risk that a given patient may encounter. An intriguing and important implication would follow. In the design of clinical trials for prevention, or reduction, of cardiac mortality in patients after a myocardial infarction, the availability of both measures may help identify patients who are more likely to die, either suddenly or not. The introduction a priori of a specific hypothesis may unmask the possibility that a given drug might effectively prevent one, but not both, types of death. This occurrence

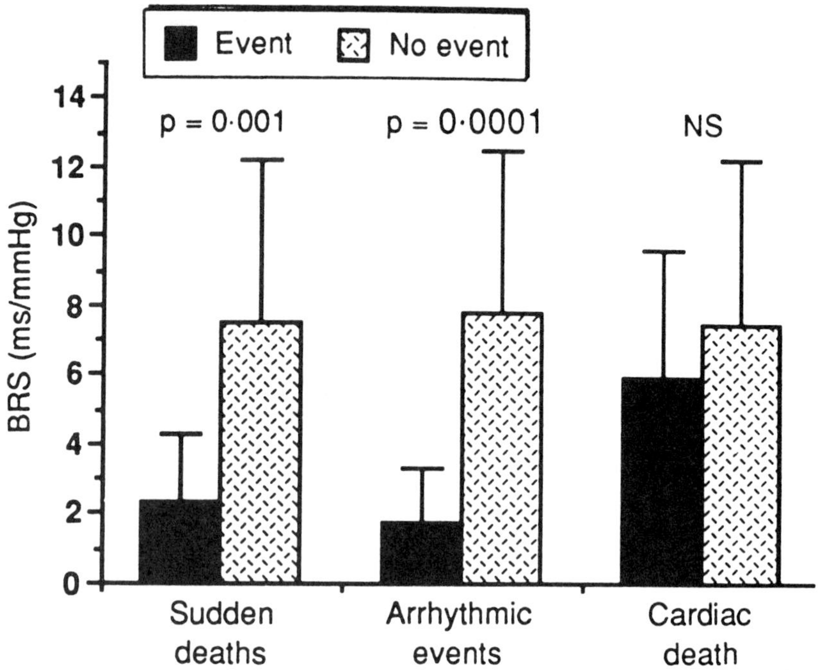

Figure 10. *Column graph (mean [SD]) of BRS according to clinical events. Arrhythmic events include sudden deaths and ventricular fibrillation. Reproduced with permission from Farrell TG, Odemuyiwa O, Bashir Y, et al: Prognostic value of baroreflex sensitivity testing after acute myocardial infarction. Br Heart J 67:129, 1992.*

may enable the testing of antiarrhythmic drugs that can interfere with one, but not with all, mechanisms of death.

The amount of progress and of data accumulation that has accrued in such a brief time is very impressive. When one examines together the pioneering study by La Rovere et al[30] and the two significant contributions by Farrell et al,[31,32] it becomes difficult to deny that the clinical use of BRS may contribute substantially to postmyocardial infarction risk stratification.

Autonomic Measures Prior to a Myocardial Infarction

So far, we have discussed the question of the potential prognostic value of autonomic measures performed in patients who have already suffered a myocardial infarction. The analysis of BRS determined in conscious dogs before and after myocardial infarction disclosed an unexpected finding that may have important practical implications. Among 68 control dogs, those that had the lower values of BRS were more likely to die (Fig. 11) either during the recovery phase after myocardial infarction or one month later during the exercise and ischemia test.[27] This finding means that the analysis of autonomic reflexes can identify a subgroup of normal individuals who would be at high risk for sudden death should they develop ischemic heart disease and suffer a myocardial infarction.

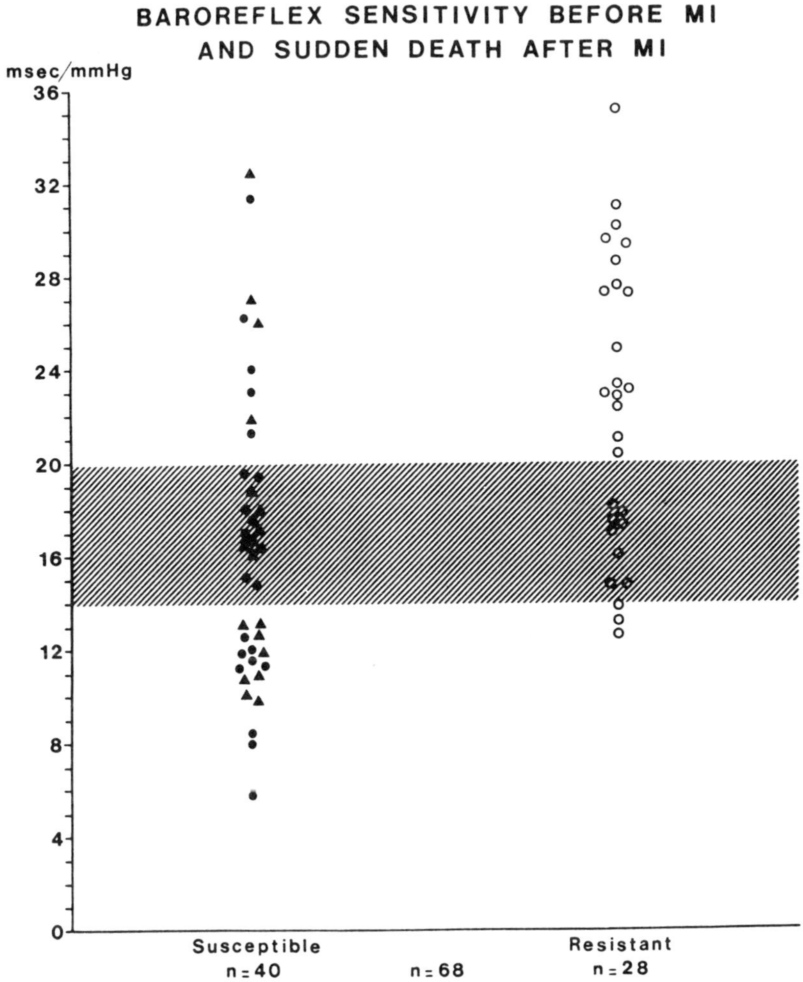

Figure 11. *Plot of BRS before myocardial infarction (MI) in 68 animals and its relation with susceptibility to sudden death after MI. In this case, the arbitrary gray zone extends from 14 to 20 msec/mm Hg. ●: Animals susceptible to sudden death during the exercise and ischemia test; ▲: Animals that died suddenly during the first four weeks after MI; and ○: Animals that survived during the exercise and ischemia test. Note how few animals have BRS less than 9 msec/mm Hg. Reproduced by permission of the American Heart Association, Inc. from Schwartz PJ, Vanoli E, Stramba-Badiale M, et al: Autonomic mechanisms and sudden death. New insights from the analysis of baroreceptor reflexes in conscious dogs with and without a myocardial infarction. Circulation 78:969, 1988.*

The individual distribution of autonomic responses has a very wide range, as exemplified by the large differences observed in BRS both in dogs and in men. In approximately 70% of dogs, BRS is decreased by a myocardial infarction.[27] Thus, myocardial infarction, besides creating an arrhythmogenic substrate, displaces the entire range of vagal reflexes (measured as BRS) toward lower values. The autonomic makeup varies greatly among different individuals. Those who are already at the lower end of the normal distribution for baroreflex responses after an infarction are likely to have very low values of BRS and may be at very high risk for sudden death.

Are the measures of heart rate variability equally effective in detecting early signs of augmented risk among normal individuals? In the same conscious animal model for sudden cardiac death,[28] Hull et al[26] examined the prognostic value of heart rate variability, measured in a 30-minute period. The internal control analysis performed in 18 resistant and in 18 susceptible dogs studied before and one month after myocardial infarction yielded an unwelcome but important answer. Prior to myocardial infarction, the heart rate variability of the susceptible dogs did not differ at all from that of the resistant animals (Fig. 12). The unavoidable conclusion is that, even though heart rate variability appropriately discriminates between high-and low-risk individuals who have already had an infarction, it does not have predictive value among normal individuals. This finding appears to be an important difference from what has been observed with BRS.

Is this difference between the two autonomic measures a real one, or does it somehow depend on the experimental preparation? To address this issue, it was considered that, when discussing heart rate variability and BRS, we may all be using only markers of tonic and reflex vagal activity. Accordingly, it was thought necessary to study vagal activity directly, i.e., by recording the activity of single vagal fibers that are mostly directed to the sinoatrial (SA)

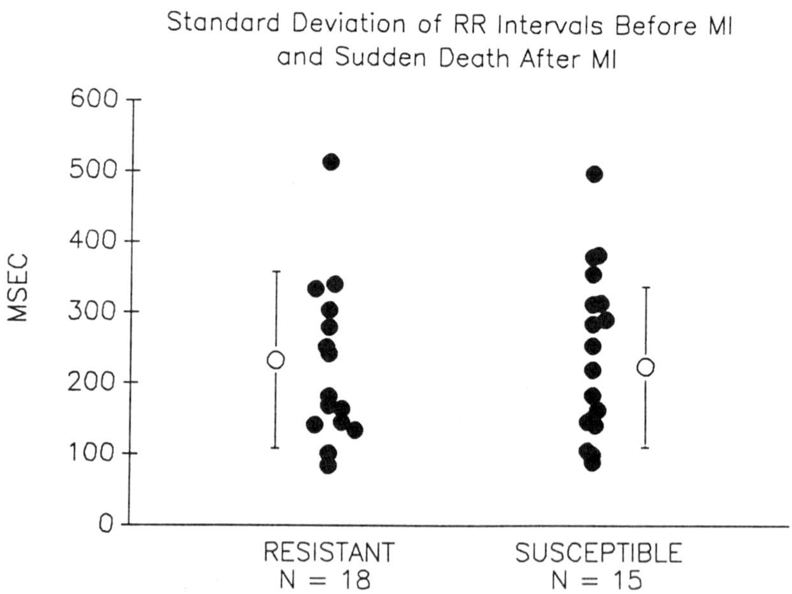

Figure 12. *Standard deviation of RR intervals before myocardial infarction (MI) and sudden death after MI measured in 15 animals that developed fibrillation during exercise and ischemia test, and in 18 animals that survived the exercise and ischemia test. It is evident that no difference existed between these two groups of animals prior to MI. Compare this figure with Figure 11 for the differences provided by determination of BRS and heart rate variability.*

node. Cerati and Schwartz[29] recorded cardiac vagal activity in 17 anesthetized cats during blood pressure increases evoked by phenylephrine (Fig. 13) and during a 60-minute occlusion of the left descending coronary artery. Within three minutes of coronary occlusion, nine cats developed ventricular fibrillation and were defined as susceptible, whereas the remaining eight cats survived and formed the resistant group.

Figure 14 shows, in the two groups, the firing rate of these single vagal fibers under resting conditions (i.e., before blood pressure increase), and in response to the blood pressure rise. The former condition can be used as a reasonable indicator of tonic vagal activity, whereas the latter constitutes a

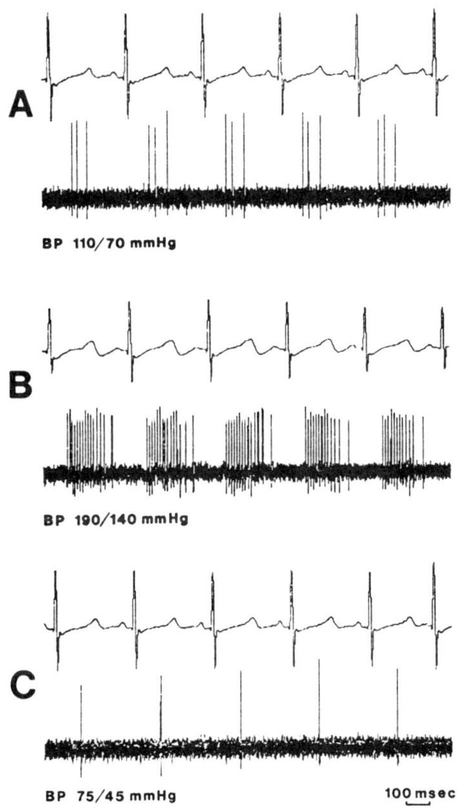

Figure 13. *Tracing showing activity of a single cardiac vagal efferent fiber at three different levels of arterial blood pressure. In each panel, the upper trace shows the electrocardiogram and the lower trace shows the electroneurogram. A: At the resting level of blood pressure, a pulse-synchronous activity, with three impulses in each burst, was present. B: When blood pressure was raised by phenylephrine, the activity of the fiber increased markedly. The activity was still synchronous with the cardiac cycle, it started 60 msec earlier, and each burst showed more impulses. C: When blood pressure was reduced by bleeding, the activity of the fiber decreased. The activity was still synchronous with the cardiac cycle, but only one impulse per cycle was present. Reproduced by permission of the American Heart Association, Inc. from Cerati D, Schwartz PJ: Single cardiac vagal fiber activity, acute myocardial ischemia, and risk for sudden death. Circ Res 69:1389, 1991.*

valid indicator of vagal reflex activity. As a matter of fact, these results represent the pure vagal component of the baroreceptor reflex. Whereas resting ("tonic") activity was similar in the two groups (1.48 ± 0.30 versus 1.58 ± 0.35 impulses/second), the reflex increase consequent to blood pressure elevation was markedly smaller in the susceptible cats (80 ± 14% versus 246 ± 66%, $p<0.05$).

The results of this study in anesthetized cats are strikingly similar to the observations made in conscious dogs. They indicate that the cats surviving coronary occlusion are those that can reflexly increase vagal activity during acute myocardial ischemia. Highly relevant here is the fact that their outcomes could be predicted by analysis of the reflex response to a baroreceptive stimulus and not by analysis of tonic activity.

Autonomic Tone and Reflexes After Myocardial Infarction Study

The data presented above indicate that the autonomic nervous system, when carefully analyzed, may provide important answers about prognosis.

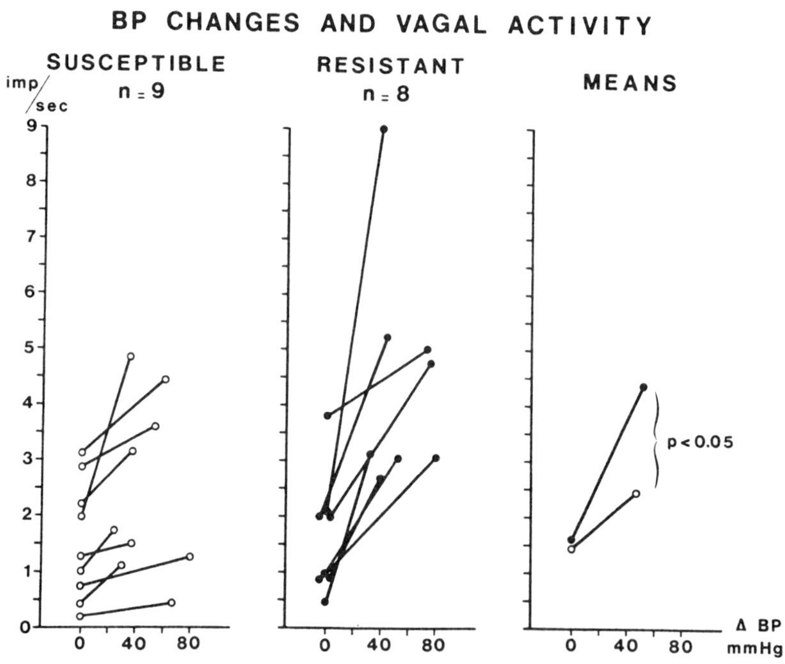

Figure 14. *Responses of cardiac vagal activity in resistant and susceptible cats, during increases in mean blood pressure following phenylephrine injection. The left and middle panels show individual responses, while the right panel shows the mean response of each group. Values are expressed as imp/sec. ○: Susceptible cats; ●: Resistant cats; and ΔBP: Changes in mean blood pressure following phenylephrine injection. Reproduced by permission of the American Heart Association, Inc. from Cerati D, Schwartz PJ: Single cardiac vagal fiber activity, acute myocardial ischemia, and risk for sudden death. Circ Res 69:1389, 1991.*

Heart rate variability is measured from a Holter recording, whereas BRS requires at least the injection of a pressor drug. Despite the proven safety of baroreflex testing, if the two tests would provide the same type of information, it would become quite logical to use only the totally noninvasive heart rate variability. A study by Bigger et al[33] has already demonstrated that this occurrence is not the case. The correlation between heart rate variability and BRS, although statistically significant, is a weak one (Fig. 15). This statement means that, for the majority of patients, one measure would not yield a satisfactory prediction of the other. Hence, heart rate variability and BRS are not redundant. This finding is not surprising, because one measure reflects

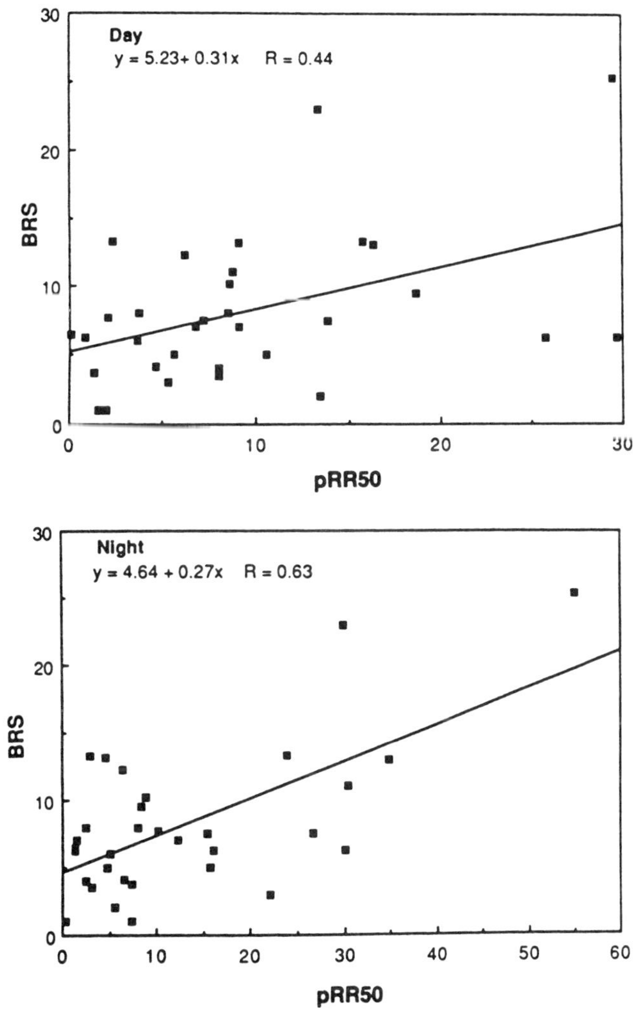

Figure 15. *Scatterplot showing correlation between BRS in msec/mm Hg and the percent of successive normal RR intervals differing >50 msec (pRR50) plotted separately for day and night. Reproduced with permission from Bigger JT Jr, La Rovere MT, Steinman RC, et al: Comparison of baroreflex sensitivity and heart period variability after myocardial infarction. J Am Coll Cardiol 14:1511, 1989.*

what can be considered vagal tone, whereas the other reflects the capability of the autonomic nervous system to respond with powerful vagal reflexes.

To provide a definitive answer about the potential value of different measures of autonomic activity, it was necessary to design a specific clinical study. This study was the background of ATRAMI. ATRAMI is the acronym for "Autonomic Tone and Reflexes After Myocardial Infarction." This prospective clinical trial was designed to test the prognostic value of BRS and of heart rate variability in a large population of patients with a myocardial infarction. Left ventricular ejection fraction and the presence of late potentials will also be determined. ATRAMI began enrollment in the summer of 1990 and is scheduled to reach the target number of 1200 enrolled patients by the spring of 1994. ATRAMI involves over 20 enrolling centers in Europe, the United States, and Japan.

Another feature of ATRAMI is that BRS is measured with two methods: the traditional invasive direct recording of arterial blood pressure through an arterial line, and a noninvasive recording by the use of digital infrared plethysmography. If the correlation between the types of measurement is sufficiently high, it would then become logical to use only the noninvasive method. This will represent a major advance in the clinical use of BRS.

Independently of the results of ATRAMI, the conduct of this large international prospective trial demonstrates the tight relationship between experimental and clinical cardiology.

References

1. Lown B, Verrier RL: Neural activity and ventricular fibrillation. N Engl J Med 294:1165, 1976.
2. Schwartz PJ, Brown AM, Malliani AE, et al: Neural mechanisms in cardiac arrhythmias. New York, NY, Raven Press, 1978, p. 442.
3. Schwartz PJ, Stone HL: The role of the autonomic nervous system in sudden coronary death. Ann NY Acad Sci 382:162, 1982.
4. Corr PB, Yamada KA, Witkowski FX: Mechanisms controlling cardiac autonomic function and their relation to arrhythmogenesis. In HA Fozzard, E Haber, RB Jennings, et al (eds): The Heart and Cardiovascular System. Vol. II. New York, NY, Raven Press, 1986, pp. 1343–1403.
5. Verrier RL, Lown B: Sympathetic-parasympathetic interactions and ventricular electrical stability. In PJ Schwartz, AM Brown, A Malliani, et al (eds): Neural Mechanisms in Cardiac Arrhythmias. New York, NY, Raven Press, 1978, pp. 75–85.
6. Schwartz PJ, Vanoli E: Cardiac arrhythmias elicited by interaction between acute myocardial ischemia and sympathetic hyperactivity: A new experimental model for the study of antiarrhythmic drugs. J Cardiovasc Pharmacol 3:1251, 1981.
7. Schwartz PJ, Priori SG: Sympathetic nervous system and cardiac arrhythmias. In DP Zipes, J Jalife (eds): Cardiac Electrophysiology. From Cell to Bedside. Philadelphia, PA, WB Saunders Co, 1990, pp. 330–343.
8. Kolman BS, Verrier RL, Lown B: The effect of vagus nerve stimulation upon vulnerability of the canine ventricle: Role of the sympathetic parasympathetic interactions. Circulation 52:578, 1976.
9. Vanoli E, De Ferrari GM, Stramba-Badiale M, et al: Vagal stimulation and prevention of sudden death in conscious dogs with a healed myocardial infarction. Circ Res 68:1471, 1991.

10. De Ferrari GM, Vanoli E, Stramba-Badiale M, et al: Vagal reflexes and survival during acute myocardial ischemia in conscious dogs with healed myocardial infarction. Am J Physiol 261:H63, 1991.
11. Yusuf S, Teo KK: Approaches to prevention of sudden death: Need for fundamental reevaluation. J Cardiovasc Electrophysiol 2(suppl):S233, 1991.
12. Schwartz PJ, Locati EH, Moss AJ, et al: Left cardiac sympathetic denervation in the therapy of the congenital long QT syndrome: A worldwide report. Circulation 84:503, 1991.
13. Schwartz PJ, Motolese M, Pollavini G, et al: Prevention of sudden cardiac death after a first myocardial infarction by pharmacological or surgical antiadrenergic interventions. J Cardiovasc Electrophysiol 3:2, 1992.
14. Billman GE, Schwartz PJ, Stone HL: Baroreceptor reflex control of heart rate: A predictor of sudden cardiac death. Circulation 66:874, 1982.
15. Wolf M, Varigos G, Hunt D, et al: Sinus arrhythmia in acute myocardial infarction. Med J Aust 2:52, 1978.
16. Myers GA, Martin GJ, Magid NM, et al: Power spectral analysis of heart rate variability in sudden cardiac death: Comparison to other methods. IEEE Trans Biomed Eng 33:1149, 1986.
17. Martin GJ, Magid NM, Myers GA, et al: Heart rate variability and sudden death secondary to coronary heart disease during ambulatory electrocardiographic monitoring. Am J Cardiol 60:86, 1987.
18. Kleiger RE, Miller JP, Bigger JT Jr, et al: Heart rate variability: A variable predicting mortality following acute myocardial infarction. J Am Coll Cardiol 3:547, 1984.
19. Kleiger RE, Miller JP, Bigger JT Jr, et al: Decreased heart rate variability and its association with increased mortality after acute myocardial infarction. Am J Cardiol 59:256, 1987.
20. Bigger JT Jr, Fleiss JL, Steinman RC, et al: Frequency domain measures of heart period variability and mortality after myocardial infarction. Circulation 85:164, 1992.
21. Bigger JT Jr, Fleiss JL, Steinman RC, et al: Correlations among time and frequency domain measures of heart period variability two weeks after acute myocardial infarction. Am J Cardiol 69:891–898, 1992.
22. The Multicenter Post Infarction Research Group: Risk stratification and survival after myocardial infarction. N Engl J Med 309:331, 1983.
23. Bigger JT Jr, Fleiss JL, Kleiger RE, et al: The relationships among ventricular arrhythmias, left ventricular dysfunction and mortality in the 2 years after myocardial infarction. Circulation 69:250, 1984.
24. Odemuyiwa O, Malik M, Farrell T, et al: Comparison of the predictive characteristics of heart rate variability index and left ventricular ejection fraction for all-cause mortality, arrhythmic events and sudden death after acute myocardial infarction. Am J Cardiol 68:434, 1991.
25. Farrell TG, Bashir Y, Cripps T, et al: Risk stratification for arrhythmic events based on heart rate variability, ambulatory electrocardiographic variables and the signal-averaged electrocardiogram. J Am Coll Cardiol 18:687, 1991.
26. Hull SS, Evans AR, Vanoli E, et al: Heart rate variability before and after myocardial infarction in conscious dogs at high and low risk of sudden death. J Am Coll Cardiol 16:978, 1990.
27. Schwartz PJ, Vanoli E, Stramba-Badiale M, et al: Autonomic mechanisms and sudden death. New insight from the analysis of baroreceptor reflexes in conscious dogs with and without a myocardial infarction. Circulation 78:969, 1988.
28. Schwartz PJ, Billman GE, Stone HL: Autonomic mechanisms in ventricular fibrillation induced by myocardial ischemia during exercise in dogs with a healed myocardial infarction. An experimental preparation for sudden cardiac death. Circulation 69:780, 1984.
29. Cerati D, Schwartz PJ: Single cardiac vagal fiber activity, acute myocardial ischemia, and risk for sudden death. Circ Res 69:1389, 1991.

30. La Rovere MT, Specchia G, Mortara A, et al: Baroreflex sensitivity, clinical correlates and cardiovascular mortality among patients with a first myocardial infarction: A prospective study. Circulation 78:816, 1988.
31. Farrell TG, Paul V, Cripps TR, et al: Baroreflex sensitivity and electrophysiological correlates in patients after acute myocardial infarction. Circulation 83:945, 1991.
32. Farrell TG, Odemuyiwa O, Bashir Y, et al: Prognostic value of baroreflex sensitivity testing after acute myocardial infarction. Br Heart J 67:129, 1992.
33. Bigger JT Jr, La Rovere MT, Steinman RC, et al: Comparison of baroreflex sensitivity and heart period variability after myocardial infarction. J Am Coll Cardiol 14:1511, 1989.

PART VI

Role in Experimental and Clinical Arrhythmias

CHAPTER 30

Respiratory Sinus Arrhythmia

J.P. Saul, R.J. Cohen

Respiratory sinus arrhythmia (RSA) can be defined simply as the variations in heart rate that occur simultaneously with respiratory activity. Although the terminology clearly implies that the phenomenon is a cardiac arrhythmia, most cardiologists and physiologists would agree that the presence of RSA is not only normal, but is actually indicative of good health. RSA is essentially ubiquitous in large mammals. Due to its ubiquitous nature, RSA has been widely investigated as both a biophysical phenomenon and, as Eckberg described it, a window on autonomic regulation.[1]

Respiration influences a large number of autonomic and hemodynamic parameters, leading to a variety of proposed physiological mechanisms for the origin of the RSA. Most investigators agree on a number of the key characteristics of RSA. First, RSA is both a frequency- and an amplitude-dependent phenomenon. That is, the amplitude of the change in heart rate at a given respiratory frequency increases as the tidal volume increases, and for a given tidal volume, the amplitude decreases as the breathing frequency increases (Fig. 1).[2–6] Second, the amplitude of the arrhythmia is a function of age, such that RSA diminishes with increasing age.[2,7–9] There is also general agreement that, at typical resting respiratory frequencies near 0.2 Hz (12 breaths/minute), the heart rate increases simultaneously with inspiration.[3,5,6,10] Most investigators have found that cardiac vagal efferents are involved in mediating the heart rate fluctuations that occur with respiration,[11–18] while some have observed that modulation of cardiac sympathetic efferents also plays a role in generating RSA at lower respiratory frequencies, below 0.15 Hz (~9 breaths/minute).[18,19] In addition, a few studies have specifically investigated the phase relationship between respiratory activity and heart rate as a function of the respiratory frequency.[3,5,18] Finally, several investigators have speculated on the question of whether RSA has a physiological function. Melcher[4] proposed that RSA is an important mechanism for transferring the increased systemic venous return produced by normal inspiration from the pulmonary to the systemic circulation.

This work was supported in part by NIH Grant #HL39291, and a grant from the Whitaker Foundation.
From *Vagal Control of the Heart: Experimental Basis and Clinical Implications* edited by MN Levy, PJ Schwartz © 1994, Futura Publishing Co. Inc., Armonk, NY.

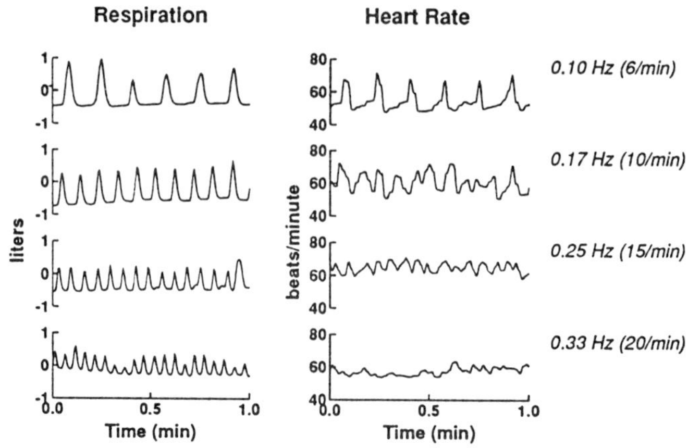

Figure 1. *Respiratory and heart rate times series from one subject breathing at four frequencies: 0.10, 0.17, 0.25, and 0.33 Hz (equivalent breathing rates 6, 10, 15, and 20 breaths per minute). Note that, at all these frequencies, heart rate tends to increase at the same time as inspiration. As frequency increases, the amplitude of the heart rate response decreases.*

Others see RSA as a physiological aberration. Regardless of its usefulness, it is clear that RSA is not a necessary component for survival.[20]

This chapter reviews the various mechanisms proposed to generate RSA, assesses the quantitative tools that have been used to characterize it, describes the physiology viewed through this window on autonomic regulation, and speculates on its clinical importance and usefulness.

Traditional Respiratory Sinus Arrhythmia Generating Mechanisms

Autonomic

By far the largest modulators of sinoatrial (SA) node rate, regardless of whether respiration is the modulation source, are the cardiac parasympathetic and sympathetic efferent nerves. Since respiration continually perturbs cardiovascular hemodynamics, it has the potential to influence cardiac autonomic efferent activity through a variety of direct and indirect mechanisms (Fig. 2) including:

1. a direct neural coupling within the central nervous system (CNS)[19,21–26];
2. central nervous modulation of arterial baroreflex sensitivity (BRS)[4,27–29];
3. central nervous modulation of arterial chemoreflex sensitivity to CO_2[29];
4. mechanical modulation of central venous volume and cardiopulmonary receptor activity (the Bainbridge reflex)[4,30–33];

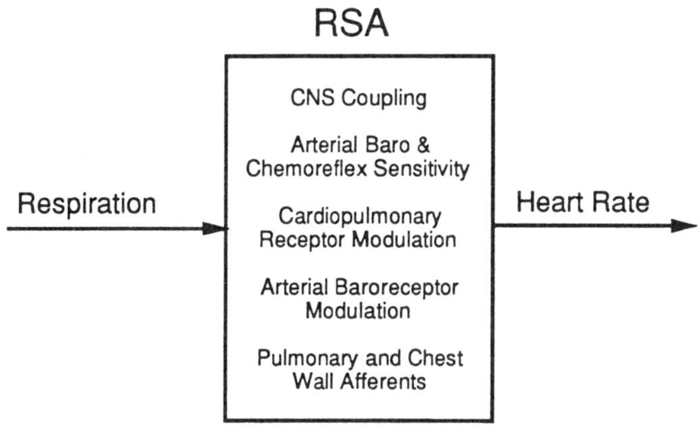

Figure 2. *Respiratory sinus arrhythmia (RSA). Respiration influences a wide range of physiological parameters through its mechanical effect and through direct links in the CNS.*

5. mechanical modulation of arterial pressure influencing heart rate through the arterial baroreflex[6,34]; and
6. stimulation of stretch receptor afferents in the lung and chest wall.[10,22,35]

Although both supportive and contrary evidence exists for most of the mechanisms listed above, it is likely that each of them plays at least some role in generating RSA.

Central

In 1865, Traube[26] proposed a central nervous origin for RSA. He observed persistence of sinus arrhythmia at or near the original respiratory frequency after complete curarization in dogs, and concluded that only a direct neural link between the respiratory and heart rate controlling centers in the brain stem could account for his observations. Although he did not directly measure phrenic nerve activity to assess central respiratory activity, others have demonstrated that a sinus arrhythmia that is synchronized with phrenic nerve activity, but not necessarily with mechanical respiratory activity, exists in various animal preparations.[19,21–25,36] Furthermore, a few investigators have demonstrated that changes in cardiac vagal efferent activity actually precede the onset of both phrenic nerve activity and mechanical inspiration.[21,37] Finally, when the phase relation between respiratory activity and changes in heart rate have been carefully investigated in humans during voluntarily controlled respiration, heart rate seems to increase just prior to the onset of inspiration at typical respiratory frequencies above approximately 0.15 Hz.[3,17,18] Together, the above data indicate clearly that the effects of afferent neural stimuli that result from the mechanical influence of respiration on the lungs, the chest wall, the heart, and the thoracic vasculature are unable to account entirely for the presence of RSA. That is, central respiratory activity directly influences heart rate in the CNS.

The exact form of this central nervous link is more difficult to establish from the available data. Using relatively large (25 to 150 mm Hg), sudden carotid baroreceptor stimuli timed to various phases of the respiratory cycle, a few investigators have demonstrated that, in both humans[4,27,28] and dogs,[29] arterial BRS decreases during late expiration and early inspiration, and increases again during late inspiration and early expiration. Eckberg[3] also found that the precise timing and amplitude of these changes were dependent on the respiratory frequency. Thus, two possible mechanisms exist to explain the central link between respiration and heart rate. The first mechanism is a direct neural link between the respiratory centers in the brain stem and the control of cardiac vagal efferent activity, such that vagal activity decreases just prior to the onset of inspiration. The second mechanism is a direct neural link to the central sensitivity of the arterial baroreflex, such that a pre-inspiratory decrease in sensitivity to baroreceptor afferent stimuli leads to a decrease in vagal efferent activity. A clear differentiation between these mechanisms has not been demonstrated experimentally. It should be noted that both of these mechanisms can account only for an inspiratory increase in heart rate, and they ignore the fact that the phase relation between heart rate and respiration varies as a function of the respiratory frequency, such that heart rate actually decreases during inspiration at low breathing rates (see below).[5,17,18] These observations may be explained partially by the often-ignored finding that cardiac sympathetic efferent activity is also modulated by respiration.[19,36,37] Many investigators of RSA in humans have chosen to discount these findings in animals because RSA seems to disappear almost completely with vagal blockade.[13,15,38,39] At respiratory frequencies below 0.15 Hz, however, it is clear that at least some RSA persists after vagal blockade with atropine[18] (Fig. 3), and has characteristics consistent with cardiac sympathetic efferent modulation of heart rate (i.e., low magnitude at frequencies above 0.15 Hz and a phase delay).[40] In addition, the findings suggest the presence of an inspiratory decrease in cardiac sympathetic efferent activity, similar to that seen for cardiac vagal activity. This finding of a simultaneous decrease in cardiac sympathetic and vagal activity is not consistent entirely with a change in arterial BRS and suggests that the central mechanism for producing RSA is at least partially direct and that it involves modulation of both vagal and sympathetic efferent activity.

Mechanical

As phrenic nerve signals are transformed into mechanical ventilation, respiration directly and indirectly influences arterial and central venous pressures and flows through mechanical thoracic coupling and changes in left and right ventricular preload.[30,41–44] These respiratory-induced changes in arterial and central venous pressure must, in turn, influence the afferent signals from the arterial and cardiopulmonary baroreceptors, respectively.

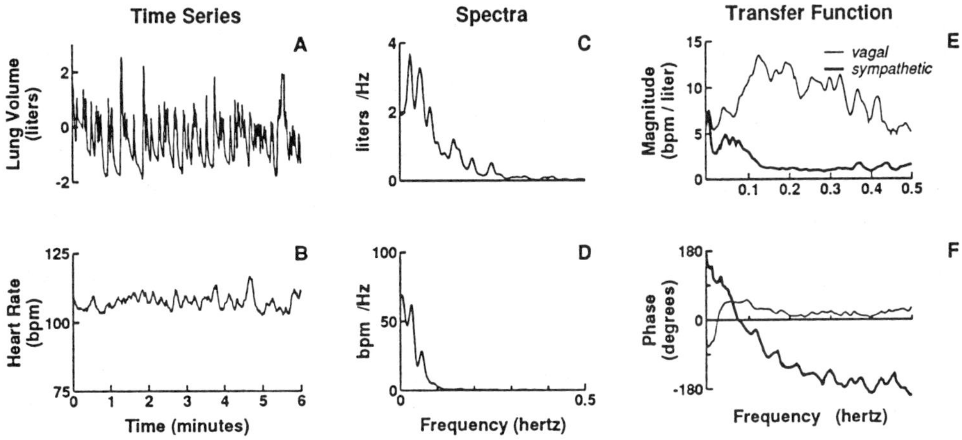

Figure 3. *Respiratory and heart rate times series (A,B) and corresponding spectra (C,D) from one patient breathing at random intervals after complete parasympathetic blockade with atropine (0.03 mg/kg) while upright. Note first that the respiratory stimulus has significant spectral content from 0 up to 0.4 Hz. In addition, note that the heart rate response is present, but only at frequencies below 0.1 Hz. The group average transfer functions between respiration and heart rate during this sympathetic state show that respiration affects heart rate with significant magnitude below about 0.12 Hz, but with an inversion at 0 Hz and a phase delay. For pure vagal heart rate control (time series and spectra not shown), respiration affects heart rate at frequencies up to 0.5 Hz with no significant phase delay.*

Bainbridge,[30] in 1915, noted that heart rate could be influenced by atrial size. He proposed a reflex linking atrial size to the firing of cardioinhibitory (vagal) fibers, such that an increase in atrial size led to a decrease in cardiac vagal efferent activity and an increase in heart rate. Since inspiration leads to an increase in the venous return to the heart and an increase in atrial stretch, he later proposed that this reflex could account for RSA.[31] Although evidence for a steady state, vagally-mediated Bainbridge reflex in humans has been difficult to substantiate,[45] other investigations have supported at least a partial role for the Bainbridge reflex in generating RSA.[4,32,33] Perhaps the best data to differentiate these mechanisms resulted from Melcher's[4] study that used continuous negative inspiratory pressure, intermittent positive pressure ventilation, and voluntarily controlled breathing to vary intrathoracic pressure and tidal volume independently. Melcher[4] found that RSA was more closely linked to intrathoracic pressure than tidal volume, regardless of the combination of these factors used to achieve a given pressure. He also found that, during these maneuvers, changes in central venous pressure were more closely linked to RSA than were changes in arterial pressure, and he concluded that RSA is due, in large part, to the effect of cardiopulmonary reflexes on heart rate. Note also that cardiopulmonary receptor activation and deactivation have profound effects on muscle sympathetic nerve activity and peripheral resistance.[45] Today, the precise role of the Bainbridge reflex in producing RSA remains unclear.

In 1958, Manzotti[34] proposed that respiratory-induced changes in venous return, which eventually lead to changes in left ventricular output, arterial pressure and, finally, heart rate, are indirectly responsible for RSA. Davies and Neilson[6] later supported this view, but other investigators discounted this view, because they found that increases in heart rate with inspiration were usually synchronous with increases in arterial pressure.[33,46] More recent investigations, using models and signal processing techniques to identify the phase relations between respiration, heart rate, and arterial pressure, have also yielded conflicting results. Akselrod et al,[47] using a combination of atrial pacing and autonomic blockade in dogs, and they found that respiratory-related fluctuations of arterial pressure result from changes in heart rate (RSA). However, deBoer et al[48] and Baselli et al[49] concluded that, in humans, the opposite was true: RSA resulted from mechanically-induced fluctuations of arterial pressure.

This conflict can probably be resolved by examining data from a very recent study,[18] shown in Figure 4. A more complete discussion of this issue is included below, after presentation of the methodology, but a brief explanation ensues here. Taken together, Figures 3 and 4 demonstrate a number of points concerning the influence of respiratory activity on both arterial pressure and heart rate. First, both of these relations are highly dependent on the frequency of respiration. Hence, data from different experiments can be compared only if the effects of the chosen respiratory frequency are taken into account. Second, total cardiac autonomic blockade changes the magnitude of the effect of respiration on arterial pressure, but does not make it zero. This finding indicates that one, respiratory-induced changes in heart rate affect arterial pressure and, two, respiratory-induced changes in arterial pressure exist independently of changes in heart rate. Third, these data indicate that the autonomic state may have a profound effect on the interplay between respiration, heart rate, and arterial pressure. Finally, these data are taken from humans, and marked species differences prevail in the magnitude of RSA, probably due to species-specific differences in mean vagal tone and differences in central nervous modulation of vagal activity by respiration. Resting supine dogs have an extremely prominent RSA, often reaching a 50-beat/minute change in heart rate with a single breath.[47]

Stretch Receptors

Finally, perhaps the earliest proposed autonomic mechanism for generating RSA is that this phenomenon is due to a reflex involving stimulation of stretch receptors in the lung and chest wall.[50] Anrep et al[22] showed that stretch receptors in the lungs and chest wall were stimulated on inspiration, and that afferent activity originating from these receptors had an inhibitory effect on vagal outflow, and this inhibitory effect led to an increase in heart rate with inspiration. Although more recent studies by Hainsworth[51] support the findings of Anrep et al,[22] there have also been contradictory or variable findings. Glick et al[52] reported a bradycardia during lung inflation, and studies in man have demonstrated increases, decreases, and biphasic responses of heart rate to inspiration or expiration.[3,5,6,10,17,18,53]

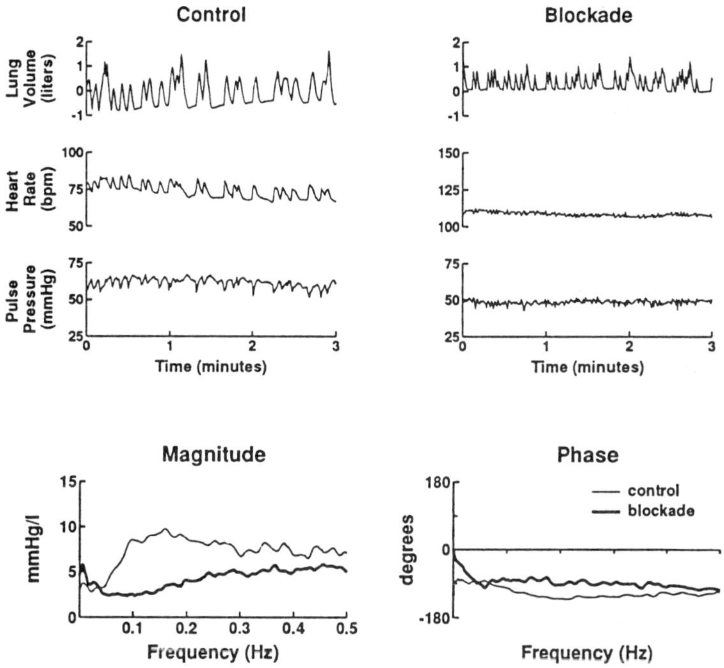

Figure 4. *Respiratory, heart rate, and pulse pressure times series over three minutes before and after complete autonomic blockade with atropine and propranolol. Group average transfer function magnitude and phase between respiration and pulse pressure are shown for 14 subjects in the same two conditions. In the time series, note that complete autonomic blockade takes away most, but not all, of the heart rate variability. A small amount of high-frequency (HF) variability remains coherent with the respiratory signal (see Fig. 5). In addition, pulse pressure variability remains after complete blockade, despite smaller breath size, indicating that there is a mechanical effect of respiration on blood pressure. The changes in blood pressure are markedly reduced, however, without the heart rate variability. This finding indicates that some RSA, probably produced through brain stem coupling, also affects blood pressure. The transfer functions show the same phenomena with disappearance of part, but not all, of the transfer magnitude during complete autonomic blockade, indicating a component for both RSA and mechanical effects of respiration on blood pressure.*

Nonautonomic

Although RSA is markedly attenuated by pharmacological or other means of vagal blockade,[13,15,18,19,22] a small RSA (~2 (beats/minute)/liter) persists even after combined pharmacological cardiac sympathetic and vagal blockade.[18] RSA of a similar magnitude has been reported in the transplanted denervated human heart.[54,55] These findings indicate that at least part of RSA originates from an intracardiac mechanism, either an intracardiac reflex or mechanical stretch of the SA node. Stretch-induced changes in SA node rate have been documented experimentally in animals,[56,57] but the magnitude of these responses is difficult to compare with data in the intact human. Saul et al[18] found that the transfer relation between respiration and heart rate after complete autonomic blockade had features that were qualitatively similar to those of a positive differentiator; i.e., increasing magnitude with frequency and a phase near 90° (Fig. 5). This finding suggests that nonautonomic RSA is related to the rate of change of lung volume, and is consistent with an atrial stretch mechanism, since respiratory air flow is related to the intrathoracic pressure changes that drive changes in atrial size.[58] Bernardi et al[54] reached similar conclusions based on the observations of Saul et al.[18] Thus, in the absence of autonomic heart rate control, the relatively small effect of respiratory-induced SA node stretch on the SA nodal firing may become evident. Note that again the dependence of nonautonomic RSA on the frequency and amplitude of respiration is critical to understanding its origin.

Quantification of the Respiratory Sinus Arrhythmia

Simple Time Domain Parameters

In 1975, Katona and Jih[13] employed a combination of vagal cooling, pharmacological cardiac autonomic blockade, and phenylephrine-induced increases in arterial pressure to hypothesize that RSA could be used as a

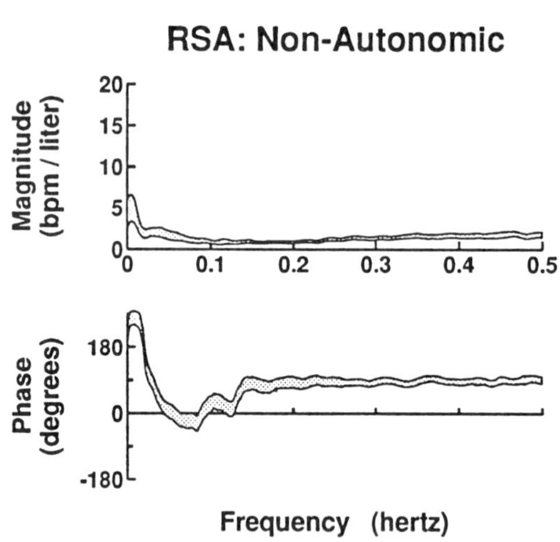

Figure 5. *After complete autonomic blockade with both propranolol and atropine, respiration still has a small effect on heart rate. Above 0.1 Hz, the effect increases with frequency and phase is very near 90°, consistent with the changes in heart rate being related to the derivative of the lung volume signal (respiratory flow). See Figure 4 for the times series showing the residual, mechanically-induced changes of heart rate. Gray stippled area indicates standard error.*

quantitative measure of parasympathetic cardiac control. Although the validity of that hypothesis is discussed below, it immediately stimulated interest in the task of quantifying RSA. Since then, numerous techniques have been used. In their report, Katona and Jih[13] derived two pertinent parameters that have been used in a variety of studies. The first parameter was what they termed the variation in heart period (VHP), defined as the peak-to-trough change in RR interval during a single breath and averaged over a certain number of breaths (Fig. 6). The second parameter, which they called parasympathetic control (PC), was the decrease in RR interval in milliseconds caused by elimination of the parasympathetic influences on the heart while sympathetic activity remained unchanged. Though heart rate is occasionally substituted for RR interval, numerous investigators have employed some variation of the VHP.[2–4,15,28,33,59] As a corollary to the VHP, Eckberg[1] proposed that the standard deviation of RR intervals (STD-RR) was closely correlated with the VHP as a quantitative measure of RSA.

The most obvious deficit of the VHP or STD-RR is that neither of these parameters take into account the respiratory stimulus characteristics, most notably the frequency of respiration and the amplitude of the breaths. In addition, both measures are subject to random errors introduced by the fact that all sinus arrhythmia is not coincident with respiration. Numerous physiological noise sources, such as central command and the arterial and cardiopulmonary baroreflexes, also contribute to sinus arrhythmia. To address the latter concern, several investigators have used the heart rate power spectrum to identify specifically the portion of the heart rate variance that is coincident with respiration, while others have simultaneously addressed both of the above issues by quantifying the frequency response of heart rate to respiratory activity.

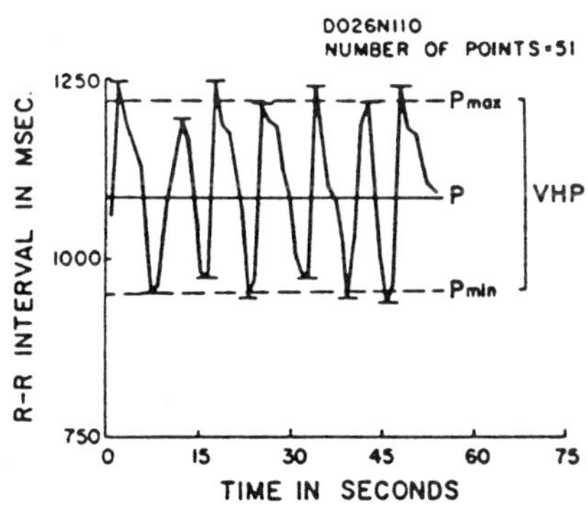

Figure 6. *Variation in heart period (VHP) is calculated as the difference between the maximum and minimum RR interval that occurs during each breath. It has often been calculated at a breathing rate of 6 breaths/min. Reproduced with permission from Fouad FM, Tarazi RC, Ferrario CM, et al: Assessment of parasympathetic control of heart rate by a noninvasive method. Am J Physiol 246:H839, 1984.*

Heart Rate Spectral Analysis

From an engineering standpoint, the variations of a periodic signal may be quantified in either the time domain or the frequency domain. The frequency domain approach, however, is often used to enhance the interpretation. One technique for transforming a time-based signal into one based on frequency is to use the power spectrum to quantify the variance as a function of frequency. Although use of such a technique now seems natural for studying the time-varying properties of physiological signals, it was not until 1971, after the availability of digital computing, that Hyndman et al[60] first used power spectral analysis to assess heart rate variability. They divided the variance of heart rate into what appeared to be three distinct physiological peaks, one of which was coincident with the frequency of respiration, usually >0.15 Hz, and two of which were at lower frequencies. The variance related to each of these peaks can be quantified by simply computing the area of the spectrum (the power) in a specific frequency range. Although the origin of the lower frequency peaks has been a topic of much investigation and debate, the presence of these peaks, even during metronomic breathing at a single high respiratory frequency (Fig. 7), makes it clear that a significant portion of the heart rate variance may not be related to respiratory activity.

Discussion of these issues are, for the most part, beyond the scope of this chapter (see Kitney and Rompelman[61] and Saul[62]). Since 1971, it has become clear, however, that when the respiratory rate is above 0.15 Hz, the peak at the respiratory frequency is strictly related to respiration, and is mediated almost entirely by modulation of vagal efferent activity.[16,18,38,40] Clearly, the above findings indicate that quantifying RSA by computing the power of the respiratory frequency peak in the heart rate power spectrum is a superior method to either the VHP or the STD-RR, because a significant portion of the heart rate

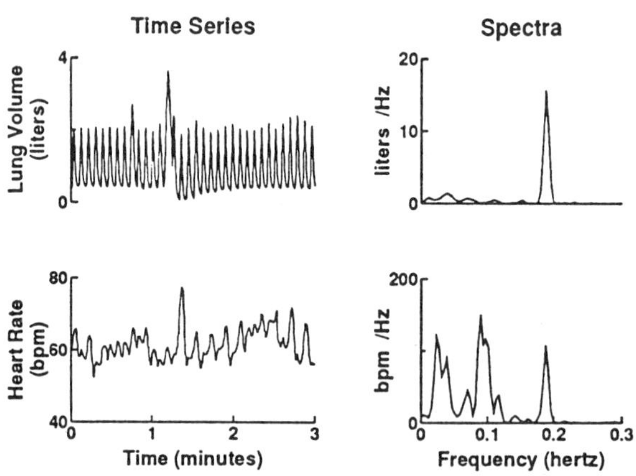

Figure 7. *Even when the respiratory rate is relatively fixed at near 0.2 Hz, heart rate fluctuations occur at lower frequencies, indicating that respiration does not explain all of the heart rate variability. Typical peaks in the heart rate power spectrum are at the respiratory frequency, near 0.1 Hz, and between 0.02 and 0.05 Hz.*

variance is not tied to respiratory activity. The findings also indicate that respiratory peaks at frequencies above 0.15 Hz specifically reflect modulation of vagal efferent activity by respiration. Some investigators have used the respiratory peak in the heart rate power spectrum as a measure of the mean level of cardiac vagal efferent activity, or tone.[39,63,64] The amplitude or area of the respiratory peak in the heart rate power spectrum, however, clearly depends not only on mean vagal activity, but also on both the frequency and tidal volume of respiration. Alternatively, the transfer function, or frequency response between respiration and heart rate which measures the gain and phase of the heart rate response to respiratory activity as a function of both the frequency and amplitude of respiration, may more accurately characterize RSA. Frequency responses are most often used to characterize the responses of physical systems, such as the transmission characteristics of an arterial catheter or the sound reproduction of a stereo speaker, but they can also be used to characterize physiological systems, such as the human ear or the autonomic nervous system.

Frequency Response

Hirsch and Bishop[2] systematically evaluated RSA as a phenomenon by having subjects breathe at a variety of frequencies and tidal volumes and quantitatively measuring the respiratory signal. They then quantified the response of heart rate to respiration as a function of the respiratory frequency between 0.015 and 1 Hz. The phase relations between respiration and heart rate were not investigated, but their magnitude data for this frequency response were plotted in the form of a Bode plot (Fig. 8), as what is known as a

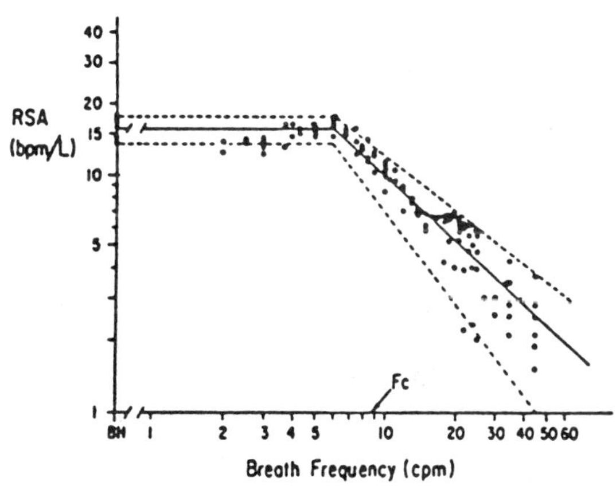

Figure 8. *Transfer function between respiration and heart rate derived by having individuals breathe at a range of frequencies from breath hold to 60 breaths/min. The corner frequency was found to be 9 breaths/min (0.15 Hz), with a roll-off of 19.6 dB/decade. The amplitude data are remarkably similar to that shown in Figure 3 for vagal heart rate control. Reproduced with permission from Hirsch JA, Bishop B: Respiratory sinus arrhythmia in humans: How breathing pattern modulates heart rate. Am J Physiol 241:H625, 1981.*

describing function. They found that, for either individuals or for a group of subjects, the phenomenon of RSA could be described well as a low-pass filter, with a corner frequency of 0.12 Hz (7.2 breaths/minute), a low-frequency (LF) maximum gain of 19.9 (beats/minute)/liter, and a high-frequency (HF) roll-off of 20.6 dB/decade.[2]

Although Hirsch and Bishop's study[2] was the first systematic investigation of the effects of both respiratory frequency and tidal volume on RSA, Angelone and Coulter[5] in 1964, performed an intriguing, but limited study of the effects of breathing frequency on heart rate. Again using a Bode plot to display the frequency response, but this time with phase information included, they arrived at results that were very similar to those of Hirsch and Bishop, but there were a few important differences. First, the peak magnitude of their response occurred at about 0.1 Hz, it decreased as frequency became either higher or lower, and a system resonance occurred at or near 0.1 Hz. Second, the phase plot demonstrated that the phase lag from respiration to heart rate changed as a function of the respiratory frequency such that, at lower frequencies, expiration and heart rate increases were in phase, whereas at higher frequencies close to a typical respiratory rate of 0.2 Hz (12 breaths/minute), inspiration and rising heart rate were in phase. Angelone and Coulter[5] also proposed that the response of respiration to heart rate, in terms of both magnitude and phase, was that of a low-pass filter, with phase characteristics suggesting that heart rate increases with expiration, but with delay increasing as a function of frequency. It may be important to note that their experimental subject was sitting. Using different analysis techniques, Eckberg[3] also determined that both the magnitude and the phase of the response of heart rate to respiration were dependent on the frequency of breathing.

Recently, Berger et al[65] devised a method for characterizing both the phase and magnitude of RSA over a broad range of physiological respiratory frequencies from zero to about 0.5 Hz. The method involves computing the frequency response (or transfer function) between a quantitative respiratory signal and heart rate during six-minute periods in which the respiratory rate is voluntarily controlled in a predetermined but erratic fashion (Fig. 3, Time Series). The method provides relatively complete characterization of RSA by providing a respiratory stimulus that contains energy over a broad range of frequencies (Fig. 3, Spectra). In addition, the method indicates relative linearity of RSA by demonstrating that the magnitude and phase of the responses are similar whether the respiratory stimulus is broad-band or fixed rate (Fig. 9), and that the coherence between the two signals is relatively high (> 0.5). The coherence function, which varies from 0 to 1, is a measure of both linearity and statistical reliability of the transfer function.

These investigators used this transfer function method in combination with maneuvers that alter the mean levels of cardiac sympathetic and parasympathetic efferent activity to investigate the individual contributions of each of the cardiac autonomic branches and arterial blood pressure fluctuations to observed RSA.[17,18] They found that:

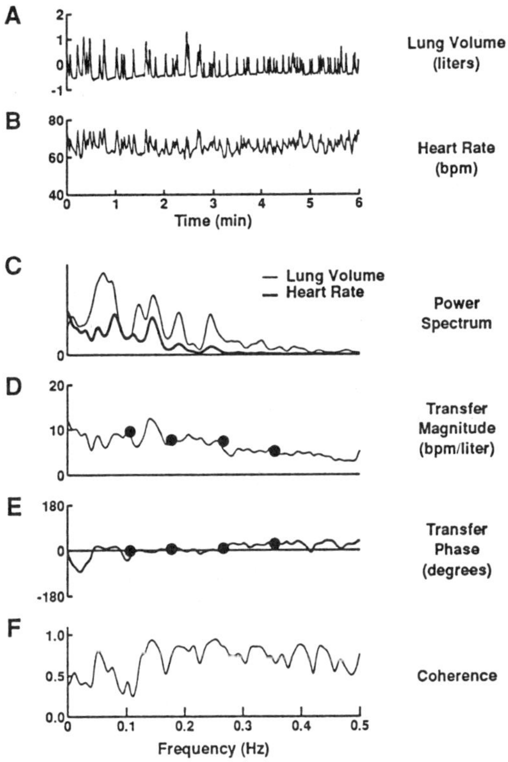

Figure 9. *Random interval breathing broadens the frequency content of the lung volume signal and the heart rate signal. This technique allows for efficient characterization of both the magnitude and phase of the transfer function between 0 and 0.5 Hz. Coherence is relatively high (>0.5) throughout the entire frequency range. Data from a subject who performed the random interval technique and breathed at the individual frequencies of 0.1, 0.17, 0.25, and 0.33 Hz shows virtual superimposition (●) using the two techniques.*

1. in agreement with previous investigators,[2,5] RSA is a frequency-dependent phenomenon with magnitude and phase characteristics of a low-pass filter;
2. RSA is dependent on modulation of both cardiac parasympathetic and sympathetic activity;
3. sympathetic RSA is characterized by markedly reduced magnitude at frequencies above 0.1 Hz and a phase delay, whereas vagal RSA is characterized by higher magnitude at all frequencies and a slight phase lead (heart rate leads respiration) (Fig. 3); and
4. RSA results from both a central link between the respiratory centers and the heart rate control centers in the brain stem, and a mechanical link between respiration and arterial pressure (Fig. 4). The role of cardiopulmonary receptors in mediating RSA was not specifically investigated in these studies.

Other Methods

A variety of other time and frequency domain techniques to quantify RSA have either been used or proposed. Porges[66] devised a method for removing LF (<0.2 Hz) heart rate oscillations that are usually below the respiratory frequency by filtering the heart rate time series with a moving polynomial. Although the method effectively eliminates heart rate fluctuations at low frequencies, it ignores the fact that respiratory activity may occur at any frequency and provides little additional information to that obtained from appropriately quantified spectral techniques. Hrushesky et al[8,9] entrained the respiratory pattern to a particular heart rate sequence and then quantified RSA as the amplitude of a cosine function that best fit the heart rate data. Their technique provides data similar to that obtained by the VHP method during fixed rate breathing, and it suffers similarly from a lack of information on respiratory volume. The method also allows respiratory rate to vary both between individuals and as a function of mean heart rate that is closely related to age, a deficit when studying a frequency-dependent phenomenon. More recently, Appel et al[67,68] have used an autoregressive moving average technique to compute the time domain impulse response function between a quantitative respiratory signal and heart rate. Their technique has been extended by Yana et al[69] by fixing the model order at two, as determined from previous experimental results on vagal and sympathetic control of heart rate.[18,40] Early results have demonstrated that vagal and sympathetic gain factors for heart rate control can be deduced by simply measuring the response of heart rate to a broad-band respiratory signal. The method must still be tested in a variety of physiological conditions.

Finally, it must be recognized that nonlinearities are present in every physiological system, and RSA is no exception. Although useful, the transfer function techniques used by Saul et al[17,18] have consistently found that, even at higher respiratory frequencies above 0.15 Hz, the coherence between respiration and heart rate is less than one. Thus, respiration does not account for all of the heart rate variance, either due to other physiological mechanisms affecting heart rate at those frequencies, system nonlinearities, or a combination of both. Eckberg[3] used Lissajous plots to demonstrate that the response of heart rate to respiration had a hysteresis, partly due to differences between the response to inspiration and expiration. The hysteresis indicated a nonlinearity in the response. Clynes,[10] using somewhat nonphysiological respiratory waveforms, demonstrated that the heart rate responses to held expiration and inspiration were similar. These responses also indicated nonlinearity. Linear analysis techniques offer significant computational and practical advantages, and appear to be adequate for the usual RSA, where respiratory activity primarily involves small fluctuations of lung volume around a mean operating point. A complete quantification of RSA, however, might need to include some information derived from nonlinear analysis techniques.

What is Respiratory Sinus Arrhythmia?

Despite the large number of studies that have been carried out to determine the mechanisms that generate RSA, only a few firm conclusions can be drawn. These conclusions, which support some role for a variety of the proposed mechanisms reviewed above, are discussed below. Alternatively, the mechanisms that directly mediate the heart rate fluctuations of RSA have been much more clearly defined.

Respiratory Sinus Arrhythmia Mediation

The available data indicate strongly that the changes in heart rate associated with respiratory activity are mediated primarily by a combination of changing levels of efferent cardiac vagal and sympathetic activity, and mechanically-induced SA node stretch with each breath. The degree of the contribution from each of these mechanisms is related to the frequency and amplitude of the respiratory signal, the mean levels of vagal and sympathetic activity, and the mechanical state of the airways.

As shown in Figure 3, in adult humans, respiratory modulation of cardiac vagal activity has the potential to influence heart rate changes at all relevant physiological frequencies between 0 and 0.5 Hz. The magnitude of the response reaches a maximum at about 0.2 Hz, and decreases as frequency either increases or decreases. Also, between 0 and 0.5 Hz, the magnitude is significantly larger than that for either modulation of sympathetic activity (Fig. 3), or the mechanical effect (Fig. 5). For subjects in the supine position, respiratory modulation of vagal activity results in an increase in heart rate just prior to the onset of inspiration (Fig. 9), and the phase characteristics suggest that a decrease in vagal efferent activity precedes inspiratory movement by approximately 0.3 to 0.5 seconds.[17,18,21]

Respiratory modulation of cardiac sympathetic activity occurs at all relevant physiological frequencies.[70,71] Due to frequency-limited adrenergic receptor responses,[72] however, it only influences heart rate significantly at frequencies below 0.15 Hz (Fig. 3).[40] In addition, even at low frequencies, the magnitude of the response is smaller than that for respiratory modulation of vagal activity. The phase characteristics of the sympathetic heart rate response demonstrate that, at low respiratory frequencies, heart rate actually decreases with inspiration. As the frequency increases to near 0.1 Hz, a phase delay makes it appear that heart rate increases with inspiration. Finally, as frequency increases above 0.1 Hz, the small heart rate increases that occur begin to lag after inspiration. These data suggest strongly that, as with vagal activity, sympathetic efferent activity decreases near the beginning of inspiration. The heart rate response is then determined entirely by the response characteristics of the SA node to modulation of sympathetic or vagal activity.[40]

The magnitude of the nonautonomic mechanical RSA reaches a minimum near 0.15 Hz. Above 0.15 Hz, it increases linearly with frequency and has a phase of almost exactly 90° degrees, but below 0.15 Hz, no obvious magnitude or phase pattern is discernable (Fig. 5). Also, at frequencies above 0.15 Hz, the magnitude is small compared to that for vagally-mediated RSA (maximum of ~2 beats/minute at 0.5 Hz), but it probably accounts for all of HF RSA under conditions of vagal blockade (Fig. 3 versus Fig. 5). Perhaps most importantly, as discussed above, the magnitude and phase characteristics of the nonautonomic transfer function at frequencies above 0.15 Hz are identical to those of a differentiator. These characteristics indicate that mechanical RSA is related to the rate of change of lung volume or respiratory flow rate. Since respiratory flow rate is closely linked to intrathoracic pressure, which is related to atrial size, mechanical RSA is likely due to SA node stretch.

Respiratory Sinus Arrhythmia Generation

The available data reviewed above (specifically including the finding that the vagally-mediated heart rate changes often precede the onset of inspiration) indicate that a direct central link exists between the respiratory and heart rate control centers in the brain stem. The data do not differentiate between a link that involves modulation of carotid–heart rate BRS and one that does not. In addition, previous investigations indicate that the mechanical effects of respiration help mediate RSA through central reflex arcs. Despite numerous studies, the contributions of afferent signals from receptors in the chest wall, the lungs, the atria and ventricles, and the carotid arteries and aorta cannot be identified precisely. Perhaps the best data to differentiate these mechanisms was derived from the study by Melcher[4] that used continuous negative inspiratory pressure and voluntarily controlled breathing to vary intrathoracic pressure and tidal volume independently. He found that RSA was more closely linked to intrathoracic pressure than to tidal volume, regardless of the combination of these factors used to achieve a given pressure.[4] Melcher[4] also found that, during these maneuvers, changes in central venous pressure were more closely linked to RSA than were changes in arterial pressure. Thus, this data suggest that the portion of RSA due to the mechanical effects of breathing is mediated primarily through modulation of cardiopulmonary volume receptors.

Together, the above data suggest a physiological snapshot of RSA. In this view, respiration simultaneously influences heart rate directly in the CNS and via SA node stretch, and indirectly through arterial and cardiopulmonary reflex stimulation. This snapshot is summarized in the model shown in Figure 10. Much of the model has been described previously in detail,[18] but the salient features for this discussion are that one, respiration enters the cardiovascular control loop both mechanically and centrally; two, the mechanical effect of respiration influences multiple systems; three, the closed loop nature of heart rate and blood pressure control makes conclusions about causality in such a system difficult to draw; and four, no matter what the stimulus, heart rate

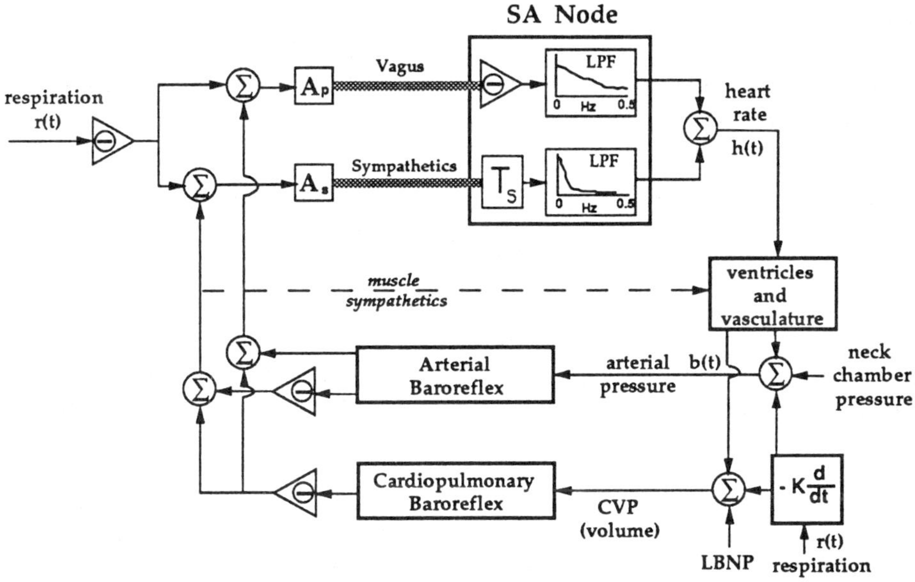

Figure 10. *Simple model of heart rate control showing respiration entering the control system mechanically and its effect on vagal and sympathetic activity in the brain stem. All baroreflex and respiratory heart rate responses are filtered through the SA node. The effect of peripheral sympathetic activity on the muscle vasculature is not accurately defined.*

changes represent a filtered version of the vagal and sympathetic signals that impinge on the SA node. Despite its apparent complexity, the analytical results of a slightly simpler version of this model have demonstrated that the model closely mimics the experimental RSA frequency response functions under the "pure" physiological vagal and sympathetic states shown in Figure 3, as well as the mixed autonomic states of supine and standing posture in control conditions.[18]

Sinus Arrhythmia: Nonrespiratory

As noted in the above section entitled "Heart Rate Spectral Analysis," respiration by no means accounts for all of the variance in the heart rate signal. Normally, respiration occurs mainly at frequencies above 0.15 Hz, whereas significant heart rate spectral peaks in a variety of settings occur at frequencies below 0.15 Hz (Fig. 7).[16,38,62,73] These lower frequency heart rate fluctuations are sinus arrhythmia, but are not part of RSA. They can occur at any frequency, but are often observed in two typical frequency bands: one near 0.1 Hz, which is considered important in arterial blood pressure control, and one between 0.01 and 0.06 Hz, which is related to a variety of physiological stimuli, including temperature fluctuations, hemorrhage, cardiac output, and LF oscillations of respiratory tidal volume (periodic breathing).[74–77] Finally, the vast majority of the variance in heart rate (sinus arrhythmia) occurs at very low frequencies less than 0.01 Hz.[78,79] These very slow fluctuations of heart rate are as yet poorly defined, but they may be related to the relatively large effects of changes in activity level throughout a normal day.

Does Respiratory Sinus Arrhythmia Measure Vagal Tone?

In 1975, Katona and Jih[13] published a study that has now become the theoretical and experimental backbone of the claim that RSA is a quantitative measure of mean cardiac vagal efferent activity. Katona et al[21] had previously found that RSA in chloralose-anesthetized dogs is due primarily to cessation of vagal efferent activity during inspiration. Hence, these investigators proposed that the VHP (see above) is linearly related to PC, defined above as the decrease in RR interval (in milliseconds) caused by elimination of the parasympathetic influences on the heart while keeping sympathetic activity unchanged. This relationship is illustrated by the following equation:

$$\mathrm{VHP} = \alpha\mathrm{PC}.$$

To substantiate their proposal, Katona et al[21] showed that the correlation coefficient between VHP and PC during combinations of propranolol, phenylephrine, and atropine averaged 0.969 in the seven dogs they studied.

Since that study, numerous investigators have used various techniques to attempt to establish a similar relationship in humans. Fouad et al[15] compared VHP during spontaneous breathing in four normotensive and nine hypertensive subjects to PC, determined by using complete muscarinic blockade with atropine. Despite the fact that respiratory rate and tidal volume were neither controlled nor accounted for, they found a highly significant correlation ($r = 0.904$) between VHP and PC across the group of subjects. Interestingly, the correlation between VHP and PC deteriorated somewhat when the subjects first underwent β-adrenergic blockade with propranolol. This finding suggested that either VHP or the PC measurement in the subjects was at least partially under the influence of cardiac sympathetic outflow. Fouad et al[15] also made no attempt to test the VHP–PC relation within subjects, as Katona and Jih[13] had done in the dog. Eckberg et al,[80] as part of a study of baroreflex changes in muscle sympathetic activity, found that VHP decreased during reductions of blood pressure and during presumed decreases in mean cardiac vagal efferent activity induced by nitroprusside. VHP did not change, however, during elevations of blood pressure or during presumed increases in mean vagal activity induced by phenylephrine. Using a nearly identical experimental protocol, Saul et al[70] found that the power of the respiratory peak in the heart rate power spectrum did not change significantly with either elevations or reductions of arterial pressure. Furthermore, in agreement with some previous data from anesthetized dogs,[81] we have observed in young healthy adults that elevations of blood pressure induced by phenylephrine may actually eliminate RSA (Fig. 11). Together, these data suggest that, in contrast to the findings of Katona and Jih[13] in anesthetized dogs, RSA may not always correlate with mean cardiac vagal efferent activity or tone in humans with high-resting levels of vagal activity.

If RSA does not necessarily reflect mean vagal outflow, what does it tell us? As discussed above, RSA results mainly from modulation of cardiac vagal and sympathetic efferent activity with respiration, and above 0.15 Hz, from modulation only of cardiac vagal activity. Given a constant link between changes in heart rate and changes in cardiac vagal activity, RSA at frequencies above 0.15 Hz specifically reflects modulation of cardiac vagal activity by respiration, and the heart's response to that modulation. Thus, by quantifying RSA, the transfer function between respiration and heart rate provides a clinical measure of the responsiveness of the heart to autonomic influences. Above 0.15 Hz, it provides a measure of parasympathetic responsiveness. Few other measures of vagal cardiac control exist, and none are so easily applicable to the study of a broad range of clinical conditions in humans.

Clinical Utility of the Respiratory Sinus Arrhythmia

As noted above, RSA is not a clinical measure of mean cardiac vagal efferent activity, but it does quantify vagal responsiveness, which is an important clinical parameter. In fact, extensive data correlate RSA with clinical outcome in a variety of disease states. Perhaps the earliest and most frequent application of RSA has been in formal autonomic testing of patients

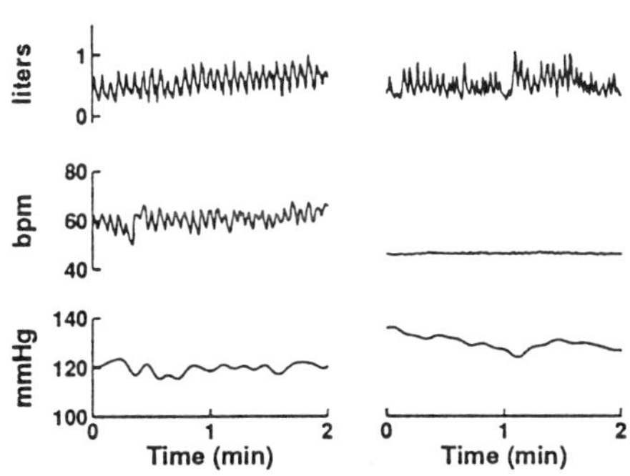

Figure 11. *Respiration (upper trace), heart rate (middle trace), and mean blood pressure (lower trace) before (left panel) and during (right panel) an infusion of phenylephrine. In this subject, RSA was quite prominent at baseline. As with a few other subjects, when mean blood pressure was raised by phenylephrine, RSA almost completely disappeared. Note mean heart rate of approximately 40, suggesting high mean vagal activity during absence of sinus arrhythmia. The data strongly suggest that the amplitude of vagal modulation and heart rate modulation are not always correlated with mean vagal activity, possibly due to saturation of the vagal or the heart rate responses.*

with suspected diabetic neuropathy. Wheeler and Watkins,[82] in 1973, may have been the first to report an absence of RSA during spontaneous and controlled (6 to 8 breaths/minute) deep breathing in diabetic patients with clinically apparent peripheral neuropathy. They postulated that the abnormality reflected vagal denervation of the heart. Although their findings have now been confirmed by other investigators[83,84] using a six breaths/minute breathing protocol, the results of these studies are difficult to interpret precisely because of the chosen respiratory rate of 0.1 Hz (6 breaths/minute). As noted above, sinus arrhythmia at frequencies <0.15 Hz is mediated by modulation of both vagal and sympathetic efferent activity. In addition, a spontaneous heart rate oscillation that is reduced significantly by either atropine or propranolol often occurs at frequencies very near 0.1 Hz,[16] bringing into question the usefulness of the commonly used 6 breaths/minute RSA test as a measure of cardiac vagal control. Nonetheless, more recent studies employing spectral analysis have demonstrated that a higher frequency RSA above 0.15 Hz is often decreased in diabetic subjects and correlates with standard tests of autonomic function.[85,86] We have demonstrated further, using the quantitative transfer function technique during random interval breathing described above, that one, RSA magnitude is less in diabetic subjects without clinical neuropathy than in normal controls; two, RSA magnitude becomes progressively smaller with increasing degree of neuropathy; and three, in agreement with Watkins and Mackay,[87] the peak magnitude of RSA shifts from around 0.1 Hz to lower frequencies as the degree of neuropathy increases. Thus, in diabetics RSA seems to provide data suggesting that cardiac vagal control of heart rate progressively decreases as the neuropathy increases.

Numerous other examples have been observed of changes in RSA magnitude as a reflection of alterations in physiological state. Hellman and Stacy[7] noted that RSA decreases as a function of age, a finding that has been confirmed in many studies.[2,8,9,39,73] Previous data from Eckberg et al[88] suggest that both vagal tone and responsiveness were decreased in patients with chronic congestive heart failure (CHF). In agreement, Saul et al[73] used spectral analysis of respiration and heart rate, and they found that RSA was less in this patient group than in normal controls. Although no correlation between RSA and mortality was found, their heart failure study group consisted of only 25 patients whose median survival was about five months.[73] No large prospective study has been performed to test the value of using RSA to predict prognosis independently in patients with moderate to severe failure. Hrushesky et al[9] recently reported that a decrease in RSA, however, actually preceded the onset of doxorubicin-induced cardiotoxicity in a group of eight adults who developed CHF. By normalizing their RSA values for patient age, Hrushesky et al[9] were able to demonstrate an 87.5% sensitivity for prediction of heart failure by a low RSA, a prediction that was significantly better than their findings for radionuclide ventricular ejection fraction. Due to the wide variance of RSA values in normal subjects, however, their specificity was only 80.8%. Despite any limitations, their data do demonstrate the clinical usefulness of RSA measurements.

A number of investigators have demonstrated that total heart rate variability, including all sinus arrhythmia, decreases after an acute myocardial infarction, and the variability may predict long-term prognosis.[89–91] Kleiger et al[89] actually found that total heart rate variability over 24 hours independently predicted mortality better than any of the traditional clinical parameters they investigated, including decreased ejection fraction, rales, and ventricular arrhythmias. Total heart rate variability, however, includes and is usually dominated by heart rate changes that are not related to respiration. In fact, as the observation period grows, less and less of heart rate variability is due to RSA.[78] Lombardi et al[63] showed that the percentage of heart rate variance related to RSA was decreased at two weeks after an acute myocardial infarction, and subsequently returned to normal over the next year. Although no predictive value was noted in their group of 70 subjects, Rosenbaum et al,[92] using a similar measure of RSA, found that a decrease in RSA was predictive of ventricular arrhythmia induction in dogs with myocardial infarction. Similarly, in humans, Myers et al[93] noted a decrease in the respiratory frequency component of the heart rate power spectrum in patients who had been previously resuscitated from sudden cardiac death and had inducible ventricular arrhythmias at electrophysiology study, compared to normal controls and noninducible patients with high-grade ventricular ectopy. In addition, using the method of Porges,[66] Billman and Hoskins[94] demonstrated that exercise elicited a significantly greater reduction in RSA during exercise in dogs that were known to be susceptible to ventricular fibrillation during brief coronary occlusions than in those dogs known to be resistant. Their data in normal dogs agreed with a previous human study, which showed that RSA decreased progressively during exercise, and eventually became less than 1% of its preexercise value at maximal exercise.[95] Also, they suggested that their data indicated a more complete withdrawal of vagal tone during exercise in the susceptible dogs and speculated on the clinical usefulness of such a test. Supporting such a hypothesis, Hayano et al[96] recently reported a significant correlation between a power spectral measure of RSA and the angiographic severity of coronary artery stenoses, independent of any changes in left ventricular function or a history of myocardial infarction. The use of RSA quantification as a clinical parameter in the management of coronary artery disease clearly deserves further investigation.

RSA has also been quantified in a number of studies investigating the role of the autonomic nervous system in pediatric diseases. Although the data are variable, the evidence suggests that RSA represents a smaller portion of the heart rate variance in normal newborn infants,[97] infants who subsequently die of sudden infant death syndrome (SIDS),[98] and in critically ill children with heart disease[99] as compared to that in normal children. The Porges technique[66] to measure RSA has been used to document changes in RSA that accompany stressful events, such as circumcision,[100] as well as to predict developmental outcome,[101] later occurrence of chronic lung disease,[102] and the duration of hospital stay.[103] Whether the authors' claims in these studies that RSA measurements reflect vagal tone is true, it is clear that the changes in RSA they document do bear a significant relation to clinical state and probably provide useful information for patient management and for understanding the underlying physiology.

The prominence of RSA as a biological phenomenon has led to many other studies of its potential clinical role, including its use in the diagnosis of familial dysautonomia and of unexplained syncope, and in monitoring the effects of digoxin in patients with CHF.[104–106] Many of these studies are preliminary, however, and often involve a small number of subjects and a variety of techniques to measure RSA.

Summary

RSA is a biological phenomenon that is nearly ubiquitous in large mammals. It reflects the complex effects of central respiratory drive on the integration of autonomic afferent signals and the production of autonomic efferent signals in the brain stem, and of respiratory mechanics on the cardiovascular structures within the thorax. The phenomenon is dependent on the frequency and amplitude of respiration, as well as on the underlying autonomic state of the organism. The magnitude and phase characteristics of RSA during different physiological states suggest that it is mediated by respiratory modulation of both cardiac sympathetic and vagal efferent activity, and mechanical stretch of the SA node. Finally, due to its complex nature, changes in RSA accompany a large variety of disease states and are potentially useful in the diagnosis and management of human disease.

References

1. Eckberg DL: Respiratory sinus arrhythmia: A window on central autonomic regulation in man. In S Hunyor, J Ludbrook, J Shaw, et al (eds): The Peripheral Circulation. Amsterdam, Elsevier Science Publishers, 1984, pp. 267–274.
2. Hirsch JA, Bishop B: Respiratory sinus arrhythmia in humans: How breathing pattern modulates heart rate. Am J Physiol 241:H620–H629, 1981.
3. Eckberg DL: Human sinus arrhythmia as an index of vagal cardiac outflow. J Applied Physiol 54:961–966, 1983.
4. Melcher A: Respiratory sinus arrhythmia in man. A study in heart rate regulating mechanisms. Acta Physiol Scand (suppl) 435:1–31, 1976.
5. Angelone A, Coulter NA: Respiratory sinus arrhythmia: A frequency dependent phenomenon. J Applied Physiol 19:479–482, 1964.
6. Davies CTM, Neilson JMM: Sinus arrhythmia in man at rest. J Applied Physiol 22:947–955, 1967.
7. Hellman JB, Stacy RW: Variation of respiratory sinus arrhythmia with age. J Applied Physiol 41:734–738, 1976.
8. Hrushesky WJM, Fader D, Schmitt O, et al: The respiratory sinus arrhythmia: A measure of cardiac age. Science 224:1001–1004, 1984.
9. Hrushesky WJM, Fader DJ, Berestka JS, et al: Diminishment of respiratory sinus arrhythmia foreshadows doxorubicin-induced cardiomyopathy. Circulation 84:697–707, 1991.
10. Clynes M: Respiratory sinus arrhythmia: Laws derived from computer simulation. J Applied Physiol 15:863–874, 1960.
11. Eckberg DL, Nerhed C, Wallin BG: Respiratory modulation of muscle sympathetic and vagal cardiac outflow in man. J Physiol (Lond) 365:181–196, 1985.

12. Barman SM, Gebber GL: Basis for synchronization of sympathetic and phrenic nerve discharges. Am J Physiol 231:1601–1607, 1976.
13. Katona PG, Jih F: Respiratory sinus arrhythmia: Noninvasive measure of parasympathetic cardiac control. J Applied Physiol 39:801–805, 1975.
14. Chess GF, Tam RMK, Calaresu FR: Influence of cardiac neural inputs on rhythmic variations of heart period in the cat. Am J Physiol 228:775–780, 1975.
15. Fouad FM, Tarazi RC, Ferrario CM, et al: Assessment of parasympathetic control of heart rate by a noninvasive method. Am J Physiol 246:H838–H842, 1984.
16. Pomeranz B, MaCaulay RJB, Caudill MA, et al: Assessment of autonomic function in humans by heart rate spectral analysis. Am J Physiol 248:H151–H153, 1985.
17. Saul JP, Berger RD, Chen MH, et al: Transfer function analysis of autonomic regulation. II. Respiratory sinus arrhythmia. Am J Physiol 25:H153–H161, 1989.
18. Saul JP, Berger RD, Albrecht P, et al: Transfer function analysis of the circulation: Unique insights into cardiovascular regulation. Am J Physiol 261:H1231–1245, 1991.
19. Levy MN, DeGeest H, Zieske H: Effects of respiratory center activity on the heart. Circ Res 18:67–78, 1966.
20. Sands KEF, Appel ML, Lilly LS, et al: Power spectrum analysis of heart rate variability in human cardiac transplant recipients. Circulation 79:76–82, 1989.
21. Katona PG, Poitras JW, Barnett GO, et al: Cardiac vagal efferent activity and heart period in the carotid sinus reflex. Am J Physiol 218:1030–1037, 1970.
22. Anrep GV, Pascual W, Rossler R: Respiratory variations of the heart rate. II. The central mechanism of the respiratory arrhythmia and the inter-relations between the central and reflex mechanisms. Proc R Soc Lond (Biol) 119:218–232, 1936.
23. Heymans C, Neil E: Reflexogenic Areas of the Cardiovascular System. Boston, MA, Little, Brown and Co, 1958.
24. Joels N, Samueloff M: The activity of the medullary centres in diffusion respiration. J Physiol (Lond) 133:360–372, 1956.
25. Hamlin RL, Smith CR, Smetzer DL: Sinus arrhythmia in the dog. Am J Physiol 210:321–328, 1966.
26. Traube L: Ueber periodische Thatigkeits-Aeusserungen des vasomotorischen und Hemmungs-Nervencentrums. Zbl Med Wiss 56:881–885, 1865.
27. Eckberg DL, Kifle YT, Roberts VL: Phase relationship between normal human respiration and baroreflex responsiveness. J Physiol (Lond) 304:489–502, 1980.
28. Melcher A: Carotid baroreflex heart rate control during the active and the assisted breathing cycle in man. Acta Physiol Scand 108:165–171, 1980.
29. Haymet BT, McCloskey DI: Baroreceptor and chemoreceptor influences on heart rate during the respiratory cycle in the dog. J Physiol (Lond) 245:699–712, 1975.
30. Bainbridge FA: The influence of venous filling upon the rate of the heart. J Physiol (Lond) 50:65–84, 1915.
31. Bainbridge FA: The relation between respiration and the pulse-rate. J Physiol (Lond) 54:192–202, 1920.
32. Kitney RI, Fulton T, McDonald AH, et al: Transient interactions between blood pressure, respiration and heart rate in man. J Biomed Eng 7:217–224, 1985.
33. Freyschuss U, Melcher A: Respiratory sinus arrhythmia in man: Relation to cardiovascular pressures. Scand J Clin Lab Invest 36:221–229, 1976.
34. Manzotti M: The effects of some respiratory manoevres on the heart rate. J Physiol (Lond) 144:541–557, 1958.
35. Angelone A, Coulter NA: Heart rate response to held lung volume. J Applied Physiol 20:464–468, 1965.
36. Gootman PM, Gootman N, Turlapaty PDMV, et al: Autonomic regulation of cardiovascular function in neonates. In G Burnstock (ed): Development of the Autonomic Nervous System. London, Pitman Medical, 1981, pp. 70–93.
37. Hukuhara T: Cross-correlation analysis of phase relation between respiratory volleys in the phrenic, sympathetic and vagus nerve activities under varied rhythm

conditions. In K Miyakawa, HP Koepchen, C Polosa (eds): Mechanism of Blood Pressure Waves. Tokyo, Japan Scientific Societies Press, 1984, pp. 65–73.
38. Akselrod SD, Gordon FA, Ubel DC, et al: Power spectrum analysis of heart rate fluctuations: A quantitative probe of beat-to-beat cardiovascular control. Science 213:220–222, 1981.
39. Pagani M, Lombardi F, Guzzetti S, et al: Power spectral analysis of heart rate and arterial pressure variabilities as a marker of sympatho-vagal interaction in man and conscious dog. Circ Res 59:178–193, 1986.
40. Berger RD, Saul JP, Cohen RJ: Transfer function analysis of autonomic regulation. I. The canine atrial rate response. Am J Physiol 25:H142–H152, 1989.
41. Olsen CO, Tyson GS, Maier GW, et al: Diminished stroke volume during inspiration: A reverse thoracic pump. Circulation 72:668–679, 1985.
42. Jurgen P, Fraser C, Stuart RS, et al: Negative intrathoracic pressure decreases independently left ventricular filling and emptying. Am J Physiol 257:H120–H131, 1989.
43. Jurgen P, Kindred MK, Robotham JL: Transient analysis of cardiopulmonary interactions. I. Diastolic events. J Appl Physiol 64:1506–1517, 1988.
44. Jurgen P, Kindred MK, Robotham JL: Transient analysis of cardiopulmonary interactions. I. Systolic events. J Appl Physiol 64:1518–1526, 1988.
45. Mark AL, Mancia G: Cardiopulmonary baroreflexes in humans. In JT Shepherd, FM Abboud (eds): Handbook of Physiology. Section 2, Vol. III, Part 2. Bethesda, MD, American Physiological Society, 1983, pp. 795–813.
46. Jennett S, McKillop JH: Observations on the incidence and mechanism of sinus arrhythmia in man at rest. J Physiol (Lond) 213:58P–59P, 1971.
47. Akselrod S, Gordon D, Madwed JB, et al: Hemodynamic regulation: Investigation by spectral analysis. Am J Physiol 249:H867–H875, 1985.
48. deBoer RW, Karemaker JM, Strackee J: Hemodynamic fluctuations and baroreflex sensitivity in humans: A beat-to-beat model. Am J Physiol 253:680–689, 1987.
49. Baselli G, Cerutti S, Civardi S, et al: Cardiovascular variability signals: Towards the identification of a closed-loop model of the neural control mechanisms. IEEE Trans Biomed Eng 35:1033–1046, 1988.
50. Hering E: Uber eine reflectorische Beziehung zwischen und Herz. Sitzber Akad Wiss Wien 64:333–353, 1871.
51. Hainsworth R: Circulatory responses from lung inflation in anesthetized dogs. Am J Physiol 226:247–255, 1974.
52. Glick G, Wechsler AS, Epstein SE, et al: Reflex cardiovascular depression produced by stimulation of pulmonary stretch receptors in the dog. J Clin Invest 48:467–473, 1969.
53. Clynes M: Computer analysis of reflex control and organization: Respiratory sinus arrhythmia. Science 131:300–302, 1960.
54. Bernardi L, Keller F, Sanders M, et al: Respiratory sinus arrhythmia in the denervated human heart. J Appl Physiol 67:1447–1455, 1989.
55. Bernardi L, Salvucci F, Suardi R, et al: Evidence for an intrinsic mechanism regulating heart rate variability in the transplanted and the intact heart during submaximal dynamic exercise? Cardiovasc Res 24:969–981, 1990.
56. James TN: The sinus node as a servomechanism. Circ Res 32:307–313, 1973.
57. Koizumi K, Ischikawa T, Nishono H, et al: Cardiac and autonomic system reactions to stretch of the atria. Brain Res 87:247–261, 1975.
58. West JB: Respiratory Physiology. Baltimore, MD, Williams & Wilkins, 1979, p. 103.
59. Ewing DJ: Cardiovascular reflexes in autonomic neuropathy. Clin Sci Mol Med 55: 321–327, 1978.
60. Hyndman BW, Kitney RI, Sayers BM: Spontaneous rhythms in physiological control systems. Nature 233:339–341, 1971.
61. Kitney RI, Rompelman O: The Study of Heart-Rate Variability. New York, NY, Oxford University Press, 1980.
62. Saul JP: Beat-to-beat variations of heart rate reflect modulation of cardiac autonomic outflow. NIPS 5:32–37, 1990.

63. Lombardi F, Sandrone G, Pernpruner S, et al: Heart rate variability as an index of sympathetic interaction after acute myocardial infarction. Am J Cardiol 60:1239–1245, 1987.
64. Izraeli S, Alcalay M, Tochner Z, et al: Pharmacological modulation of parasympathetic cardiac control: Dose-dependent effect of atropine on the power spectrum of heart rate fluctuations. Comp in Cardiol 16:57–60, 1989.
65. Berger RD, Saul JP, Cohen RJ: Assessment of autonomic response by broad-band respiration. IEEE Trans Biomed Eng BME-36:1061–1065, 1989.
66. Porges SW: Method and apparatus for evaluating rhythmic oscillations in periodic response systems. Patent number 4,510,944: April 16, 1985.
67. Appel ML, Berger RD, Saul JP, et al: Beat-to-beat variability in cardiovascular parameters: Noise or music? J Am Coll Cardiol 14:1139–1148, 1989.
68. Appel ML, Saul JP, Berger RD, et al: Closed loop identification of cardiovascular regulatory mechanisms. Comp in Cardiol 16:3–7, 1989.
69. Yana K, Saul JP, Berger RD, et al: Fluctuation analysis of the heart rate related to instantaneous lung volume: A time domain approach. Proc IEEE EMBS 790–792, 1990.
70. Saul JP, Rea RF, Eckberg DL, et al: Heart rate and muscle sympathetic nerve variability during reflex changes of autonomic activity. Am J Physiol 258:H713–H721, 1990.
71. Ninomiya I, Kujime K, Nishiura N, et al: Discharge pattern of sympathetic nerve to the heart in the conscious cat. In K Miyakawa, HP Koepohen, C Polosa (eds): Mechanisms of Blood Pressure Waves. Tokyo, Japan Scientific Societies Press, 1984, pp. 57–63.
72. Hill-Smith I, Purves RD: Synaptic delay in the heart: An ionophorctic study. J Physiol (Lond) 279:31–54, 1978.
73. Saul JP, Arai Y, Berger RD, et al: Assessment of autonomic regulation in chronic congestive heart failure by heart rate spectral analysis. Am J Cardiol 61:1292–1299, 1988.
74. Saul JP, Kaplan DT, Kitney RI: Nonlinear interactions between respiration and heart rate: A phenomenon common to multiple physiologic states. Comp in Cardiol 15:1988.
75. Kitney RI: An analysis of the nonlinear behaviour of the human thermal vasomotor control system. J Theor Biol 52:231–248, 1975.
76. Madwed JB: Dynamic Analysis of Arterial Blood Pressure and Heart Rate During Baseline Conditions and Hemorrhage in the Conscious Dog. Cambridge, MA, Harvard University, 1986. Thesis
77. Preiss G, Iscoe S, Polosa C: Analysis of a periodic breathing pattern associated with Mayer waves. Am J Physiol 228:768–774, 1975.
78. Saul JP, Albrecht P, Berger RD, et al: Analysis of long term heart rate variability: Methods, 1/f scaling and implications. Comp in Cardiol 14:419–422, 1987.
79. Kobayashi M, Musha T: 1/f fluctuation of heartbeat period. IEEE Trans Biomed Eng BME-29:456–457, 1982.
80. Eckberg DL, Rea RF, Anderson OK, et al: Baroreflex modulation of sympathetic activity and sympathetic neurotransmitters in man. Acta Physiol Scand 133:221–231, 1988.
81. Anrep GV, Pascual W, Rossler R: Respiratory variations of the heart rate. I. The reflex mechanism of the respiratory arrhythmia. Proc R Soc Lond (Biol) B 119:191–217, 1936.
82. Wheeler T, Watkins PJ: Cardiac denervation in diabetics. Brit Med J 4:584–586, 1973.
83. Ewing DJ, Clark BF: Autonomic neuropathy: Its diagnosis and prognosis. Clin Endocrinol Metab 15:855–888, 1986.
84. Ewing DJ: Practical bedside investigation of autonomic failure. In R Bannister (ed): Autonomic Failure: A Textbook of Clinical Disorders of the Autonomic Nervous System. Oxford, England, Oxford University Press, 1983, pp. 371–405.

85. Pagani M, Malfatto G, Pierini S, et al: Spectral analysis of heart rate variability in the assessment of autonomic diabetic neuropathy. J Auton Nerv Sys 23:143–153, 1988.
86. Freeman R, Saul JP, Roberts MS, et al: Spectral analysis of heart rate in diabetic autonomic neuropathy. Arch Neurol 48:185–190, 1991.
87. Watkins PJ, Mackay JD: Cardiac denervation in diabetes neuropathy. Ann Intern Med 92:304–307, 1980.
88. Eckberg DL, Drabinsky M, Braunwald E: Defective cardiac parasympathetic control in patients with heart disease. N Engl J Med 285:877–883, 1971.
89. Kleiger RE, Miller JP, Bigger JT, et al: Decreased heart rate variability and its association with increased mortality after acute myocardial infarction. Am J Cardiol 59:256–262, 1987.
90. Bigger JT, Kleiger RE, Fleiss JL, et al: Components of heart rate variability measured during healing of acute myocardial infarction. Am J Cardiol 61:208–215, 1988.
91. Wolf MW, Varigos GA, Hunt D, et al: Sinus arrhythmia in acute myocardial infarction. Med J Aust 2:52–53, 1978.
92. Rosenbaum DS, Saul JP, Cohen RJ: Sympathovagal imbalance and arrhythmogenicity during the evolving canine myocardial infarction. Circulation 78:II–639, 1988. Abstract.
93. Myers GA, Martin GJ, Magid NM, et al: Power spectral analysis of heart rate variability in sudden cardiac death: Comparison to other methods. IEEE Trans Biomed Eng BME–33:1149–1156, 1986.
94. Billman GE, Hoskins RS: Time-series analysis of heart rate variability during submaximal exercise. Evidence for reduced cardiac vagal tone in animals susceptible to ventricular fibrillation. Circulation 80:146–157, 1989.
95. Arai Y, Saul JP, Albrecht P, et al: Modulation of autonomic activity during and immediately after exercise. Am J Physiol 25:H132–H141, 1989.
96. Hayano J, Sakakibara Y, Yamada M, et al: Decreased magnitude of heart rate spectral components in coronary artery disease. Its relationship to angiographic severity. Circulation 81:1217–1224, 1990.
97. Dykes FD, Ahmann PA, Baldzer K, et al: Breath amplitude modulation of heart rate variability in normal full term neonates. Pediatr Res 20:301–308, 1986.
98. Kitney RI, Ong HG: An analysis of cardiorespiratory control in babies and its relation to sudden infant death syndrome. Automedica 7:105, 1986.
99. Gordon D, Herrera VL, McAlpine L, et al: Heart rate spectral analysis: A noninvasive probe of cardiovascular regulation in critically ill children with heart disease. Ped Cardiol 9:69–77, 1988.
100. Porter FL, Porges SW, Marshall RE: Newborn pain cries and vagal tone: Parallel changes in response to circumcision. Child Devel 59:495–505, 1988.
101. Fox NA, Porges SW: The relation between neonatal heart period patterns and developmental outcome. Child Devel 56:28–37, 1985.
102. Porter F, Ultmann M, Miller JP, et al: Vagal tone in preterm infants at risk for chronic lung disease. Pediatr Res 25:227A, 1989. Abstract.
103. DiPietro JA, Porges SW: Vagal responsiveness to gavage feeding as an index of preterm status. Pediatr Res 29:231–236, 1991.
104. Maddens M, Lipsitz LA, Wei JY, et al: Impaired heart rate response to cough and deep breathing in elderly patients with unexplained syncope. Am J Cardiol 60:1368–1372, 1987.
105. Maayan C, Axelrod FB, Akselrod S, et al: Evaluation of autonomic dysfunction in familial dysautonomia by power spectral analysis. J Auton Nerv Syst 21:51–58, 1987.
106. Binkley PF, Nunziata E, Cody RJ: Digoxin mediated reduction of sympathetic tone contributes to vasodilation in dilated cardiomyopathy. Circulation 82 (suppl. III): 316, 1990. Abstract.

CHAPTER 31

Role of the Vagus in Isorhythmic Atrioventricular Dissociation

M.N. Levy

The principal function of the arterial baroreceptor reflex is the short-term regulation of arterial blood pressure (P_A). This control is achieved mainly by regulating both peripheral vascular resistance via the sympathetic nervous system and heart rate via both divisions of the autonomic nervous system. One little recognized consequence of the baroreceptor regulation of heart rate is that when two independent pacemakers are active simultaneously in the heart, the baroreceptor reflex tends to synchronize those automatic foci. The best example of this subsidiary function of the baroreceptor reflex is the pacemaker synchronization that occurs in isorhythmic atrioventricular (AV) dissociation, but a similar mechanism also operates in parasystole. This chapter describes the synchronizing effect of the baroreceptor reflex in these two arrhythmias, and the predominance of the vagus nerves in this action is documented.

Isorhythmic Atrioventricular Dissociation

In isorhythmic AV dissociation, the atria and ventricles are each controlled by separate pacemakers that are presumed to be independent. Atrial activity is initiated usually by an impulse that originates in sinoatrial (SA) node pacemaker cells, and the ventricles are activated by an impulse that originates in pacemaker cells in the AV junction or in the ventricular conduction system.[1–3] Yet, despite the anatomical separation of these automatic foci, a distinct interaction is often evident between them.[1–3] The strongest evidence of such an interaction is that the dissociated pacemakers may generate impulses at the same mean frequency, either briefly or persistently. Such a brief synchronization is termed accrochage (from accrocher, to hook together). A longer synchronization is termed isorhythmic dissociation (IRD).

If one of the interacting pacemaking sites initiates atrial activation and

From *Vagal Control of the Heart: Experimental Basis and Clinical Implications* edited by MN Levy, PJ Schwartz © 1994, Futura Publishing Co. Inc., Armonk, NY.

the other initiates ventricular activation, persistent synchronization of the two sites is termed isorhythmic AV dissociation. Even though the atria and ventricles might beat at precisely the same mean frequency, no direct communication need exist between their respective pacemakers. For example, isorhythmic AV dissociation may be induced in patients who have complete heart block and have had an artificial pacemaker installed.[4,5] When the ventricles of such patients are paced at a constant frequency that is close to the spontaneous firing frequency of the SA node, the automatic cells in the SA node assume the same mean firing frequency as that of the artificial ventricular pacemaker (Fig. 1). If the frequency of ventricular pacing is changed slightly, the mean firing frequency of the SA node changes by an equal amount. This entrainment of the natural pacemaker by the artificial pacemaker cannot be ascribed to a surreptitious spread of the artificial pacemaker current to the atria, because the P wave of the electrocardiogram oscillates slowly back and forth across the QRS complex (Fig. 1). Hence, the atrial frequency is, at times, slightly less than the ventricular pacing frequency (top tracing) and, at other times, slightly greater than the ventricular pacing frequency (bottom panel), although the mean frequencies are identical. If the artificial pacemaker current had indeed spread and paced the atria as well as the ventricles, the temporal relationship of the P wave to the QRS complex would have remained constant from cycle to cycle.

Experiments on Animals

In an effort to elucidate the mechanisms responsible for isorhythmicity, we developed an animal model to simulate the clinical condition.[6] We produced complete heart block in anesthetized dogs by injecting ethanol into the region of the AV node, and we attached a stimulating electrode to the external surface

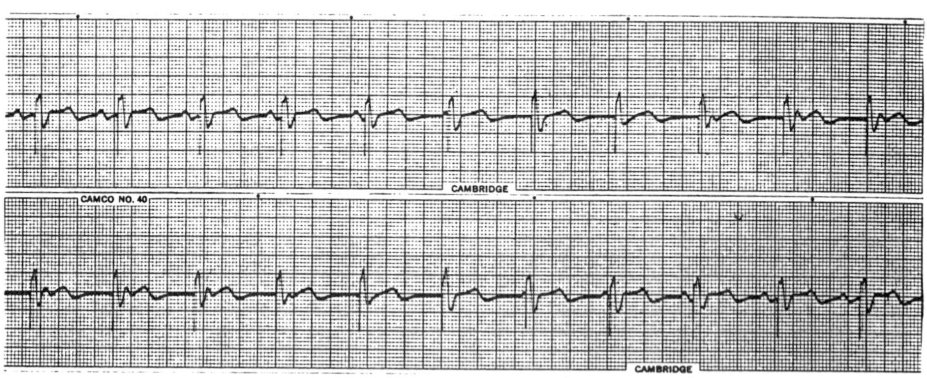

Figure 1. *Electrocardiogram (lead II) recorded from a patient who had complete heart block and whose ventricles were being artificially paced at a constant frequency of 65 pulses/min. The two strips are continuous. Reproduced by permission of the American Heart Association, Inc. from Levy MN, Edelstein J: The mechanism of synchronization in isorhythmic A-V dissociation. II. Clinical studies. Circulation 42:689, 1970.*

of the right ventricle so that we could pace the ventricles at any desired frequency.

When the cardiac nerves were intact, isorhythmic AV dissociation could be induced in every animal when we paced the ventricles at a frequency close to the spontaneous SA node firing frequency. The changes in the P-St intervals (which parallel the PR intervals) during IRD were very characteristic. They mimicked the changes in PR intervals observed in patients with complete heart block and ventricular pacing (Fig. 1).

In the experimental animals with isorhythmic AV dissociation, the P wave of the electrocardiogram wandered rhythmically back and forth across the ventricular pacing artifact (St) and subsequent QRS complex, just as in the human patients. The hallmark of isorhythmicity was the configuration of the P-St tracings. In Figure 2A, note that the P-St tracings to the left of arrow 1 and to the right of arrow 2 comprise alternating sequences of upright and inverted U-shaped deflections, separated by vertical lines. Each inverted U represents the temporal changes in positive P-St intervals (i.e., P precedes St), whereas each upright U represents the temporal changes in negative P-St intervals (i.e., St precedes P). The intervening vertical lines denote the times at which P crosses St from either direction. Thus, the alternating upright and inverted U deflections denote isorhythmic AV dissociation, because the numbers of P waves and St artifacts (and QRS complexes) are precisely equal.

Figure 2A shows that the P_A (upper tracing) varied with the pattern of the P-St intervals. When P-St became positive (inverted U configuration), the P_A rose, whereas when P-St became negative (upright U configuration), the blood pressure declined. The positive P-St signifies that atrial depolarization precedes ventricular depolarization, whereas the negative P-St signifies that atrial depolarization follows ventricular depolarization. Presumably, atrial contraction contributes to ventricular filling and, thereby, augments stroke volume (S.V.), when P-St is positive but not when P-St is negative.

To determine whether the synchronization of the atrial and ventricular pacemakers was causally related to the large oscillations in P_A, we attenuated the pressure oscillations transiently in these animals.[6] In each animal, we connected a blood reservoir to a femoral artery via rubber tubing, and adjusted the reservoir to a hydrostatic level approximately equal to the animal's mean arterial pressure. At the beginning of the experiment shown in Figure 2A (to the left of arrow 1), the rubber tubing was clamped and IRD prevailed.

When the clamp was removed from the tubing (Fig. 2A, between the arrows), the blood pressure oscillations were markedly attenuated. Concomitantly, the rhythmic oscillation of the P wave about the St deflection ceased. The P-St interval tracing assumed a saw-tooth pattern. This new pattern denotes that the P waves marched steadily through consecutive cardiac cycles; i.e., a finite and sustained difference prevailed between the frequencies of SA node firing and of ventricular pacing. The AV dissociation was no longer isorhythmic.

We postulated that the synchronization of the SA nodal and ventricular pacemakers was mediated reflexly, principally by the baroreceptor reflex. To test this hypothesis, we interrupted the cardiac vagal and sympathetic fibers

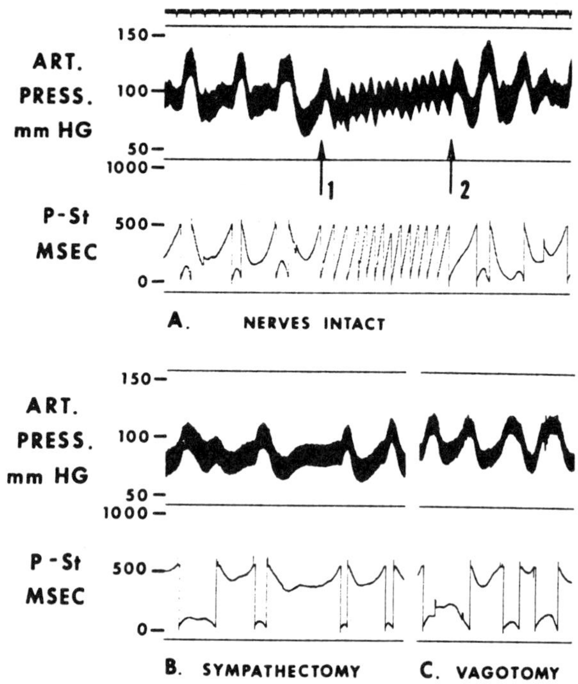

Figure 2. *Record obtained from an anesthetized dog in which complete AV block had been induced and in which the ventricles were being paced at a constant frequency. A: The cardiac neural pathways were intact, and the ventricles were paced at 120 pulses/min. At arrow 1, the tubing that connected a cannula in the left subclavian artery with an elevated blood reservoir was unclamped. At arrow 2, the tubing was clamped again. B and C: The ventricles were paced at 111 pulses/min. Between A and B, both stellate ganglia were excised. Between B and C, both cervical vagi were cut. Downward deflections of the time marker, 10-s intervals. Reproduced by permission of the American Heart Association, Inc. from Levy MN, Zieske H: Mechanism of synchronization in isorhythmic dissociation. I. Experiments on dogs. Circ Res 27:429, 1970.*

involved in this reflex in eight anesthetized dogs.[6] In some animals (as in Fig. 2), we severed the sympathetic pathways first, and then the vagal. In other animals, we reversed the sequence. When the fibers from just one division were interrupted, isorhythmic AV dissociation could still be induced. The vagal pathways appeared to be the more important, however, as judged by the range of ventricular pacing frequencies that could entrain the SA node pacemaker cells (unpublished observations from the experiments described in Levy and Zieske[6]). When the vagus nerves were intact but the stellate ganglia were excised, the ventricular pacemaker could entrain the SA node automatic cells over approximately the same range of pacing frequencies as when both autonomic divisions were intact. When the sympathetic pathways were intact but the vagi were transected, however, the range of ventricular pacing frequencies that could induce isorhythmicity was much narrower. When the pathways of both divisions were interrupted, isorhythmicity could still be induced (e.g., Fig. 2C), but in only half of the animals.[6] In these annimals, the range of pacing frequencies that could induce isorhythmicity was extremely narrow. These results suggest that reflex mechanisms play an important role in synchronizing the two separate cardiac pacemakers, but other, nonneural mechanisms must also operate. This contention is discussed more fully below.

Baroreceptor Control System

The putative control system[7] that synchronizes the atrial and ventricular pacemakers is illustrated in Figure 3. The ventricular pacemaker (which generates the RR interval) in this model represents an artificial pacemaker and, hence, is not influenced by the baroreceptor reflex. Had the RR generator been an AV junctional or idioventricular pacemaker (as in spontaneous isorhythmic AV dissociation), the control system diagrammed in Figure 3 would still be applicable, so long as the influence of the baroreceptor reflex on the natural ventricular pacemaker differed quantitatively from its influence on the SA node (which generates the PP interval). The disparity in the firing times of the atrial and ventricular pacemakers defines the PR interval (Fig. 3).

The PR interval strongly influences the atrial contribution to ventricular filling and, therefore, affects the S.V. In Brockman's[8,9] experiments on dogs with induced complete heart block, the S.V. sharply increased as the time between the beginnings of atrial and ventricular systole (A_s-V_s interval) progressively increased from 0 to 0.1 seconds (Fig. 4). A further increase in the A_s-V_s interval to about 0.3 seconds led to a progressive decrease in S.V. Over the remaining range of A_s-V_s intervals, changes in that interval had no appreciable effect on S.V.

The relation between S.V. and the time difference between atrial and ventricular excitation (PR interval) is represented in Figure 3 by the block

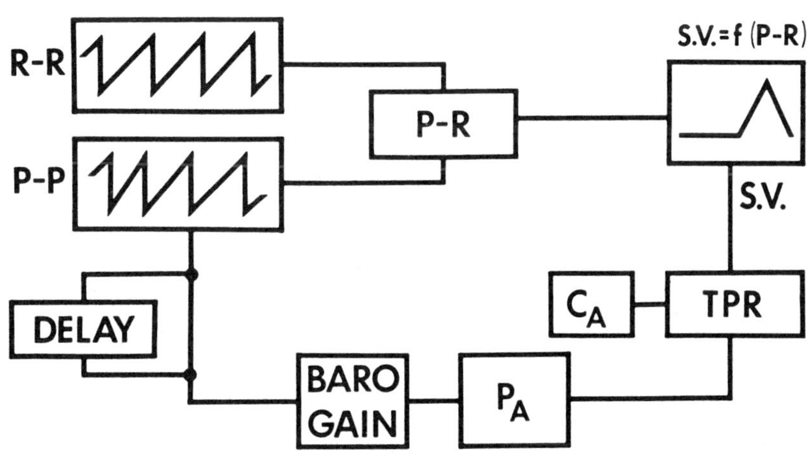

Figure 3. *The biological control system that produces AV synchronization in isorhythmic AV dissociation. S.V.: stroke volume; TPR: total peripheral resistance; and BARO GAIN: gain of baroreceptor reflex. Reproduced by permission of the American Heart Association, Inc. from Levy MN, Zieske H: Mechanism of synchronization in isorhythmic A-V dissociation. III. Computer model. Circ Res 28:23, 1971.*

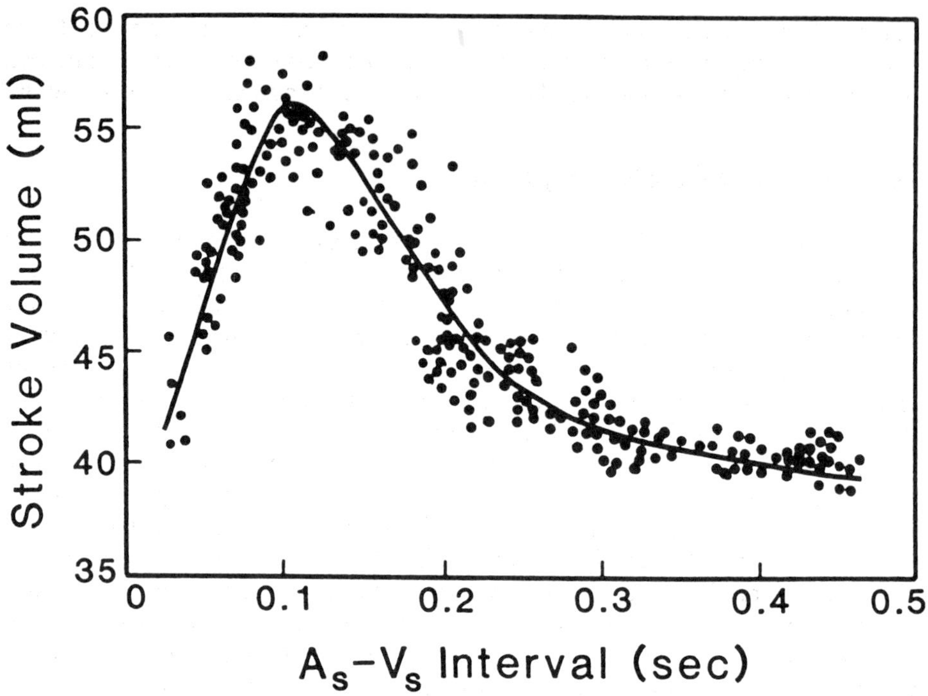

Figure 4. *Effect of the time delay (A_S-V_S interval) between atrial and ventricular contractions on S.V. in dogs with complete AV block. Reproduced with permission from Brockman SK: Dynamic function of atrial contraction in regulation of cardiac performance. Am J Physiol 204:597, 1963.*

labelled S.V. = f(P-R). The transfer function in this block has a configuration like that found experimentally by Brockman[8,9] (Fig. 4). In patients or experimental animals with a constant ventricular rate, the S.V. and total peripheral resistance (TPR) determine the level of the P_A, as represented in Figure 3. A time lag exists between any change in S.V. and the resulting change in P_A; the time constant for this lag is the product of TPR and the arterial compliance (C_A). Finally, the P_A reflexly affects the firing rate of the SA node, via the arterial baroreceptors (Fig. 3). Substantial time elapses from a given change in PR interval until the resultant change in cardiac sympathetic and vagal activity affects the firing of the SA node pacemaker cells. This time lag, plus the hemodynamic lag related to C_A and TPR, are responsible for the rhythmic oscillations of the P wave about the QRS complex in isorhythmic AV dissociation, as explained below.

Stabilization by Negative Feedback

The timing diagrams shown in Figure 5 explain how the baroreceptor reflex synchronizes the firing of the SA node pacemaker cells with the artificial ventricular pacemaker.[7] The model above (Fig. 3) indicates that S.V. is a function of the PR interval. The timing diagram in Figure 5 shows that when P precedes R by an interval such that P falls on the negative slope region of that function, negative feedback prevails. This negative feedback synchronizes the atrial pacemaker cells with the ventricular pacemaker. Over the negative slope region of this function (from 0 to about 100 milliseconds in Fig. 4), the S.V. becomes greater as the PR interval increases.

To illustrate how negative feedback operates when the P wave falls within the negative slope portion of the S.V. function, consider an example in which the dissociated atria and ventricles have been beating at the same frequency (regardless of the reason). Consider also that the PR interval is such that the P wave occurs at a time (P_S, Fig. 5) in the cardiac cycle such that the S.V. function has a negative slope. Since the slope is negative (i.e., because S.V. varies directly with PR), the timing diagrams described below show that the time from P_S to R tend to be stable (hence the subscript $_S$). During such stable synchronization, the PR interval remains constant from beat to beat. Thus, in diagram A (Fig. 5), $P_1R_1 = P_2R_2 = P_3R_3$.

Now consider a perturbation, such that a P wave (P_A, Fig. 5) occurs prematurely during the fourth beat. P_AR_4 then exceeds the previous constant PR intervals. If P_A still falls on the negative slope region of the function, then S.V. is augmented, arterial pressure rises, and the baroreceptor reflex prolongs the next PP interval. If the next P wave does not occur at P_S, but it is still slightly premature (e.g., at P_B), the S.V. would still be greater than that which would yield the stable P_SR interval. Therefore, the next PP interval (P_B-P_6) would be slightly greater than the stable PP interval (e.g., P_1-P_2). This process would continue until the P waves fell at the stable point (P_S) in the cardiac cycle. Timing diagram B shows that if a P wave (e.g., P_C) occurs later than expected, S.V. would diminish, and the baroreceptor reflex would tend to correct this by briefly shortening the PP intervals until the P waves again occur at the stable position, P_S. Diagrams A and B show, therefore, that a perturbation that shortens a PP interval immediately tends to lengthen the next cycle and, conversely, a perturbation that lengthens a PP interval tends to shorten the next cycle.

Furthermore, timing diagrams C and D in Figure 5 show that synchronization cannot persist while the P waves arise during the positive slope region of the S.V. function, because positive feedback prevails.[7] Hence, an aberrant short PP interval generates a still shorter one, and an aberrant long PP interval generates an even longer one. Therefore, the relation of the P wave to the R wave continues to change until the P wave occurs during the negative-slope portion of the S.V. function. Negative feedback then prevails, and SA node firing then tends to be synchronized with the firing of the artificial ventricular pacemaker.

Oscillations in PR Intervals

The synchronization achieved by the negative feedback mechanism illustrated in Figure 5 would tend to be steady rather than oscillatory. Our

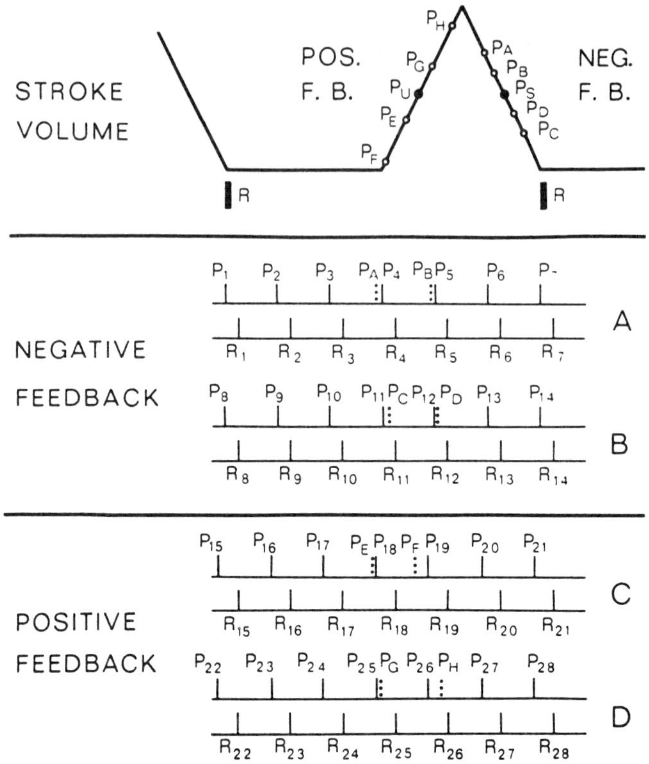

Figure 5. *Schema to illustrate the feedback that results because the S.V. of the heart varies with the time between atrial and ventricular excitation (i.e., with the PR interval). A stable equilibrium exists when the P wave (P_S) falls during the negative slope region of the function, because negative feedback prevails, as shown by timing diagrams A and B. An unstable equilibrium exists when the P wave (P_U) falls during the positive slope region of the function, because positive feedback prevails, as shown by diagrams C and D. Reproduced by permission of the American Heart Association, Inc. from Levy MN, Zieske H: Mechanism of synchronization in isorhythmic A-V dissociation. III. Computer model. Circ Res 28:23, 1971.*

experiments on animals and our observations in human subjects, however, reveal that, although the mean frequency of SA node firing equals the constant frequency of the ventricular pacemaker, the SA node pacemaker cells actually fire in an oscillatory pattern. The SA node sometimes fires at a greater frequency than does the ventricular pacemaker, and sometimes at a lower frequency.

We therefore designed experiments[6] on anesthetized dogs to test the hypothesis that the oscillatory nature of SA node activity in isorhythmic AV block reflects the substantial delays inherent in the physiological control system (Fig. 3). The principal delays are in the translation of a change in S.V. into a change in P_A and in the baroreceptor reflex (Fig. 3). To diminish the delays in the system, we first eliminated the time lag involved in translating S.V. changes into blood pressure changes by holding the P_A constant at 120 mm Hg by a specially constructed servo system.[6] We circumvented the delay in the baroreceptor reflex by relating changes in P-St interval directly to changes in efferent vagal activity. To achieve this result, we applied electrodes to the cardiac ends of both transected vagi, and we modulated the frequency of vagal stimulation by a function of the P-St interval that resembled the S.V. function displayed in the top panel of Figure 5. The frequency control was such that, as the P-St interval increased from 0 to 100 milliseconds, the vagal stimulation frequency was raised proportionately. As the P-St interval increased from 100 to 200 milliseconds, the vagal stimulation frequency was decreased proportionately. Finally, as the P-St interval was increased above 200 milliseconds, vagal stimulation frequency remained at a constant low level. We could control the gain of this control system by adjusting the change in vagal stimulation frequency that would be produced per unit change in P-St interval.

The results of a representative experiment on a dog with complete AV block are shown in Figure 6. In this experiment, the basal vagal stimulation period (reciprocal of frequency) was 870 milliseconds whenever the P-St interval exceeded 200 milliseconds. Whenever P-St passed through the range

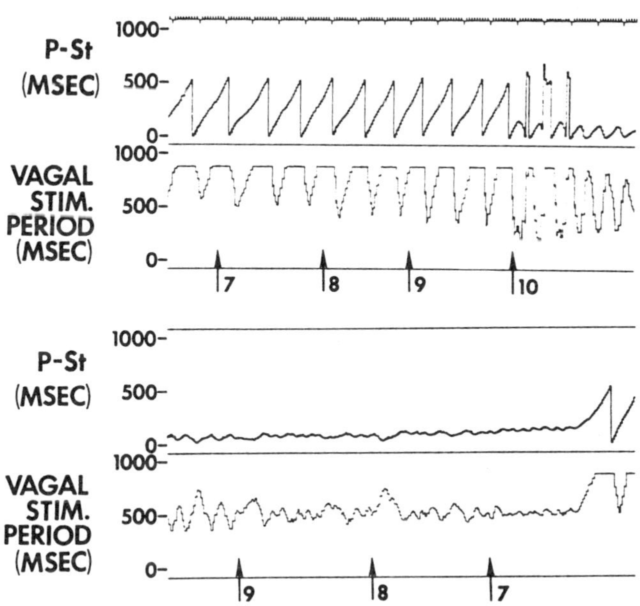

Figure 6. *The effects of diminishing the delays in the control system that produces AV synchronization. The frequency of efferent vagal stimulation was varied as a function of the P-St interval. The gain setting (in arbitrary units) of the controller that was used to vary the change in vagal stimulus period (reciprocal of frequency) per unit change in P-St interval is denoted by the arrow numbers. Synchronization (denoted at first by the alternating positive and negative P-St periods) was not achieved until the gain was increased to 10 (upper panel). Once achieved, synchronization persisted at lower gain settings (lower panel); the two panels are continuous. During sustained synchronization (lower panel), the P-St interval fluctuated only slightly, principally because the delay in the control system had been minimized. Reproduced by permission of the American Heart Association, Inc. from Levy MN, Zieske H: Mechanism of synchronization in isorhythmic dissociation. I. Experiments on dogs. Circ Res 27:429, 1970.*

of 0 to 200 milliseconds, however, the vagal stimulation period varied as a triangular function. Figure 6 (top half) discloses that as the function gain (reflected by the heights of the inverted triangles) was increased from 6 to 7, 8, and 9 arbitrary units, a greater and greater maximum frequency of vagal stimulation was delivered, as indicated by the decreasing minima in the vagal stimulus period tracing. At these gains, the SA node pacemaker cells did not synchronize with the ventricular pacemaker, as indicated by the saw-tooth appearance of the P-St interval tracing.

When we increased the function gain setting to 10 units (Fig. 6, top half), synchronization was finally achieved, manifested at first by some oscillation of the P wave around the St. After about 25 seconds, synchronization consisted of a sinusoidal oscillation of the P-St interval between 0 and +50 milliseconds. The amplitude of this oscillation then diminished substantially; i.e., the P-St interval remained quite steady (Fig. 6, bottom half). When the function gain setting was subsequently decreased to 9 and then to 8 units, synchronization persisted and the P-St interval remained steady. Subsequent reduction of the gain setting to 7 units was associated with persistence of synchronization for over 30 seconds, but isorhythmicity ceased eventually (near the right border of the tracing). It was not reestablished until the function gain setting was increased again to 10 units (not shown).

Thus, when most of the delay has been removed from the physiological control system, isorhythmicity can be achieved via neural control, and the P-St interval may remain quite steady. The rhythmic fluctuations of SA node firing ordinarily seen in isorhythmic AV dissociation is characteristic of the "hunting behavior" of negative feedback control systems with long time delays.[7] Due to the substantial delays in the physiological control system (Fig. 3) that evoke isorhythmicity, the level of cardiac efferent neural activity that determines the sinus rate at a given moment is appropriate not to the P-St interval that prevails at that same moment, but to the P-St interval that prevailed at some previous time (equal to the delay in the system). Thus, the system hunts for the appropriate P-St interval and, in the process, it alternately overshoots and undershoots the appropriate level of neural activity.

The observations described above strongly support the hypothesis that it is the baroreceptor reflex that tends to synchronize the firing of SA node cells with the firing of a ventricular pacemaker. Nevertheless, other synchronizing mechanisms probably also operate. The experiment illustrated in Figure 2 shows that isorhythmicity may still prevail even after the efferent limbs of the baroreceptor reflex have been effectively interrupted.[6] Synchronization could still be induced in half the animals after bilateral vagotomy and stellate ganglionectomy, although the range of ventricular pacing frequencies that could still induce isorhythmicity was restricted markedly. The ability to induce isorhythmicity at all, however, does indicate that ancillary synchronizing mechanisms must also operate.

Heart rate has been shown to vary inversely with the perfusion pressure in the isolated SA node artery in anesthetized dogs.[10,11] This mechanism thus constitutes a nonneural baroreceptor control system that is intrinsic to the heart. Another auxiliary mechanism in AV dissociation may be the tendency for mechanical stretch of the SA node region to initiate firing of the sinus pacemaker cells as the atrial contract against closed AV valves.[12] A third ancillary system resides in the strong tendency for periodic bursts of vagal activity to synchronize the firing of SA node automatic cells.[13–15] When complete AV block prevails, each ventricular pacing stimulus initiates a ventricular contraction. The consequent ejection of blood into the systemic arteries stimulates the arterial baroreceptors and reflexly induces a burst of action potentials, first in afferent fibers to the medulla oblongata and, then, after a brief delay, in efferent vagal fibers to the heart. Thus, each ventricular contraction is followed by a burst of action potentials in the efferent cardiac vagal fibers. By virtue of the strong synchronizing action of such bursts of efferent vagal activity, the SA node pacemaker cells tend to fire at the identical frequency.[13–15] This ancillary synchronizing mechanism does involve the baroreceptor reflex, but not in the classical sense that a change in blood pressure evokes a parallel change in efferent vagal activity. This ancillary mechanism would operate even if the arterial systolic and diastolic pressure levels remained constant from beat to beat.

Studies on Human Subjects

Isorhythmic AV dissociation occurs most commonly when the AV junctional rhythm accelerates as a consequence of such processes as acute rheumatic fever, digitalis toxicity, and anesthesia.[3,5,16,17] IRD induced by acceleration of a junctional pacemaker tends to be transient. As long as the pathways between the SA node and AV junction conduct normally, the slower pacemaking center becomes dominated by the faster center usually within several beats. If the conducting pathways between the two automatic foci are functionally blocked, however, and if the two foci tend to fire at frequencies that are not too disparate, isorhythmic AV dissociation may be very persistent.[4,5] This type of isorhythmicity, therefore, is more appropriate for studies of the mechanism of synchronization.

The cardiovascular responses in human subjects[4,5] who have complete AV block and who have an artificial ventricular pacemaker resemble the responses in the animal models. For example, in a 69-year-old man who had complete AV block and who was studied by Kaplinsky et al,[5] the basal sinus rate varied only slightly (between 97 and 100 beats/minute). When the ventricular pacing rate (VPR) in this person was set at either 87 or 91 pulses/minute, the atrial and ventricular rhythms remained completely dissociated (CD), and a graph of the sequential PR intervals (Fig. 7) resembled the saw-tooth pattern of the P-St interval tracings in our animal experiments (Fig. 2). When the VPR was increased to 94 pulses/minute (which was less than the basal atrial rate in this patient), however, the mean atrial rate then decreased to equal the VPR; that is, IRD now prevailed. The atrial rhythm now consisted of an oscillation of cardiac cycle lengths such that the atrial rate at times exceeded VPR and at times was less than VPR. The time-course of PR intervals (Fig. 7) reflected these oscillations in atrial rate. The PR interval tracing in this patient was

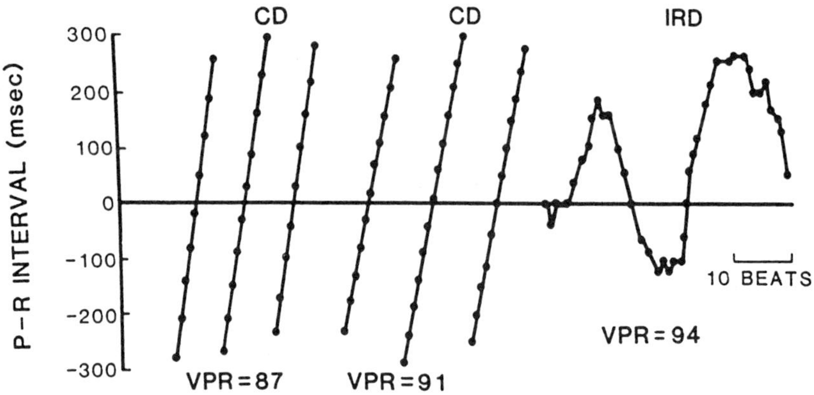

Figure 7. *The sequential changes in the PR intervals of the electrocardiogram in a 69-year-old man with complete heart block. When the ventricular pacing rates (VPRs) were 87 and 91 pulses/min, the atria and ventricles were completely dissociated (CD). When the pacing rate was increased to 94 pulses/min, however, isorhythmic dissociation (IRD) prevailed. Reproduced with permission from Kaplinsky E, Aronson R, Neufeld HN: Isorhythmic dissociation—a "physiological" arrhythmia. J Electrocardiol 10:179, 1977.*

equivalent to the alternating sequence of upright and inverted U deflections in the P-St tracings in our animal experiments when isorhythmicity prevailed (Fig. 2).

When the P_A was measured in patients with isorhythmic AV dissociation,[4,5,18] isorhythmicity was accompanied by oscillations in blood pressure that closely resembled the oscillations in our experimental animals. In the patient whose electrocardiogram is reproduced in Figure 1, the variations in PR interval were paralleled by blood pressure changes (Fig. 8). When the P wave was obscured by the QRS complex or was partially evident just behind it (left half of the tracing), the patient's blood pressure was about 115/60 mm Hg. When the P wave moved in front of the QRS complex, however, the blood presssure rose to 160/85 mm Hg within a few heartbeats. Furthermore, in the patients studied by Kaplinsky et al,[5] the P_A was similarly correlated with the PR intervals. Thus, the mechanism responsible for isorhythmicity appears to be similar in human subjects and in experimental animals.

Parasystole

In electrocardiograms recorded from human subjects, the most common type of ventricular extrasystole is characterized by a fixed coupling interval between the normal sinus beat and the extrasystolic beat. One of the principal features that distinguishes parasystole from the more common variety of extrasystoles is that, in parasystole, the coupling interval between the preceding sinus beat and the parasystolic beat is very variable. In some instances of well-established parasystole, however, the coupling interval may become fixed temporarily.[19–25]

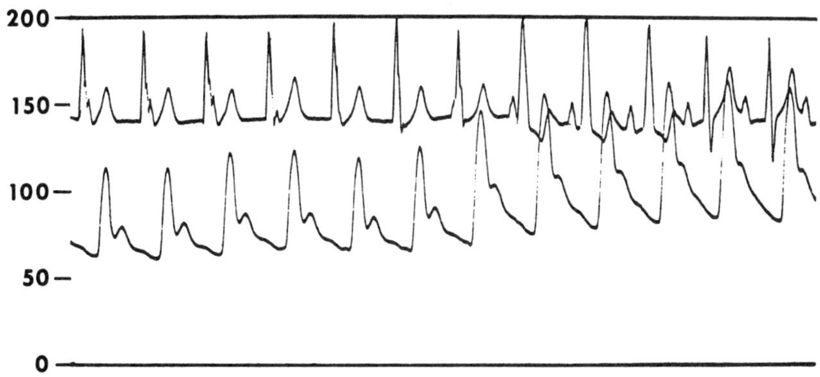

Figure 8. *Correlation between the electrocardiogram and the P_A (mm Hg) in the patient from whom the electrocardiogram in Figure 1 was recorded. The right ventricle was paced at 67 pulses/min. Note that the blood pressure rises substantially when the P wave moves in front of the QRS complex. Reproduced by permission of the American Heart Association, Inc. from Levy MN, Edelstein J: The mechanism of synchronization in isorhythmic A-V dissociation. II. Clinical studies. Circulation 42:689, 1970.*

To investigate the mechanisms responsible for fixed coupling in parasystole, we conducted a series of experiments on anesthetized dogs.[26] We instituted artificial respiration, opened the chest, and introduced an electrode catheter into the right ventricular cavity to register the ventricular electrogram. We also attached a bipolar stimulating electrode to the epicardial surface of the left ventricle. The ventricular electrogram and the stimulus signal served as inputs to a computer that was programmed to measure the intervals between consecutive ventricular activations (RR intervals) and the times from the beginning of an R wave to the beginning of a stimulus (St) delivered to the left ventricle (R-St intervals).

In order to mimic ventricular parasystole, we stimulated the left ventricle electrically at frequencies that were approximately half the prevailing firing frequency of the SA node. Thus, whenever ventricular stimuli (e.g., stimuli 1 to 6 in Fig. 9) were delivered while the ventricles were refractory, no response was evoked. If the stimuli were delivered when the ventricles were excitable (e.g., stimuli 7 to 17), however, premature depolarizations were induced. Since the stimuli were delivered at a frequency that was close to (but not precisely equal to) half the prevailing sinus frequency, stimuli that fell during the ventricular excitable period induced a transient bigeminal pattern of ventricular extrasystoles. Note that in the RR interval tracing that corresponds to stimuli 7 to 17, the pattern consists of an alternating pattern of short and long RR intervals. The short RR intervals are the coupling intervals, and they are of almost uniform duration. The long RR intervals are the compensatory pauses, and they are also of almost uniform duration. Thus, the pattern closely resembles the bigeminal pattern often observed in patients that have the common variety of fixed coupled extrasystoles.

Figure 10 provides more detail about the responses of this same animal.[26] The tracings were recorded at a slower paper speed and, thus, the responses are

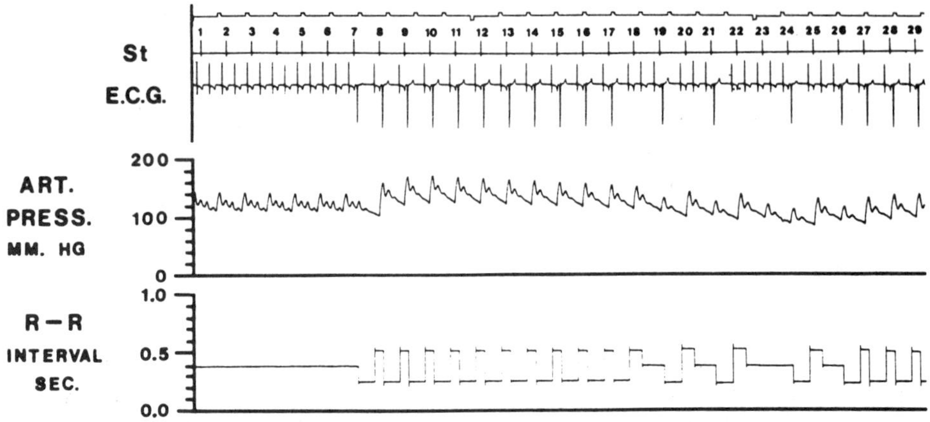

Figure 9. *The changes in the right ventricular electrogram (E.C.G.), the P_A, and the R-R intervals in an anesthetized dog in which the ventricles were stimulated electrically at the times (St) indicated in the top tracing. The normally conducted depolarizations are indicated in the ECG by the upward spikes of the electrogram, whereas the electrically-induced ectopic depolarizations are identified by the inverted spikes. The time marker deflections denote 1-s intervals. Reproduced by permission of the American Heart Association, Inc. from Levy MN, Lee MH, Zieske H: A feedback mechanism responsible for fixed coupling in parasystole. Circ Res 31:846, 1972.*

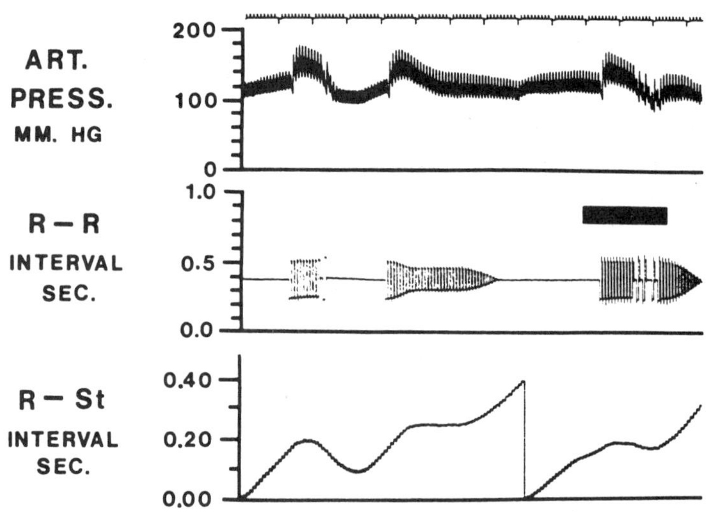

Figure 10. *An experiment on an anesthetized dog (same animal as that from which Fig. 9 was derived) in which three bursts of electrically-induced ectopic activity (manifested by the alternating short and long R-R intervals) were attended by elevations of the P_A. Ectopic beats were evoked when the R-St interval (time from the QRS complex to the pacing stimulus) exceeded 0.17 s. The left ventricle was paced at 66 beats/min. In view of the constant pacing frequency, any change in slope of the R-St tracing signifies a change in the natural heart rate. The horizontal bar in the middle of the figure indicates the portion of the experiment that is displayed in Figure 9 at a faster paper speed. The downward deflections of the time marker denote 10-s intervals. Reproduced by permission of the American Heart Association, Inc. from Levy MN, Lee MH, Zieske H: A feedback mechanism responsible for fixed coupling in parasystole. Circ Res 31:846, 1972.*

displayed over a longer time. The horizontal bar in the middle tracing indicates the segment from which Figure 9 was derived. Near the left border of Figure 10, the spontaneous sinus rate was 133 minutes^{-1}. The frequency of left ventricular stimulation was fixed at 66 minutes^{-1} throughout the experiment. Thus, the ventricular stimulation frequency was slightly less than half the spontaneous sinus firing frequency. Therefore, the slope of the R-St tracing was positive, which denotes that each stimulus is delivered a little later in the cardiac cycle than was the preceding stimulus. At the beginning of this portion of the experiment, the pacing stimulus occurred very shortly after the beginning of the R wave (i.e., the R-St interval was only slightly greater than 0) and, hence, the ventricle was refractory. As the R-St interval approached 0.20 seconds, however, the stimuli began to induce premature beats, as manifested by the alternating short and long RR intervals. Concomitantly, the P_A increased abruptly. The rise in blood pressure is a manifestation of postextrasystolic potentiation.[27,28]

The increased P_A was associated with a reduction in the SA nodal firing frequency. This change in sinus rate was probably mediated by the baroreceptor reflex. The reduction in the spontaneous sinus rate is reflected by the initial peaking and subsequent decline of the R-St interval tracing (Fig. 10). The spontaneous heart rate continued to decline for several seconds, as manifested by the progressive reduction in R-St intervals. As the R-St interval diminished, the stimuli were again delivered during the ventricular refractory period, and extrasystoles ceased. The P_A declined, and this result induced (probably reflexly) an increase in the sinus rate.

Two additional episodes of ectopic beats are evident in Figure 10. In both sequences, the ventricular stimulus proceeded through the alternate cardiac cycles at progressively longer R-St intervals. The positive slope indicates that the ventricular pacemaker did not entrain the SA node firing during these periods. The pronounced reduction in the slope of the R-St tracing with the advent of the ectopic beats, however, demonstrates a strong synchronizing tendency. Indeed, the slope approximated 0 for several seconds during the second and third episodes of ectopic activity. This occurrence is analogous to the accrochage that is often observed during AV dissociation,[6] which has been discussed in the preceding section of this chapter.

When we used a slightly greater ventricular stimulation frequency (not shown) in this same dog, we observed periods of synchronization that persisted for one to six minutes.[26] Each episode of ectopic beats was accompanied by a pronounced elevation of blood pressure that was, in turn, attended by a temporary reversal of the slope of the R-St tracing. This behavior was not appreciably modified by β-receptor blockade with propranolol. Bilateral cervical vagotomy, however, completely abolished the synchronizing tendency.

The left panel of Figure 11 illustrates the fixation of the coupling (R-St) interval in a dog that responded to ventricular pacing on alternate sinus cycles with late premature depolarizations.[26] Note that when the ectopic activity appeared, the R-St intervals were about 400 milliseconds, in contrast to the R-St intervals of about 200 milliseconds that prevailed during the ectopic depolarizations in the preceding experiment (Figs. 9 and 10).

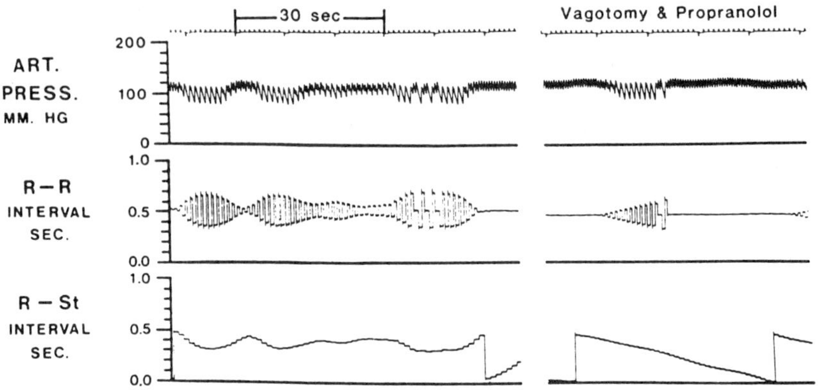

Figure 11. *An experiment on an anesthetized dog in which the onset of electrically-induced ectopic beats was attended by a reduction in* P_A*. Left: The cardiac autonomic pathways were intact, and the SA node was entrained by the ventricular parasystolic focus throughout most of this record. Right: Propranolol was administered and both vagi were transected. The absence of synchronization is manifested by a steady decline in R-St interval, despite the pressure change associated with the burst of ectopic beats. Reproduced by permission of the American Heart Association, Inc. from Levy MN, Lee MH, Zieske H: A feedback mechanism responsible for fixed coupling in parasystole. Circ Res 31:846, 1972.*

At the left margin of Figure 11, the slope of the R-St tracing was negative, which denotes that the constant ventricular pacing frequency exceeded half the spontaneous sinus rate. Rhythmic changes in the R-St interval were paralleled by variations in the P_A. For example, as the pacing stimuli fell progressively earlier in the cardiac cycle, the P_A diminished. The spontaneous sinus rate quickly accelerated and soon exceeded twice the fixed pacing frequency (the slope of the R-St tracing became positive temporarily). This change in heart rate was probably induced mainly by the baroreceptor reflex. As the slope of the R-St tracing became positive, the pacing stimuli began to occur progressively later in the cardiac cycle, and the blood pressure again rose. Throughout most of the tracing shown in the left panel of Figure 11, the R-St interval oscillated slowly between 400 and 500 milliseconds.

In this experiment, propranolol did not appreciably alter the response to ventricular stimulation.[26] Subsequent bilateral cervical vagotomy, however, did abolish the tendency for fixation of the coupling interval, as shown in the right panel of Figure 11. Despite the ectopic beats and the concomitant drop in blood pressure displayed in the right panel of Figure 11, the slope of the R-St tracing did not change substantially.

In the nine animals that we studied, propranolol did not appreciably attenuate the tendency for the coupling interval to be fixed in our model of ventricular parasystole.[26] In seven of these animals, subsequent transection of both vagus nerves did abolish this tendency. In two animals, however, the fixation tendency was still evident (although weakened) even after the effects of the sympathetic and vagal pathways had been abrogated. Fixation of the

R-St interval denotes entrainment of the SA node pacemaker cells by the artificial pacemaker used to stimulate the ventricles.

Entrainment appears to be mediated by a feedback control system similar to that which operates in isorhythmic AV dissociation (Fig. 3). In the control system that we believe operates in parasystole,[26] the two pacemaking sites that tend to be synchronized are the SA node and the parasystolic focus (Fig. 12). The SA node is responsive to various neural and humoral influences, whereas the ventricular parasystolic focus is relatively independent of such influences (and entirely independent when the "parasystolic focus" is an electronic stimulator). The phase difference between the SA node firing and the parasystolic firing is, by definition, the coupling interval (R-R, in Fig. 12) between the conducted and the ectopic beats. The coupling interval, in turn, determines the S.V. of the premature and the postextrasystolic beats. S.V., heart rate, and peripheral resistance then determine the P_A. Finally, the blood pressure affects the SA nodal firing frequency, mainly via the baroreceptor reflexes. A finite time is required for a change in coupling interval to alter the heart rate, and this delay accounts for the rhythmic oscillations in the coupling (R-St) intervals in Figure 11 (left panel). The influence of this delay is analogous to that which induces the periodic oscillations in PR intervals in isorhythmic AV dissociation.

Abrogation of the influence of the efferent autonomic pathways of the baroreceptor reflex attenuates markedly, but does not entirely eliminate, the tendencies toward entrainment in isorhythmic AV dissociation or in ventricular parasystole. Thus, the baroreceptor reflex probably plays an important role in these arrhythmias, but it is certainly not the only synchronizing mechanism.

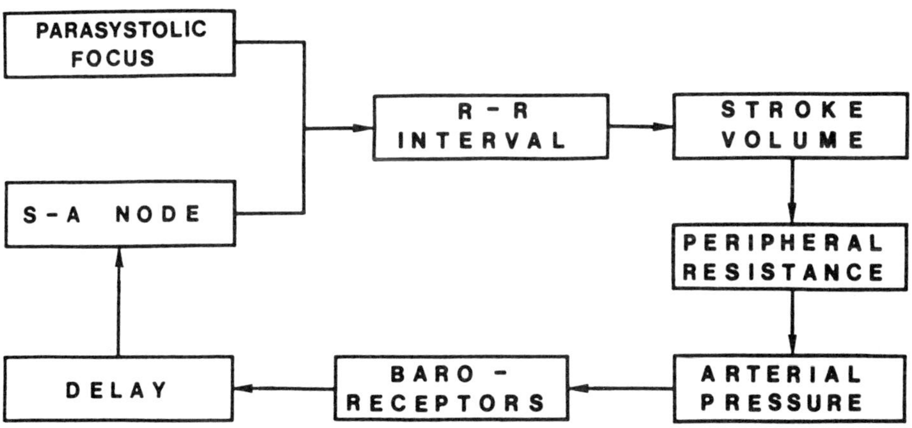

Figure 12. *Block diagram of the negative feedback control system that acts to synchronize the SA node pacemaker cells with a constantly discharging parasystolic ventricular focus. Reproduced by permission of the American Heart Association, Inc. from Levy MN, Lee MH, Zieske H: A feedback mechanism responsible for fixed coupling in parasystole. Circ Res 31:846, 1972.*

References

1. Lewis T: Mechanism and Graphic Registration of the Heart Beat. 3rd ed. London, Shaw & Sons Ltd, 1925, p. 178.
2. Segers M, Lequime L, Denolin H: Synchronization of auricular and ventricular beats during complete heart block. Am Heart J 33: 685, 1947.
3. Marriott HJL: Atrioventricular synchronization and accrochage. Circulation 14:38, 1956.
4. Levy MN, Edelstein J: The mechanism of synchronization in isorhythmic A-V dissociation. II. Clinical studies. Circulation 42:689, 1970.
5. Kaplinsky E, Aronson R, Neufeld HN: Isorhythmic dissociation—a "physiological" arrhythmia. J Electrocardiol 10:179, 1977.
6. Levy MN, Zieske H: Mechanism of synchronization in isorhythmic dissociation. I. Experiments on dogs. Circ Res 27:429, 1970.
7. Levy MN, Zieske H: Mechanism of synchronization in isorhythmic A-V dissociation. III. Computer model. Circ Res 28:23–33, 1971.
8. Brockman SK: Dynamic function of atrial contraction in regulation of cardiac performance. Am J Physiol 204:597, 1963.
9. Brockman SK: Cardiodynamics of complete heart block. Am J Cardiol 16:72, 1965.
10. Hashimoto K, Tanaka S, Hirata M, et al: Responses of the sino-atrial node to change in pressure in the sinus node artery. Circ Res 21:297, 1967.
11. James TN: Pulse and impulse in the sinus node. Henry Ford Hosp Med J 15:275, 1967.
12. Diederich KW, Djonlagic H: Mechanism of synchronization in isorhythmic dissociation. Cardiology 58:129, 1973.
13. Levy MN, Martin PJ, Iano T, et al: Paradoxical effect of vagus nerve stimulation on heart rate in dogs. Circ Res 25:303, 1969.
14. Levy MN, Iano T, Zieske H Jr: Effects of repetitive bursts of vagal activity on heart rate. Circ Res 30:186, 1972.
15. Michaels DC, Slenter VAJ, Salata JJ, et al: A model of dynamic vagus-sinoatrial node interactions. Am J Physiol 245: H1043, 1983.
16. Chander S: Isorhythmic atrioventricular dissociation during enflurane anesthesia. Southern Med J 75:945, 1982.
17. Hill RF: Treatment of isorhythmic A-V dissociation during general anesthesia with propranolol. Anesthesiology 70:141, 1989.
18. Duncan E, Silverman I, Swiryn S: Left posterior escape rhythm with isorhythmic atrioventricular dissociation. Arch Intern Med 147:977, 1987.
19. Langendorf R, Pick A: Parasystole with fixed coupling. Circulation 35:304, 1967.
20. Watanabe Y: Reassessment of parasystole. Am Heart J 81:451, 1971.
21. Jalife J, Moe GK: Biologic model of parasystole. Am J Cardiol 43:761, 1979.
22. El-Sherif N: The ventricular premature complex: Mechanisms and significance. In WJ Mandel (ed): Cardiac Arrhythmias. Their Mechanisms, Diagnosis, and Management. Philadelphia, PA, JB Lippincott Co, 1980, p. 288.
23. Chung EK: Principles of Cardiac Arrhythmias. 4th ed. Baltimore, MD, Williams & Wilkins, 1989, p. 446.
24. Courtemanche M, Glass L, Rosengarten MD, et al: Beyond pure parasystole: Promises and problems in modeling complex arrhythmias. Am J Physiol 257:H693, 1989.
25. Hoshino K, Ikeda N, Tanakadate A, et al: Computer-based model of parasystolic activity modulated by ventricular activation in the open chest dog. J Electrocardiol 22:277, 1989.
26. Levy MN, Lee MH, Zieske H: A feedback mechanism responsible for fixed coupling in parasystole. Circ Res 31:846, 1972.

27. Wohlfart B, Noble MIM: The cardiac excitation-contraction cycle. Pharmac Ther 16:1, 1982.
28. Schouten VJA: Interval dependence of force and twitch duration in rat heart explained by Ca^{2+} pump inactivation in sarcoplasmic reticulum. J Physiol (Lond) 431:427, 1990.

CHAPTER 32

Central Nervous System and Behavioral Factors in Vagal Control of Cardiac Arrhythmogenesis

R.L. Verrier, L.W. Dickerson

This chapter focuses on the mechanisms whereby the brain affects cardiac electrical stability through alterations in vagus nerve activity. Historically, this relationship has been explored by stimulating various structures within the central nervous system (CNS) using stereotaxic positioned electrodes or by local delivery of neuroactive drugs. With the advent of methods for evaluating cardiac vulnerability in conscious animals, it became possible to examine the influence of diverse behavioral states, such as anger and fear, on the electrophysiological function of the heart. This approach has been combined with pharmacological, surgical, and cryogenic neural ablation techniques to provide insights into neurocardiac mechanisms of arrhythmogenesis. The investigation of sleep states has also been informative because of its diversity of autonomic nervous system activity. With the introduction of power spectrum analysis of heart rate variability, progress has been accelerated in defining sympathetic-parasympathetic interactions in health and disease. The final topic to be discussed in the chapter is the state-dependent modulatory influence of opioids on cardiac rhythm. This avenue of research is particularly exciting because of the potential for therapeutic intervention.

Central Nervous System Stimulation Studies

Over 70 years ago, it was demonstrated that significant arrhythmias, including ventricular tachycardia (VT), can be evoked in normal animals by stimulating certain areas in the hypothalamus.[1] This finding was subsequently confirmed in a variety of species. Hockman and colleagues,[2] using

Supported by Grant HL-33567 from the National Heart, Lung and Blood Institute, National Institutes of Health, Bethesda, Maryland
From *Vagal Control of the Heart: Experimental Basis and Clinical Implications* edited by MN Levy, PJ Schwartz © 1994, Futura Publishing Co. Inc., Armonk, NY.

stereotaxic techniques, showed that cerebral stimulation and hypothalamic activation elicited a spectrum of ventricular arrhythmias. These observations are consistent with clinical reports that cerebral vascular disease, and especially intracranial hemorrhage, can produce pronounced cardiac repolarization abnormalities and life-threatening arrhythmias.[3,4]

The posterior hypothalamus is a site of particular importance in CNS-induced arrhythmogenesis. Stimulation of this structure increased 10-fold the incidence of ventricular fibrillation (VF) associated with acute coronary artery occlusion.[5] Enhanced vulnerability was due to increased sympathetic activity because β-adrenergic receptor (β-AR) blockade, but not vagotomy, prevented it.[6] Arrhythmias that developed immediately following cessation of diencephalic or hypothalamic stimulation required intact vagi and stellate ganglia.[7,8] The likely basis for the arrhythmogenic effect of vagal activity is that during CNS stimulation, automaticity of cardiac Purkinje fibers is enhanced by adrenergic discharge, and upon cessation of stimulation, the rapid recovery of high vagal tone slows heart rhythm, exposing the increased automaticity of the fibers and leading to ventricular premature beats and tachyarrhythmias.

Insights into the CNS pathways involved in behaviorally induced arrhythmias have been provided by Skinner and Reed.[9] Cryogenic blockade of the thalamic gating mechanism or its output from the frontal cortex to the brain stem delayed or prevented the occurrence of VF during stress in pigs. Recently, Carpeggiani and colleagues[10] showed that cryogenic blockade of the amygdala is also capable of preventing stress-induced VF. Thus, these distinct pathways within the CNS appear to play a critical role in mediating arrhythmogenesis due to intense behavioral arousal. CNS regulation of cardiovascular function has been discussed in detail by Smith and DeVito,[11] Gutterman and colleagues,[12] Jordan,[13] Cechetto and Saper,[14] LeDoux,[15] and McCloskey (see Ch. 5).

Behavioral Stress, Vagal Activation, and Arrhythmias

Models have been developed to study the impact of behavioral state on cardiac electrical stability.[16–19] These models have included both aversive behavioral conditioning paradigms and the elicitation of natural emotions, including anger and fear.[16–19] Quantification of changes in cardiac electrical stability in the normal as well as in the ischemic heart was achieved by means of the repetitive extrasystole (RE) threshold technique.[17,20] Aversive conditioning of dogs in a Pavlovian sling with mild chest shock on three consecutive days showed that subsequent exposure to the environment without shock elicited a reduction in the RE threshold greater than 30% (Fig. 1).[17,21] The same paradigm elicited a threefold increase in the occurrence of spontaneous VF when occlusion was carried out in the aversive sling compared to the nonaversive cage environment. A primary role of the sympathetic nervous system in stress-induced changes in cardiac vulnerability was indicated by the fact that

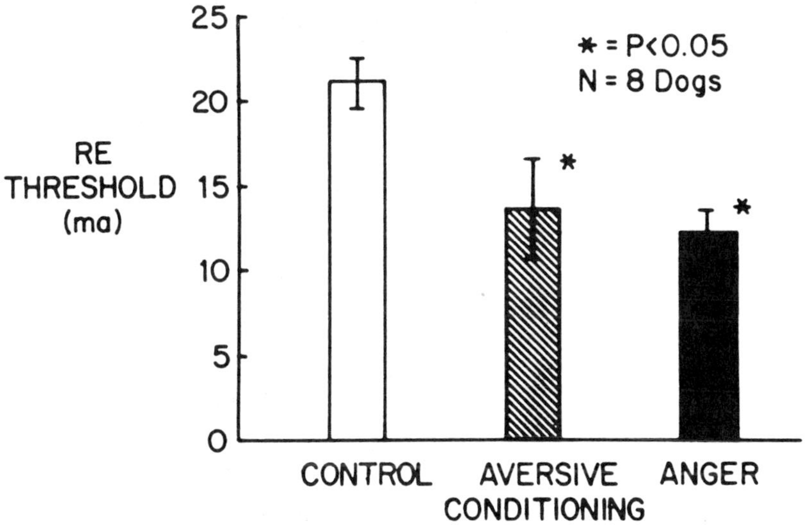

Figure 1. *Effects of behavioral stress on the repetitive extrasystole (RE) threshold in normal dogs. Both passive aversive conditioning using a mild electric shock and induction of an anger-like state by denial of access to food produced significant reductions in the vulnerable period threshold. Heart rate was maintained constant during cardiac electrical testing by ventricular pacing. Reproduced, with permission, from Verrier RL, Lown B: Behavioral stress and cardiac arrhythmias. Annu Rev Physiol 46:158, 1984. Copyright © 1984 by Annual Reviews Inc.*

β-adrenergic blockade with propranolol or the cardioselective drugs tolamolol and metoprolol completely prevented these adverse effects.[22,23]

An important role of vagal tone in the aversive stress paradigm was also demonstrated. Specifically, when relatively small doses of atropine (0.05 mg/kg) were given to block vagal influences on the heart, vulnerability in the aversive environment was markedly enhanced (Fig. 2).[21] That vagal influences on vulnerability in conscious animals are contingent on the level of adrenergic tone is suggested by the observation that the administration of atropine in the nonstressful cage environment did not alter the RE threshold. Furthermore, catecholamines were markedly elevated in the aversive environment but not in the nonstressful cage environment.[24] Finally, when β-adrenergic blockade was induced in the aversive environment, atropine failed to alter the RE threshold (Fig. 3).[25]

These observations suggest that accentuated antagonism of the profibrillatory effects of enhanced adrenergic activity by muscarinic stimulation operates in conscious animals undergoing alterations in behavior[21] as well as in the anesthetized state.[26–29] Stramba-Badiale, Vanoli, Schwartz and their coworkers[30,31] have characterized sympathetic-parasympathetic interactions during ischemia and infarction in the conscious state. Even during intense stress, there may be sufficient vagal tone to inhibit presynaptically the amount of norepinephrine (NE) released at sympathetic nerve endings and to oppose the effects of adrenergic receptor stimulation by muscarinic opposition of second messenger formation (Table 1).

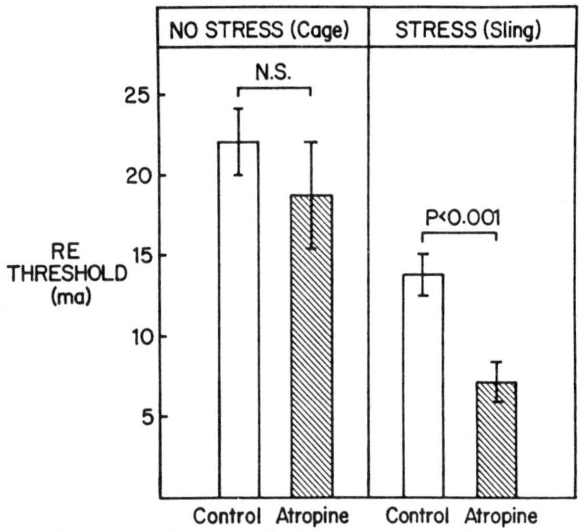

Figure 2. *Influence of atropine (0.05 mg/kg) on the repetitive extrasystole (RE) threshold in conscious dogs exposed to nonaversive and aversive environments. In the aversive setting, blockade of vagal efferent activity with atropine substantially reduced the vulnerable period threshold, indicating an enhanced propensity for VF. In the nonstressful setting, where adrenergic activity was low, no effect of the drug was evident. Heart rate was maintained constant during cardiac electrical testing by ventricular pacing. Reproduced, with permission, from Verrier RL, Lown B: Behavioral stress and cardiac arrhythmias. Annu Rev Physiol 46:158, 1984. Copyright © 1984 by Annual Reviews Inc.*

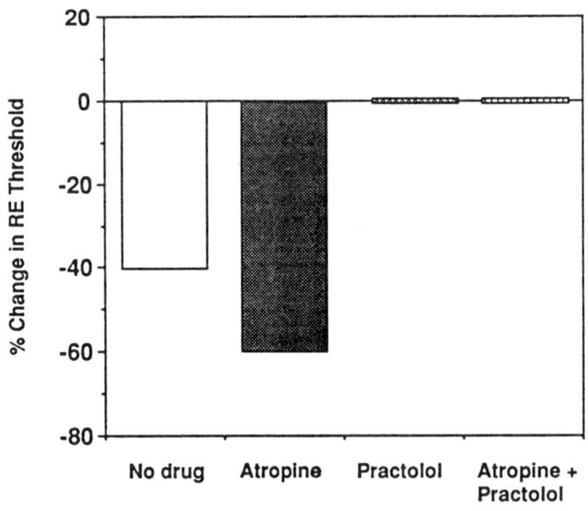

Figure 3. *Effect of β-adrenergic blockade with practolol (1 mg/kg, I.V.) on atropine-induced (0.05 mg/kg) changes in the repetitive extrasystole (RE) threshold during aversive conditioning in six dogs.[25] In the absence of drugs, the aversive environment resulted in a 40% reduction in RE threshold. Following muscarinic receptor (mAChR) blockade, the stress-induced reduction in threshold increased by another 20%. When β_1-receptors were blocked by practolol, however, atropine no longer exerted an effect on the RE threshold during stress. Thus, the cardioprotective effect of vagal activity during behavioral stress is contingent on the prevailing level of adrenergic stimulation.*

Table 1.
Sympathetic-Parasympathetic Interactions and Myocardial Electrical Stability

Vagal tone increases myocardial electrical stability and protects against VF during myocardial ischemia.

Vagally induced reduction in heart rate plays an important role during both myocardial ischemia and reperfusion, because it increases diastolic perfusion time and reduces cardiac metabolic demand.

Enhanced vagal activity has an additional antifibrillatory effect due to antagonism of adrenergic influences.

The bases for sympathetic–parasympathetic interactions are:

- inhibition of NE release from nerve endings
- attenuation of response to catecholamines at receptor sites.

Beneficial effects of vagal activity may be vitiated if profound bradycardia and hypotension ensue.

Myocardial infarction may alter autonomic influences by damaging neural fibers.

Adapted from Verrier RL: Autonomic control of cardiac arrhythmias. In BN Singh, HJJ Wellens, M Hiraoka (eds): Electropharmacologic Control of Cardiac Arrhythmias: To Delay Conduction or to Prolong Refractoriness. Mt. Kisco, NY, Futura Publishing Co, 1994, pp. 135–150.

In the future, it will be important to study the role of the vagus in arrhythmogenesis during natural states such as anger and fear.[18] We anticipate that during anger there may be residual vagal tone that is cardioprotective. Vagus nerve activity may be particularly intense during fear, as suggested by the well-described phenomenon of vasovagal syncope.[13–15,32] Such intense bursting of vagal activity could be arrhythmogenic either by inducing abrupt changes in cycle length, which favor triggered activity, or by reducing heart rate and, thereby, exposing latent enhanced automaticity due to elevated catecholamines.

T Wave Alternans and Vagal Activation

While interest in T wave alternans stems from the pioneering work of Sir Thomas Lewis,[33] appreciation of its modulation by the sympathetic[34] and parasympathetic[35] nervous systems has been relatively recent. Schwartz and Malliani[34] focussed attention on the role of the sympathetic nervous system in provoking alternans by stimulating nerves in cats and reporting alternans in association with a fearful response to an exercise treadmill in a patient with the long QT syndrome. A resurgence in interest[36–42] has been prompted by the demonstration that computerized analysis of the T wave provides a quantitative means for assessing susceptibility to VF.[38] Adam and colleagues[36] and

Smith and coworkers[37] demonstrated a statistically significant correlation between fluctuations in overall energy of the T wave and the ventricular fibrillation threshold (VFT) during coronary artery occlusion and hypothermia in dogs. Subsequently, it was shown in humans that there is a close relationship between the magnitude of T wave alternans and the inducibility of arrhythmias using programmed electrical stimulation.[39]

We applied the analytical technique of complex demodulation of the T wave to track cardiac vulnerability dynamically during both myocardial ischemia and reperfusion.[38] We found that the magnitude of changes in T wave alternans parallelled precisely the time-course of changes in VFT and that of spontaneous susceptibility to VF. Furthermore, the effects of stellectomy and of stellate ganglion stimulation were also detectable.

Recently, we demonstrated that vagal influences on vulnerability could likewise be quantified using complex demodulation of the T wave. Vagus nerve stimulation was also shown to exert a significant effect on T wave alternans in the occlusion-release model.[43] Specifically, we found that the surge in T wave alternans that occurs during acute left anterior descending (LAD) coronary artery occlusion can be markedly suppressed by electrical stimulation of the left vagus nerve. Vagus nerve excitation, however, was ineffectual in preventing alternans during reperfusion. These findings concur with reports from several laboratories indicating an important antifibrillatory effect of vagus nerve stimulation during acute myocardial ischemia. Such an effect did not occur during reperfusion when heart rate was kept constant, as in our study.[44–47] As discussed above, the likely basis for these differing effects of vagal activity on alternans during occlusion and reperfusion is that the antifibrillatory influence of this pathway is dependent on accentuated antagonism of adrenergic activity (Table 1).

An observation from the clinical literature suggests that vagal activation may suppress T wave alternans and, consequently, reduce susceptibility to ventricular tachyarrhythmias. Navarro-Lopez et al[35] reported the case of a 60-year-old woman with acute gastroenteritis who experienced recurring ventricular tachyarrhythmias. During bilateral carotid sinus massage, she exhibited momentary interruption of chronic T wave alternans (Fig. 4). Since this maneuver is known to elicit profound vagotonia, this report provides an enticing suggestion of a correspondence between the animal and human studies.

Sleep States and Vagal Control of Heart Rhythm

Autonomic Tone During Sleep

Sleep is associated with dramatic changes in autonomic nervous system activity.[48–50] These changes are particularly evident during rapid eye movement (REM) or active sleep, when the CNS may operate in an "open-loop" mode, independent of feedback control.[49] During non-REM sleep, the system

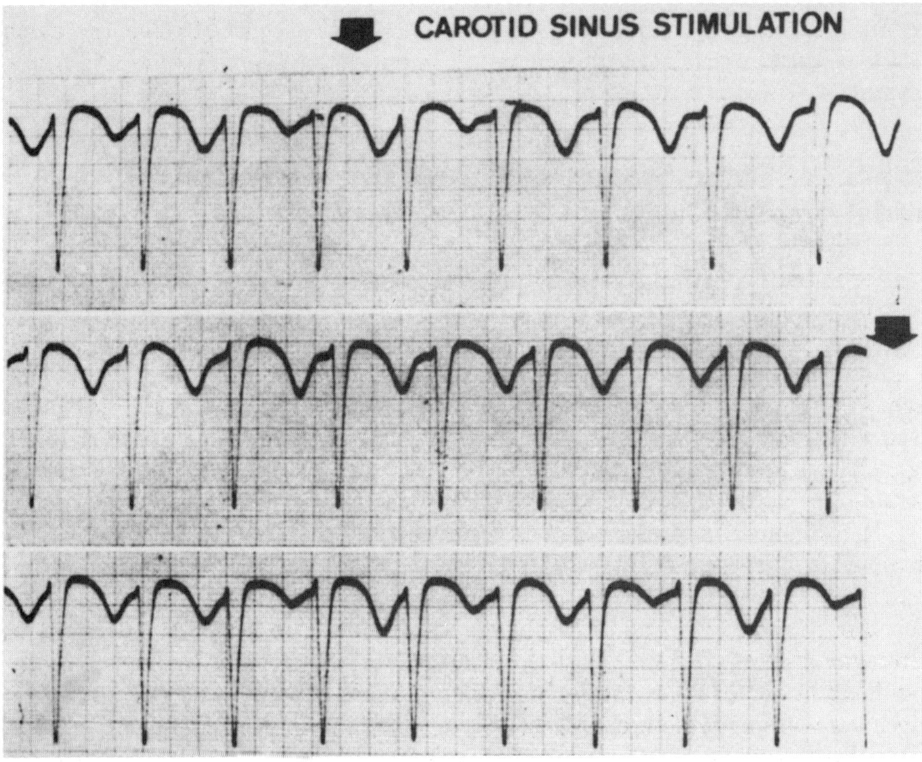

Figure 4. *Continuous tracing of lead V_2 in a 60-year-old woman with a significant level of T wave alternans and recurring ventricular fibrillation in association with acute gastroenteritis. Carotid sinus stimulation interrupted T wave alternans. Arrows point to the beginning and the end of the stimulation. Reproduced with permission from Navarro-Lopez F, Cinca J, Sanz G, et al: Isolated T wave alternans. Am Heart J 95:372, 1978.*

operates in a "closed-loop" fashion, being highly regulated as a result of end-organ feedback. An alternative view is that autonomic control may alternate between a mode resembling wakefulness during phasic REM sleep and a mode resembling non-REM sleep during tonic REM sleep.[51] The apparent transient disruption of homeostatic mechanisms during REM sleep can result both in major surges in cardiac sympathetic activity and in suppression of the usual vagal tone of sleep. Such effects can have an adverse impact on the stability of cardiac rhythm and myocardial perfusion. Surges in sympathetic nervous system activity, particularly during phasic REM sleep, may be responsible for the prevalent but poorly understood phenomenon of nocturnal angina. The significant increase in baroreceptor gain during non-REM sleep is also likely to play an important role in cardiovascular homeostasis in health and disease.[52]

Deep non-REM sleep (slow wave sleep) is associated with marked stability of autonomic regulation.[49] Marked respiratory sinus arrhythmia (RSA) is present, indicating a high degree of parasympathetic tone. Sympathetic nervous system activity is relatively stable during this stage and its cardiovascular input is reduced. During transitions from non-REM to REM sleep, however, bursts of vagus nerve activity may result in pauses in heart rhythm and frank asystole.

Impact of Sleep States on Myocardial Perfusion and Arrhythmias

Ischemic events and arrhythmias during the nocturnal period[53–56] have been documented in patients with advanced coronary disease[53] or Prinzmetal's variant angina.[54] The REM phase of sleep is especially conducive of ST segment changes and perfusion abnormalities.[53,54] In fact, 8% to 10% of ischemic attacks occur during sleep.[57,58] The high incidence of ischemic events associated with nocturnal arousal[59] may be due in part to increased platelet aggregation exacerbated by assumption of the upright posture.[60,61] Other factors regulating coronary vascular tone must also be considered.[62–64]

Recent experimental studies have shed light on fundamental mechanisms involved in sleep-induced changes in myocardial perfusion and arrhythmogenesis.[65–68] Both REM sleep and slow wave sleep significantly increase the effective refractory period (ERP) of the ventricles,[69] an effect independent of alterations in heart rate. The increased excitability of the heart is largely mediated by increases in cardiac vagal tone, since it is abolished by muscarinic blockade with atropine methylnitrate but is not abolished by bilateral stellectomy. Furthermore, even low-intensity electrical scanning of the cardiac cycle induced VF during REM sleep but not during slow wave sleep.

Subsequent investigations revealed that sympathetic activity periodically surges during REM sleep, an action that could destabilize the heart electrophysiologically.[65,66] The experiments involved chronically instrumented dogs in which heart rate, arterial blood pressure (P_A), coronary arterial blood flow, and electroencephalographic data were recorded simultaneously. Coronary stenosis was set to reduce baseline flow by 60%. During REM sleep, there were transient increases in heart rate with concomitant reductions in coronary flow (Fig. 5).[66] Since this surge phenomenon is abolished by bilateral stellectomy, it is assumed that increased adrenergic discharge is responsible for the flow deficit. The heart rate surges occur predominantly during those periods of REM sleep marked by intense phasic activity.[67] The increase in adrenergic discharge could lead to a coronary blood flow decrement by at least two mechanisms: stimulation of α-adrenergic receptors on the coronary vascular smooth muscle and/or decrease in diastolic coronary perfusion time as a result of the bursts in heart rate. A significant correlation between the magnitude of the increase in heart rate and the decrease in coronary blood flow supports the latter possibility.[66]

The link between REM sleep-induced changes in heart rate and coronary insufficiency appears to be consistent with clinical reports of patients with advanced coronary heart disease. In particular, Nowlin and coworkers[53] found in patients with advanced coronary artery disease that attacks of nocturnal angina occurred predominantly (32 of 39 episodes in four patients) during REM sleep and were associated with heart rate acceleration (Fig. 6).

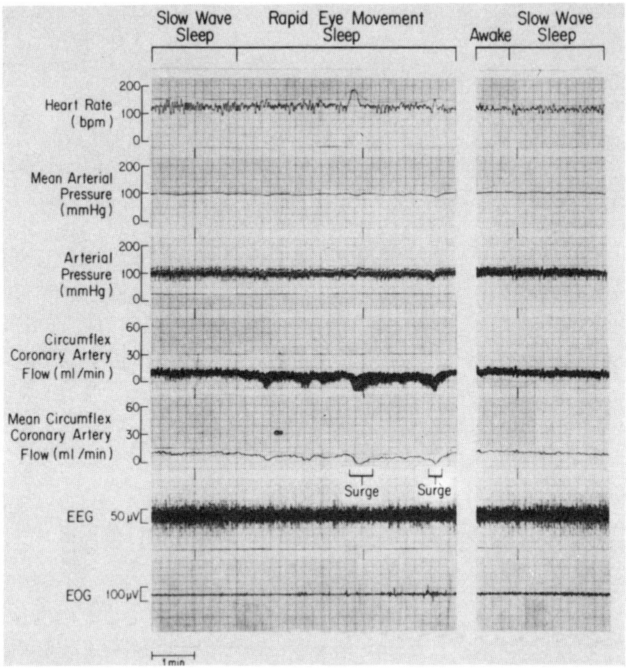

Figure 5. *Recordings of effects of sleep stage on heart rate, mean and phasic arterial pressures, and mean and phasic circumflex coronary artery flows in a typical dog during stenosis. Note phasic decreases in coronary flow occurring during heart rate surges while the dog is in REM sleep. EEG: electroencephalogram; EOG: electro-oculogram. Reprinted with permission from Kirby DA, Verrier RL: Differential effects of sleep stage on coronary hemodynamic function during stenosis. Physiol Behav 45:1018, 1989. Copyright 1989, Pergamon Press Ltd.*

Heart Rhythm Pauses and Arrhythmogenesis During Sleep

We recently observed, in chronically instrumented dogs, prolonged pauses in heart rhythm during transitions from slow wave sleep to periods marked by desynchronized EEG rhythms.[70,71] These pauses persisted from one to eight seconds and were followed by dramatic increases in coronary blood flow averaging 30% and ranging up to 84% (Fig. 7).[18] An intense burst of vagal activity appeared to produce the phenomenon, since the pauses developed against a background of marked RSA, varying degrees of heart block with nonconducted P waves, and low heart rate. Furthermore, the phenomenon, including the postpause surge in coronary flow, was emulated by electrical stimulation of the vagus nerve.

These observations carry important implications for diagnosing and treating neurogenically induced ischemia and arrhythmias.[72,73] Nocturnal asystolic events have been reported in both young adults[74] and individuals with obstructive sleep apnea.[75,76] Pauses in heart rhythm could set the stage for triggered activity, as abrupt changes in cycle length are conducive to early and late afterdepolarizations.[77] An intriguing possibility is that, in individuals who

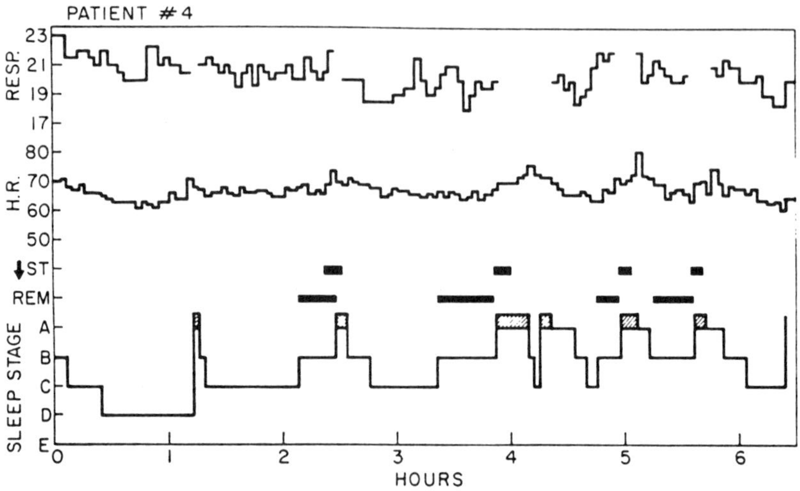

Figure 6. *Composite graph of a night of sleep in a patient with nocturnal angina pectoris. Note association between REM-related surges in heart rate and occurrence of ST segment changes. RESP: respirations; H.R.: heart rate; ST: periods of significant ST segment depression on electrocardiogram. Reproduced, with permission, from Nowlin JB, Troyer WG Jr, Collins WS, et al: The association of nocturnal angina pectoris with dreaming. Ann Intern Med 63:1043, 1965.*

may be sensitized by proarrhythmic medications, sleep-induced pauses may initiate severe ventricular arrhythmias.

Clinically, vagal-sympathetic interactions during the course of an apnea are sometimes expressed as a bradycardia-tachycardia sequence. The bradycardia or asystole in some apnea patients is associated with increases in the QT interval that may predispose them to serious ventricular arrhythmias such as torsades de pointes, particularly if the bradycardia is terminated by a ventricular premature beat.[78] It is important to note, however, that prolonged QT intervals are observed in a variety of other conditions besides sleep apnea, such as in some patients with ventricular arrhythmias, and the prolongation of QT interval is enhanced by sleep, with no difference observed between REM and non-REM stages.[79] Furthermore, nocturnal asystoles lasting up to nine seconds or bradycardias can occur during sleep in otherwise healthy young adults[74] and may not be an uncommon expression of the enhanced vagotonia of sleep.

Power Spectrum Analysis of Heart Rate Variability During Sleep

During the past few years, heart rate variability has been analyzed to assess autonomic neural patterning during human sleep.[48,51,80–82] The most commonly employed technique to study heart rate variability is power spectrum analysis, which identifies interbeat fluctuations by separating the signal into its fundamental frequencies (see Ch. 30).[83] Accordingly, vagus nerve activity expresses itself as a high-frequency peak (0.4 Hz range in dogs and

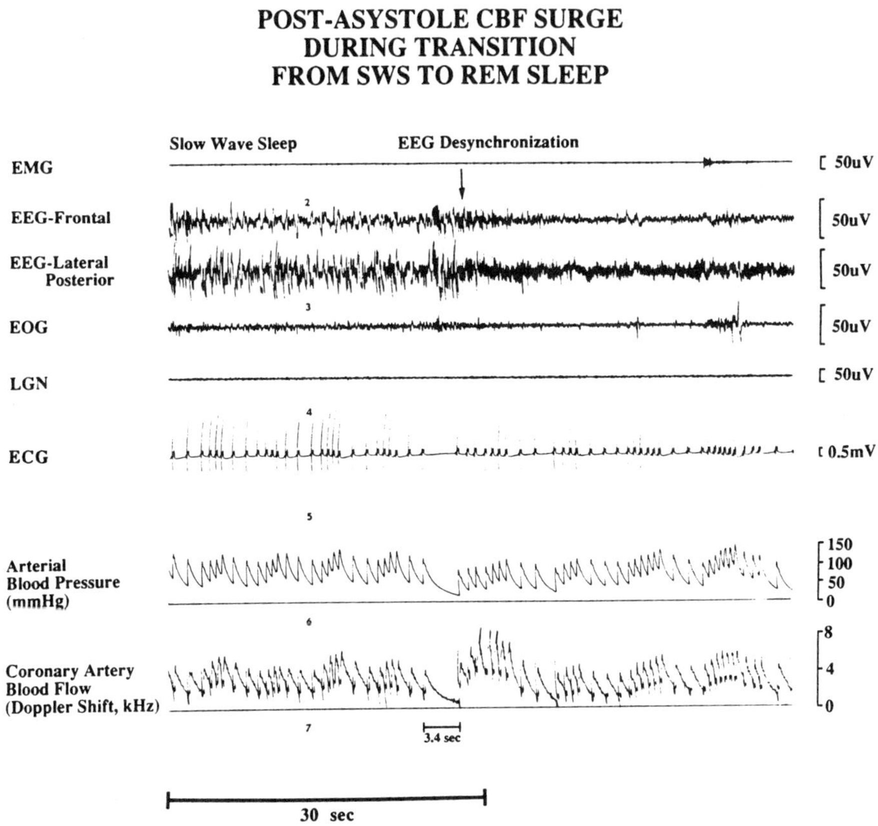

Figure 7. *Coronary blood flow (CBF) surge during deep slow wave sleep (SWS) interrupted by EEG desynchronization. This response pattern is common and represents a transition to REM sleep. The 3.4-s pause in heart rhythm was followed by a brief increase of 41% in average peak CBF and a decrease of 8% in the product of heart rate times systolic blood pressure, an indicator of myocardial metabolic demand. EMG: electromyogram; EEG: electroencephalogram; EOG: electro-oculogram; LGN: lateral geniculate nucleus field potential recordings.*

0.25 Hz range in humans) coinciding with respiration.[84] Another major peak occurs in a mid-frequency bandwidth and represents sympathetic-parasympathetic interactions and baroreceptor responsiveness. A third, low-frequency peak is thought to reflect activity of the renin-angiotensin system and changes in vasomotor tone associated with thermoregulation.

Zemaityte and coworkers[81] used power spectrum analysis in conjunction with autonomic nervous system blockers such as atropine and propranolol to define autonomic function during sleep in normal subjects. They found a marked decrease in heart rate and increase in RSA during non-REM sleep. The sympathetic input remained relatively constant throughout all stages of sleep except for an initial decrease during drowsy sleep. REM sleep was characterized by irregular fluctuations in autonomic activity on a background of an average increase in heart rate and a decrease in RSA relative to non-REM sleep. The authors concluded that the periodic structure of the heart rate changes, especially those in RSA during sleep, is related to the baseline level of autonomic activity during wakefulness. These studies, while informative, should be interpreted with some caution, since both atropine and propranolol cross the blood-brain barrier.

That coronary disease can alter the periodicity of heart rate and blood pressure fluctuations during sleep and dreaming was recognized by the pioneering work of MacWilliam.[85] These early insights have been corroborated and extended in a number of recent studies. Bigger and coworkers[80] compared baroreflex sensitivity (BRS) and heart period variability after myocardial infarction during both day and night. They found that BRS and tonic vagal activity reflected by heart rate spectral patterns were more greatly reduced in patients with inferior myocardial infarction than in those with anterior myocardial infarction. They also observed that BRS and the heart period variability were significantly more concordant during night than day. This finding is consistent with the perception that slow wave sleep has a generally stabilizing effect on heart rhythm and may also enhance maximal dynamic vagal responsiveness, as indicated by the BRS test.[86]

Furlan and coworkers[82] raised the intriguing possibility that circadian variations in neural regulation may play a key role in the extensively documented occurrence of early morning cardiovascular mortality.[60,87–89] Using spectral analysis, they observed a pronounced and consistent decrease in markers of sympathetic activity and an increase in vagal activity during the night. At about 6:00 A.M., however, patients, lying in bed quietly awake, experienced a progressive rise in spectral indicators of sympathetic activity and a concomitant decrease in markers of vagal tone. The authors proposed that important changes in autonomic function in addition to the putative rise in platelet aggregability[88] may contribute to the circadian fluctuations in cardiovascular events, including stroke, myocardial infarction, and sudden death.[87]

Neuromodulatory Role of Opioids on Vagal Function

Two major themes have emerged from recent studies of the effects of opioids on cardiac electrical stability. The first theme is that their mechanism of action is dependent on the particular type of stress that impinges on the heart. The second is that μ-receptors are the primary mediators of opioid-induced changes in arrhythmogenesis. These principles are discussed with reference to the clinically relevant conditions of acute behavioral stress and myocardial ischemia.

Role During Behavioral Stress

In our initial studies, we examined the effects of morphine on behaviorally induced changes in cardiac electrical stability. Morphine was selected because it is the prototypical opioid and because of its widespread clinical use.[90–92] We focused on behavioral stress as an experimental model that would render a relatively comprehensive picture of opioid influences on neurocardiac interactions. The experimental paradigm consisted of the aversive sling/nonaversive cage sequence discussed above.[93] Administration of intravenous morphine (0.25 mg/kg) did not alter the threshold in the absence of stress but did completely prevent the stress-induced changes in vulnerability. As we had previously established that the aversive setting results in high plasma levels of epinephrine and NE,[24] it is likely that morphine exerts its protective action by opposing the profibrillatory influence of enhanced adrenergic activity.

A major component of morphine's protective effect on cardiac electrical stability appears to derive from an increase in vagal efferent tone, since the electrophysiological changes are largely abolished by muscarinic receptor (mAChR) blockade with atropine sulfate (Fig. 8).[93] It is likely that the vagomimetic action of morphine protects the heart during behavioral stress through vagal antagonism of adrenergic inputs.[94] This influence is likely to be due to both presynaptic inhibition of NE release from sympathetic nerve endings and to a direct muscarinic opposition of catecholamine-induced second messenger release at myocardial receptor sites.[26,27] The net effect of these actions is to increase cardiac electrical stability.[47,95]

It is important to note, however, that even after blockade of mAChRs with

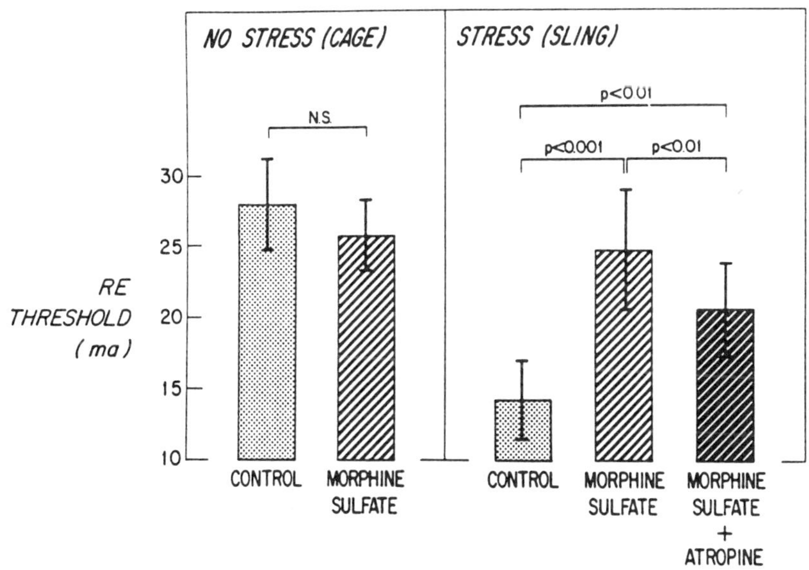

Figure 8. *Effect of morphine sulfate (MS) on repetitive extrasystole (RE) threshold in the two environments in 12 dogs. Morphine (0.25 mg/kg) significantly elevated RE threshold in the sling environment by 40% ($p<0.001$). Administration of atropine sulfate (0.2 mg/kg) following MS partially annulled this effect, but RE threshold still remained significantly above the control level in the sling ($p<0.01$). MS was without effect on RE threshold in the cage environment. Values are expressed as means ± SEM. Reproduced with permission from DeSilva RA, Verrier RL, Lown B: The effects of psychological stress and vagal stimulation with morphine on vulnerability to ventricular fibrillation (VF) in the conscious dog. Am Heart J 95:201, 1978.*

atropine, a significant component of morphine's effects during behavioral stress remained.[93] Two major possibilities that must be considered are decreased perception of the noxious stimuli and sympathoinhibition resulting from resetting of the sensitivity of the baroreceptor reflex arc.[96] With respect to the former, it is well established that morphine has a profound influence on behavioral affect and could well have ameliorated the apprehension and anxiety associated with aversive conditioning.

The relative contributions of morphine's multiple effects, namely, enhanced vagal efferent input and altered perception, may vary depending on the particular stress involved. Based on the facts that morphine is a potent μ-receptor agonist, and on structure-activity data discussed below, it is likely that this receptor is the primary mediator of the observed cardiac electrophysiological changes. Other subtypes, however, such as δ-receptors that are activated by morphine, must be considered in future studies of stress-induced arrhythmias.

Role During Myocardial Ischemia

The pioneering studies of Lowenstein and colleagues[90,91] demonstrated that the administration of high-dose opioids exerts a remarkable stabilizing effect on cardiac rhythm during major surgery in patients with coronary artery disease. Notwithstanding this extensive clinical experience, there has been a relative paucity of experimental work to define the influence of opioids on cardiac excitable properties during acute myocardial ischemia.

To address this issue, we examined the effects of μ-receptor activation on cardiac electrical properties during acute coronary artery occlusion in the canine model. The effects of full and partial μ-agonism were compared, using fentanyl and buprenorphine, respectively.[97,98] Fentanyl was chosen because it is a relatively pure μ-agonist with demonstrated efficacy in the surgical and coronary care unit setting. Buprenorphine is of clinical interest because it has 25 to 50 times the analgesic potency of morphine sulfate but exhibits a ceiling on respiratory depression. The drug causes only a moderate reduction in heart rate and P_A in humans and canines. Our study demonstrated that fentanyl significantly reduced vulnerability to VF during coronary artery occlusion (Fig. 9).[98] The protective effect of the drug appears to be due mainly to increased vagal efferent activity, as it was abolished by the administration of atropine. Buprenorphine was found to be completely without effect on vulnerability during coronary artery occlusion.[98] Thus, partial μ-agonism does not appear to be sufficient to protect the heart from the profibrillatory influence of acute ischemia. Nevertheless, this agent may be protective against arrhythmias associated with myocardial infarction. Pant and coworkers[99] found that injection of buprenorphine reduced the spontaneous ventricular ectopic activity 24 hours after myocardial infarction in dogs. These findings are not inconsistent with our observations, as the drug may be antiarrhythmic but not antifibrillatory. Indeed, it is well known that the arrhythmias that develop within the first 24 hours after infarction are the result of enhanced auto-

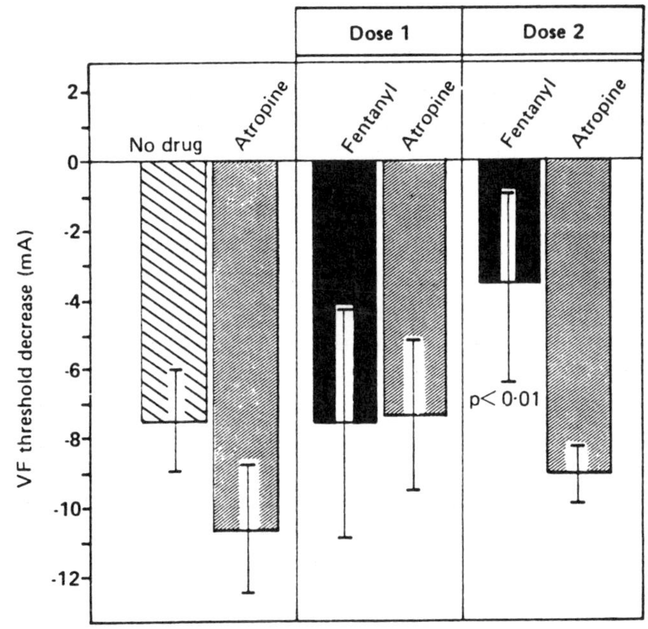

Figure 9. *The effect of fentanyl on the decline in VF threshold during acute coronary artery occlusion in six dogs. In the absence of any drug, VF threshold fell by 7.5 mA. After the second dose of fentanyl (30 mcg/kg/dose), this decline was significantly reduced to 3.6 mA. Atropine pretreatment increased this decline to 10.6 mA prior to fentanyl administration and prevented the antifibrillatory effect of the second dose of the opioid. Values are expressed as means ± SEM. Reproduced with permission from Saint V, Carr DB, Verrier RL: Comparative effects of the opioids fentanyl and buprenorphine on ventricular vulnerability during acute coronary artery occlusion. Cardiovasc Res 23:1003, 1989.*

maticity of Purkinje fibers.[100,101] By comparison, susceptibility to VF in response to acute myocardial ischemia is thought to be due to increased dispersion of refractoriness and microreentry.[100,102] Collectively, these results not only demonstrate the potent stabilizing influence of opioids on cardiac rhythm but also the stress-specificity of the intermediary mechanisms.

Conclusions and Future Directions

An impressive body of information attests to the pivotal role vagus nerve activity plays in CNS regulation of cardiac electrical stability. The parasympathetic nervous system exerts its influence largely by blunting the heart rate response to acute myocardial ischemia and by antagonizing the deleterious effects of catecholamines on the heart. It is evident that multiple intermediary mechanisms are involved, including direct effects on myocardial excitable properties and indirect influences mediated through changes in myocardial perfusion and platelet aggregability.

Among the most exciting prospects for the future is the definition of the modulatory role of neuroactive peptides, which are likely to be essential to fine tuning sympathetic-parasympathetic interactions. The continued application of heart rate variability analytical techniques in conjunction with selective autonomic blocking agents also constitutes a powerful investigative tool.

In the future, the role of various brain stem nuclei in integrating the cardiovascular response to alterations in behavioral state needs to be investigated. Experiments using selective ablation of the nucleus tractus solitarius (NTS) and either cryogenic blockade of the amygdala or of the thalamic gating mechanism or its output have yielded valuable insights into the role of baroreflex integration in the development of behaviorally induced hypertension.[9,10,103,104] Application of these techniques to the study of behaviorally induced arrhythmias is likely to be fruitful. Localized drug injection techniques, if adapted to the freely-moving conscious animal, could also be useful. This method would allow the investigation of specific neurotransmitter systems at specific brain sites and may open new avenues for the pharmacotherapy of arrhythmias.

In the domain of cardiac electrophysiology, sophisticated mapping techniques will make it possible to pinpoint alterations in neural patterning that conduce to life-threatening arrhythmias due to inhomogeneous activation of the sympathetic and parasympathetic nervous systems.[105–110] Finally, dynamic tracking of cardiac vulnerability by complex demodulation of the T wave offers a powerful tool to study vagal influences in both animals and humans.[38] The technique is able to detect the influence of both sympathetic and parasympathetic activity and, thus, may provide an important probe to elucidate fundamental nervous system interactions in arrhythmogenesis in both the normal and ischemic hearts.

Acknowledgment: The authors thank Sandra S. Verrier for her editorial contributions.

References

1. Levy AG: The exciting causes of ventricular fibrillation in animals under chloroform anesthesia. Heart 4:319, 1912.
2. Hockman CH, Mauck HP, Hoff EC: ECG changes resulting from cerebral stimulation. II. A spectrum of ventricular arrhythmias of sympathetic origin. Am Heart J 68:98, 1966.
3. Cropp GJ, Manning GW: Electrocardiographic changes simulating myocardial ischemia and infarction associated with spontaneous intracranial hemorrhage. Circulation 22:25, 1960.
4. Hugenholtz PG: Electrocardiographic abnormalities in cerebral disorders: Report of six cases and review of the literature. Am Heart J 63:451, 1962.
5. Satinsky J, Kosowsky B, Lown B, et al: Ventricular fibrillation induced by hypothalamic stimulation during coronary occlusion. Circulation 44:II-60, 1971. Abstract.
6. Verrier RL, Calvert A, Lown B, et al: Effect of acute blood pressure elevation on the ventricular fibrillation threshold. Am J Physiol 226:893, 1974.
7. Manning JW, Cotten M de V: Mechanism of cardiac arrhythmias induced by diencephalic stimulation. Am J Physiol 203:1120, 1962.
8. Korteweg GCJ, Boeles TF, Tencate J: Influence of stimulation of some subcortical areas on electrocardiogram. J Neurophysiol 20:100, 1957.

9. Skinner JE, Reed JC: Blockade of frontocortical-brain stem pathway prevents ventricular fibrillation of ischemic heart. Am J Physiol 240:H156, 1981.
10. Carpeggiani C, Landisman C, Montaron M-F, et al: Cryoblockade in limbic brain (amygdala) prevents or delays ventricular fibrillation after coronary artery occlusion in psychologically stressed pigs. Circ Res 70:600, 1992.
11. Smith OA, DeVito JL: Central neural integration for the control of autonomic responses associated with emotion. Ann Rev Neurosci 7:43, 1984.
12. Gutterman DD, Bonham AC, Arthur JM, et al: Central neural regulation of coronary blood flow. In JP Buckley, CM Ferrario (eds): Brain Peptides and Catecholamines in Cardiovascular Regulation. New York, NY, Raven Press, 1987, p. 125.
13. Jordan D: Autonomic changes in affective behavior. In AD Loewy, KM Spyer (eds): Central Regulation of Autonomic Functions. New York, NY, Oxford University Press, 1990, pp. 349–366.
14. Cechetto CF, Saper CB: Role of the cerebral cortex in autonomic function. In AD Loewy, KM Spyer (eds): Central Regulation of Autonomic Functions. New York, NY, Oxford University Press, 1990, pp. 208–223.
15. LeDoux JE: Emotion. In VB Mountcastle, F Plum, SR Geiger (eds): Handbook of Physiology. Vol. 5, Part 1: Higher Functions of the Brain. Bethesda, MD, American Physiological Society, 1987, pp. 419–459.
16. Verrier RL, Hagestad EL, Lown B: Delayed myocardial ischemia induced by anger. Circulation 75:249, 1987.
17. Lown B, Verrier RL, Corbalan R: Psychologic stress and threshold for repetitive ventricular response. Science 182:834, 1973.
18. Verrier RL, Dickerson LW: Autonomic nervous system and coronary blood flow changes related to emotional activation and sleep. Circulation 83(suppl. II):II-81, 1991.
19. Skinner JE: Regulation of cardiac vulnerability by the cerebral defense system. J Am Coll Cardiol 5:88B, 1985.
20. Matta RJ, Verrier RL, Lown B: Repetitive extrasystole as an index of vulnerability to ventricular fibrillation. Am J Physiol 230:1469, 1976.
21. Verrier RL, Lown B: Behavioral stress and cardiac arrhythmias. Annu Rev Physiol 46:155–176, 1984.
22. Matta RJ, Lawler JE, Lown B: Ventricular electrical instability in the conscious dog. Effects of psychological stress and beta adrenergic blockade. Am J Cardiol 38:594, 1976.
23. Verrier RL, Lown B: Influence of neural activity on ventricular electrical stability during acute myocardial ischemia and infarction. In E Sandoe, DC Julian, JW Bell (eds): Management of Ventricular Tachycardia: Role of Mexiletine. Amsterdam, Excerpta Medica (International Congress Series #458), 1978, p. 133.
24. Liang B, Verrier RL, Melman J, et al: Correlation between circulating catecholamine levels and ventricular vulnerability during psychological stress in conscious dogs. Proc Soc Exp Biol Med 161:266, 1979.
25. Verrier RL, Lown B: Vagal tone and ventricular vulnerability during psychological stress. Circulation 62:III-176, 1980. Abstract.
26. Levy MN, Warner MR: Autonomic interactions in cardiac control: Role of neuropeptides. In DP Zipes, J Jalife (eds): Cardiac Electrophysiology: From Cell to Bedside. Philadelphia, PA, WB Saunders, 1990, p. 305.
27. Löffelholz K, Muscholl E: Inhibition by parasympathetic nerve stimulation of the release of the adrenergic transmitter. Naunyn-Schmiedebergs Arch Pharmacol 267:181, 1970.
28. Revington ML, McCloskey DI: Sympathetic-parasympathetic interactions at the heart, possibly involving neuropeptide Y, in anaesthetized dogs. J Physiol (Lond) 428:359, 1990.
29. Kolman BS, Verrier RL, Lown B: The effect of vagus nerve stimulation upon vulnerability of the canine ventricle: Role of sympathetic-parasympathetic interactions. Circulation 52:578, 1975.

30. Stramba-Badiaie M, Vanoli E, DeFerrari GM, et al: Sympathetic-parasympathetic interaction and accentuated antagonism in conscious dogs. Am J Physiol 260:H335-H340, 1991.
31. Vanoli E, DeFerrari GM, Stramba-Badiale M, et al: Vagal stimulation and prevention of sudden death in conscious dogs with a healed myocardial infarction. Circ Res 68:1471, 1991.
32. Zanchetti A, Baccelli G, Mancia G: Cardiovascular effects of emotional behaviour. In C Bartorelli, A Zanchetti (eds): Cardiovascular Regulation in Health and Disease. Milano, Istituto di Richerche Cardiovasculari, 1970, pp. 17–32.
33. Lewis T: Notes upon alternation of the heart. Quart J Med 4:141–145, 1911.
34. Schwartz PJ, Malliani A: Electrical alternation of the T-wave: Clinical and experimental evidence of its relationship with the sympathetic nervous system and with the long Q-T syndrome. Am Heart J 89:45–50, 1975.
35. Navarro-Lopez F, Cinca J, Sanz G, et al: Isolated T wave alternans. Am Heart J 95:369, 1978.
36. Adam DR, Smith JM, Akselrod S, et al: Fluctuations in T-wave morphology and susceptibility to ventricular fibrillation. J Electrocardiol 17:209, 1984.
37. Smith JM, Clancy EA, Valeri CR, et al: Electrical alternans and cardiac electrical instability. Circulation 77:110, 1988.
38. Nearing BD, Huang AH, Verrier RL: Dynamic tracking of cardiac vulnerability by complex demodulation of the T wave. Science 252:437, 1991.
39. Rosenbaum DS, Jackson L, Leigh A, et al: Repolarization alternans: An electrocardiographic marker of arrhythmia vulnerability in man. Circulation 84:II-J, 1991. Abstract.
40. Surawicz B, Fisch C: Cardiac alternans: Diverse mechanisms and clinical manifestations. J Am Coll Cardiol 20:483–499, 1992.
41. Zipes DP: Sudden cardiac death: Future approaches. Circulation 85(suppl I):I160-I166, 1992.
42. Rosenbaum MB, Acunzo RS: Pseudo 2:1 atrioventricular block and T wave alternans in the long QT syndromes. J Am Coll Cardiol 18:1363–1366, 1991.
43. Nearing BD, Verrier RL: Evaluation of antifibrillatory interventions by complex demodulation of the T-wave. Circulation 84:II-499, 1991. Abstract.
44. Kent KM, Smith ER, Redwood DR, et al: Electrical stability of acutely ischemic myocardium. Influences of heart rate and vagal stimulation. Circulation 47:291, 1973.
45. Verrier RL: Neurogenic aspects of cardiac arrhythmias. In N El-Sherif, P Samet (eds): Cardiac Pacing and Electrophysiology. Philadelphia, PA, WB Saunders, 1991, p. 77.
46. Zuanetti G, DeFerrari GM, Priori SG, et al: Protective effect of vagal stimulation on reperfusion arrhythmias in cats. Circ Res 61:429, 1987.
47. Zipes DP, Miyazaki T: The autonomic nervous system and the heart: Basis for understanding interactions and effects on arrhythmia development. In DP Zipes, J Jalife (eds): Cardiac Electrophysiology: From Cell to Bedside. Philadelphia, PA, WB Saunders, 1990, p. 312.
48. Harper RM, Frysinger RC, Zhang J, et al: Cardiac and respiratory interactions maintaining homeostasis during sleep. In R Lydic, JF Biebuyck (eds): Clinical Physiology of Sleep. Bethesda, MD, American Physiological Society, 1988, p. 67.
49. Parmeggiani PL, Morrison AR: Alterations in autonomic functions during sleep. In AD Loewy, KM Spyer (eds): Central Regulation of Autonomic Functions. New York, NY, Oxford University Press, 1990, pp. 367–386.
50. Baust W, Bohnert B: The regulation of heart rate during sleep. Exp Brain Res 7:169, 1969.
51. Raetz SL, Richard CA, Garfinkel A, et al: Dynamic characteristics of cardiac R-R intervals during sleep and waking states. Sleep 14:526, 1992.
52. Smyth HS, Sleight P, Pickering GW: Reflex regulation of arterial pressure during sleep in man. Circ Res 24:109, 1969.

53. Nowlin JB, Troyer WG Jr, Collins WS, et al: The association of nocturnal angina pectoris with dreaming. Ann Intern Med 63:1040, 1965.
54. King MJ, Zir LM, Kaltman AJ, et al: Variant angina associated with angiographically demonstrated coronary artery spasm and REM sleep. Am J Med Sci 265:419, 1973.
55. Murao S, Harumi K, Katayama S, et al: All-night polygraphic studies of nocturnal angina pectoris. Jpn Heart J 13:295, 1972.
56. Quyyumi AA, Wright CA, Mockus LJ, et al: Mechanisms of nocturnal angina pectoris: Importance of increased myocardial oxygen demand in patients with severe coronary artery disease. Lancet 1:1207, 1984.
57. Barry J, Selwyn AP, Nabel EG, et al: Frequency of ST-segment depression produced by mental stress in stable angina pectoris from coronary artery disease. Am J Cardiol 61:989, 1988.
58. Campbell S, Barry J, Rebecca GS, et al: Active transient myocardial ischemia during daily life in asymptomatic patients with positive exercise tests and coronary artery disease. Am J Cardiol 57:1010, 1986.
59. Barry J, Campbell S, Yeung AC, et al: Waking and rising at night as a trigger of myocardial ischemia. Am J Cardiol 67:1067, 1991.
60. Muller JE, Stone PH, Turi ZG, et al: Circadian variation in the frequency of onset of acute myocardial infarction. N Engl J Med 313:1313, 1985.
61. Brezinski DA, Tofler GH, Muller JE, et al: Morning increase in platelet aggregability: Association with assumption of the upright posture. Circulation 78:35, 1988.
62. Yasue H, Ogawa H, Okumura K: Coronary artery spasm in the genesis of myocardial ischemia. Am J Cardiol 63:29E, 1989.
63. Ludmer PL, Selwyn AP, Shook TL, et al: Paradoxical vasoconstriction induced by acetylcholine in atherosclerotic coronary arteries. N Engl J Med 315:1046, 1986.
64. Maseri A, L'Abbate A, Chierchia S, et al: Significance of spasm in the pathogenesis of ischemic heart disease. Am J Cardiol 44:788, 1979.
65. Kirby DA, Verrier RL: Differential effects of sleep stage on coronary hemodynamic function. Am J Physiol 256 (Heart Circ Physiol 25):H1378, 1989.
66. Kirby DA, Verrier RL: Differential effects of sleep stage on coronary hemodynamic function during stenosis. Physiol Behav 45:1017, 1989.
67. Dickerson LW, Huang AH, Schryver T, et al: Distribution of heart rate and coronary blood flow surges during tonic and phasic REM sleep. Sleep Res 19:37, 1990. Abstract.
68. Verrier RL: Behavioral state and cardiac arrhythmias. In R Lydic, JF Biebuyck (eds): Clinical Physiology of Sleep. Bethesda, MD, American Physiological Society, 1988, p. 31.
69. Francis GC, Hagestad EL, Verrier RL: Influence of sleep stage on ventricular refractoriness. Physiologist 29:163, 1986. Abstract.
70. Dickerson LW, Huang AH, Nearing BD, et al: Primary coronary vasodilation associated with pauses in heart rhythm during sleep. Am J Physiol 264:R186–196, 1993.
71. Dickerson LW, Verrier RL: Asystole linked to EEG desynchronization during sleep: Is the initiating event of CNS or cardiovascular origin? Sleep Res 20A:83, 1991. Abstract.
72. Hung J, Whitford EG, Parsons RW, et al: Association of sleep apnoea with myocardial infarction in men. Lancet 336:261, 1990.
73. De Olazabal JR, Miller MJ, Cook WR, et al: Disordered breathing and hypoxia during sleep in coronary artery disease. Chest 82:548, 1982.
74. Guilleminault CP, Pool P, Motta J, et al: Sinus arrest during REM sleep in young adults. N Engl J Med 311:1006, 1984.
75. Guilleminault C, Connolly SJ, Winkle RA: Cardiac arrhythmia and conduction disturbances during sleep in 400 patients with sleep apnea syndrome. Am J Cardiol 52:490, 1983.
76. Shaw TRD, Corrall RJM, Craib IA: Cardiac and respiratory standstill during sleep. Br Heart J 40:1055, 1978.

77. Rosen MR: The concept of afterdepolarizations. In MR Rosen, MJ Janse, AL Wit (eds): Cardiac Electrophysiology: A Textbook. Mt. Kisco, NY, Futura Publishing Co, 1990, p. 267.
78. Gillis AM, Stoohs R, Guilleminault C: Changes in the QT interval during obstructive sleep apnea. Sleep 14:346, 1991.
79. Gillis AM, MacLean KE, Guilleminault C: The QT interval during wake and sleep in patients with ventricular arrhythmias. Sleep 11:333, 1988.
80. Bigger JT, La Rovere MT, Steinman RC, et al: Comparison of baroreflex sensitivity and heart period variability after myocardial infarction. J Am Coll Cardiol 14:1511, 1989.
81. Zemaityte D, Varoneckas G, Sokolov E: Heart rhythm control during sleep. Psychophysiology 21:279, 1984.
82. Furlan R, Guzzetti S, Crivellar W, et al: Continuous 24-hour assessment of neural regulation of systemic arterial pressure and RR variabilities in ambulant subjects. Circulation 81:537, 1990.
83. Pagani M, Lombardi F, Guzzetti S, et al: Power spectral analysis of heart rate and arterial pressure variabilities as a marker of sympatho-vagal interaction in man and conscious dog. Circ Res 59:178, 1986.
84. Akselrod S, Gordon D, Ubel A, et al: Power spectrum analysis of heart rate fluctuation: A quantitative probe of beat-to-beat cardiovascular control. Science 213:220, 1981.
85. MacWilliam JA: Blood pressure and heart action in sleep and dreams: Their relation to haemorrhages, angina, and sudden death. Br Med J 22:1196, 1923.
86. Conway J, Boon N, Jones JV, et al: Involvement of the baroreceptor reflexes in the changes in blood pressure with sleep and mental arousal. Hypertension 5:746, 1983.
87. Muller JE, Tofler GH, Stone PH: Circadian variation and triggers of onset of acute cardiovascular disease. Circulation 79:733, 1989.
88. Tofler GH, Brezinski D, Schafer AI, et al: Concurrent morning increase in platelet aggregability and the risk of myocardial infarction and sudden cardiac death. N Engl J Med 316:1514, 1987.
89. Kleiger RE, Miller JP, Bigger JT, et al: Decreased heart rate variability and its association with increased mortality after acute myocardial infarction. Am J Cardiol 59:256, 1987.
90. Lowenstein E, Hallowell P, Levine FH, et al: Cardiovascular responses to large doses of intravenous morphine in man. N Engl J Med 281:333, 1969.
91. Lowenstein E, Whiting RB, Bittar DA, et al: Local and neurally mediated effects of morphine on skeletal muscle vascular resistance. J Pharmacol Exp Ther 180:359, 1972.
92. Carr DB: Opioids. In L Firestone (ed): Molecular Basis of Drug Action in Anesthesia (Intern Anesth Clin, Vol. 26). Boston, MA, Little, Brown, 1988, p. 273.
93. DeSilva RA, Verrier RL, Lown B: The effects of psychological stress and vagal stimulation with morphine on vulnerability to ventricular fibrillation (VF) in the conscious dog. Am Heart J 95:197, 1978.
94. Verrier RL: Behavioral stress, myocardial ischemia, and arrhythmias. In DP Zipes, J Jalife (eds): Cardiac Electrophysiology: From Cell to Bedside. Philadelphia, PA, WB Saunders, 1990, p. 343.
95. Schwartz PJ, Priori SG: Sympathetic nervous system and cardiac arrhythmias. In DP Zipes, J Jalife (eds): Cardiac Electrophysiology: From Cell to Bedside. Philadelphia, PA, WB Saunders, 1990, p. 330.
96. Holaday JW: Cardiovascular effects of endogenous opiate systems. Annu Rev Pharmacol Toxicol 23:541, 1983.
97. Saini V, Carr DB, Hagestad EL, et al: Antifibrillatory action of the narcotic agonist fentanyl. Am Heart J 115:598, 1988.
98. Saini V, Carr DB, Verrier RL: Comparative effects of the opioids fentanyl and buprenorphine on ventricular vulnerability during acute coronary artery occlusion. Cardiovasc Res 23:1001, 1989.

99. Pant KK, Gurtu S, Saxena RC, et al: Antiarrhythmic activity of buprenorphine against cardiac arrhythmia following coronary artery ligation. Indian J Med Res 80:487, 1984.
100. Wit AL, Rosen MR, Hoffman BF: Electrophysiology and pharmacology of cardiac arrhythmias. II. Relationship of normal and abnormal electrical activity of cardiac fibers to the genesis of arrhythmias. B. Reentry. Am Heart J 88:799, 1974.
101. Lazzara R, El-Sherif N, Scherlag BJ: Early and late effects of coronary artery occlusion on canine Purkinje fibers. Circ Res 35:391, 1974.
102. Surawicz B: Dispersion of refractoriness in ventricular arrhythmias. In DP Zipes, J Jalife (eds): Cardiac Electrophysiology: From Cell to Bedside. Philadelphia, PA, WB Saunders, 1990, p. 377.
103. Nathan MA, Reis DJ: Chronic labile hypertension produced by lesions of the nucleus tractus solitarii in the cat. Circ Res 40:72, 1977.
104. Nathan MA, Tucker LW, Severini WH, et al: Enhancement of conditioned arterial pressure responses in cats after brainstem lesions. Science 201:71, 1978.
105. Smith WM, Wharton JM, Blanchard SM, et al: Direct cardiac mapping. In DP Zipes, J Jalife (eds): Cardiac Electrophysiology: From Cell to Bedside. Philadelphia, PA, WB Saunders, 1990, p. 849.
106. Pogwizd SM, Corr PB: Reentrant and nonreentrant mechanisms contribute to arrhythmogenesis during early myocardial ischemia: Results of three-dimensional mapping. Circ Res 61:352, 1987.
107. Burgess MJ: Ventricular repolarization and electrocardiographic T wave form and arrhythmia vulnerability. In MN Levy, M Vassalle (eds): Excitation and Neural Control of the Heart. Bethesda, MD, American Physiological Society, 1982, p. 181.
108. Kleber AG, Janse MJ: Impulse propagation in myocardial ischemia. In DP Zipes, J Jalife (eds): Cardiac Electrophysiology: From Cell to Bedside. Philadelphia, PA, WB Saunders, 1990, p. 156.
109. Kramer JB, Saffitz JE, Witkowski FX, et al: Intramural reentry as a mechanism of ventricular tachycardia during evolving canine myocardial infarction. Circ Res 56:736, 1985.
110. Wit AL, Dillon SM: Anisotropic reentry. In DP Zipes, J Jalife (eds): Cardiac Electrophysiology: From Cell to Bedside. Philadelphia, PA, WB Saunders, 1990, p. 353.
111. Verrier RL: Autonomic control of cardiac arrhythmias. In BN Singh, HJJ Wellens, M Hiraoka (eds): Electropharmacologic Control of Cardiac Arrhythmias: To Delay Conduction or to Prolong Refractoriness? Mt. Kisco, NY, Futura Publishing Co, 1994, pp. 135–150.

CHAPTER 33

Vagal Activity and Ventricular Tachyarrhythmias

M.B. Waxman, D. Cameron, R.W. Wald

The last 30 years have witnessed an unprecedented growth in our understanding of the mechanisms and treatment of cardiac arrhythmias.[1] There has been a parallel expansion of our knowledge of the role played by the autonomic nervous system in cardiac arrhythmias.[2–11] By interacting with the anatomical and electrophysiological substrate of an arrhythmia, autonomic tone may be instrumental in initiating the arrhythmia, and once started, the arrhythmia may accelerate, slow, terminate, or transform to another arrhythmia because of additional changes in the autonomic nervous system.[4–6,11]

The participation of the autonomic nervous system and, in particular, of the parasympathetic system in human tachycardias was first documented in 1913, when Cohn and Fraser[12] published two cases of paroxysmal supraventricular tachycardia that were repeatedly terminated by carotid sinus pressure. The ability of vagal stimulation to terminate paroxysms of rapid heart actions was originally reported in separate papers by Bensen and Priesendorff in 1880.[12] Cohn and Fraser, however, provided the first electrocardiographic proof of the tachycardia and its termination. While vagal tone is most conspicuously involved in modulating supraventricular arrhythmias, it may also, in a less obvious way, significantly affect ventricular arrhythmias.[4–6] This finding was first demonstrated in classical experiments performed by Levy.[13] In cats whose hearts were sensitized by the anesthetic chloroform, he showed that vagal tone protected against the development of ventricular arrhythmias, including ventricular fibrillation, in response to epinephrine.[13,14]

In recent years, it has been shown that enhanced vagal tone can terminate some forms of ventricular tachycardia in man.[15–22] These observations have been reinforced by different experiments that have disclosed:

1. the presence of nerve fibers containing acetylcholinesterase (AChE) in the ventricles of cats, dogs, and man[23,24];

Supported in part by grants-in-aid from the Heart and Stroke Foundation of Ontario.

2. that muscarinic receptors (mAChRs) are present in ventricular muscle preparations[25];
3. that vagal stimulation and acetylcholine (ACh) administration slows the idioventricular rhythm in dogs with experimentally-induced heart block[26,27];
4. that ACh reduces automaticity of isolated Purkinje fibers of dogs in vitro[28,29];
5. that ACh reverses the stimulatory action of isoproterenol on the slow response in Purkinje fibers[30];
6. that vagal stimulation antagonizes the adrenergically-mediated shortening of ventricular effective refractory period (ERP)[31,32]; and
7. that ACh and vagal stimulation depress left ventricular contractile force.[33]

This chapter discusses the role of vagal tone in clinical and experimental ventricular arrhythmias. Some of the concepts derived from work on the interaction between the autonomic nervous system and supraventricular arrhythmias[4–6,11,34–36] are, where applicable, incorporated in this chapter.

Physiological and Pharmacological Methods of Manipulating Vagal Tone

Spontaneous or purposeful pertubations of vagal tone invariably result in complex direct and reflex responses in cardiovascular function. These responses can enhance or diminish the actual effect of the intervention. Of these, heart rate, blood pressure, and ventricular volume appear to be of greatest significance. The complexity of the effects of vagal maneuvers and of their interpretation are illustrated at several levels, as follows (Table 1).

Activation of efferent vagal tone in man mainly involves methods that elevate the blood pressure by phenylephrine or the Valsalva maneuver, and direct stimulation of baroreceptors by carotid sinus massage or negative pressure around the carotid sinuses.[5] These maneuvers activate afferent activity from the baroreceptors, and this activity then reflexly increases vagal tone and decreases sympathetic tone.[37,38] As a consequence, activation of baroreceptors by carotid sinus massage slows the heart rate and reduces the blood pressure. Phenylephrine also activates baroreceptors, but despite the resultant sympathetic withdrawal, the vasoconstrictor effect of phenylephrine maintains an elevated blood pressure. Since baroreceptor stimulation affects both vagal and sympathetic tone, it is important to sort out which action predominates. For example, in one experiment phenylephrine increased the blood pressure and raised the ventricular fibrillation threshold in dogs.[39] Since vagotomy has no effect, but carotid sinus nerve interruption abolished the action, this protective effect was attributed to sympathetic withdrawal. In other experiments, dogs underwent coronary artery occlusion and release. In these studies, blood pressure elevation by phenylephrine also raised the

Table 1.
Effects of Common Vagal Interventions During Normal Sinus Rhythm

Maneuver	*Sympathetic Tone*	*Heart Rate*	*Blood Pressure*	*End Diastolic Volume*	*Contractility*	*Vagal Tone*
CSM	D	D	D	I	D	I
Valsalva-Phase 2	I	I	D	D	I	D
Valsalva-Phase 4	I	D	I	I	I	I
Supine Position	D	D	I	I	D	I
Phenylephrine	D	D	I	I	I	I
Edrophonium	D	D	NC	I	D	I
Atropine	NC	I	NC	D	I	D

This table summarizes the major effects of the following maneuvers: carotid sinus massage (CSM); phase 2 and phase 4 of the Valsalva maneuver; the supine position; phenylephrine; edrophonium; and atropine on sympathetic tone, heart rate, blood pressure, end diastolic volume, contractility, and vagal tone. Symbols: I: increased; D: decreased; and NC: no change.

ventricular fibrillation threshold through its effect on sympathetic tone.[40] In addition to the neural effects of baroreceptor stimulation as well as of the means of stimulating the baroreceptors, the accompanying blood pressure elevation or blood pressure reduction can exert arrhythmogenic or antiarrhythmic effects, respectively.[41–43] Likewise, heart rate slowing can exert a powerful antiarrhythmic effect.[44–47] These processes have to be considered whenever vagal tone is modified via the baroreceptors. By contrast, the administration of edrophonium increases the concentration of ACh and, thereby, increases vagal tone without any noticeable alteration in blood pressure. Edrophonium has other widespread effects, however, including autonomic ganglionic stimulation and bronchonconstriction, and these effects may interact with its cardiac effect.[5,48]

Right- and left-sided carotid sinus massage can have qualitatively and quantitatively different effects on sinoatrial (SA) node slowing, atrioventricular (AV) conduction, and blood pressure both experimentally[49] and clinically.[50,51] The basis for these differences has not been elucidated. Vagal innervation of the mammalian ventricle has been established,[23–25,52] but the anatomical and functional distribution of the right and left vagus nerve remains largely unknown. Depending on the site of origin of ventricular tachycardia, the effects created by carotid sinus massage may be lateralized.

Clinically and experimentally, the effects of vagal tone on the heart are measured by changes in sinus rate or AV nodal conduction time.[4–6,53–55] Although efferent vagus nerve stimulation consistently affects the refractory period and other properties of ventricular muscle,[31,56] we lack a noninvasive marker for the effect of vagal tone on ventricular tissue. Due to this circumstance, we must infer vagal effects on the ventricles by observing rate and conduction changes in supraventricular structures. This process may be less than satisfactory, because it remains to be established whether, and to what degree, the response of supraventricular structures to alterations in vagal tone correlates with changes in ventricular tissues.

The Valsalva maneuver activates autonomic reflexes in a complex fashion.[57–59] At the onset of the strain, the blood pressure and vagal tone rise transiently (phase 1). This is followed by decreases in venous return, cardiac dimensions, blood pressure, and pulse pressure, while sympathetic tone increases (phase 2). Upon release of the strain, there is a marked transient fall in blood pressure (phase 3), which is then followed by increases in venous return, cardiac dimensions, and blood pressure, and the latter activates vagal tone (phase 4). Thus, vagal tone is activated as a result of high sympathetic tone and an elevated blood pressure after release of the strain. The relatively slower response of onset and offset of sympathetic tone compared to vagal tone is crucial to the development of the overshoot in blood pressure and the resultant reflex increase in vagal tone. Despite the fact that autonomic tone changes in different directions during the various phases of the Valsalva maneuver, many believe that the Valsalva maneuver is synonymous with increased vagal tone. Therefore, if a change in heart rhythm occurs during or after a Valsalva maneuver, the change is often ascribed to increased vagal tone. The assumption may be incorrect, because vagal tone is reduced during most of the Valsalva maneuver (see the section below that discusses the effect of cardiac dimensions).

As is true for any intervention, when one measures the effect of autonomic tone on arrhythmias, one must select appropriate conditions. For example, it would be difficult to observe a heart rate response to isoproterenol if the sinus rate is already near maximal as a result of, for example, exercise. Similarly, to demonstrate the effects of vagal stimulation on a host of ventricular electrophysiological changes, one may require heightened background adrenergic tone.[32,60,61]

In the face of heart disease, whether at an early or advanced stage, baroreceptor function and the ability to enhance vagal tone through baroreceptor stimulation is significantly attenuated.[62,63] This feature of altered baroreflex sensitivity (BRS), has been widely used by Schwartz and coworkers[64–66] to predict ventricular fibrillation in animals with experimental coronary artery occlusion,[64,65] and mortality in man after myocardial infarction.[66]

Atropine administration nullifies the effects of vagal tone by competitive blockade of mAChRs.[67] The interpretation of atropine's action is complex, however, because: one, it causes significant hypotension when administered to subjects in the upright position,[68] possibly as a result of its ganglionic blocking properties[69]; two, it accelerates the sinus rate[67]; and three, it blocks presynaptic mAChRs on postganglionic sympathetic nerve terminals,[70] and thus removes an inhibitory influence on the release of norepinephrine (NE). As an example, in experimental and clinical acute myocardial infarction, atropine may cause ventricular fibrillation by its direct action on ventricular mAChRs, as well as by any of the above modulating influences.[71–75]

The actions of ACh are complex and difficult to study in isolation. For example, when administered intravenously, ACh dramatically decreases blood pressure because of arteriolar vasodilatation.[76] ACh not only stimulates mAChRs, but it is also the ganglionic neurotransmitter for the sympathetic and parasympathetic nervous system. Accordingly, its administration systemically, or even in isolated tissue preparations, may result in complex interactions between both divisions of the autonomic nervous system. The direct actions of ACh on atrial and ventricular muscle, as well as on Purkinje fibers, are significantly influenced by background adrenergic tone.[30,77]

At the level of the neuroeffector junction and beyond, the parasympathetic and sympathetic systems interact in four ways[78]: vagal stimulation inhibits the release of NE at sympathetic nerve terminals[79]; sympathetic stimulation releases neuropeptide Y (NPY), which, in turn, interferes with the actions of vagal stimulation, possibly by inhibiting the release of ACh[80,81]; α stimulation with phenylephrine attenuates the bradycardia induced by direct vagus nerve stimulation[82]; and ACh antagonizes the intracellular production of adenosine 3'5'-cyclic phosphate (cyclic AMP) by catecholamines in ventricular tissue.[77,83,84]

Heart Rate as the Major Mediator of the Action of Vagal Tone on Ventricular Arrhythmias

Heart rate changes, the most obvious manifestation of altered vagal tone, can induce, exacerbate, terminate, or reduce ventricular arrhythmias by a variety of mechanisms.[85–89] An increase in rate may slow conduction within zones critical to ventricular reentry by encroaching upon the refractory period within such zones.[90,91] Alternatively, a rapid rate may lead to ventricular tachycardia by enhancing automaticity.[92,93] Slowing, on the other hand, may increase the temporal dispersion of recovery of excitability,[94] as well as depress conduction through diastolic depolarization.[95,96] Both factors may influence the ventricular arrhythmogenic effects of bradycardia experimentally and clinically.[97–100] For these reasons, a rate increase may at times have antiarrhythmic effects.

Premature ventricular beat frequency in man may be greatly reduced during spontaneous or induced rate slowing.[101–103] Suppression of premature ventricular beats by carotid sinus massage or other vagotonic maneuvers is largely abolished by simultaneous atrial pacing, which prevents concomitant slowing in heart rate (Fig. 1).[104] Experimentally, vagal stimulation abolishes premature ventricular beats generated by the combination of cyclopropane and epinephrine.[42,105] As in man, this antiarrhythmic effect is also largely mediated through a decrease in rate.[106] As will be covered in the section that discusses myocardial infarction, heart rate slowing secondary to vagal stimulation is paramount to the prevention of ventricular fibrillation in the setting of experimental coronary artery occlusion/reperfusion.[8,107] The influence of heart rate on premature ventricular beats may, in some cases, be related to an electrotonic influence of sinus beats on protected automatic foci within the ventricular conduction system.[108] Some antiarrhythmic drugs, such as β-receptor blocking drugs and amiodarone, which produce prominent slowing,

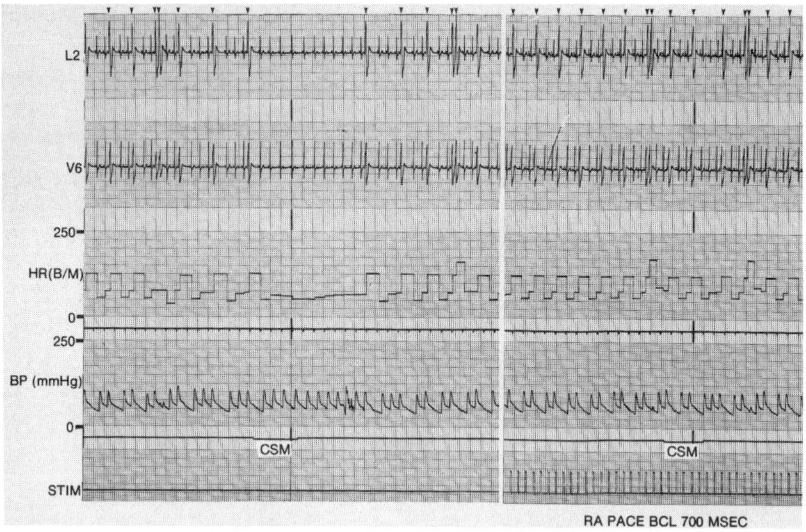

Figure 1. *Suppression of premature ventricular beats (PVBs) by carotid sinus massage. Simultaneous recording of ECG leads L2 and V6, beat-to-beat heart rate (HR), blood pressure (BP), and atrial stimulus code (STIM) in a man with frequent PVBs (see arrows) who has right ventricular dysplasia. In the left panel, PVBs are eliminated for nine seconds following carotid sinus massage (CSM), and they reappear as the background rate reaccelerates. In the right panel, the atria are paced at a cycle length of 700 msec and now CSM fails to stop the PVBs. Reproduced with permission from Waxman MB, Cameron DA, Wald RW: The influence of the autonomic nervous system on arrhythmias. In DP Zipes (ed): Cardiology Clinics, Arrhythmias-II. Philadelphia, PA, WB Saunders Co., 1983, pp. 143–185.*

may ameliorate or abolish ventricular arrhythmias and, thereby, reduce mortality.[109,110]

Exercise induces ventricular arrhythmias by a complex interaction of rate, sympathetic stimulation, and vagal withdrawal, as well by major alterations in cardiac volume and afterload. Most of the focus has been in patients with coronary artery disease, where it is difficult to separate the effects of ischemia from the actions of altered autonomic tone.[111] Exercise and other interventions that increase rate, however, can also induce ventricular arrhythmias in patients without ischemic heart disease. In some cases, such as in patients with complete AV block, exercise can induce ventricular arrhythmias with little or no change in heart rate.[112]

Cardiac Volume and Arterial Blood Pressure Changes: Integral Components of the Maneuvers Used to Alter Vagal Tone

Cardiac pressure, dimensions, and stretch play a crucial role in modulating electrophysiological properties, both in the atria and ventricles.[41,42,105,113–121]

Direct Effects of Blood Pressure on Ventricular Arrhythmias

Blood pressure elevation has direct and reflex actions on ventricular arrhythmias. Acute blood pressure elevation increases ventricular arrhythmias after coronary occlusion,[43] and it is an essential component of the inhalational hydrocarbon-catecholamine model of ventricular arrhythmias.[41,42,105] Even the denervated heart develops ectopic activity during unilateral outflow tract obstruction, and these arrhythmias arise from the afterloaded ventricle.[122] These findings suggest that increased ventricular afterload may induce ventricular arrhythmias by mechanical stretch, a factor known to enhance Purkinje fiber automaticity.[123]

Certain subsets of patients with premature ventricular beats may exhibit a characteristic response to blood pressure elevation. In patients with mitral valve prolapse and who exhibit spontaneous premature ventricular beats, blood pressure elevation by phenylephrine infusion elicits or increases these beats. This effect prevails even in the face of β-adrenergic receptor (β-AR) blockade, or of pacing, which prevents the reflex slowing in heart rate. Reversal of the phenylephrine-induced hypertension by amyl nitrite inhalation or nitroprusside immediately abolishes the premature ventricular beats (Fig. 2).[124]

Effects of Ventricular Dimension on Ventricular Arrhythmias

Ventricular tachycardia has been terminated in nine patients during the strain phase of the Valsalva maneuver at a time when there was marked reduction in heart size, arterial blood pressure, and pulse pressure.[117] Adrenergic and cholinergic blockade did not interfere with the termination (Fig. 3). Standing or the administration of nitroglycerin independently reduced ventricular volume and enhanced the potency of the Valsalva maneuver in terminating the tachycardias. By contrast, the dependent position increased ventricular volume, and this reduced the potency of the Valsalva maneuver in terminating ventricular tachycardia (Fig. 4). It was concluded that an abrupt reduction in cardiac dimensions can interrupt ventricular tachycardia irrespective of any changes in autonomic tone. Two cases of ventricular tachycardia terminating during retching[125] and one case of ventricular tachycardia terminating by strong coughing[126] may be explained by a similar mechanism, because these maneuvers have hemodynamic effects similar to those of a strong Valsalva strain.[59]

In a related vein, the Valsalva strain phase, passive upright tilting, as well as the expiratory phase of respiration, shorten the cycle length of atrial flutter in man by a mechanism that is independent of autonomic tone.[119] The change in cycle length was ascribed to a decrease in cardiac volume. Other reports in man have shown that atrial stretch can affect the rate of atrial flutter[118,120,121] or the refractory period of the atria.[115,116] Thus, the Valsalva and other

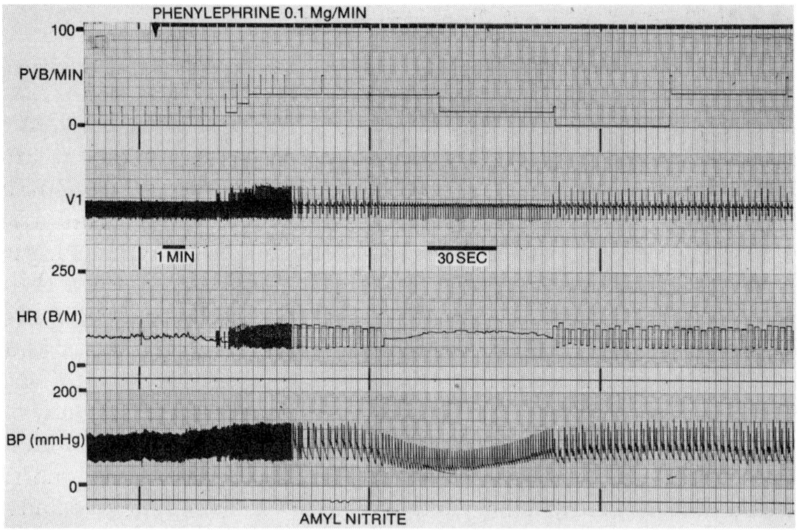

Figure 2. *Induction and elimination of PVBs through alterations in blood pressure in a woman with mitral valve prolapse. This is a simultaneous record of average PVB count per min (PVB/min), ECG lead V1, beat-to-beat heart rate (HR), and blood pressure (BP). The PVB/min count is expressed every 30 s and the vertical pips signify the sampling periods. During control conditions, there are very rare PVBs (upgoing complexes). During an infusion of phenylephrine (0.1 mg/min), systolic blood pressure rises by 25 mm Hg and PVBs are induced with an average count of 32/min. Amyl nitrite inhalation transiently reduces the blood pressure, and the PVBs totally stop for 75 s. The PVBs resume when the pressure returns to the elevated levels. Reproduced with permission from Waxman MB, Cameron DA, Wald RW: The influence of the autonomic nervous system on arrhythmias. In DP Zipes (ed): Cardiology Clinics, Arrhythmias-II. Philadelphia, PA, WB Saunders Co, 1983, pp. 143–185.*

autonomic maneuvers that alter vagal tone,[38] also may have other effects that alter the electrophysiological properties of cardiac tissue.

As noted earlier, when measuring the effects of autonomic tone on the heart, one must select suitable conditions. Since the original publication,[117] four other cases of ventricular tachycardia were studied that initially showed no response to Valsalva strains up to 60 mm Hg. However, by following pretreatment with procainamide in doses that slowed but did not terminate the tachycardia, it was possible to reproducibly interrupt or stop ventricular tachycardia with Valsalva strains of 30 mm Hg or greater in each case.[4]

The importance of blood pressure and cardiac dimension in ventricular arrhythmias is illustrated by the effects of angiotension-converting enzyme (ACE) inhibitors on arrhythmias and mortality. Patients with hypertension[127] or heart failure[128] of diverse etiologies often have ventricular arrhythmias, and an increased incidence of sudden cardiac death. Captopril and other ACE inhibitors reduce afterload, ameliorate heart failure, lower mortality, and reduce the incidence of ventricular arrhythmias.[129,130] The extent to which their antiarrhythmic action accounts for the improvement in mortality is not known, but one preliminary report showed a reduction in sudden death.[131]

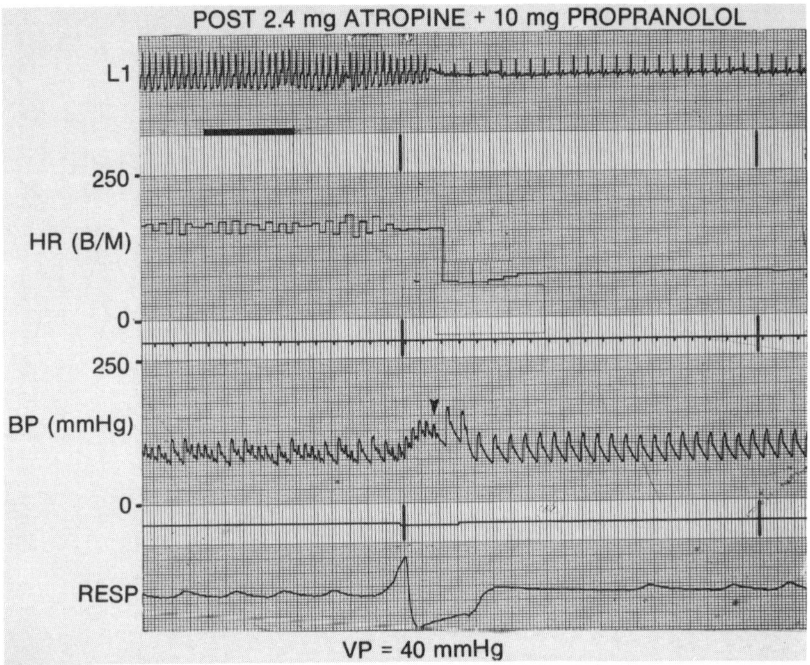

Figure 3. *Valsalva maneuver termination of ventricular tachycardia (VT) following autonomic blockade. Simultaneous recording of ECG lead V1, beat-to-beat heart rate (HR), blood pressure (BP), and respiratory activity (RESP) during VT. A Valsalva pressure (VP) of 40 mm Hg is held and VT ends during the strain when the systolic blood pressure and pulse pressure just begin to fall (see arrow). Valsalva strains also terminated VT prior to autonomic blockade (not shown). Reproduced by permission of the American Heart Association, Inc. from Waxman MB, Wald W, Finley JP, et al: Valsalva termination of ventricular tachycardia. Circulation 62:843–851, 1980.*

Physiological Activation of Vagal Tone During Tachycardias

During tachycardia, vagal tone may be activated, either spontaneously or as a consequence of maneuvers a patient may perform, voluntarily or involuntarily. Patients with paroxysmal supraventricular tachycardia frequently manifest spontaneous automatic termination of the tachycardia within the first minute of the onset of their paroxysms. In a systemic study of this phenomenon, the following sequence of events took place. The blood pressure fell dramatically at the onset of the tachycardia. In response to this occurrence, sympathetic tone increased, the tachycardia rate rose, and the blood pressure recovered markedly. These responses led to activation of vagal tone, tachycardia slowing, and, ultimately, termination of the tachycardia (Fig. 5).[36] Interventions that interfered with the sympathetic response or its effects prevented spontaneous termination of the tachycardia. Such interventions include the dependent position (by blunting the initial hypotension), upright position (by countering the effectiveness of the compensatory sympathetic

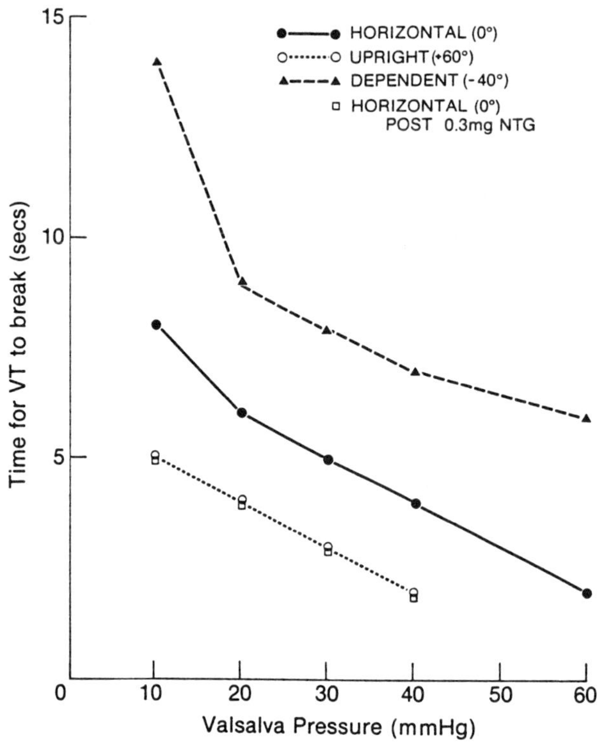

Figure 4. *A plot of the time for ventricular tachycardia (VT) to break against the Valsalva pressure generated. Episodes of VT were repeatedly restarted and the time for different Valsalva strains to break VT is measured in the horizontal (0°, •——•), dependent (−40°; ▲——▲), and upright (+60°, ○——○) position as well as after nitroglycerin at 0° (□). Under each condition, there is an inverse relationship between the Valsalva pressure and the time needed for VT to break. Thus, VT terminates sooner with a stronger Valsalva strain. The upright position and nitroglycerin increase the Valsalva potency, while the dependent position reduces the potency of the Valsalva maneuver. Note that nitroglycerin at 0° has an identical effect to the upright position (+60°, ○——○) on the potency of the Valsalva maneuver in terminating VT. Reproduced by permission of the American Heart Association, Inc. from Waxman MB, Wald W, Finley JP, et al: Valsalva termination of ventricular tachycardia. Circulation 62:843–851, 1980.*

response), or β-adrenergic receptor (β-AR) blockers (by reducing the initial hypotension and the sympathetic compensation). Thus, one mechanism of activation of vagal reflexes during tachycardia is a reflex increase in blood pressure as a consequence of the initial hypotension.[4,6,11,36,132–134]

In patients with paroxysmal supraventricular tachycardia, a deep inspiration markedly augments the blood pressure. At times, this inspiration is sufficient to terminate the tachycardia through an increase in vagal tone.[35] The precise mechanism of the blood pressure increase is unknown, but it likely is secondary to the increase in venous pressure observed during the tachycardia. This occurrence prevents collapse of the inferior vena cava as it enters the thorax during an increased inspiratory effort.[135,136] Thus, another mechanism of augmenting vagal tone during a tachycardia is a deep breath.

Although assuming a dependent body position has only a minimal effect on

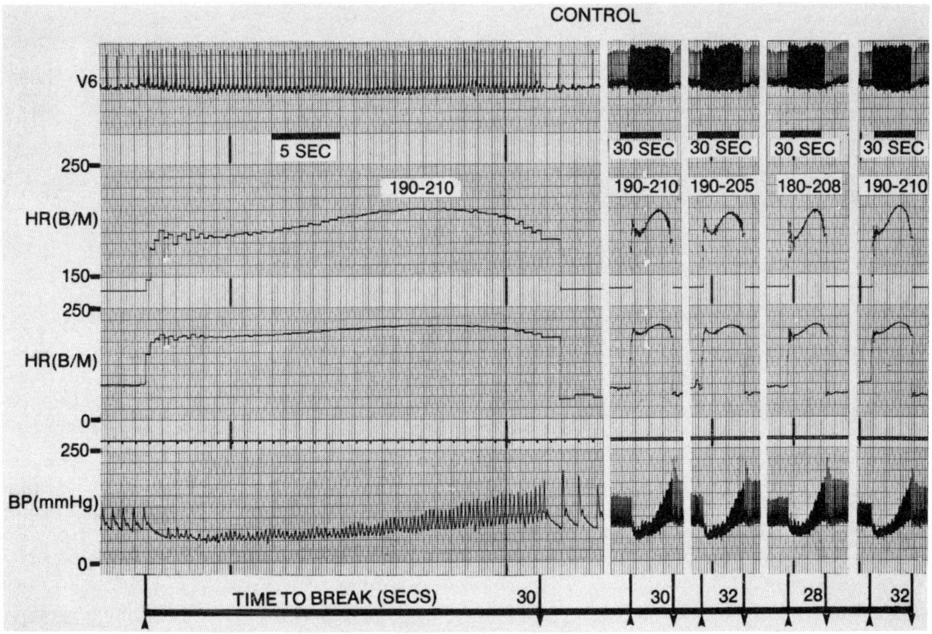

Figure 5. *A simultaneous recording of ECG lead V6, beat-to-beat heart rate (HR) on two scales, and blood pressure (BP) from a patient with paroxysmal supraventricular tachycardia. The up arrows denote the administration of a premature atrial beat, while the down arrows denote spontaneous termination of the induced tachycardia. Five consecutive episodes of paroxysmal supraventricular tachycardia were initiated, all of which terminated spontaneously within 32 s or less. Each episode of tachycardia was accompanied by considerable hypotension. As the blood pressure recovered, the rate initially accelerated and then slowed, leading to termination. There is a remarkably uniform pattern of response of the heart rate, blood pressure, as well as the time for spontaneous termination to occur in the five episodes of paroxysmal supraventricular tachycardia. Modified with permission from Waxman MB, Sharma AD, Cameron DA, et al: Reflex mechanisms responsible for early spontaneous termination of paroxysmal supraventricular tachycardia. Am J Cardiol 49:259–272, 1982.*

blood pressure during normal rhythm,[137] it can markedly augment the blood pressure during paroxysmal supraventricular tachycardia by increasing venous return.[35] The increased blood pressure during a dependent position activates vagal tone that, in turn, frequently terminates the tachycardia. The larger increase in blood pressure in response to a shift to a dependent body position is likely the result of a requirement for a higher venous pressure to overcome the impediment to diastolic filling during tachycardia.[11]

A Valsalva maneuver during tachycardia is followed by a marked overshoot in blood pressure, and this response requires intact sympathetic reflexes and cardiac function.[55,63] The increased vagal tone that ensues often terminates paroxysmal supraventricular tachycardia.[4–6,34]

The combination of a reduction in venous return by passive upright tilting and I.V. isoproterenol can cause a dramatic paradoxic bradycardia in individuals who are susceptible to vasodepressor reactions and have a history of fainting (Fig. 6).[138] Like Sharpey-Schafer and his colleagues[139] in 1958, as well

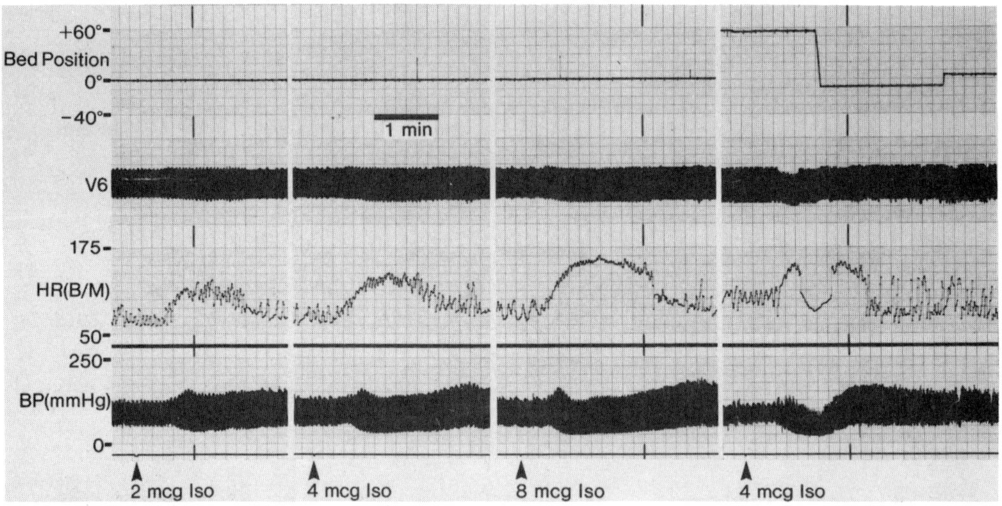

Figure 6. *Simultaneous recording of bed position surface electrocardiographic lead V6, beat-to-beat heart rate (HR) expressed as beats per minute (B/M), and blood pressure (BP) in a patient with a history of classical vasodepressor episodes (fainting). The first three panels show the response to incremental doses of isoproterenol (Iso) at 0°, and one observes that 2, 4, and 8 μg produced a smooth rise and fall in heart rate. Coincident with the rate increase the mean blood pressure falls. The patient did not experience untoward symptoms during these injections, but was conscious of rapid forceful heart beating. The right-hand panel shows the response to 4-μg isoproterenol at +60°. Before isoproterenol was administered, a heart rate increase, a reduction of the systolic blood pressure by 15 to 20 mm Hg, and an increased diastolic pressure of 5 mm Hg compared to 0° are seen. Fifty-four s after 4-μg isoproterenol administration the heart rate, which had reached a value of 150 beats/min^{-1}, abruptly fell to 80 beats/min^{-1}, and the blood pressure was reduced to 90/25 mm Hg. The patient complained of feeling profoundly faint. Following rotation of the bed position to -10°, the heart rate returned almost immediately to 155 beats/min^{-1}. Then over the next 60 s, the rate returned toward normal, followed by wide rate swings over several minutes. The faintness subsided within seconds of the return to a horizontal position. The blood pressure rapidly rose to 175/50 mm Hg. Reproduced with permission from Waxman HB, Yao L, Cameron D, et al: Isoproterenol induction of vasodepressor-type reaction in vasodepressor-prone persons. Am J Cardiol 63:58–65, 1989.*

as Oberg and Thoren[140] in 1972, we concluded that adrenergic stimulation by means of isoproterenol, coupled with a reduced cardiac volume, leads to an overly powerful cardiac contraction. In turn, this process activates cardiac afferent C-fibers, reflexly increases efferent vagal tone, and slows the heart rate.[141] In complementary experiments in rats, the inferior vena cava was occluded for 60 seconds during an infusion of isoproterenol. This action causes a marked paradoxical bradycardia that, like the clinical situation, is mediated by activation of cardiac vagal afferents.[142,143] Experiments in dogs have yielded similar results.[144,145] It is likely that tachycardias could provide the ingredients needed to activate cardiac C-fibers, i.e., reduced venous return combined with marked sympathetic activation.[145,146]

Transient activation of vagal tone during paroxysmal supraventricular tachycardia may produce a slowing that outlasts the original stimulus. The augmented blood pressure after the rate slowing reduces background sympathetic tone and allows the tachycardia to stabilize at a slower steady state level for protracted periods.[11]

Impaired Activation of Vagal Tone in Heart Disease

The response of the diseased heart to manipulations of vagal and sympathetic tone is diminished.[62,63,147,148] In addition, activation of vagal tone requires normal responsiveness to sympathetic tone. The diseased heart is unable to achieve a significant increase in vagal tone, in part because of impaired sympathetic responsiveness.[11] The blunted overshoot in blood pressure following a Valsalva maneuver in patients with heart failure illustrates this point.[55,58,59,149,150]

There is an inverse relationship between the rate of a tachycardia and the cardiac output or blood pressure.[4,6,11] Even a modest tachycardia may greatly reduce cardiac output and blood pressure in the face of ventricular dysfunction.[151] Where coronary perfusion is limited, the reduction in ventricular compliance during tachycardia is exaggerated, causing further reduction in cardiac output and blood pressure[152] and, therefore, an even larger increase in sympathetic tone. Moreover, the diseased heart exhibits minimal hemodynamic improvement in response to sympathetic tone because of cardiac denervation[153] and reduced responsiveness to autonomic tone and other stimuli.[154] The failure of hemodynamic compensation maintains high sympathetic tone, and this occurrence may accelerate or transform the tachycardia, as in the transformation of ventricular tachycardia to ventricular fibrillation.[64,65] For similar reasons, vagal tone remains depressed and cannot be activated. In turn, the restraint that vagal tone imposes on sympathetic tone is impaired. As in the case of atropine-induced ventricular fibrillation in acute myocardial infarction, this impairment of vagal tone may also contribute to the transformation of ventricular tachycardia to fibrillation.[71–75]

Although most of the information about the autonomic reflex response during a tachycardia is derived from paroxysmal supraventricular tachycardia,[4–6,11,34–36,132,133] it seems logical that similar reflex events might transpire during ventricular tachycardia.[134,155] However, in contrast to paroxysmal supraventricular tachycardia, where increased vagal tone terminates the tachycardia, activation of vagal tone may have a different or less obvious effect on ventricular tachycardia.

Termination of Ventricular Tachycardia by Increased Vagal Tone

Despite ample evidence of cholinergic sensitivity of the ventricular myocardium, documented cases illustrating the effects of parasympathetic nervous

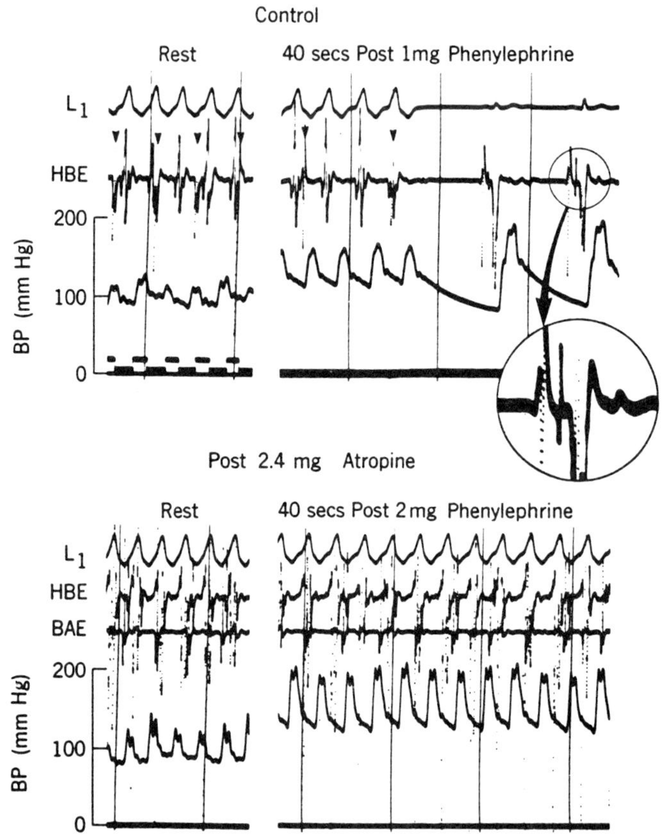

Figure 7. *Effect of phenylephrine on VT before and after atropine. The top panel is a simultaneous recording of ECG lead L1, His bundle electrogram (HBE), and blood pressure in a woman with VT. The arrows point to the dissociated atrial activity. Forty sec after 1.0-mg phenylephrine, the VT and atrial rates that were 180 and 110 beats/min, respectively, slow to 160 and 60 beats/min and conversion to sinus rhythm occurs. A clear His bundle potential precedes ventricular depolarization during sinus rhythm, but not during VT. The bottom panel is recorded during a second episode of VT following pretreatment with atropine. A bipolar right atrial electrocardiogram (BAE) has been added and the arrows again point to the dissociated atrial activity. Following atropine, the VT rate speeds to 230 beats/min, while the atrial rate rises to 155 beats/min. Despite 2-mg phenylephrine and a much higher pressor response, the tachycardia fails to terminate, although the VT and atrial rates slow to 180 and 150 beats/min, respectively. Reproduced by permission of the American Heart Association, Inc. from Waxman WB, Wald RW: Termination of ventricular tachycardia by an increase in cardiac vagal drive. Circulation 56:385–391, 1977.*

system influences on ventricular arrhythmias in man are sparse.[15–22] Twelve cases of idiopathic paroxysmal ventricular tachycardia that were terminated by phenylephrine were described in two reports.[15,17] Detailed studies in four of these cases led to the conclusion that phenylephrine terminated ventricular tachycardia by a reflex increase in cardiac vagal drive.[17] Pretreatment of these cases with atropine at least doubled the dose of phenylephrine and increased the pressure rise needed to stop the tachycardia and, in two of these individuals, the tachycardia could not be interrupted after atropine (Fig. 7). Moreover, pretreatment with the cholinesterase (ChE) inhibitor edrophonium greatly reduced the dose of phenylephrine and the magnitude of the blood pressure rise needed to end the tachycardia. Carotid sinus massage, by itself, irrespective of its intensity or duration, could not interrupt the tachycardia. However, after pretreatment with edrophonium, carotid sinus massage interrupted the tachycardia in all four cases and after adrenergic blockade with propranolol in two of the cases. The interplay between the vagotonic and sympatholytic actions of phenylephrine[38] is further illustrated by more recent observations in two additional cases of ventricular tachycardia. The dose of phenylephrine and the magnitude of the corresponding blood pressure rise that terminated ventricular tachycardia was reduced by pretreatment either with edrophonium or propranolol (Fig. 8).[4]

These observations suggest that the vagotonic and sympatholytic effects of carotid sinus massage and those of phenylephrine[37,38,54] are additive in terminating ventricular tachycardia. An increase in the intensity of either effect may reduce the requirement for the other. The electrophysiological mechanism of ventricular tachycardia termination by an increase in vagal tone and withdrawal of sympathetic tone remains to be elucidated. Both of these changes, however, can prolong the ventricular refractory period[31,32,61] and abolish slow channel-dependent action potentials,[30] which may participate in the tachycardia circuit.

Since its original description,[15,17] termination of ventricular tachycardia by vagal maneuvers has been corroborated in several additional publications.[16,18–22] In one report, four cases were described in whom the Valsalva maneuver (all cases) and carotid sinus massage (one case) could terminate ventricular tachycardia.[21] In each of these cases, adenosine had a similar effect. These patients had no evidence of structural heart disease. All patients were exercise-inducible, and in three patients isoproterenol facilitated the induction of tachycardia. β-adrenergic blockade prevented the induction and/or terminated the tachycardia in all cases. Within the same report, adenosine failed to terminate ventricular tachycardia in any of a parallel series of 14 patients with structural heart disease. Vagal maneuvers were also tested in 11 of these 14 cases with the same negative result. The relationship between the cholinergic and adenosine sensitivity illustrated by these cases may, as the authors suggest, rest with a mechanism mediated by cyclic adenosine monophosphate, although other possibilities could not be ruled out.[84]

Morphine, the cardiac glycosides, and fentanyl are drugs that enhance vagal tone. Morphine sulphate exerts a protective effect on ventricular vulnerability in both the anesthetized dog[156] and in the awake dog subjected to psychological stress.[157] Since much of this action is blocked by atropine, its mechanism is likely mediated by an increase in vagal tone. That component of the action of morphine that is not blocked by atropine may be ascribed to a central sympatholytic action.[157] Acetylstrophanthidin reduces ventricular premature beat frequency in some patients.[158] Although the beneficial effect of this agent may well be mediated by an increase in vagal tone,[159] indirect vagal or sympatholytic effects on heart rate may be equally responsible for these

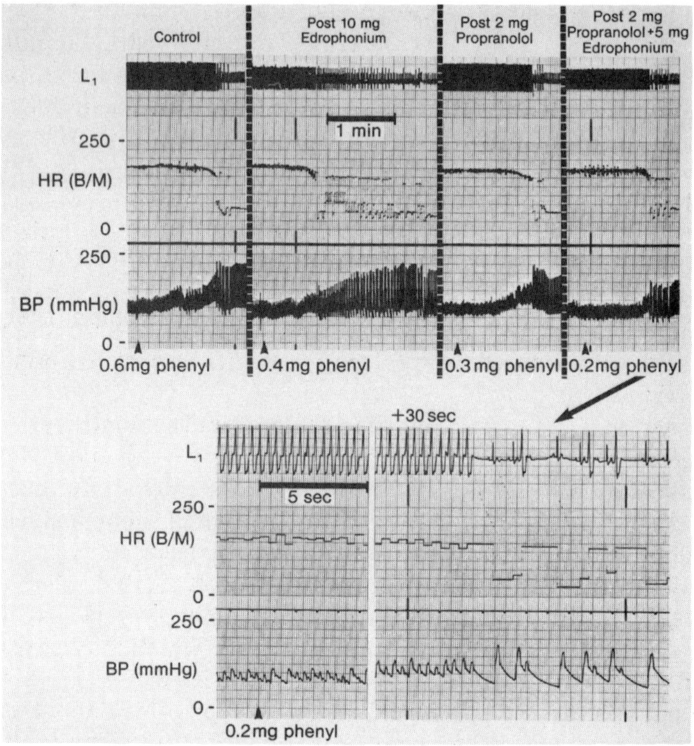

Figure 8. *Phenylephrine termination of VT by vagal and sympathetic interactions. Simultaneous recording of ECG lead L1, beat-to-beat heart rate (HR), and blood pressure (BP) in a patient with VT. The minimum doses of phenylephrine (phenyl) capable of terminating the tachycardia are shown in each of the upper four panels. During control conditions, it is 0.6 mg; following pretreatment with 10-mg edrophonium, it is 0.4 mg; following 2-mg propranolol it is 0.3 mg; and following 2-mg propranolol and 5-mg edrophonium it is 0.2. The lower expanded record is a replay of the panel on the right. Following the reversions, there are variable numbers of PVBs with a morphology identical to the tachycardia, and these PVBs disappear within several seconds. Reproduced with permission from Waxman MB, Cameron DA, Wald RW: The influence of the autonomic nervous system on arrhythmias. In DP Zipes (ed): Cardiology Clinics, Arrhythmias-II. Philadelphia, PA, WB Saunders Co, 1983, pp. 143–185.*

observations. Fentanyl exerts a protective effect against ventricular fibrillation in dogs with experimental coronary artery occlusion.[160]

Induction of Ventricular Tachycardia by Withdrawal of Vagal Tone

mAChR blockade with atropine can cause ventricular arrhythmias, including ventricular tachycardia and ventricular fibrillation in experimental animals and in man. Most commonly, this occurrence has been reported in the setting of an acute myocardial infarction.[71–75] The mechanism of atropine-induced ventricular tachyarrhythmias is unknown, but several possibilities have been proposed. One of these, the increase in heart rate, can have multiple direct electrophysiological effects (see the section above entitled "Heart Rate as the Major Mediator of the Action of Vagal Tone on Ventricular Arrhythmias"),[85–89] or act by intensification of myocardial ischemia. Another mechanism is by withdrawal of the vagal restraint on sympathetic tone.[70,78,79,161] Differentiation between the foregoing mechanisms is difficult, because a rate increase usually precedes atropine-induced tachyarrhythmias.[99,100]

An important exception to the above findings occurred in the case of a patient with complete heart block and no coronary artery disease. The patient was given atropine to increase the escape rate. After atropine, there was no change in heart rate, but the patient developed ventricular fibrillation.[162] After electroconversion, the patient continued to exhibit runs of ventricular tachycardia while the atropine was eliminated. In this case, atropine induced ventricular fibrillation without a background of myocardial infarction or ischemia and without a change in background heart rate. Presumably, ventricular fibrillation developed because of either a direct arrhythmogenic action of vagal tone withdrawal or a decreased muscarinic inhibition of NE release.[161]

Induction of ventricular tachycardia or fibrillation by vagal withdrawal is infrequently reported outside of the setting of acute myocardial infarction.[162] An example of this occurrence was illustrated by the following case in which deep inspiration induced ventricular tachycardia.[18] This observation could be explained either by the hemodynamic effects of a deep inspiration (i.e., an increase in venous return and an increase in left ventricular afterload) or by a reduction in efferent vagal tone. In an effort to distinguish between these possibilities, a number of interventions were studied, as described below.

First, Müller's maneuver replicates the effects of inspiration on preload and afterload[163,164] but, unlike inspiration,[165,166] it does not lead to pulmonary inflation and, hence, does not reduce vagal tone.[167] To replicate the effect of Müller's maneuver, the patient was instructed to inspire deeply against a closed valve. Whereas during normal inspiration ventricular tachycardia was consistently elicited, closure of the valve (Müller's maneuver) prevented the development of the arrhythmia (Fig. 9). This experiment suggested that the induction of ventricular tachycardia by a deep inspiration was not related to preload or afterload changes but, rather, to vagal withdrawal.[165–167]

Second, carotid sinus massage was applied during an increased inspiratory effort in order to counteract the reduction in vagal tone resulting from the inspiration. Carotid sinus massage inhibited the provocation of tachycardia by inspiration. This observation suggested that deep inspiration induces ventricular tachycardia by withdrawal of vagal tone.

Finally, the relationship between the tidal volume during an exaggerated inspiratory effort and the number of beats of induced ventricular tachycardia was linear. This finding allowed an opportunity to test the role of efferent vagal tone in this process by examining the relationship between tidal volume and the number of beats of ventricular tachycardia during control conditions, after edrophonium and after atropine.[5] In all three conditions, the linear relationship between tidal volume and the number of beats of ventricular tachycardia

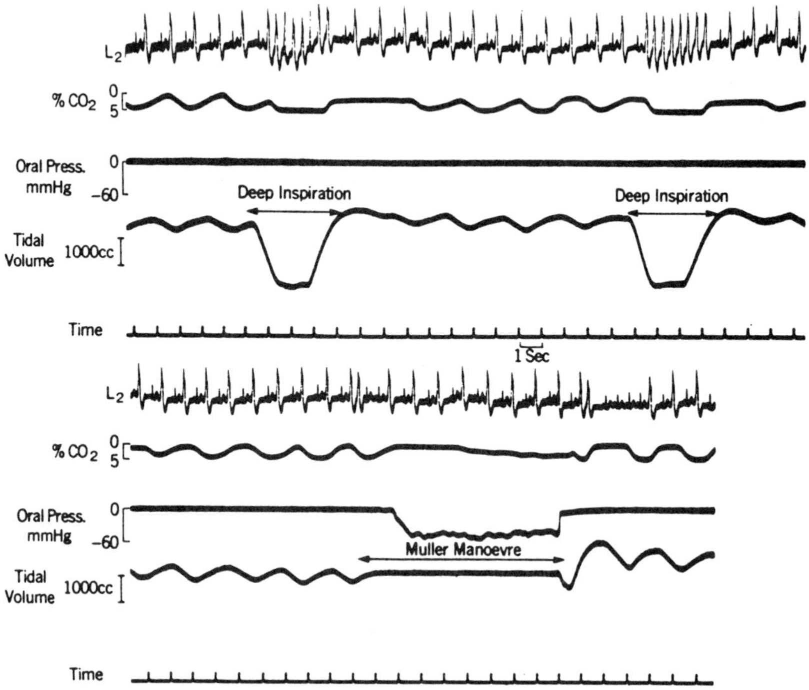

Figure 9. *Induction of VT by a deep inspiration. Continuous recording of ECG lead L2, airway CO_2 concentration, oral mouthpiece pressure (Oral Press.), tidal volume, and 1-sec time marks in a patient with sinus rhythm and bigeminal PVBs. Two successive deep inspirations (top record) provoke runs of VT lasting eight cycles. A strong Müller maneuver (bottom record) of −40 mm Hg does not evoke VT. Reproduced with permission from Waxman MB, Staniloff H, Wald RW: Respiratory and vagal modulation of ventricular tachycardia. J Electrocardiol 14:83–90, 1981. Copyright © 1981, Churchill Livingstone, New York.*

persisted. The effect of any given inspiratory volume, however, was attenuated by edrophonium and enhanced by atropine (Fig. 10).

This case illustrates the induction of nonsustained ventricular tachycardia through withdrawal of vagal tone by a deep inspiratory effort.

Slowing of Idioventricular Pacemakers by Vagal Tone

Recently, we examined the effects of enhanced vagal tone on the rate of a stable idioventricular rhythm in a young man without evident heart disease.[168] Careful mapping localized the origin of the rhythm to the junction of the posterior septum and the posterior wall of the left ventricle, just under the mitral valve annulus. Enhancement of vagal tone by carotid sinus massage, the Valsalva maneuver, phenylephrine, or edrophonium significantly slowed the rate of the idioventricular rhythm. In fact, because these maneuvers often

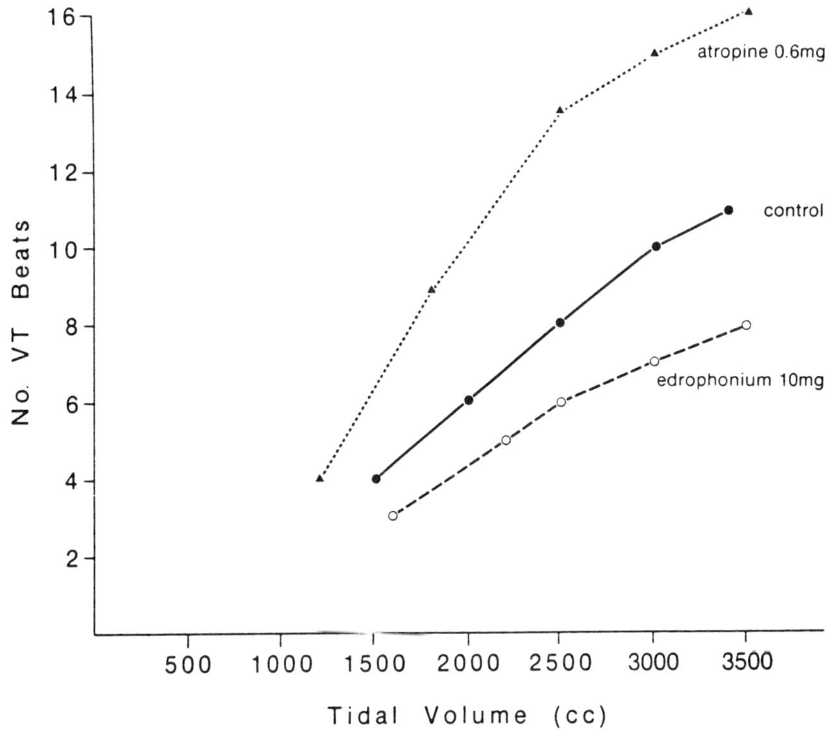

Figure 10. *Plot of number of induced VT beats against various tidal volumes. The background rhythm is sinus with bigeminal PVBs. The control curve shows that at tidal volumes of 1500 cc or greater, VT is evoked and the duration of tachycardia rises proportionally to the inspired volume. Following edrophonium 10-mg I.V., larger inspired volumes are needed to evoke VT, which lasts for shorter periods of time. Atropine, 0.6-mg I.V. shifts the relationship in the opposite direction, so that smaller inspired volumes evoke longer runs of VT. Reproduced with permission from Waxman MB, Staniloff H, Wald RW: Respiratory and vagal modulation of ventricular tachycardia. J Electrocardiol 14:83–90, 1981. Copyright © 1981, Churchill Livingstone, New York.*

slowed the ventricular rhythm more than the sinus rate, they allowed emergence of sinus rhythm (Fig. 11).

We considered whether the rate depressant effect of the various vagal maneuvers on the idioventricular pacemaker may have been due to presynaptic or postsynaptic sympathetic inhibition.[169,170] A dependence of the resting idioventricular rate on the baseline level of sympathetic tone would be implicit to this hypothesis. The arguments against this hypothesis were persuasive, because propranolol did not affect the basal pacemaker rate, and it did not interfere with the rate depressant effects of carotid sinus massage or phenylephrine (Fig. 11). Also, propranolol did not alter the acceleration of the idioventricular pacemaker after mAChR blockade with hyoscine butylbromide.[67]

This case has major implications with respect to the effects of vagal tone on ventricular premature beats that arise by a mechanism of automatic-

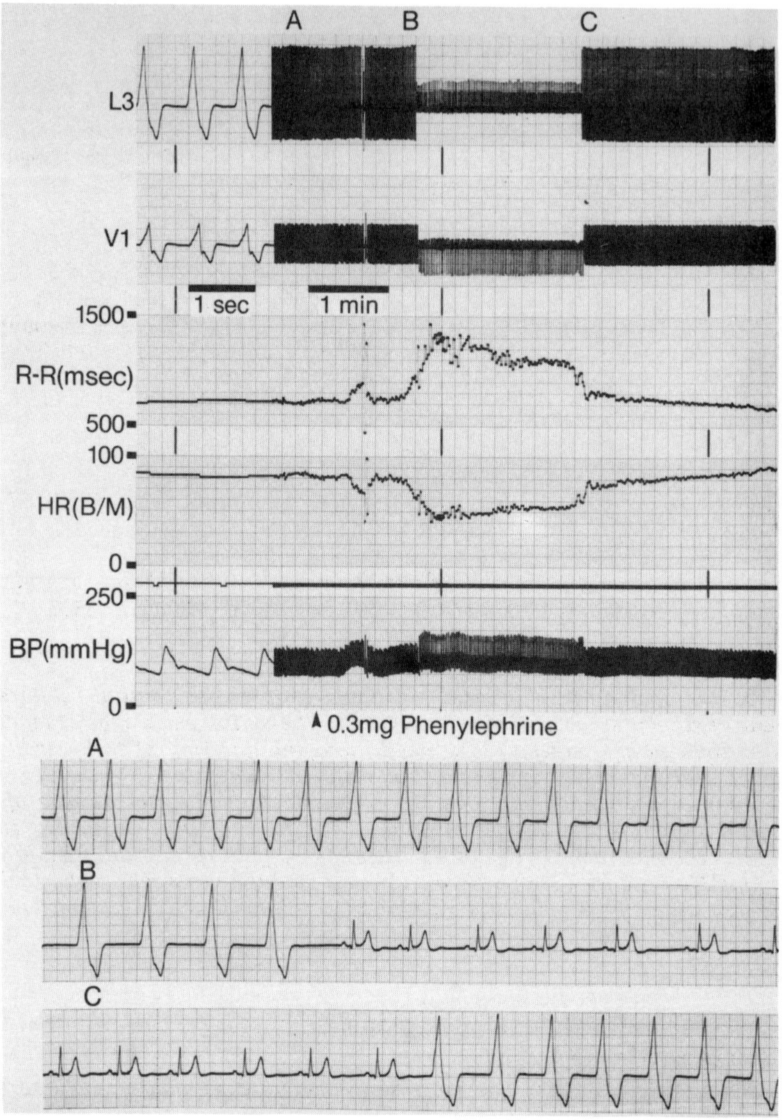

Figure 11. *Simultaneous recording of surface electrocardiographic L3, atrial electrogram, and RR interval following the prior administration of propranolol, 10-mg I.V. Phenylephrine 0.3 mg raises the arterial blood pressure and prolongs the RR interval from 700 to 900 msec, at which points sinus rhythm ensues with cycle intervals of up to 1400 msec. The bottom three panels are recordings of select segments of lead III of the sequence at 25 mm/sec. When the pressor effects of phenylephrine disappear, the idioventricular rhythm reappears. Reprinted with permission from the American College of Cardiology from Waxman MB, Cupps CL, Cameron DA: Modulation of an idioventricular rhythm by vagal tone. J Am Coll Cardiol 11:1052–1060, 1988.*

ity,[92,93,108,171] as well as with respect to the rate of ventricular escape pacemakers in complete distal heart block.[1]

Prevention of the Induction of Ventricular Fibrillation of Vagal Tone

Ventricular Fibrillation Secondary to Inhalational Anesthetics and Catecholamines

For nearly a century, it has been known that activation of the sympathetic nervous system or the injection of cathecholamines into mammals that are anesthetized with inhalational anesthetics can lead to premature ventricular beats, ventricular tachycardia, or ventricular fibrillation.[172] This interaction between the sympathetic nervous system and the anesthetic chloroform led to an extremely high surgical mortality rate at the end of the last century and the beginning of this century, when chloroform was the primary anesthetic used.[13,14] The myocardial sensitization by inhalational anesthetics to catecholamines remains a feature of later generations of inhalational anesthetics, such as cyclopropane, halothane, fluorane, and others.[172]

Levy's[13,14] pioneering work, which showed that vagal tone was protective against these arrhythmias, was subsequently confirmed by others.[42,105] Although the mechanism of its antiarrhythmic effect in this setting remains to be elucidated, vagal stimulation was postulated to act primarily by lowering the heart rate.[106]

Encouraged by our clinical observations of vagally-sensitive ventricular tachycardia[15,17,18] and those of others,[16,19–22] we used this model to further examine the potential protective effect of efferent vagal stimulation against ventricular fibrillation.[173] In halothane-sensitized dogs, paced at a constant rate, we administered increasing doses of NE or epinephrine to establish the minimum doses needed to induce ventricular fibrillation. Observations were made during control conditions and during maximal bilateral vagus nerve stimulation before and after mAChR blockade with atropine. The major findings were as follows:

1. the doses of NE and epinephrine that caused ventricular fibrillation were increased by 100% and 50%, respectively, during vagal stimulation;
2. after atropine, vagal stimulation was not protective;
3. the time to onset of ventricular fibrillation in response to NE was increased by 25% during vagal stimulation;
4. vagal stimulation attenuated the rise in blood pressure in response to NE and epinephrine; and
5. withdrawal of resting vagal tone through vagotomy did not alter the basal dose of either catecholamine needed to induce ventricular fibrillation (Fig. 12).[173]

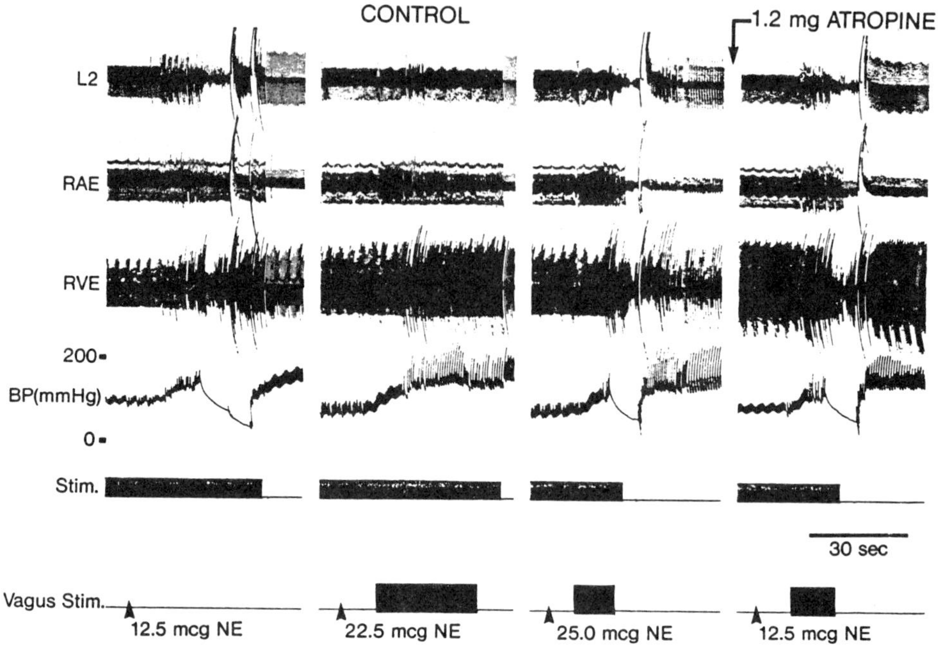

Figure 12. *A typical record from a dog in whom ventricular fibrillation was induced with norepinephrine (NE). The figure contains a simultaneous record of ECG lead 2 (L2), right atrial electrogram (RAE), right ventricular electrogram (RVE), aortic blood pressure (BP), AV sequential stimulus code marker (Stim.), and bilateral vagal nerve stimulation code marker (Vagus Stim.). In the first panel, 12.5 μg of NE was administered in the absence of vagal stimulation, and it caused a marked rise in arterial blood pressure and ventricular fibrillation (denoted by the falling blood pressure). The animal was cardioverted back to sinus rhythm. In the second panel, 22.5-μg NE was given, and 8 sec later, bilateral vagal nerve stimulation was started and maintained for 30 sec. Ventricular fibrillation did not occur. In the third panel, 25.0-μg NE was given and, 5 sec later, vagal nerve stimulation was started but ventricular fibrillation developed, after which the nerve stimulation was terminated. The fourth panel was recorded 5 min after 1.2-mg atropine was administered. 12.5-μg NE was given and, 6 sec later, vagal nerve stimulation was started, but despite this, ventricular fibrillation developed. Thus, vagal nerve stimulation prevented the induction of ventricular fibrillation from a control threshold of 12.5 to a protected level of 22.5-mcg of NE. Following atropine, however, vagal nerve stimulation did not raise the dose of NE needed to cause ventricular fibrillation. Reproduced with permission from Waxman MB, Sharma AD, Lascault GR, et al: The protective effect of vagus nerve stimulation on catecholamine-halothane induced ventricular fibrillation in dogs. Can J Physiol Pharmacol 67:801–809, 1989.*

The protective action of vagal stimulation in this case presumably is mediated at a postjunctional level.[170] At this level, vagal stimulation counters the actions of sympathetic nerve stimulation or catecholamine infusion on the mechanical and electrophysiological properties of mammalian ventricular muscle and Purkinje fibers.[30,32,54,169,170,174] Furthermore, because atropine blocked the protective action of vagal stimulation, we concluded that the protective effect of the vagus nerve stimulation is mediated through mAChRs.[84] These receptors may be diffusely located throughout the ventricle, or localized to regions such as ventricular endocardium and septum, where cholinergic fibers have been demonstrated.[24]

Vagotomy did not lower the dose of epinephrine required to induce ventricular fibrillation. Thus, despite the beneficial effect of maximal vagal stimulation, resting vagal tone did not protect against epinephrine-induced fibrillation. Therefore, it appears that large increases in vagal tone, such as those caused by direct nerve stimulation, are needed to protect against catecholamine-induced ventricular fibrillation in this model. In related experiments not involving halothane, vagal stimulation greatly attenuated the effects of isoproterenol on the multiple extrasystole threshold in dogs. In these experiments, resting vagal tone also failed to affect the threshold dose of isoproterenol.[175]

Blood pressure elevation and increased rate play essential roles in the arrhythmogenic action of catecholamines in hearts sensitized by volatile anesthetics.[41,42,105,106,176] In order to eliminate a rate-related effect,[106] the heart was controlled throughout the experiments. The blood pressure, however, was not controlled and vagal stimulation blunted the blood pressure response to NE and epinephrine. This blunting is probably accomplished through a negative inotropic effect of vagal stimulation on ventricular myocardium, an effect which is greatly enhanced by an elevated sympathetic tone.[54] Additional studies are required to determine whether the protective action of vagal stimulation depends on its effect on blood pressure.

To understand how vagal stimulation is protective, first we need to clarify the mechanisms by which catecholamines interact with halothane to induce ventricular fibrillation. Two speculations are offered. First, catecholamines shorten the refractory period of Purkinje fibers and ventricular muscle tissue.[30,31] This effect could be additive with that of halothane, which also decreases the refractory period of Purkinje fibers and ventricular muscle.[177] Second, catecholamines enhance diastolic depolarization in Purkinje tissue and this result, in turn, may depress conduction.[95] This effect could be additive to that of halothane, which also depresses conduction.[178] Thus, catecholamines and halothane provide two of the major ingredients needed for reentry, namely, a short refractory period and slow conduction.[90,179] Vagal stimulation may protect by antagonizing the adrenergic effects on the refractory period of ventricular muscle and Purkinje fibers,[32,174,180] or by a direct effect on cardiac electrophysiological properties. Vagal stimulation and ACh slow ventricular automaticity in dogs,[26,27] and in man,[168] depress Purkinje fiber automaticity,[28,29] prolong Purkinje fiber action potential duration,[181] and increase the refractory period of ventricular muscle even in the absence of background adrenergic stimulation.[31]

In summary, vagal stimulation protects the dog heart exposed to halothane from NE- and epinephrine-induced ventricular fibrillation. This action is mediated in part via a mAChR.[173]

Effects of Vagal Tone on Ventricular Arrhythmias in Acute Myocardial Infarction

During acute myocardial infarction, both limbs of the autonomic nervous system are significantly disturbed.[2] The apparent increase in sympathetic drive in some individuals or the increase in vagal tone in others are probably the net result of the overactivity in each.[182] Compromised left ventricular contractility can evoke peripheral hemodynamic changes. It also leads to ventricular distention and activation of the powerful Bezold-Jarisch reflex,[183] which results in marked bradycardia, a feature frequently observed during the earliest phase of myocardial infarction in man.[182] Other receptors within the ventricles, atria, pericardium, lungs, and peripheral circulation also contribute to the complex autonomic responses in acute myocardial infarction.[184]

Vagal stimulation is protective against ventricular fibrillation in experimental coronary artery occlusion and reperfusion.[71,72,107,185–187] Most of this protective effect may be due to rate slowing.[8,72,188] Some of this protective effect against ventricular fibrillation, however, is independent of rate slowing. This finding has been demonstrated in dogs in which the ventricular fibrillation threshold was increased[24,107,186] and the incidence of spontaneous ventricular fibrillation was decreased[185] after acute coronary occlusion, independent of rate changes. Moreover, edrophonium hydrochloride restored the ventricular fibrillation threshold that is lowered by acute ischemia[189] and reduced the incidence of spontaneous ventricular fibrillation during acute coronary occlusion, also independent of rate changes.[185]

Although maximal vagal stimulation may be protective, resting vagal tone may be insufficient to protect against ventricular arrhythmias. In a study in cats with coronary artery occlusion/reperfusion-induced complex ventricular arrhythmias, efferent vagal nerve stimulation protected against these arrhythmias, but vagotomy alone did not affect the development of serious ventricular arrhythmias.[187] In other experiments, vagotomy or atropine in cats[73] or atropine in dogs[71,72,186] increased the incidence of spontaneous ventricular fibrillation after left anterior descending (LAD) coronary artery occlusion. Atropine has also been reported to cause ventricular tachycardia and fibrillation in the setting of acute myocardial infarction in man.[74,75] Similarly, resting vagal tone was ineffective in its protective effect in other canine models of ventricular arrhythmias, such as ventricular fibrillation induced by catecholamines and halothane,[173] and repetitive extrasystoles induced by isoproterenol.[175]

In dogs, BRS predicted susceptibility to ventricular fibrillation during acute coronary artery ligation (see also Ch. 34).[64,65] Recently, it was found that cardiac vagal efferent activity increased after experimental coronary artery occlusion in cats.[190] The extent of the increase was greater among animals that did not succumb to ventricular fibrillation than in those that did. In these same experiments, heightened BRS also identified cats that were resistant to ventricular fibrillation.[190] The BRS can also predict mortality postmyocardial infarction in man.[66]

Aside from its direct effects on heart rate, blood pressure, and contractility, vagal nerve stimulation antagonizes adrenergic end-organ effects at multiple levels: presynaptic, postsynaptic, receptor, membrane, and intracellular (cyclic AMP). Vagal nerve stimulation may protect against ventricular arrhythmias at any of these levels. Multiple trials in man have shown that β-AR blocking drugs protect against sudden death after myocardial infarction.[109] Given the extent to which vagal stimulation modulates adrenergic effects, it is generally believed that the benefits of vagal nerve stimulation on ventricular arrhythmias in the setting of myocardial infarction may well be mediated through the sympathetic nervous system.[191] Although this finding is supported by many experiments in which vagal stimulation had little or no effect in the absence of sympathetic influences, recent work in man suggests a significant action of the vagus in prolonging the ventricular ERP, even after β blockade.[192,193] This hypothesis, together with other clinical data[15–22] suggests that extrapolation of the conclusions from experimental work to man must be done cautiously. Ultimately, the importance and the mechanism of cholinergic protection against ventricular arrhythmias in man is yet to be explored.

Summary

This chapter presents an integrated overview of the interaction between vagal tone and ventricular arrhythmias, while bearing in mind that a disturbance of vagal tone invariably involves sympathetic tone as well as changes in heart rate, blood pressure, and cardiac dimensions. We did not attempt to be all inclusive but, instead focused on a few important principles as well as a select number of clinical and experimental examples. In making these choices, we hope to add clinical relevance to our observations and speculations.

Most ventricular arrhythmias are not caused by a primary disturbance of autonomic tone and, more particularly, vagal tone. The extent to which vagal tone may be an important component of ventricular arrhythmias, however, has not been systematically explored and the tools needed to make such an assessment are still in their infancy. With newer, evolving techniques of assessing vagal tone, such as analyzing heart rate variability,[194] it may be possible in the future to begin to answer this question (see Chs. 26 through 29). For the time being, the clinician and the basic researcher will have to devise clever experiments to disturb and analyze the effects of the multiple components of vagal tone on cardiac arrhythmias.

Acknowledgments: The authors gratefully recognize the skill and devotion of Mr. John Asta in carrying out the animal experiments and analyzing much of the data from our laboratory. We also thank Miss Diana Kratis for her able secretarial assistance.

References

1. Zipes DP: Genesis of cardiac arrhthmias: Electrophysiological considerations. In E Braunwald (ed): Heart Disease: A Textbook of Cardiovascular Medicine. 3rd edition. Philadelphia, PA, WB Saunders Co, 1988, p. 581–620.
2. Corr PB, Gillis RA: Autonomic neural influences on the dysrhythmias resulting from myocardial infarction. Circ Res 43:1–9, 1978.
3. Coumel P, Leclercq JF: Role of the autonomic nervous system in the genesis of clinical arrhythmias. In MB Rosenbaum, MV Elizari (eds): Frontiers in Cardiac Electrophysiology. Boston, MA, Martinus Nijhoff, 1983, p. 552–581.
4. Waxman MB, Cameron DA, Wald RW: The influence of the autonomic nervous system on arrhythmias. In DP Zipes (ed): Cardiology Clinics, Arrhythmias-II. Philadephia, PA, WB Saunders Co, 1983, pp. 143–185.
5. Waxman MB, Cameron DA, Wald RW, et al: The use of autonomic maneuvers for diagnosis and treatment of cardiac arrhythmias. In GS Wagner, RA Waugh, BW Ramo (eds): Cardiac Arrhythmias. New York, NY, Churchill Livingstone, 1983, pp. 57–108.
6. Waxman MB, Wald RW: The effects of autonomic tone on tachycardias. In B Surawicz, CP Reddy, EN Prystowsky (eds): Tachycardias. Boston, MA, Martinus Nijhoff, 1984, pp. 67–102.
7. Corr PB, Yamada KA, Witkowski FX: Mechanisms controlling cardiac autonomic function and their relation to arrhythmogenesis. In HA Fozzard, E Haber, RB Jennings, et al (eds): The Heart and Cardiovascular System. New York, NY, Raven Press, 1986, pp. 1343–1403.
8. Schwartz PJ, Priori SG: Sympathetic nervous system and cardiac arrhythmias. In DP Zipes, J Jalife (eds): Cardiac electrophysiology: From Cell to Bedside. Philadelphia, PA, WB Saunders Co, 1990, pp. 330–343.
9. Verrier RL: Behavioral stress, myocardial ischemia and arrhythmias. In DP Zipes, J Jalife (eds): Cardiac Electrophysiology: From Cell to Bedside. Philadelphia, PA, WB Saunders Co, 1990, pp. 330–352.
10. Zipes DP, Miyazaki T: The autonomic nervous system and the heart: Basis for understanding interactions and effects on arrhythmia development. In DP Zipes, J Jalife (eds): Cardiac Electrophysiology: From Cell to Bedside. Philadelphia, PA, WB Saunders Co, 1990, pp. 312–330.
11. Waxman MB, Cameron DA: The reflex effects of tachycardias on autonomic tone. Ann NY Acad Sci 601:378–393, 1990.
12. Cohn AE, Fraser FR: Paroxysmal tachycardia and the effect of stimulation of the vagus nerves by pressure. Heart 5:93–108, 1913–1914.
13. Levy AG: The exciting causes of ventricular fibrillation in animals under chloroform anaesthesia. Heart 4:319–378, 1912–1913.
14. Levy AG: The genesis of ventricular extrasystoles under chloroform as the special reference to consecutive ventricular fibrillation. Heart 5:299–334, 1913–1914.
15. Waxman MB, Downar E, Berman ND, et al: Phenylephrine (neosynephrine) terminated ventricular tachycardia. Circulation 50:656–664, 1974.
16. Lorentzen D: Pacemaker induced ventricular tachycardia: Reversion to normal sinus rhythm by carotid sinus massage. JAMA 235:282–283, 1976.
17. Waxman MB, Wald RW: Termination of ventricular tachycardia by an increase in cardiac vagal drive. Circulation 56:385–391, 1977.
18. Waxman MB, Staniloff H, Wald RW: Respiratory and vagal modulation of ventricular tachycardia. J Electrocardiol 14:83–90, 1981.
19. Hess DS, Hanlon T, Scheinman M, et al: Termination of ventricular tachycardia by carotid sinus massage. Circulation 65:627–633, 1982.
20. Stern EH, Schweitzer P: Termination of ventricular tachycardia by carotid sinus massage. Chest 83:564–565, 1983.

21. Lerman BB, Belardinelli L, West A, et al: Adenosine-sensitive ventricular tachycardia: Evidence suggesting cyclic AMP-mediated triggered activity. Circulation 74:270–280, 1986.
22. Grubb BP: Termination of ventricular tachycardia by carotid sinus stimulation. Int J Cardiol 23:397–399, 1989.
23. Jacobowitz D, Cooper T, Barner HB: Histochemical and chemical studies of the localization of adrenergic and cholinergic nerves in normal and denervated cat hearts. Circ Res 20:289–298, 1967.
24. Kent DM, Epstein SE, Cooper T, et al: Cholinergic innervation of the canine and human ventricular conducting system. Anatomic and electrophysiologic correlations. Circulation 50:948–955, 1974.
25. Birdsall NJM, Hulme EC: Biochemical studies on muscarinic acetylcholine receptors. J Neurochem 27:7–16, 1976.
26. Eliakim M, Bellet S, Tawil E, et al: Effect of vagal stimulation and acetylcholine on the ventricle. Studies in dogs with complete heart block. Circ Res 9:1372–1379, 1961.
27. Danilo P Jr, Rosen MR, Hordof AJ: Effects of acetylcholine on the ventricular specialized conduction system of neonatal and adult dogs. Circ Res 43:777–784, 1978.
28. Bailey JC, Greenspan K, Elizari MV, et al: Effects of acetylcholine on automaticity and conduction in the proximal portion of the His-Purkinje specialized conduction system of the dog. Circ Res 30:210–216, 1972.
29. Gadsby DC, Wit AL, Cranefield PF: The effects of acetylcholine on the electrical activity of canine cardiac Purkinje fibres. Circ Res 43:29–35, 1978.
30. Bailey JC, Watanabe AM, Besch HR Jr, et al: Acetylcholine antagonism of the electrophysiological effects of isoproterenol on canine cardiac Purkinje fibers. Circ Res 44:378–383, 1979.
31. Martins JB, Zipes DP: Effects of sympathetic and vagal nerves on recovery properties of the endocardium and epicardium of the canine left ventricle. Circ Res 46:100–110, 1980.
32. Nattel S, Euler DE, Spear JF, et al: Autonomic control of ventricular refractoriness. Am J Physiol 241: H878–H882, 1981.
33. De Geest H, Levy MN, Zieske H, et al: Depression of ventricular contractility by stimulation of the vagus nerves. Circ Res 17:222–235, 1965.
34. Waxman MB, Wald RW, Sharma AD, et al: Vagal techniques for termination of paroxysmal supraventricular tachycardia. Am J Cardiol 46:655–664, 1980.
35. Waxman MB, Bonet JF, Finley JP, et al: Effects of respiration and posture in paroxysmal supraventricular tachycardia. Circulation 62:1011–1020, 1980.
36. Waxman MB, Sharma AD, Cameron DA, et al: Reflex mechanisms responsible for early spontaneous termination of paroxysmal supraventricular tachycardia. Am J Cardiol 49:259–272, 1982.
37. Smyth HR, Sleight P, Pickering G: Reflex regulation of arterial pressure during sleep in man: A quantitive method of assessing baroreflex sensitivity. Circ Res 24:109–121, 1969.
38. Eckberg DL, Sleight P: Human Baroreflexes in Health and Disease. Oxford, Oxford University Press, 1992, pp. 61–299.
39. Verrier R, Calvert A, Lown B, et al: Effect of acute blood pressure elevation on the ventricular fibrillation threshold. Am J Physiol 226:893–897, 1974.
40. Blatt C, Verrier RL, Lown B: Acute blood pressure elevation and ventricular fibrillation threshold during coronary occlusion and reperfusion in the dog. Am J Cardiol 39:523–528, 1977.
41. Moe GK, Malton SD, Rennick BR, et al: The role of arterial pressure in the induction of idioventricular rhythm under cyclopropane anesthesia. J Pharmacol Exp Ther 94:319–327, 1948.
42. Dresel PE, Sutter MC: Factors modifying cyclopropane–epinephrine cardiac arrhythmias. Circ Res 9:1284–1290, 1961.

43. Harris AS, Ohshima H, Boggs PB: Changes in infarction arrhythmias resulting from changes in arterial pressure. Am J Physiol 210:526–534, 1966.
44. Cope RL: Suppressive effect of carotid sinus stimulation on premature ventricular beats in certain instances. Am J Cardiol 6:314–320, 1959.
45. Weiss T, Lattin GM, Engelman K: Vagally mediated suppression of premature ventricular contractions in man. Am Heart J 89:700–707, 1975.
46. Pickering TG, Johnson J, Honour AJ: Comparison of the effects of sleep, exercise and autonomic drugs on ventricular extrasystoles using ambulatory monitoring of electrocardiogram and electroencephalogram. Am J Med 65:575–583, 1978.
47. Winkle RA: The relationship between ventricular ectopic beat frequency and heart rate. Circulation 66:439–446, 1982.
48. Day MD: Anticholinesterase agents. In Autonomic Pharmacology: Experimental and Clinical Aspects. Edinburgh, Churchill and Livingstone, 1979, pp. 53–64.
49. Wang SC, Borison HL: Decussation of the pathways in the carotid sinus cardiovascular reflex: An example of the principle of convergence. Am J Physiol 150:722–728, 1947.
50. Probst P, Muhlberger V, Lederbauer M, et al: Electrophysiologic findings in carotid sinus massage. PACE 6:689–696, 1983.
51. Peretz DI, Abdulla AL: Management of cardioinhibitory hypersensitive carotid sinus syncope with permanent cardiac pacing—a seventeen year prospective study. Can J Cardiol 1:86–91, 1985.
52. Joo F, Csillik B: Cholinesterase activity of intercalated discs in mammalian heart muscle. Nature (London) 193:1192–1193, 1962.
53. Levy MN, Zieske H: Autonomic control of cardiac pacemaker activity and atrioventricular transmission. J Appl Physiol 27:465–470, 1969.
54. Levy M, Martin PJ: Neural control of the heart. In RB Berne, N Sperelakis, SR Geiger (eds): Handbook of Physiology. Section 2: The Cardiovascular System - the Heart, Vol. I. Bethesda, MD, American Physiological Society, 1979, pp. 581–620.
55. Eckberg DL: Parasympathetic cardiovascular control in human disease: A critical review of methods and results. Am J Physiol 239:H581–593, 1980.
56. Takahashi N, Barber MJ, Zipes DP: Efferent vagal innervation of canine ventricle. Am J Physiol 248 (Heart Circ Physiol 17):H89–H97, 1985.
57. Korner PI, Tonkin AM, Uther JB: Reflex and mechanical circulatory effects of graded Valsalva maneuvers in normal man. J Appl Physiol 40:434–440, 1976.
58. Sharpey-Schafer EP: Effects of Valsalva's maneuver on the normal and failing circulation.Br Med J 1:693–695, 1955.
59. Sharpey-Schafer EP: Effect of respiratory acts on the circulation. In WF Hamilton, P Dow (eds): Handbook of Physiology. Vol. 3. Washington, DC, American Physiological Society, 1965, pp. 1875–1886.
60. Kolman BS, Verrier RL, Lown B: The effect of vagus nerve stimulation upon vulnerability of the canine ventricle. Role of sympathetic-parasympathetic interactions. Circulation 52:578–585, 1975.
61. Kolman BS, Verrier RL, Lown B: Effect of vagus nerve stimulation upon excitability of the canine ventricle. Role of sympathetic-parasympathetic interactions. Am J Cardiol 37:1041–1045, 1976.
62. Eckberg DL, Drabinsky M, Braunwald E: Defective cardiac parasympathetic control in patients with heart disease. N Engl J Med 285:877–883, 1971.
63. Eckberg DL, Sleight P: Baroreflex malfunction in cardiovascular patients: General principles. In Human Baroreflexes in Health and Disease. Oxford, Oxford University Press, 1992, pp. 303–326.
64. Billman GE, Schwartz PJ, Stone HL: Baroreceptor reflex control of heart rate: A predictor of sudden cardiac death. Circulation 66:874–880, 1982.
65. Schwartz PJ, Vanoli E, Stramba-Badiale M, et al: Autonomic mechanisms and sudden death: New insights from analysis of barorecptor reflexes in conscious dogs with and without a myocardial infarction. Circulation 78:969–979, 1988.
66. La Rovere MT, Specchia G, Mortara A, et al: Baroreflex sensitivity, clinical

correlates and cardiovascular mortality among patients with a first myocardial infarction: A prospective study. Circulation 78:816–824, 1988.
67. Day MD: Muscarinic receptor blocking agents (antimuscarinics). In Autonomic Pharmacology. Edinburgh, Churchill and Livingstone, 1979, pp. 65–85.
68. Kalser MH, Frye CW, Gordon AS: Postural hypotension induced by atropine sulphate. Circulation 10:413–422, 1954.
69. Brown AM: Cardiac sympathetic adrenergic pathways in which synaptic transmission is blocked by atropine sulphate. J Physiol (Lond) 191:271–288, 1967.
70. Langer SZ: Presynaptic regulation of the release of catecholamines. Pharmacol Rev 32:337–361, 1981.
71. Epstein SE, Redwood DR, Smith ER: Atropine and acute myocardial infarction. Circulation 45:1273–1278, 1972.
72. Goldstein RE, Karsh RB, Smith ER, et al: Influence of atropine and of vagally mediated bradycardia on the occurrence of ventricular arrhythmias following acute coronary occlusion in closed-chested dogs. Circulation 47:1180–1190, 1973.
73. Corr PB, Gillis RA: Role of the vagus nerves in the cardiovascular changes induced by coronary occlusion. Circ Res 49:86–97, 1974.
74. Massumi RA, Mason DT, Amsterdam EA, et al: Ventricular fibrillation and tachycardia after intravenous atropine for treatment of bradycardia. N Engl J Med 287:336–338, 1972.
75. Scheinman MM, Thorburn D, Abbott JA: Use of atropine in patients with acute myocardial infarction and sinus bradycardia. Circulation 52:627–633, 1975.
76. Day MD: Acetylcholine and parasympathomimetic agents. In Autonomic Pharmacology. Edinburgh, Churchill and Livingstone, 1979, pp. 13–64.
77. Lindemann JP, Watanabe AM: Muscarinic cholinergic inhibition of β-adrenergic stimulation of phospholamban phosphorylation and Ca^{2+} transport in guinea pig ventricles. J Biol Chem 260:13122–13129, 1985.
78. Löffelholz K, Pappano AJ: The parasympathetic neuroeffector junction of the heart. Pharmacol Rev 37:1–24, 1985.
79. Löffelholz K, Muscholl E: A muscarinic inhibition of the noradrenaline release evoked by sympathetic nerve stimulation. Naunyn Schmiedebergs Arch Pharmacol 265:1–15, 1969.
80. Potter EK: Presynaptic inhibition of cardiac vagal postganglionic nerves by neuropeptide Y. Neurosci Lett 83:101–106, 1987.
81. Warner MR, Levy MN: Inhibition of cardiac vagal effects of neurally released and exogenous neuropeptide Y. Circ Res 65:1536–1546, 1989.
82. McGrattan PA, Brown JH, Brown MO: Parasympathetic effects on in vivo rat heart can be regulated through an alpha 1-adrenergic receptor. Circ Res 60:465–471, 1987.
83. Brown JH: Cholinergic inhibition of catecholamine-stimulable cyclic AMP accumulation in murine atria. J Cyclic Nucleotide Res 5:423–433, 1979.
84. Watanabe AM: Cholinergic agonists and antagonists. In MR Rosen, BF Hoffman (eds): Cardiac Therapy. Boston, MA Martinus Nijhoff, 1983, pp. 95–144.
85. Klein HO: Rate-dependence premature beats in man. Chest 69:441–444, 1976.
86. Yusuf S, Lopez R, Sleight P: Heart rate and ectopic prematurity in relation to sustained ventricular arrhythmias. Br Heart J 44:233–239, 1980.
87. Lederman SN, Wenger TL, Harrell FE, et al: Effects of different paced heart rates on canine coronary occlusion and reperfusion arrhythmias. Am Heart J 13:1365–1369, 1987.
88. Coumel P: Rate dependence and adrenergic dependence of arrhythmias. Am J Cardiol 64:41J–45J, 1989.
89. Bernier M, Curtis MJ, Hearse DJ: Ischemia-induced and reperfusion-induced arrhythmias: Importance of heart rate. Am J Physiol 256 (Heart Circ Physiol 25):H21–H31, 1989.
90. Moe GK: Evidence for reentry as a mechanism of cardiac arrhythmias. Rev Physiol Biochem Pharmacol 72:56–81, 1975.

91. El-Sherif N: Reentrant ventricular arrhythmias in the late myocardial infarction period. 6. Effect of the autonomic system. Circulation 58:103–110, 1978.
92. Vassale M, Knob RE, Cummins M, et al: An analysis of fast idioventricular rhythm in the dog. Circ Res 41:218–226, 1977.
93. Wald RW, Waxman MB: Pacing-induced automaticity in sheep Purkinje fibers. Circ Res 48:531–538, 1981.
94. Han J, Millet K, Chizzonitti B, et al: Temporal dispersion of recovery of excitability in atrium and ventricle as a function of heart rate. Am Heart J 71:481–487, 1966.
95. Singer DH, Lazzara R, Hoffman BF: Interrelationships between automaticity and conduction in Purkinje fibers. Circ Res 21:537–558, 1967.
96. Rosenbaum MB, Elizari MV, Lazzari JO, et al: The mechanisms of intermittent bundle brunch block: Relationship to prolonged recovery, hypopolarization and spontaneous diastolic depolarization. Chest 63:666–677, 1973.
97. Chadda KD, Banka V, Helfant RH: Rate dependent ventricular ectopia following acute coronary occlusion: The concept of an optimal antiarrhythmic heart rate. Circulation 49:654–658, 1974.
98. Scherlag BJ, Kabell G, Harrison L, et al: Mechanisms of bradycardia induced ventricular arrhythmias in myocardial ischemia and infarction. Circulation 65:1429–1434, 1982.
99. Pantridge JF, Adgey AAJ: Prehospital coronary care: Mobile care unit. Am J Cardiol 24:666–673, 1969.
100. Adgey AAJ, Geddes JS, Webb SW, et al: Acute phase of myocardial infarction. Lancet 2:501–504, 1971.
101. Lown B, Tykocinski M, Gaufein A, et al: Sleep and ventricular premature beats. Circulation 48:691–701, 1973.
102. Pickering TG, Johnson J, Honour AJ: Comparison of the effects of sleep, exercise and autonomic drugs on ventricular extrasystoles using ambulatory monitoring of electrocardiogram and electroencephalogram. Am J Med 65:575–583, 1978.
103. Cope RL: Suppressive effect of carotid sinus stimulation on premature ventricular beats in certain instances. Am J Cardiol 6:314–320, 1959.
104. Weiss T, Mancia G, Del Bo A, et al: The role of heart rate in the phenylephrine-induced suppression of premature ventricular beats. Eur J Clin Invest 9:9, 1979. Abstract.
105. Dresel PE, MacConnell KL, Nickerson M: Cardiac arrhythmias induced by minimal doses of epinephrine in cyclopropane-anesthetized dogs. Circ Res 8:948–955, 1960.
106. Vick RL: Effects of altered heart rate on chloroform-epinephrine cardiac arrhythmias. Circ Res 18:316–322, 1966.
107. Kent KM, Epstein SE: Neural basis for the genesis and cotrol of arrhythmias associated with myocardial infarction. Cardiology 61:61–74, 1976.
108. Jalife J, Moe GK: A biological model of parasystole. Am J Cardiol 43:761–772, 1979.
109. Yusuf S, Peto R, Lewis J, et al: Beta blockade during and after myocardial infarction: An overview of the randomized trials. Prog Cardiovasc Dis 27:335–371, 1985.
110. Burkhart F, Pfisterer M, Kiowski W, et al: Effect of antiarrhythmic therapy on mortality in survivors of myocardial infarction with asymptomatic complex ventricular arrhythmias: Bassel Antiarrhythmic Study of Infarct Survival (BASIS). J Am Coll Cardiol 16:1711–1718, 1990.
111. Baltazar R, Mower MM, Salomon J, et al: Exertional ventricular tachycardia. Am Heart J 101:354–355, 1981.
112. Winkler RB, Freed MD, Nadas AS: Exercise-induced ventricular ectopy in children and young adults with complete heart block. Am Heart J 99:87–92, 1980.
113. Lab MJ: Contraction-excitation feedback in myocardium: Physiological basis and clinical relevance. Circ Res 50:757–766, 1982.

114. Reiter MJ, Synhorst DP, Mann DE: Electrophysiological effects of acute ventricular dilatation in the isolated rabbit heart. Circ Res 62:554–562, 1988.
115. Kaseda S, Zipes DP. Contraction-excitation feedback in the atria: A cause of changes in refractoriness. J Am Coll Cardiol 11:1327–1336, 1988.
116. Klein LS, Miles WM, Zipes DP: Effect of atrioventricular interval during pacing or reciprocating tachycardia on atrial size, pressure, and refractory period: Contraction-excitation feedback in human atrium. Circulation 82:60–68, 1990.
117. Waxman MB, Wald W, Finley JP, et al: Valsalva termination of ventricular tachycardia. Circulation 62:843–851, 1980.
118. Waxman MB, Kirsh JA, Cameron DA, et al: The mechanisms of flutter interval alternans. PACE 13:138–143, 1990.
119. Waxman MB, Yao L, Cameron DA, et al: Effect of posture, the Valsalva maneuver and respiration on atrial flutter rate: An effect mediated through cardiac volume. J Am Coll Cardiol 17:1545–1552, 1991.
120. Waxman MB, Kirsh JA, Yao L, et al: Slowing of the atrial flutter rate during 1:1 atrioventricular conduction in humans and dogs: An effect mediated through atrial pressure and volume. Cardiovasc Electrophysiol 3:544–557, 1992.
121. Lammers WJEP, Ravelli F, Disertori M, et al: Variations in human atrial flutter cycle length induced by ventricular beats: Evidence of a reentrant circuit with a partially excitable gap. J Cardiovasc Electrophysiol 2:375–387, 1991.
122. Wehrmacher WH, Euler DE, Talano JV, et al: Experimental cardiac arrhythmias in the unbalanced heart. Am J Cardiol 37:181, 1976. Abstract.
123. Kaufmann R, Theophile U: Automatic-fornende Dehnungseffekte an Purkinjefaden, Papillarmuskeln und Vorhoftrabekeln von Rhesus–Affen. Pflugers Arch 297:174–189, 1967.
124. Finely JP, Wald RW, Bonet JF, et al: The mechanism of premature ventricular beat initiation in mitral valve prolapse. Proceedings of the 31st Annual Canadian Cardiovascular Society Meeting, Vancouver, British Columbia, October, 1979.
125. Lyon LJ, Nevins MA: Retching and termination of ventricular tachycardia, report of two cases. Chest 74:110–113, 1978.
126. Wei JY, Greene HL, Weisfeldt ML: Cough-facilitated conversion of ventricular tachycardia. Am J Cardiol 45:174–176, 1980.
127. Ghali JK, Kadakia S, Cooper RS, et al: Impact of left ventricular hypertrophy on ventricular arrhythmias in the absence of coronary artery disease. J Am Coll Cardiol 17:1277–1282, 1991.
128. De Maria R, Gavazzi A, Caroli A, et al: Ventricular arrhythmias in dilated cardiomyopathy as an independent prognostic hallmark. Am J Cardiol 69:1451–1457, 1992.
129. Webster MWI, Fitzpatrick A, Nicholls G, et al: Effects of enalapril on ventricular arrhythmias in congestive heart failure. Am J Cardiol 56:566–569, 1985.
130. SOLVD Investigators: Effect of enalapril on survival in patients with reduced left ventricular ejection fractions and congestive heart failure. N Engl J Med 325:293–302, 1991.
131. Fonarow G, Chelimsky-Fallick, Stevenson LW, et al: Impact of vasodilator regimen on sudden death in advanced heart failure: A randomized trial of angiotensin-converting-enzyme inhibition and direct vasodilation. J Am Coll Cardiol 17:92A, 1991.
132. Curry PVL, Rowland E, Fox KM, et al: The relationship between posture, blood pressure and electrophysiological properties in patients with paroxysmal supraventricular tachycardia. Arch Mal Coeur 1:293–299, 1978.
133. Schlepper M, Weppner HG, Merle H: Hemodynamic effects of supraventricular tachycardias and their alteration by electrically and Verapamil induced termination. Cardiovasc Res 12:28–33, 1978.
134. Feldman T, Carroll JD, Munkenbeck F, et al: Hemodynamic recovery during simulated ventricular tachycardia: Role of adrenergic receptor activation. Am Heart J 115:576–587, 1983.

135. Abel FL, Waldhausen JA: Respiratory and cardiac effects on venous return. Am Heart J 78:266–275, 1969.
136. Berne RM, Levy MN: Control of cardiac output: Coupling of heart and blood vessels. In Cardiovascular Physiology. 5th edition. St. Louis, MO, CV Mosby, 1986, pp. 176–196.
137. Blomquist GC, Stone HL: Cardiovascular adjustments to gravitational stress. In JT Shepherd, FM Abboud (eds): Handbook of Physiology. The Cardiovascular System. Volume 3: Peripheral Circulation and Organ Blood Flow, Part 2. Bethesda, MD, The American Physiological Society, 1983, pp. 1025–1063.
138. Waxman MB, Yao L, Cameron D, et al: Isoproterenol induction of vasodepressor-type reaction in vasodepressor-prone persons. Am J Cardiol 63:58–65, 1989.
139. Sharpey-Schafer EP, Hayter CJ, Barlow ED: Mechanism of acute hypotension from fear or nausea. Br Med J 2:878–880, 1958.
140. Oberg B, Thoren P: Increased activity in left ventricular receptors during hemorrhage or occlusion of caval veins in the cat. A possible cause of vasovagal reaction. Acta Physiol Scand 85:164–173, 1972.
141. Thoren P: Role of cardiac vagal C-fibers in cardiovascular control. Rev Physiol Biochem Pharmacol 86:1–94, 1979.
142. Waxman MB, Asta JA, Cameron DA: Vasodepressor reaction induced by inferior vena cava occlusion and isoproterenol. Can J Physiol Pharmacol 70:872–881, 1992.
143. Waxman MB, Asta JA, Cameron DA: Localization of the reflex pathway responsible for the vasodepressor reaction induced by inferior vena cava occlusion and isoproterenol. Can J Physiol Pharmacol 70:882–889, 1992.
144. Holmberg MJ, Gorman AJ, Cornish KG, et al: Intracoronary epinephrine attenuates baroreflex control of heart rate in the conscious dog. Am J Physiol 247:R237–R245, 1984.
145. Huikuri HV, Zaman L, Castellano A, et al: Changes in spontaneous sinus node rate as an estimate of cardiac autonomic tone during stable and unstable ventricular tachycardia. J Am Coll Cardiol 13:646–652, 1989.
146. Leitch JW, Klein GJ, Yee R, et al: Syncope associated with supraventricular tachycardia. Circulation 85:1064–1071, 1992.
147. Higgins CB, Vatner SF, Eckberg DL, et al: Alterations in the baroreceptor reflex in conscious dogs with heart failure. J Clin Invest 51:715–724, 1972.
148. Vatner SF, Higgins CB, Braunwald E: Sympathetic and parasympathetic components of reflex tachycardia induced by hypotension in conscious dogs with and without heart failure. Cardiovasc Res 8:153–161, 1974.
149. Sarnoff SJ, Hardenbergh E, Whittenberger JL: Mechanism of the arterial pressure response to the Valsalva test: The basis for its use as an indicator of the intractness of the sympathetic outflow. Am J Physiol 145:316–327, 1948.
150. Elisberg EI, Miller G, Weinberg SL, et al: The effect of the Valsalva maneuver in the circulation. II. The role of the autonomic nervous system in the production of the overshoot. Am Heart J 45:227–236, 1953.
151. Lima JAC, Weiss JL, Guzman PA, et al: Incomplete filling and incoordinate contraction as mechanisms of hypotension during ventrcular tachycardia in man. Circulation 68:928–938, 1983.
152. Fifer MA, Bourdillon PD, Lorell BH: Altered left ventricular diastolic properties during pacing induced angina in patients with aortic stenosis. Circulation 74:675–683, 1986.
153. Chidsey CA, Braunwald E: Sympathetic activity and neurotransmitter depletion in congestive heart failure. Pharmacol Rev 18:685–700, 1966.
154. Bristow MR, Ginsburg R, Umans V, et al: β_1-β_2-Adrenergic-receptor subpopulation in nonfailing and failing human ventricular myocardium: Coupling of both receptor subtypes to muscle contraction and selective β_1-receptor down-regulation in heart failure. Circ Res 59:297–309, 1986.
155. Nakano J: Effects of atrial and ventricular tachycardia on the cardiovascular dynamics. Am J Physiol 206:547–552, 1964.

156. De Silva RA, Verrier RL, Lown B: Effect of morphine sulfate on vulnerability of the canine ventricle. Clin Res 24:214A, 1976.
157. De Silva RA, Verrier RL, Lown B: The effects of psychological stress and vagal stimulation with morphine on vulnerability to ventricular fibrillation (VF) in the conscious dog. Am Heart J 95:197–203, 1978.
158. Lown B, Graboys TB, Podrid PJ, et al: Effect of a digitalis drug on ventricular premature beats. N Engl J Med 296:301–306, 1977.
159. Gillis RA, Quest JA: The role of the nervous system in the cardiovascular effects of digitalis. Pharmacol Rev 31:19–97, 1980.
160. Saini V, Carr DB, Verrier RL: Comparative effects of the opioids fentanyl and buprenorphine on ventricular vulnerability during acute coronary artery occlusion. Cardiovasc Res 23:1001–1006, 1989.
161. Levy MN, Blattberg B: Effect of vagal stimulation on the overflow of norepinephrine into the coronary sinus during cardiac sympathetic nerve stimulation in the dog. Circ Res 38:81–85, 1976.
162. Lazzari JO, Benchuga EG, Elizari MV, et al: Ventricular fibrillation after intravenous atropine in a patient with atrioventricular block. PACE 5:196–207, 1982.
163. Robotham JL, Rabson J, Permutt S, et al: Left ventricular hemodynamics during respiration. J Appl Physiol 47:1295–1303, 1979.
164. Hausknecht MJ, Brin KP, Weisfeldt ML, et al: Effects of left ventricular loading by negative intrathoracic pressure in dogs. Circ Res 62:620–631, 1988.
165. Anrep GV, Pascual W, Rossler R: Respiratory variations of heart rate. 1. The reflex mechanism of respiratory arrhythmia. Proc R Soc Lond (Biol)119:218–230, 1936.
166. Hellman JB, Stacy RW: Variations of respiratory sinus arrhythmia with age. J Appl Physiol 41:734–738, 1976.
167. Widdicombe JC, Nadel JA: Reflex effects of lung inflation on tracheal volume. J Appl Physiol 44:681–686, 1963.
168. Waxman MB, Cupps CL, Cameron DA: Modulation of an idioventricular rhythm by vagal tone. J Am Coll Cardiol 11:1052–1060, 1988.
169. Vanhoutte PM, Levy MN: Prejunctional cholinergic modulation of adrenergic neurotransmission in the cardiovascular system. Am J Physiol 238:H275–H281, 1980.
170. Rardon DP, Bailey JC: Parasympathetic effects of electrophysiologic properties of cardiac ventricular tissue. J Am Coll Cardiol 2:1200–1209, 1983.
171. Nau GJ, Acunzo RS, Aldariz AE, et al: Electrocardiographic observations on the mechanisms of ventricular premature beats. Clin Prog Electrophysiol Pacing 4:14–30, 1986.
172. Reynolds AK: On the mechanism of myocardial sensitization to catecholamines by hydrocarbon anesthetics. Can J Physiol Pharmacol 62:183–198, 1984.
173. Waxman MB, Sharma AD, Lascault GR, et al: The protective effect of vagus nerve stimulation on catecholamine-halothane induced ventricular fibrillation in dogs. Can J Physiol Pharmacol 67:801–809, 1989.
174. Inoue H, Zipes DP: Changes in atrial and ventricular refractoriness and in atrioventricular nodal conduction produced by combinations of vagal and sympathetic stimulation that result in a constant spontaneous sinus cycle length. Circ Res 60:942–951, 1987.
175. Furey SA, Levy MN: Interactions among heart rate, autonomic activity and arterial blood pressure upon the multiple repetitive extrasystole threshold in the dog. Am Heart J 106:1112–1120, 1983.
176. Zink J, Sasyniuk BI, Dresel PE: Halothane- epinephrine-induced cardiac arrhythmias and the role of heart rate. Anaesthesiology 43:548–555, 1975.
177. Hauswirth O: Effects of halothane on single atrial, ventricular and Purkinje fibers. Circ Res 24:745–750, 1969.
178. Atlee JL, Alexander SG: Halothane effects on conductivity on the AV node and His-Purkinje system in the dog. Anaesth Analg 56:378–386, 1977.

179. Surawicz B: Ventricular fibrillation. II. Progress report since 1971. Clin Prog Pacing Electrophysiol 2:395–419, 1984.
180. Gilmour RF Jr, Zipes DP: Evidence for prejunctional and postjunctional antagonism of the sympathetic neuroeffector and junction by acetylcholine in canine cardiac Purkinje fibers. J Am Coll Cardiol 3:760–765, 1984.
181. Lipsius SL, Gibbons WR: Acetylcholine lengthens action potential of sheep cardiac Purkinje fibers. Am J Physiol 238:H237–243, 1980.
182. Webb SW, Adgey AAJ, Partridge JF: Autonomic disturbance at onset of acute myocardial infarction. Br Med J 3:89–92, 1972.
183. Mark AL: The Bezold-Jarisch reflex revisited: Clinical implications of inhibiting reflexes originating in the heart. J Am Coll Cardiol 1:90–102, 1983.
184. Hainsworth R, Kidd C, Linden RJ (eds): Cardiac Receptors. Cambridge, MA, Cambridge University Press, 1979.
185. Myers RW, Pearlman AS, Hyman RM, et al: Beneficial effects of vagal stimulation and bradycardia during experimental acute myocardial ischemia. Circulation 49:934–947, 1974.
186. Kent KM, Smith ER, Redwood DR, et al: Electrical stability of acute ischemic myocardium. Circulation 47:291–298, 1973.
187. Zuanetti G, De Ferrari GM, Priori SG, et al: Protective of vagal stimulation on reperfusion arrhythmias in cats. Circ Res 61:429–435, 1987.
188. Kent KM: Cholinergic innervation of the heart: Electrical stability during acute ischemia and during congestive heart failurre. In PJ Schwartz, AM Brown, A Malliani, et al (eds): Neural Mechanisms in Cardiac Arrhythmias. New York, NY, Raven Press, 1978, pp. 99–106.
189. Harrison LA, Harrison LH, Kent KM, et al: Enhancement of electrical stability of acutely ischemic myocardium by edrophonium. Circulation 50:99–102, 1974.
190. Cerati D, Schwartz PJ: Single cardiac vagal fiber activity, acute myocardial ischemia, and the risk for sudden death. Circ Res 69:1389–1401, 1991.
191. Verrier RL: Autonomic substrates for arrhythmias. Prog Cardiol 1:65–85, 1988.
192. Prystowsky EN, Jackman WM, Rinkenberger RL, et al: Effects of autonomic blockade on ventricular refractoriness and atrioventricular nodal conduction in humans. Evidence supporting a direct cholinergic action on ventricular muscle refractoriness. Circ Res 49:511–518, 1981.
193. Morady F, Kou WH, Nelson SD, et al: Accentuated antagonism between β-adrenergic and vagal effects on ventricular refractoriness in humans. Circulation 77:289–297, 1988.
194. Akselrod S, Gordon D, Ubel FA, et al: Power spectrum analysis of heart rate fluctuation: A quantitative probe of beat-to-beat cardiovascular control. Science 213:220–223, 1981.

CHAPTER 34

Vagal Activity and Ventricular Fibrillation

G.M. De Ferrari, E. Vanoli, P.J. Schwartz

The relationship between acute myocardial ischemia, the autonomic nervous system, and lethal arrhythmias is not only a complex one, but also one that has important practical implications.[1–5] As illustrated schematically in Figure 1, acute myocardial ischemia can elicit both sympathetic and vagal reflexes. The evidence for the existence of a cardiocardiac sympathetic excitatory reflex[6] and the subsequent demonstration of its involvement in the onset of life-threatening arrhythmias[7] contributed significantly to the concept that the incidence of sudden cardiac death among patients with ischemic heart disease might be reduced by antiadrenergic interventions. Its clinical counterpart has been the successful use of β-adrenergic blocking agents in post-myocardial infarction patients. While the picture seems rather clear on the sympathetic side, where there is a consensus for the arrhythmogenic action of sympathetic activity in the setting of an ischemic myocardium, the situation seems far more complex on the parasympathetic side. Indeed, it has been proposed that vagal activity may be either beneficial or detrimental, according to its intensity and, possibly, to its concomitant effects on both heart rate and, thereby, on myocardial perfusion. A series of relatively recent studies, however, has brought some clarity in this area as well and allows a comprehensive discussion.

This chapter examines the relationship between vagal activity and malignant ventricular arrhythmias, at both the experimental and clinical levels. Previous experimental studies are discussed first, beginning from those involving direct interventions on the vagi and continuing with pharmacological interactions with the parasympathetic nervous system. Data gathered in a conscious animal model conclude the discussion of the experimental studies and introduce the limited, direct clinical experience in this area.

From *Vagal Control of the Heart: Experimental Basis and Clinical Implications* edited by MN Levy, PJ Schwartz © 1994, Futura Publishing Co. Inc., Armonk, NY.

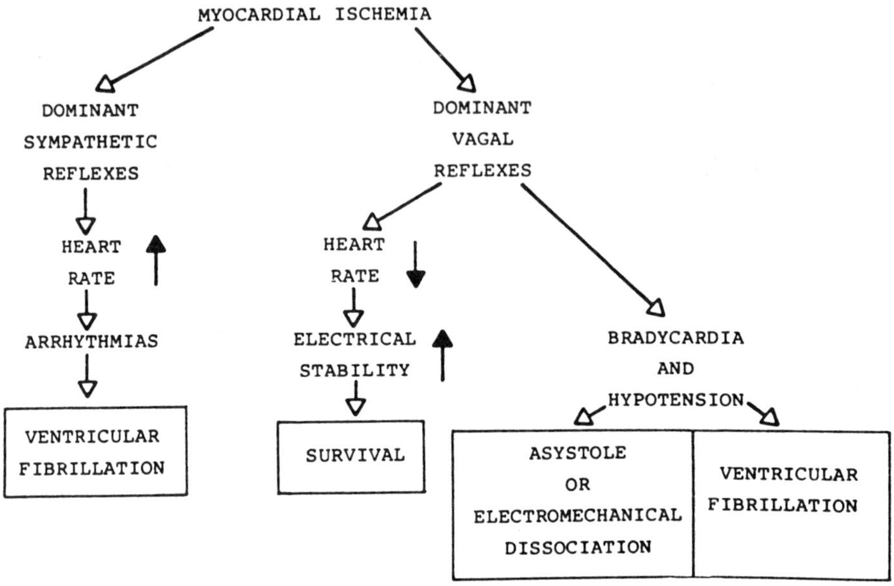

Figure 1. *Effects on cardiac rhythm of the autonomic reflexes produced by acute myocardial ischemia. If sympathetic reflexes are dominant, this action results in an increase in heart rate. The detrimental effects of sympathetic hyperactivity and of the consequent higher heart rate on the ischemic myocardium markedly increase the likelihood for the occurrence of malignant arrhythmias and, ultimately, of ventricular fibrillation. Conversely, when vagal activity is dominant, heart rate decreases and the electrical stability of the ischemic myocardium increases. When vagal reflexes are excessive, however, this occurrence may produce bradycardia and hypotension, with a further underperfusion of the ischemic myocardium that may lead to asystole or to ventricular fibrillation. Reproduced with permission from Schwartz PJ, Stone HL: The analysis and modulation of autonomic reflexes in the prediction and prevention of sudden death. In DP Zipes, J Jalife (eds): Cardiac Arrhythmias: Mechanisms and Management. New York, NY, Grune & Stratton, 1985, pp. 165–176.*

Neural Modulation Studies

The first studies on the effect of vagal stimulation were made more than 100 years ago. Einbrodt[8] used an inductorium to provoke ventricular fibrillation (VF). He noticed that during vagal stimulation, the distance among the coils could be markedly reduced, thereby increasing the current delivered before VF occurred.[8] Despite this pioneering observation, dating back to 1859, the dominant view for a long time has been that vagal hyperactivity is proarrhythmic and favors the occurrence of VF. In 1901, Hering[9] reported that a sudden rise in left ventricular pressure in the isolated heart did not produce extrasystoles, unless the vagus nerve was stimulated at the same time. In 1929, Scherf[10] injected aconitine I.V. in dogs and showed that stimulation of either vagus reproducibly elicited a bigeminal ventricular rhythm at a dose of aconitine otherwise insufficient to produce extrasystoles. More than 30 years later, Scherf et al[11] confirmed the facilitating effect of vagal stimulation on ventricular arrhythmias. For example, fast couplets were provoked, by focal application of a hypertonic solution of sodium chloride on the exposed heart of the dog.[11]

Even though few studies were available to suggest a potential protective effect of vagal stimulation,[12,13] it was widely accepted, until the 1970s, that the bradycardia caused by vagal hyperactivity facilitated ventricular ectopic activity, and possibly, VF. This concept was strengthened by the observation, made in the first coronary care units, that in patients with acute myocardial infarction, marked bradycardia was often followed by ventricular arrhythmia.[14] Experimental studies also indicated that bradycardia increased temporal dispersion of refractory periods and decreased significantly the ventricular fibrillation threshold (VFT).[15]

In 1970, Scherlag et al[16] investigated the potential electrophysiological mechanisms underlying malignant arrhythmias in the early phase of a coronary artery occlusion in dogs. They performed vagal stimulation to cause sinus arrest and to estimate ventricular automaticity, and found that intense vagal stimulation abolished ventricular ectopy and could, in one animal, repeatedly interrupt ventricular tachycardia (VT) (Fig. 2). They interpreted this fact as the result of sinus rate slowing.

In 1973, Kerzner et al[17] investigated the potential proarrhythmic effect of vagal stimulation in dogs with an anterior myocardial ischemia and infarction. They concluded that vagal activation did not induce VF in the early phase of myocardial ischemia, but that it caused ventricular arrhythmias several hours after the onset of ischemia. This study may be considered a transition point in the prevailing views of the effects of vagal stimulation. It confirms a proarrhythmic effect, but it confines it mainly to a late time period in the course of myocardial ischemia. It also suggests that these arrhythmias may result from enhanced automaticity, similarly to clinical accelerated idioventricular rhythms, and that they are unlikely to lead to VF.

Shortly thereafter, one group of investigators[18–20] seriously questioned, with three studies, the concept of a proarrhythmic action of vagal stimulation and suggested an opposite effect. In one study, Kent et al[18] evaluated the effect of heart rate and of vagal stimulation on cardiac electrical stability in dogs with anterior myocardial ischemia. They suggested that, during ischemia, the dispersion of refractoriness and the propensity to VF actually *increased* with heart rate increases, contrary to what occurred in the absence of ischemia.[15] Vagal stimulation that reduced heart rate from 90 to 50 beats/minute markedly increased the VFT. This effect was considered to be heart rate-independent, because an increase in rate from 50 to 90 beats/minute, induced by pacing in a few dogs, had no effect on VFT. Also, in the same study, vagal stimulation increased VFT almost threefold in the nonischemic myocardium paced at a constant rate.

In the second of these studies, Goldstein et al[19] found that vagal stimulation did not change the incidence of ventricular arrhythmias during anterior myocardial ischemia in closed-chest dogs. It should be mentioned that the animals received very high doses of morphine, which has vagotonic actions (see below); that none of the control dogs had VF; and that vagal stimulation was started 10 minutes after the onset of ischemia.

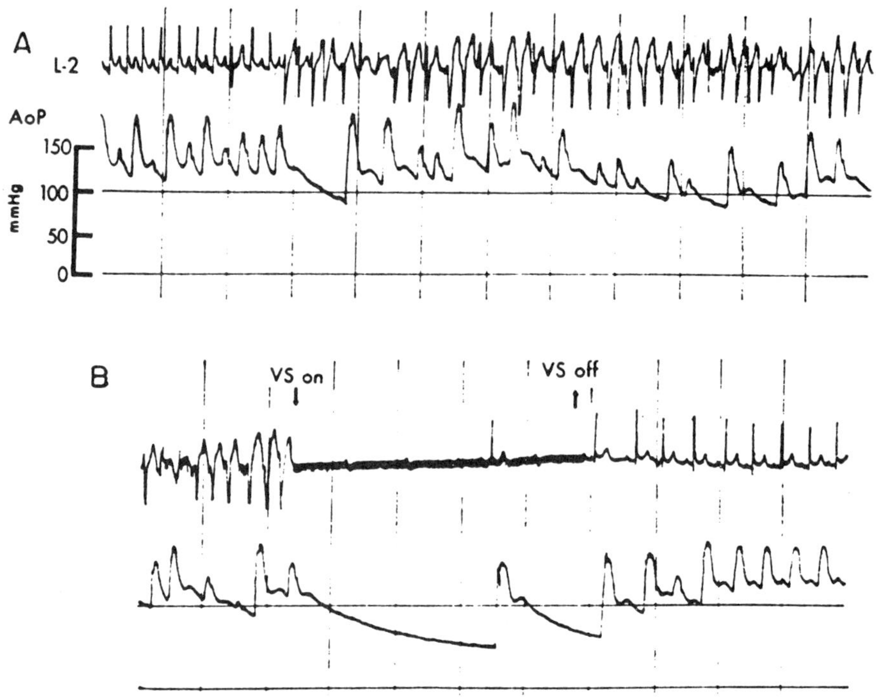

Figure 2. *Effects of vagal stimulation on ventricular arrhythmias and VT after acute coronary artery ligation in an anesthetized dog. In the two panels, the upper trace (L-2) is the electrocardiogram (lead II) and the lower trace (AoP) is the aortic blood pressure. Vagal stimulation (VS on) at the time of a long run of VT interrupts the tachycardia and produces complete AV block. After cessation of vagal stimulation (VS off), sinus rhythm resumes. Reproduced with permission from Scherlag BJ, Helfant RH, Haft JI, et al: Electrophysiology underlying ventricular arrhythmias due to coronary ligation. Am J Physiol 29:1668, 1970.*

Finally, Myers et al[20] assessed the effects of vagal stimulation, initiated before the onset of anterior myocardial ischemia, on the occurrence of VF in barbiturate-anesthetized dogs. The time of onset of VF was delayed and the incidence of VF was significantly reduced, both when the heart rate was allowed to decrease and also when it was kept constant by right ventricular pacing. The authors indicate that the stimulation of the decentralized nerve elicited an effect similar to that evoked by the intact vagus.[20] A significant improvement was found, however, only in survival time, whereas the reduction in the incidence of VF was not significant (Fig. 3).

Corr and Gillis[21] have approached several of these questions in the chloralose-anesthetized cat. Bilateral vagotomy increased the incidence of VF produced by occlusion of the left anterior descending (LAD) coronary artery from 20% to 55%. This effect was not mediated by the increase in heart rate. In a subsequent similar study, these investigators[22] found that vagal stimulation did not reduce the incidence of VF below that (20%) of the control group. They suggested that cats have a significant reflex vagal activation during anterior ischemia, such that additional electrical stimulation would not influence the

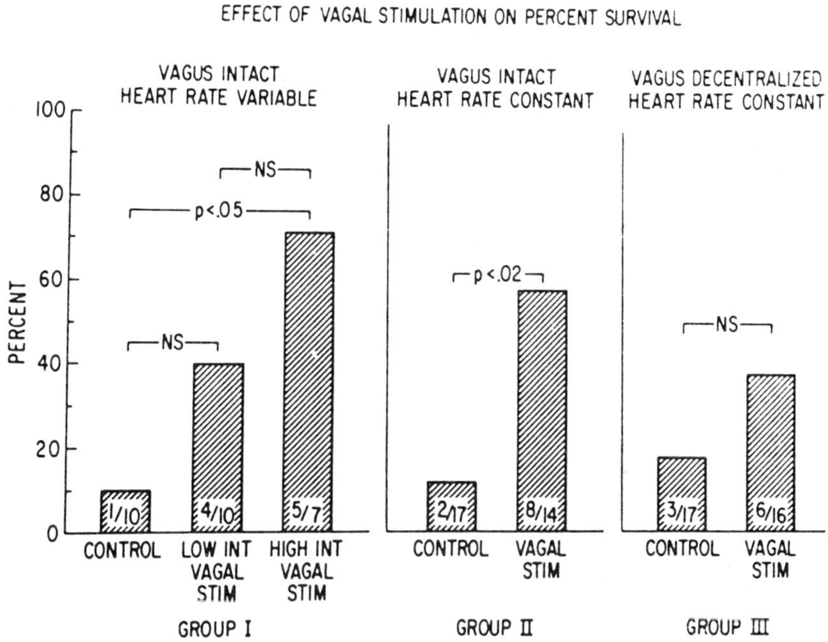

Figure 3. *Effect of vagal stimulation on survival during a 30-minute occlusion of the LAD and of the first septal coronary arteries in anesthetized dogs. The three groups described here were differently treated during the coronary artery occlusion. In group I, heart rate was allowed to fall during vagal stimulation (to 80 to 100 beats/min in the low-intensity vagal stimulation, and to 55 to 77 beats/min in the high-intensity vagal stimulation). In groups II and III, heart rate was kept constant by right ventricular pacing. In group III, the vagus was decentralized before the beginning of the stimulation. When heart rate was allowed to decrease, high-intensity vagal stimulation significantly improved the survival. When heart rate was kept constant (at 180 beats/min), only the stimulation of the intact vagus significantly reduced mortality. Reproduced by permission of the American Heart Association, Inc. from Myers RW, Pearlman AS, Hyman RM, et al: Beneficial effects of vagal stimulation and bradycardia during experimental acute myocardial ischemia. Circulation 49:945, 1974.*

incidence of VF, whereas removal of this activity by vagotomy would increase the likelihood of VF. They have also studied the effects of vagotomy (and of atropine) on arrhythmias following occlusion of the right coronary artery.[23] They found that, contrary to their previous study with anterior myocardial ischemia, removal of vagal effects did not increase the occurrence of VF.[23] These interventions did not inhibit the decrease in heart rate after coronary artery occlusion. Therefore, it is possible that the reduction in heart rate has been due to direct sinoatrial (SA) node ischemia.

Kolman et al[24] used the single pulse technique to study the effect of vagal stimulation on ventricular irritability in anesthetized dogs. They indicated that vagus nerve stimulation alone does not affect the VFT, but it does prevent the decrease in VFT induced by simultaneous left stellate ganglion stimulation. Similar conclusions were drawn by Furey and Levy,[25] who evaluated the repetitive extrasystole threshold, which is strongly related to VFT.[26] They showed that vagal stimulation also counteracted the effect of isoproterenol infusion.[25] Hence, part of the antagonism was occurring postjunctionally. These two studies, therefore, differ from the previous one of Kent et al,[18] because the latter showed an increase in VFT independent of sympathetic stimulation. Kent et al[18] used trains of electrical stimuli for the determination of the threshold. This may have released an amount of endogenous norepinephrine (NE) from ventricular tissue[27] that was sufficient to set the stage for sympathetic–parasympathetic antagonism. Also, the stimulation of the nondecentralized vagus (in the study by Kent et al,[18] but not in the two following studies) may have activated vagal afferent fibers and produced a reflex withdrawal of cardiac efferent sympathetic activity.[28] Independently from these theoretical explanations, the question of the direct effect versus only the antiadrenergic effect of vagal hyperactivity is not yet settled, as is mentioned in the last part of this chapter.

A different way to investigate the relationship between vagal activity and VF may be to assess the actual firing of the vagus during episodes of acute myocardial ischemia and to correlate the neural activity with the spontaneous occurrence of arrhythmia. In our laboratories, we recorded vagal activity from the cardiac branch of the right vagus (single fiber recording) in anesthetized cats. Therefore, we have assessed directly the tonic and reflex vagal activity and the susceptibility to sudden death.[29] In 17 anesthetized cats, cardiac vagal activity was recorded in control conditions and during a 60-minute occlusion of the LAD coronary artery. VF occurred within a few minutes of occlusion in nine cats, defined as susceptible, whereas the remaining eight cats survived, and were defined as resistant.

An example of neural recording during the first minutes of ischemia in a resistant cat is shown in Figure 4. Resting activity prior to coronary occlusion was similar in the two groups. During the first two minutes of myocardial ischemia, however, vagal activity did not change in the susceptible animals (−18%), but it increased in the resistant animals (+48%, $p<0.01$) (Fig. 5). These results suggest that survival is associated with a greater vagal response.

Experimental studies have demonstrated that the reperfusion of ischemic myocardium very often leads to malignant arrhythmias, including VF.[30,31] The effect of parasympathetic activation on this type of arrhythmias has been examined less intensively. We evaluated the effects of bilateral vagotomy and of vagal stimulation on reperfusion arrhythmias in cats.[32] In control animals, the incidence of VF was 62%, and that of sustained ventricular tachycardia (sVT) was 31%. Similar results occurred in vagotomized animals. These findings indicate that tonic vagal activity does not have a protective role in reperfusion arrhythmias. Vagal stimulation strikingly decreased the incidence of VF to 7%, when heart rate was allowed to decrease, but it only caused a nonsignificant reduction (48%) in VF incidence when heart rate was kept constant by ventricular pacing. The overall incidence of malignant arrhythmias (including both VF and sVT), however, was significantly reduced in the paced cats, due to the prevention of sustained VT, as shown in Figure 6.

Studies involving modulation of the vagal activity, performed in the last 15 to 20 years, suggest that vagal hyperactivity may exert antiarrhythmic

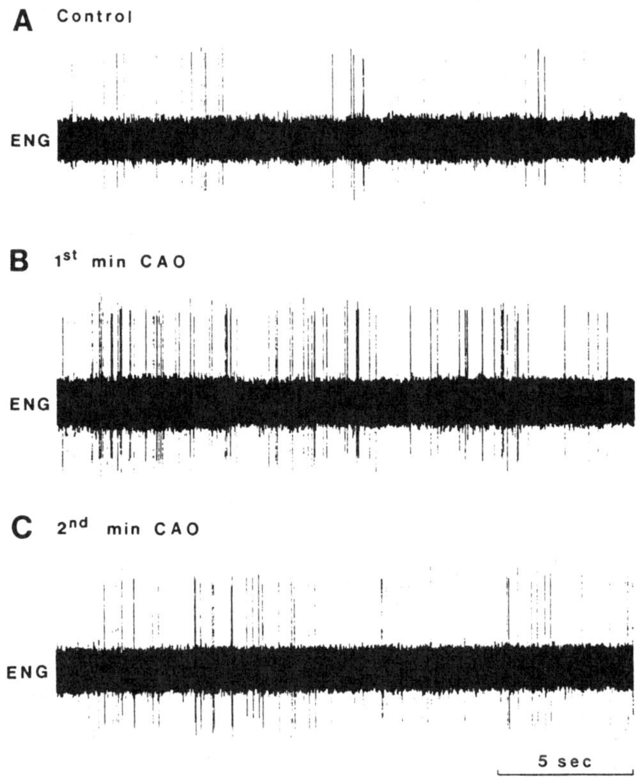

Figure 4. *Electroneurogram (ENG) of the single cardiac vagal efferent in the control condition and during the first two minutes of coronary artery occlusion. Panel A: Control conditions. Panel B: Beginning of the first minute of coronary artery occlusion (CAO). Panel C: After 90 sec of coronary artery occlusion (and min CAO). Modified by permission of the American Heart Association, Inc. from Cerati D, Schwartz PJ: Single cardiac vagal fibers activity, acute myocardial ischemia, and risk for sudden death. Circ Res 69:1393, 1991.*

effects in most experimental conditions and, particularly, when significant sympathetic activity is also present.

Pharmacological Studies

Muscarinic receptor (mAChR) blockers, such as atropine, are commonly used to antagonize the effects of cardiac parasympathetic activity. Enhancement of the vagal responses can be obtained by various mechanisms. These mechanisms include: direct stimulation by muscarinic agonists; block of the degradation of the naturally released acetylcholine (ACh) by inhibition of acetylcholinesterase (AChE); and reflexly-induced increase in vagal outflow and further pharmacological interactions at the central or peripheral level, resulting in increased ACh release.

In 1943, LeRoy et al[33] published the results of the administration of atropine

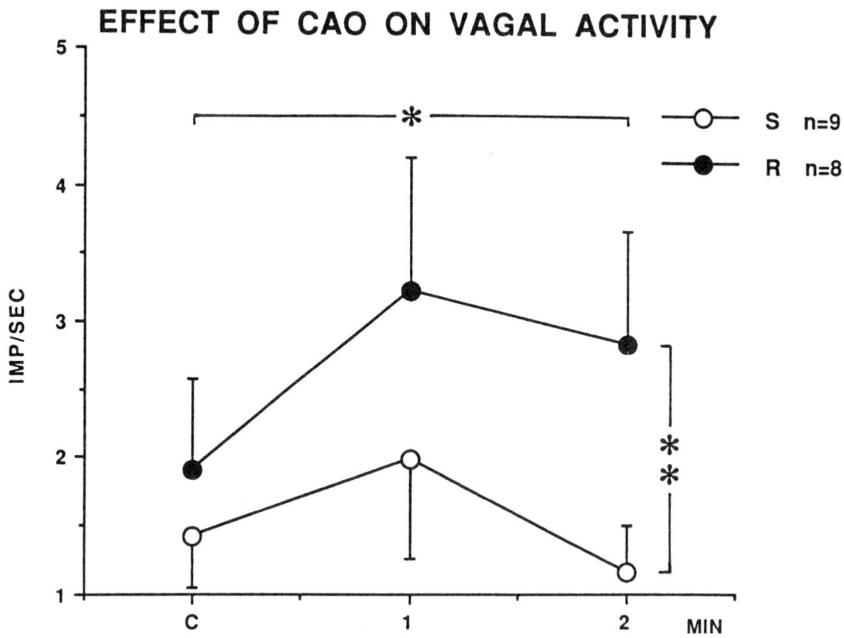

Figure 5. *Graph showing cardiac vagal activity in control conditions and during the first two minutes of coronary artery occlusion (CAO) in resistant (R = 8) and susceptible cats (S = 9). Data are expressed as imp/sec. It is evident that the resistant animals had a significantly higher neural response than the susceptible. *: p<0.01: **: p<0.09. Reproduced by permission of the American Heart Association, Inc. from Cerati D, Schwartz PJ: Single cardiac vagal fibers activity, acute myocardial ischemia, and risk for sudden death. Circ Res 69:1395, 1991.*

sulphate I.M. on the incidence of sudden death in the 24 hours after circumflex coronary artery occlusion in conscious and anesthetized dogs. They concluded that atropine decreased the incidence of sudden death in both conditions, from 70% to 34% and 50%, respectively.[33] Although they did not analyze their data statistically, they interpreted this occurrence to be due to the block of the "inhibition of the vagal reflex coronary vasoconstriction that is the chief cause of early sudden death." A subsequent chi-square test of the published data, however, does not show a significant difference in the mortality rates.

Subsequent studies have suggested either no effect or an increase in the incidence of malignant ischemic arrhythmias after atropine administration. Goldstein et al[19] administered atropine I.V. to closed-chest dogs subjected to LAD coronary occlusion. They found increases in the incidence of both total ventricular arrhythmias and of extrasystoles with short coupling intervals and a slight increase in the occurrence of VF. It is possible that part of the discrepancy with the preceding study may be explained on the basis of the different ischemic area. Indeed, Corr et al[23] have suggested such a possibility in acute feline experiments. Atropine did not influence malignant arrhythmias associated with myocardial ischemia induced by right coronary artery occlusion.[23] Atropine, however, significantly increased the incidence of VF caused by anterior myocardial ischemia, independent of heart rate changes.[21] In the

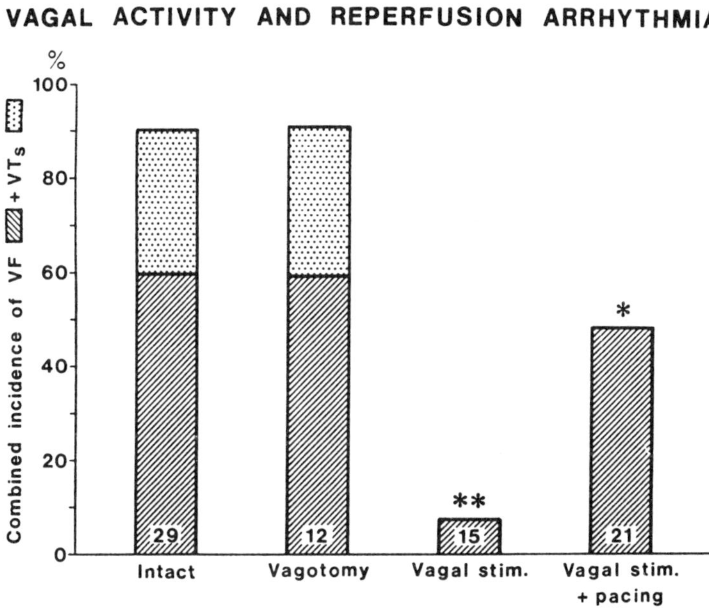

Figure 6. *Incidence of reperfusion ventricular fibrillation (stippled area, VF) and sustained ventricular tachycardia (dotted area, VT) in the four groups of animals. Significance refers to the combined incidence of the two arrhythmias: *: p<0.005 vs neurally intact and p<0.05 vs vagotomy; **: p<0.001 vs neurally intact and vagotomy. Reproduced by permission of the American Heart Association, Inc. from Zuanetti G, De Ferrari GM, Priori SG, et al: Protective effect of vagal stimulation on reperfusion arrhythmias in cats. Circ Res 61:432, 1987.*

absence of myocardial ischemia, the use of atropine as a preanesthetic drug in dogs is accompanied by a higher incidence of frequent ventricular arrhythmias.[34]

Das and Bhattacharya[35] showed that the anticholinesterase agent physostigmine significantly reduced the incidence of VF caused by hypothermia or by the combination of hypothermia and anterior myocardial ischemia in dogs. The mechanisms responsible for this beneficial effect was thought to be the preservation of myocardial glycogen content. Edrophonium, another anticholinesterase agent, increased the VFT markedly in closed-chest dogs, both under nonischemic conditions and after the occlusion of the LAD coronary artery.[36] This result agreed with the findings obtained by the same group when they used vagal stimulation.[18] Their results did not depend on a decrease in heart rate. The repetitive extrasystole threshold, which is linked to VFT,[26] was significantly increased by morphine in anesthetized dogs.[37] The vagotonic action of the opiate was shown to be responsible for this effect, because it was completely blocked by atropine or vagotomy (Fig. 7).

Rabinowitz et al[38] studied the effect of the muscarinic agonist methacholine on the repetitive extrasystole threshold in anesthetized dogs. The I.V. infusion of this drug, at doses ranging from 1 to 5 mcg/kg•min, caused a significant blood pressure decrease, but had no effect on heart rate. It induced

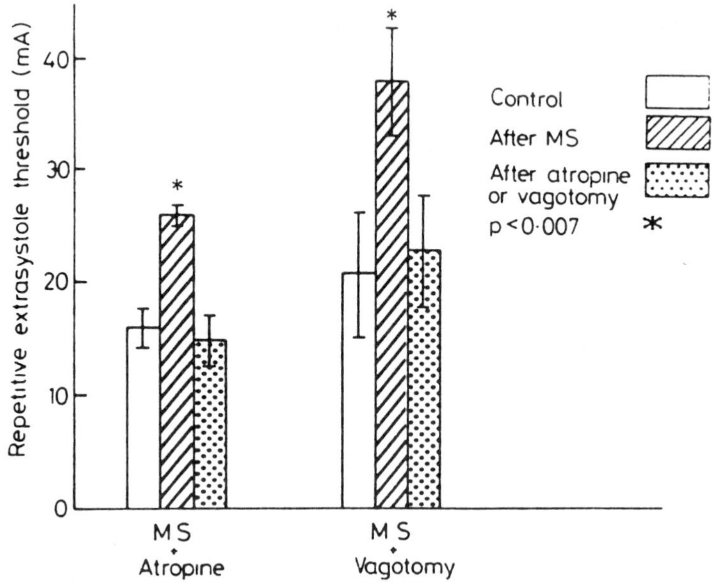

Figure 7. *Effects of atropine and vagotomy on the repetitive extrasystole threshold changes associated with morphine sulphate (MS, 0.25 mg/kg) in two groups of anesthetized dogs. The increase in repetitive extrasystole threshold induced by morphine sulphate was completely abolished by either atropine (200 μg/kg I.V.) (third histogram of the left group of columns) or by bilateral cervical vagotomy (third histogram of the right group of columns). Reproduced with permission from DeSilva RA, Verrier RL, Lown B: Protective effect of the vagotonic action on morphine sulphate on ventricular vulnerability. Cardiovasc Res 12:170, 1978.*

a marked increase in the repetitive extrasystole threshold, which appeared to be greater than the one caused by cervical vagosympathetic trunk stimulation, although the two interventions were not directly compared. Actually, this finding was not completely new, because it had been suggested in 1935 that the susceptibility to VF from alternating current shock was reduced by methacholine.[39] Rabinowitz et al[38] showed that propranolol produced similar effects, and the addition of methacholine did not allow any further increase in the repetitive extrasystole threshold. The same group investigated the effects of muscarinic and adrenergic receptor stimulation on serum potassium concentration and VFT.[40] Methacholine infusion (3 mcg/kg•min), increased VFT by 30%, and it completely prevented the decrease in VFT (also about 30%) caused by the infusion of adrenaline (1 mcg/kg•min), although it did not oppose the attendant decrease in serum potassium concentration.

Recently, Meesman et al[41] assessed the effect of enhanced vagal activity on spontaneous VTs occurring 24 to 72 hours after an anterior myocardial infarction, and on the inducible sustained VT four to seven days after myocardial infarction. Both the anticholinesterase agent edrophonium and the muscarinic agonist methacholine had no significant effect on either type of tachycardia. These types of arrhythmias, however, are generally considered to be different from those that lead to VF and sudden death.

We have used an acute feline animal model in which malignant arrhythmias are elicited by the combination of acute myocardial ischemia and sympathetic hyperactivity to assess the antiarrhythmic potential of oxotremorine, a muscarinic agonist with powerful peripheral cardiac effects.[42] An advantage of this model is that is has been used for analysis of the efficacy of several antiarrhythmic drugs,[43] so that comparisons between different drugs are possible and meaningful. In order to perform a quantitative analysis, ventricular arrhythmias are arbitrarily graded as follows: 0: no premature ventricular contractions (PVCs); 1: 1 to 10 PVCs; 2: 11 to 50 PVCs; 3: VT; and 4: VF. Oxotremorine produced a significant heart rate decrease and a striking antiarrhythmic effect. It completely abolished VF and clearly reduced the arrhythmia grade from 3.29 ± 0.16 to 0.76 ± 0.26 (mean $\pm$ SEM, $p<0.001$). The severity index was still significantly reduced, from 3.27 ± 0.17 to 1.53 ± 0.34 ($p = 0.002$) when heart rate was controlled by atrial pacing (Fig. 8). Figure 9

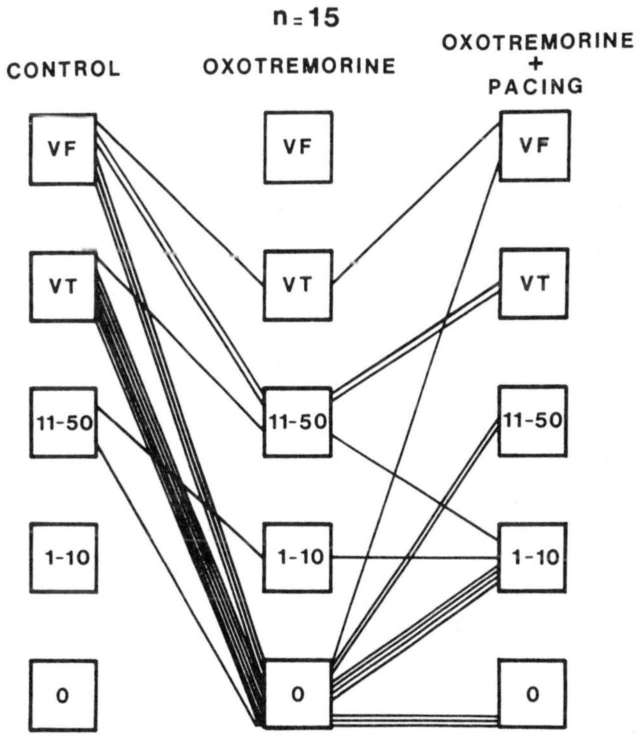

Figure 8. *Effects of oxotremorine on the occurrence of ventricular arrhythmias in 15 anesthetized cats. Each line represents the mean response of one cat over three consecutive trials. Left: The arrhythmia observed in the control condition. Middle: The arrhythmias observed with oxotremorine. Right: The arrhythmia observed when, after administration of oxotremorine, the trials were repeated with the prevention of the heart rate reduction by atrial pacing. VF: ventricular fibrillation; VT: ventricular tachycardia; 11–50 and 1–10: numbers of PVCs (not in VT); 0: no arrhythmias. Reproduced with permission from De Ferrari GM, Vanoli E, Curcuruto P, et al: Prevention of life-threatening arrhythmias by pharmacologic stimulation of the muscarinic receptors with oxotremorine. Am Heart J 124:883–890, 1992.*

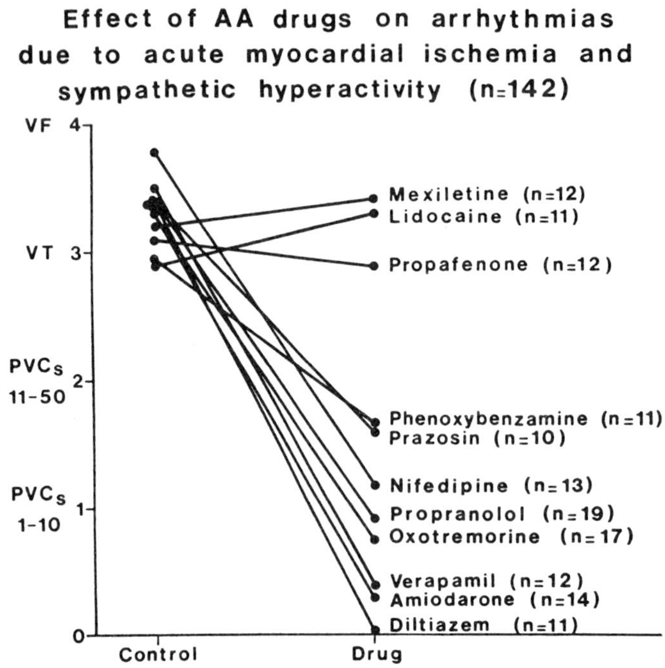

Figure 9. *Effects of different drugs on the occurrence of ventricular arrhythmias in 142 cats studied with this experimental protocol. Mean values of the severity of arrhythmias for each single drug, following the grading system as in Figure 8, before and after the treatment are shown. In this model, oxotremorine provided a protection similar to that obtained with propranolol. Reproduced with permission from De Ferrari GM, Vanoli E, Curcuruto P, et al: Prevention of life-threatening arrhythmias by pharmacologic stimulation of the muscarinic receptors with oxotremorine. Am Heart J 124:883–890, 1992.*

shows a comparison of the antiarrhythmic efficacy of oxotremorine and several other agents used in this animal model.

Pharmacological studies in anesthetized animals suggest that muscarinic blockade may have a modest effect during inferior or posterior myocardial ischemia, but is likely to favor arrhythmias during anterior ischemia. Direct muscarinic stimulation has antifibrillatory effects, especially in the presence of increased sympathetic drive. Inhibition of AChE may lead to similar results, although the data are not unequivocal.

A Chronic Animal Model for Sudden Cardiac Death

To gain insights into the pathophysiology of sudden cardiac death and to explore specifically the influence of the autonomic nervous system, we developed, in the early 1980s, an experimental preparation in which conscious dogs with a healed anterior myocardial infarction undergo a submaximal exercise stress test coupled with a two-minute occlusion of the circumflex coronary artery.[44] This clinically relevant combination of transient myocardial ischemia at the time of physiologically elevated sympathetic activity results in VF in approximately 55% of the animals. The outcome during the exercise and ischemia test (VF in susceptible animals, but not in "resistant" animals) is highly reproducible for several months and, hence, allows internal control studies.

We observed that, in response to myocardial ischemia during exercise, the susceptible dogs further increased an already physiologically elevated heart rate, whereas the resistant animals tended to show a heart rate decrease.[44,45] These findings generated the hypothesis that the presence of dominant vagal reflexes might be associated with a greater likelihood of survival. Accordingly, we examined the relationship between baroreflex sensitivity (BRS), a marker of vagal reflexes, and susceptibility to sudden cardiac death. Specifically, a study was performed in a population of 192 dogs after myocardial infarction.[46] That study constitutes the experimental rationale for the use of BRS in risk stratification after myocardial infarction. The results of this study, together with other measures of autonomic balance, are discussed in detail in Ch. 29.

The available data, therefore, suggested a tight relationship between indexes of elevated vagal activity and a decreased risk for sudden death. They did not provide, however, direct evidence for vagally-mediated protection from VF. To address this issue, we have recently performed three different studies.

In the first of these studies, atropine was given to 45 resistant animals to test whether removal of muscarinic effects would induce ventricular arrhythmias.[47] Atropine caused the novel occurrence of arrhythmia or a worsening of the pattern in 51% of the dogs, notably the occurrence of VF in 11 dogs (24%, $p = 0.001$), as shown in Figure 10. These 11 animals were characterized, in the control test, by a marked heart rate decrease that was absent in the other dogs. The changes suggested the presence of a very powerful vagal reflex following myocardial ischemia (Fig. 11). In 5 of 7 dogs (71%), the deleterious effect was mainly due to the heart rate effect of atropine, as indicated by the pacing experiments. This study indicates that a low sympathetic activation primarily characterizes the resistant animals. In approximately 25% of the animals undergoing transient myocardial ischemia, however, the presence of adequate vagal tone and reflexes is essential for survival from sudden death.

A new technique for direct electrical stimulation of the vagus nerve in the conscious animal[48] was used in a further study.[49] Two groups of susceptible dogs underwent either a further exercise and ischemia test with no additional intervention (control group), or a trial in which right vagal stimulation was started a few seconds after the beginning of the occlusion. VF occurred in 23 of 25 (92%) control animals, but occurred only in 3 of 26 (11.5%) vagally-stimulated dogs (Fig. 12). An example of vagally-mediated protection is shown in Figure 13. In the vagal stimulation test, heart rate during ischemia was 85 beats/minute lower than in the control test (170 ± 36 versus 255 ± 33 beats/minute). When heart rate was kept, by atrial pacing, at the level attained in the control tests, 5 of the 9 animals (55%) remained protected from VF.

In this study, we stimulated the intact cervical vagus. Both the efferent and the afferent vagal fibers were stimulated. As already mentioned, vagal afferent stimulation produces a reflex withdrawal of sympathetic efferent activity.[28] In theory, this withdrawal might have significantly influenced our

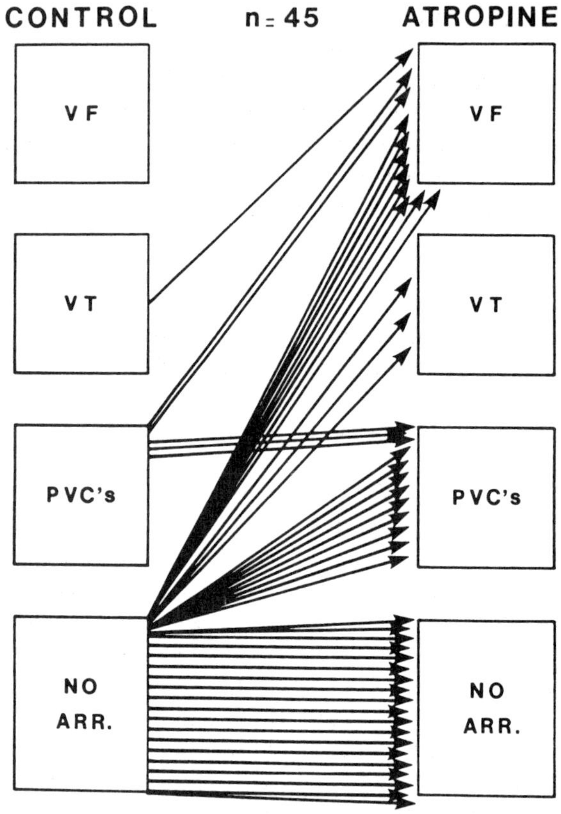

Figure 10. *Effect of atropine on the incidence of arrhythmias during the exercise and ischemia test. In control conditions, one animal had a single episode of three consecutive premature ventricular beats and was assigned to the ventricular tachycardia group (VT), five had scattered isolated premature ventricular contractions (less than 10, PVCs), and the remaining animals had no arrhythmias (NO ARR.). Atropine caused a worsening in 23 of 45 dogs (51%). Reproduced with permission from De Ferrari GM, Vanoli E, Stramba-Badiale M, et al: Vagal reflexes and survival during acute myocardial ischemia in conscious dogs with a healed myocardial infarction. Am J Physiol 261:H65, 1991.*

results. This was not the case, however, as indicated by three lines of evidence. One, atropine completely blocks the chronotropic effects of vagal stimulation performed during high sympathetic activity induced by a similar exercise protocol.[48] In this condition, if activation of afferent vagal fibers had importantly inhibited the sympathetic outflow, vagal stimulation would still have reduced heart rate. Two, the protective effect of vagal stimulation was completely prevented by atropine. This finding indicates that protection was dependent on efferent vagal stimulation. Finally when stimulation was limited to vagal efferent fibers by surgical decentralization in one dog, thus eliminating central activation and potential sympathetic withdrawal, the animal was still protected from VF.

Sympathetic efferent activity can certainly be influenced by vagal afferent stimulation, but the relevance of this effect in our exercising dogs is highly

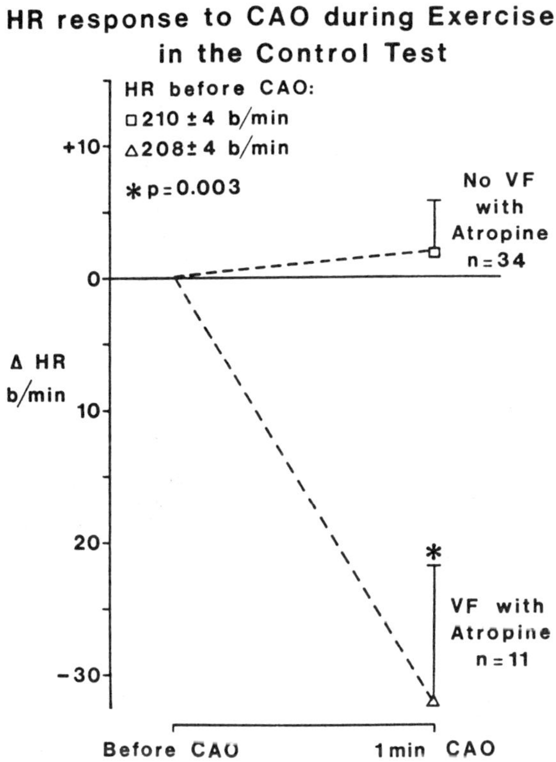

Figure 11. *Heart rate (HR) response to coronary artery occlusion (CAO) during the control exercise and ischemia test. The dogs that develop ventricular fibrillation (VF) in the atropine test show, in the control test, a marked decrease in heart rate that was not observed in the other dogs, suggesting more powerful vagal reflexes. Data are expressed as mean ±SEM. Reproduced with permission from De Ferrari GM, Vanoli E, Stramba-Badiale M, et al: Vagal reflexes and survival during acute myocardial ischemia in conscious dogs with a healed myocardial infarction. Am J Physiol 261:H66, 1991.*

questionable. Indeed, during exercise, the level of circulating catecholamines is so high that a transient decrease in the firing of sympathetic nerves is quite unlikely to affect cardiac electrophysiology. Conversely, in resting individuals who may experience ischemic episodes, the simultaneous sympathetic withdrawal may very well contribute to the antifibrillatory effect of vagal stimulation. This possibility adds to the validity of the rationale for stimulating the intact vagus. The study indicates that electrically produced vagal hyperactivity can drastically reduce the incidence of lethal arrhythmia in this conscious animal model and that the reduction in heart rate is not a crucial component in half of the protected animals.

Finally, we have assessed the hemodynamic and antiarrhythmic effects of two muscarinic agonists and compared them with those of β-adrenergic blockade.[50] Eleven susceptible dogs underwent exercise and ischemia tests with the following treatments: saline, propranolol, methacholine, and oxotremorine. Saline never prevented VF, whereas propranolol was effective in 90% of the dogs ($p<0.001$), methacholine was effective in 40% of the dogs ($p = 0.035$), and

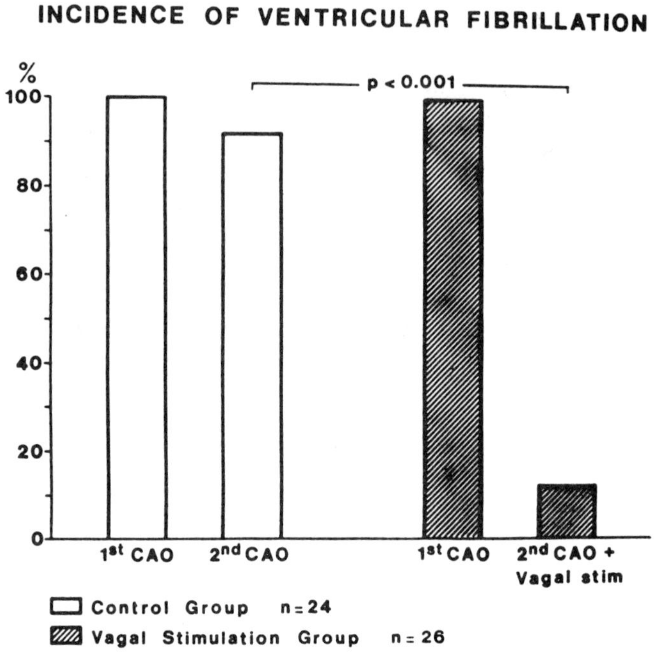

Figure 12. *Incidence of VF in two consecutive exercise and ischemia tests in the control group and in the group in which vagal stimulation was performed during the second coronary artery occlusion (2nd CAO). Reproduced by permission of the American Heart Association, Inc. from Vanoli E, De Ferrari GM, Stramba-Badiale M, et al: Vagal stimulation and prevention of sudden death in conscious dogs with a healed myocardial infarction. Circ Res 68:1474, 1991.*

oxotremorine was effective in 62.5% of the dogs ($p = 0.005$). Propranolol and oxotremorine significantly reduced heart rate, compared to saline, but methacholine did not. Propranolol significantly reduced left ventricular dP/dt max, particularly during myocardial ischemia, when dP/dt max values after propranolol were approximately half of those observed after the other treatments. Therefore, compared to β-blockade, methacholine and oxotremorine provide a less marked, but still valid protection and impair contractility significantly less.

The studies in a clinically relevant chronic animal model confirm an important role for vagal activity in the protection from VF. They suggest that direct electrical stimulation or activation of the mAChR may reduce the incidence of sudden death, and that part of this effect is heart rate-independent.

Clinical Studies

Acute myocardial ischemia activates both sympathetic and parasympathetic fibers (see Ch. 27).[51–53] This occurrence elicits sympathetic excitatory[6] and vagal depressor[53] reflexes. The pioneering studies of Pantridge and

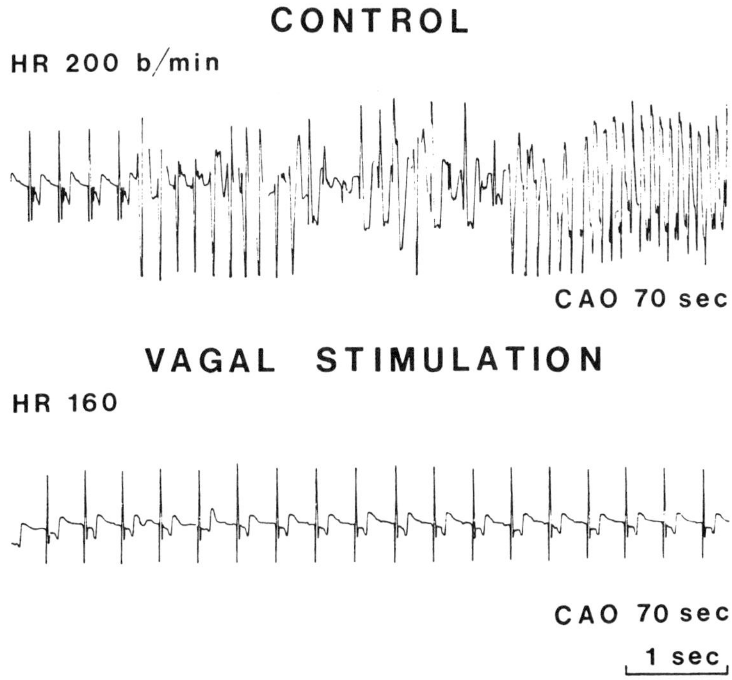

Figure 13. *ECG recording in the same dog, during the exercise and ischemia test. Upper trace: Control test. Lower trace: Test with vagal stimulation. Ten seconds after cessation of exercise, VT, which degenerated into fibrillation, occurred in the control test. When vagal stimulation was performed during coronary artery occlusion (CAO), this animal had no ventricular arrhythmia. Reproduced by permission of the American Heart Association, Inc. from Vanoli E, De Ferrari GM, Stramba-Badiale M, et al: Vagal stimulation and prevention of sudden death in conscious dogs with a healed myocardial infarction. Circ Res 68:1473, 1991.*

colleagues[54,55] have indicated that the majority of patients have signs of autonomic imbalance within the first 30 minutes of acute myocardial infarction.

Excessive parasympathetic activation leads to marked bradycardia, atrioventricular (AV) block, and hypotension, and is more common in inferior and posterior myocardial infarction. Atropine has always been considered the treatment of choice for this clinical syndrome. The experimental findings on the possible adverse effects of atropine and increased heart rate during acute myocardial ischemia (see above), as well as clinical reports that suggest possible proarrhythmic effects of atropine,[56,57] stimulated several retrospective analyses in the mid-1970s.[58–60] These studies suggested the overall safety of atropine, provided that proper attention is paid to the dosage and its administration in a coronary care setting. Malignant arrhythmias were uncommon. It should, however, be mentioned that approximately 70% of the patients in these retrospective analyses had inferior myocardial infarctions. The majority received atropine several hours after the onset of symptoms, a time period that would not correspond to the most dangerous for the occurrence of VF.

In 1935, Nathanson[61] induced the appearance of polymorphic and repetitive ventricular arrhythmias in six elderly subjects by I.V. administration of 0.1 mg of adrenaline. This proarrhythmic effect was prevented by the previous subcutaneous administration of 20 mg of methacholine, provided the first reaction to methacholine had subsided and the ensuing decrease in heart rate occurred. After this report, only a very limited number of clinical studies has dealt with the effects of parasympathetic activation on ventricular arrhythmias. Miller et al[62] evaluated the effects of the infusion of edrophonium in 11 patients with acute myocardial infarction, within 24 hours from the onset of symptoms. The anticholinesterase agent caused a slight decrease in heart rate, but not in cardiac output and stroke work index. The authors indicate a trend toward a decrease in potentially malignant PVCs and in VT, but the results were not significant.[62]

Waxman and colleagues,[63] have provided evidence that VTs could respond to vagal activation, contrary to the traditional and general belief. They showed that phenylephrine could terminate episodes of VT.[63] They indicated that reflex vagal activation was the mechanism, because the ability of phenylephrine to terminate sustained VT was potentiated by edrophonium and reduced by atropine.[64] They have also shown that ventricular automaticity, as expressed by idioventricular rhythm, is decreased by vagal activity.[65]

We have recently assessed the antiarrhythmic effect of baroreflex activation in patients with frequent, stable PVCs.[66] When heart rate was allowed to decrease, phenylephrine completely abolished ectopic activity in 9 of 10 patients. During atrial pacing at the predrug rate, PVCs reappeared in most subjects, as shown in Figure 14. Their mean number, however, was still significantly less than the control values, which indicates that the antiarrhythmic effect of reflex vagal activation is only partially rate-dependent.

Most of these clinical studies could not assess the potential effect of vagomimetic interventions on the occurrence of VF. Recent studies, however, confirm the experimental findings of a tight correlation between indexes of high vagal tone and powerful vagal reflexes and a reduced incidence of malignant ventricular arrhythmia and sudden cardiac death (see Ch. 29).[67,68] This evidence, albeit indirect, supports the hypothesis that vagal activity may protect patients with ischemic heart disease from VF.

Mechanisms of Protective Effect

Several mechanisms are likely to participate in the reduction of malignant arrhythmias afforded by moderate vagal hyperactivity. The heart rate decrease induced by vagomimetic interventions is beneficial, particularly in the setting of acute myocardial ischemia. Heart rate is a major determinant of myocardial oxygen demand, and higher rates are accompanied by greater degrees of myocardial ischemia during acute coronary artery occlusion in both anesthetized[69] and conscious[20] dogs. Also, lower heart rates may decrease the likelihood of both reentrant arrhythmias[70] and nonreentrant arrhythmias, such as triggered activity caused by delayed afterdepolarizations.[71] Indeed, in

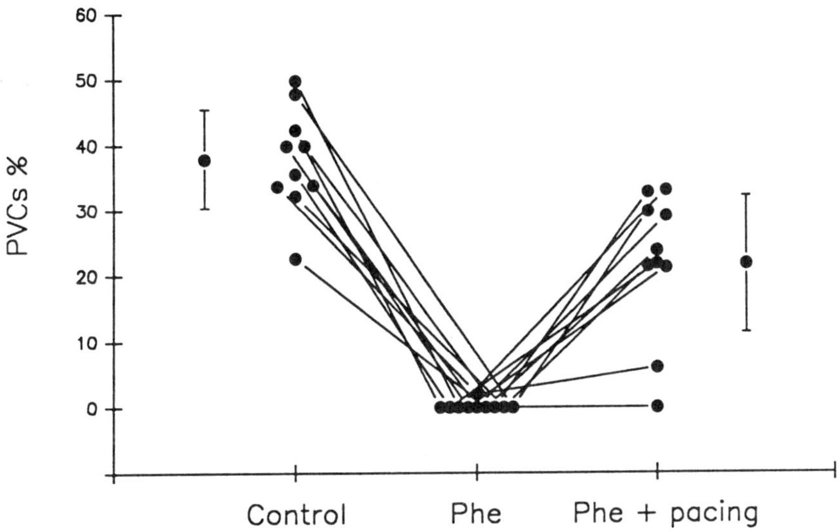

Figure 14. *Effect of phenylephrine (Phe) infusion on premature ventricular complexes (PVCs) in patients with chronic stable VPCs that decrease heart rate in response to phenylephrine. ●: Represents the number of PVCs/100 beats in the single patient during baseline (control), after phenylephrine infusion when heart rate is allowed to both decrease (Phe) and is held constant by pacing (Phe + pacing). —●—: Represents the mean values ±standard deviation in control conditions and during pacing. Reproduced with permission from Facchini M, De Ferrari GM, Bonazzi O, et al: Effect of reflex vagal activation on frequency of ventricular premature complexes. Am J Cardiol 63:349–354, 1991.*

anesthetized dogs with a coronary artery occlusion, an increase in pacing rates above 150 beats/minute causes a marked increase in premature ventricular beats, tachycardia, and fibrillation.[72]

The relative importance of a heart rate decrease in the different studies that have shown a protective effect of vagomimetic interventions is not unequivocal. Few studies indicate it as the sole cause of the antiarrhythmic effect, whereas several others suggest that it does not play a relevant role. We believe that, on the basis of the available literature, and on our own studies, heart rate modulation plays a significant role, but that other mechanisms are also important in the prevention of malignant arrhythmias.

The question of direct muscarinic effects on the electrophysiological properties of ventricular myocardium is still debated. Certainly, vagomimetic interventions profoundly counteract the effects of catecholamines. This marked antagonism, occurring both at presynaptic and at postsynaptic levels, is discussed in Ch. 11. Although most studies indicate that vagal activity acts through inhibition of sympathetic effects, experimental[73] and clinical data[74] suggest direct electrophysiological effects, likely to be more marked at the epicardial level.[75] Ch. 16 deals specifically with vago-sympathetic interactions and ventricular refractoriness. We believe that the antagonism of sympathetic effects is an important mechanism for the protection from VF, and that, with the likely exception of the effects on the epicardium[75] described above, primary muscarinic modulation of the working ventricular myocardium is of minor importance.[76]

The effect of muscarinic activation on coronary arteries is controversial. Although vasoconstriction has been described, especially in baboons,[77] it was recently shown that ACh produces coronary vasodilation both in dogs and baboons, independently of the interaction with the sympathetic nervous system.[78] These studies, however, were performed in animals with an intact endothelial layer. The presence of the endothelium is likely to play a relevant role, through the release of relaxing factors. Also, when the endothelial layer is absent or damaged, a vasoconstrictor effect is unmasked,[76] which has also been observed in humans.[79,80] Overall, it is unlikely that coronary vasodilation plays a major role in the beneficial effect of vagal hyperactivity.

Conclusions

The data presented above provide what we believe to be convincing evidence that vagal activation, particularly at the outset of an episode of acute myocardial ischemia, has an important antifibrillatory effect. When these data are combined with the abundant evidence that individuals with signs of either reduced vagal tone or vagal reflexes are at significantly greater risk for cardiovascular mortality and for sudden death, it appears logical to attempt to increase vagal activity or to enhance the ability to respond to ischemia with strong vagal reflexes.

From the data available, four main approaches seem worthy of serious consideration. The first, and most attractive because of its physiological basis and lack of negative side effects, is exercise training. The second, which still requires considerable pharmacological efforts, is the development of a cardioselective M_2 mAChR agonist. The third consists of a pharmacological intervention indirectly causing an increased release of ACh, and thus a vagomimetic effect.[76,81] The fourth, which may appear today as somewhat futuristic but which is actually within current technical possibilities, is the development of a chronically implantable electrode that would allow a patient to activate his own vagus whenever he perceives the occurrence of cardiac pain. Whatever plan will be implemented, it is satisfactory to see that, from the diversity of experimental studies that have shed some light on the pathophysiology underlying the link between vagal activity and malignant arrhythmias, a novel therapeutic strategy for the reduction of sudden cardiac death is now surfacing.

References

1. Schwartz PJ, Brown AM, Malliani A, et al (eds): Neural Mechanisms in Cardiac Arrhythmias. New York, NY, Raven Press, 1978, p. 442.
2. Schwartz PJ, Stone HL: The role of the autonomic nervous system in sudden coronary death. Ann NY Acad Sci 382:162–181, 1982.
3. Lown B, Verrier RL: Neural activity and ventricular fibrillation. N Engl J Med 294:1165, 1976.

4. Corr PB, Yamada KA, Witkowski FX: Mechanisms controlling cardiac autonomic function and their relation to arrhythmogenesis. In HA Fozzard, E Haber, RB Jennings, et al (eds): The Heart and Cardiovascular System. New York, NY, 1986, pp. 1343–1403.
5. Schwartz PJ, Priori SG: Sympathetic nervous system and cardiac arrhythmias. In DP Zipes, J Jalife (eds): Cardiac Electrophysiology: From Cell to Bedside. Philadelphia, PA, WB Saunders Co, 1990, pp. 330–343.
6. Malliani A, Schwartz PJ, Zanchetti A: A sympathetic reflex elicited by experimental coronary occlusion. Am J Physiol 217:703–709, 1969.
7. Schwartz PJ, Foreman RD, Stone HL, et al: Effect of dorsal root section on the arrhythmias associated with coronary occlusion. Am J Physiol 231:923–928, 1976.
8. Einbrodt: Ueber Herzeizung und ihr Verhaeltnis zum Blutdruck. Akademie der Wissenschaften (Vienna). Sitzungsberichte 38:345, 1859.
9. Hering HE: Die Myoerethischen Unregelmaessigkeiten des Herzens. Praeger Medizinische Wochenschrift 26:7, 1901.
10. Scherf D: Untersuchungen ueber die Entstehungweise der Extrasystolen und der extrasystolischen Allorhythmien. Z Exp Med 65:198, 1929.
11. Scherf D, Blumenfeld S, Yildiz M: Experimental study on ventricular extrasystoles provoked by vagal stimulation. Am Heart J 62:670–675, 1961.
12. Garrey WE: Some effects of cardiac nerves upon ventricular fibrillation. Am J Physiol 21:283, 1908.
13. Shumacker HB, Riberi A, Boone RD, et al: Ventricular fibrillation in the hypothermic state. IV. The role of extrinsic cardiac innervation. Ann Surg 143:223, 1954.
14. Lown B, Fakhro A, Hood WB, et al: The coronary care unit. JAMA 199:188, 1967.
15. Han J, Millet D, Chizzonitti B, et al: Temporal dispersion of recovery of excitability in atrium and ventricle as a function of heart rate. Am Heart J 71:481, 1966.
16. Scherlag BJ, Helfant RH, Haft JI, et al: Electrophysiology underlying ventricular arrhythmias due to coronary ligation. Am J Physiol 291:1665–1671, 1970.
17. Kerzner J, Wolf M, Kosowsky BK, et al: Ventricular ectopic rhythms following vagal stimulation in dogs with acute myocardial infarction. Circulation 47:44–50, 1973.
18. Kent KM, Smith ER, Redwood DR, et al: Electrical stability of acutely ischemic myocardium: Influences of heart rate and vagal stimulation. Circulation 47:291–298, 1973.
19. Goldstein RE, Karsh RB, Smith ER, et al: Influence of atropine and of vagally mediated bradycardia on the ocurrence of ventricular arrhythmias following acute coronary occlusion in closed-chest dogs. Circulation 47:1180–1190, 1973.
20. Myers RW, Pearlman AS, Hyman RM, et al: Beneficial effects of vagal stimulation and bradycardia during experimental acute myocardial ischemia. Circulation 49:943–947, 1974.
21. Corr PB, Gillis RA: Role of the vagus nerves in the cardiovascular changes induced by coronary occlusion. Circulation 49:86–97, 1974.
22. Corr PB, Gillis RA: Effect of autonomic neural influences on the cardiovascular changes induced by coronary occlusion. Am Heart J 89:766–774, 1975.
23. Corr PB, Pearle DL, Gillis RA: Coronary occlusion site as a determinant of the cardiac rhythm effects of atropine and vagotomy. Am Heart J 92:741–749, 1976.
24. Kolman BS, Verrier RL, Lown B: The effect of vagus nerve stimulation upon vulnerability of the canine ventricle: Role of the sympathetic parasympathetic interactions. Circulation 52:578–585, 1976.
25. Furey SA III, Levy MN: Interactions among heart rate, autonomic activity, and arterial pressure upon the multiple repetitive extrasystole threshold in the dog. Am Heart J 106:1112–1120, 1983.
26. Matta RJ, Verrier RL, Lown B: Repetitive extrasystole as an index of vulnerability to ventricular fibrillation. Am J Physiol 230:1469–1473, 1976.
27. Vincenzi F, West TC: Release of autonomic mediators in cardiac tissue by direct subthreshold stimulation. J Pharmacol Exp Ther 141:185–189, 1963.

28. Schwartz PJ, Pagani M, Lombardi F, et al: A cardio-cardiac sympatho-vagal reflex in the cat. Circ Res 32:215–220, 1973.
29. Cerati D, Schwartz PJ: Single cardiac vagal fibers activity, acute myocardial ischemia, and risk for sudden death. Circ Res 69:1389–1401, 1991.
30. Corbalan R, Verrier RL, Lown B: Differing mechanisms for ventricular vulnerability during coronary artery occlusion and release. Am Heart J 92:223–230, 1976.
31. Murdock DK, Loeb JM, Euler DE, et al: Electrophysiology of coronary reperfusion. A mechanism for reperfusion arrhythmias. Circulation 61:175–181, 1980.
32. Zuanetti G, De Ferrari GM, Priori SG, et al: Protective effect of vagal stimulation on reperfusion arrhythmias in cats. Circ Res 61:429–435, 1987.
33. LeRoy GV, Fenn GK, Gilbert NC: The influence of xanthine drugs and atropine on the mortality rate after experimental occlusion of a coronary artery. Am Heart J 23:637–643, 1942.
34. Muir WW: Effects of atropine on cardiac rate and rhythm in dogs. JAVMA 172:917–921, 1978.
35. Das PK, Bhattacharya SK: Studies on the effect of physostigmine on experimental cardiac arrhythmias in dogs. Br J Pharmacol 44:397–403, 1972.
36. Harrison LA, Harrison LH, Kent KM, et al: Enhancement of electrical stability of acutely ischemic myocardium by edrophonium. Circulation 50:99–102, 1974.
37. DeSilva RA, Verrier RL, Lown B: Protective effect of the vagotonic action of morphine sulphate on ventricular vulnerability. Cardiovasc Res 12:167–172, 1978.
38. Rabinowitz SH, Verrier RL, Lown B: Muscarinic effects of vagosympathetic trunk stimulation on the repetitive extrasystole (RE) threshold. Circulation 53:622–627, 1976.
39. Hoff HE, Nahum LH: The nature of ventricular fibrillation following electrical shock and its prevention by acetyl-beta-methyl choline chloride. Am J Physiol 110:675, 1935.
40. Hohnloser SH, Verrier RL, Lown B: Effects of adrenergic and muscarinic receptor stimulation on serum potassium concentrations and myocardial electrical stability. Cardiovasc Res 20:891–896, 1986.
41. Meesmann M, Karagueuzian HS, Ino T, et al: The role of enhanced vagal activity on ischemic ventricular tachycardia: Pharmacologic basis of inefficiency. Am Heart J 121:1703–1713, 1991.
42. De Ferrari GM, Vanoli E, Curcuruto P, et al: Prevention of life-threatening arrhythmias by pharmacologic stimulation of the muscarinic receptors with oxotremorine. Am Heart J 124:883–890, 1992.
43. Schwartz PJ, Vanoli E, Zaza A, et al: The effect of antiarrhythmic drugs on life-threatening arrhythmias induced by the interaction between acute myocardial ischemia and sympathetic hyperactivity. Am Heart J 109:937–948, 1985.
44. Schwartz PJ, Billman GE, Stone HL: Autonomic mechanisms in ventricular fibrillation induced by myocardial ischemia during exercise in dogs with a healed myocardial infarction. An experimental preparation for sudden cardiac death. Circulation 69:780–790, 1984.
45. Schwartz PJ, Stone HL: The analysis and modulation of autonomic reflexes in the prediction and prevention of sudden death. In DP Zipes, J Jalife (eds): Cardiac Arrhythmias: Mechanisms and Management. New York, NY, Grune & Stratton, 1985, pp. 165–176.
46. Schwartz PJ, Vanoli E, Stramba-Badiale M, et al: Autonomic mechanisms and sudden death. New insights from the analysis of baroreceptor reflexes in conscious dogs with and without a myocardial infarction. Circulation 78:969–973, 1988.
47. De Ferrari GM, Vanoli E, Stramba-Badiale M, et al: Vagal reflexes and survival during acute myocardial ischemia in conscious dogs with a healed myocardial infarction. Am J Physiol 261:H63–H69, 1991.
48. Stramba-Badiale M, Vanoli E, De Ferrari GM, et al: Sympathetic-parasympathetic

interaction and accentuated antagonism in conscious dogs. Am J Physiol 260:H335–H340, 1991.
49. Vanoli E, De Ferrari GM, Stramba-Badiale M, et al: Vagal stimulation and prevention of sudden death in conscious dogs with a healed myocardial infarction. Circ Res 68:1471–1481, 1991.
50. De Ferrari GM, Salvati P, Grossoni M, et al: Pharmacologic modulation of the autonomic nervous system in the prevention of sudden cardiac death. A study with propranolol, methacholine and oxotremorine in conscious dogs with a healed myocardial infarction. J. Am Coll Cardiol 22:283, 1993.
51. Malliani A, Recordati G, Schwartz PJ: Nervous activity of afferent cardiac sympathetic fibres with atrial and ventricular endings. J Physiol (Lond) 229:457–469, 1973.
52. Recordati G, Schwartz PJ, Pagani M, et al: Activation of cardiac vagal receptors during myocardial ischemia. Experientia 27:1423–1424, 1971.
53. Thoren P: Vagal reflexes elicited by left ventricular C-fibers during myocardial ischemia in cats. In PJ Schwartz, AM Brown, A Malliani, et al (eds): Neural Mechanisms in Cardiac Arrhythmias. New York, NY, Raven Press, 1978, pp. 179–190.
54. Webb SW, Adgey AAJ, Pantridge JF: Autonomic disturbance at onset of acute myocardial infarction. Br Med J 3:89–92, 1972.
55. Pantridge JF: Autonomic disturbance at the onset of acute myocardial infarction. In PJ Schwartz, AM Brown, A Malliani, et al (eds): Neural Mechanisms in Cardiac Arrhythmias. New York, NY, Raven Press, 1978, pp. 7–17.
56. Massumi RA, Mason DT, Amsterdam EA, et al: Ventricular fibrillation and tachycardia after intravenous atropine for treatment of bradycardias. N Engl J Med 287:336, 1972.
57. Zipes DP, Knoebel SB: Rapid rate-dependent ventricular ectopy. Adverse responses to atropine-induced rate increase. Chest 62:255, 1972.
58. Chadda KD, Lichstein E, Gupta PK, et al: Bradycardia–hypotension syndrome in acute myocardial infarction. Am J Med 59:158–164, 1975.
59. Scheinman MM, Thorburn D, Abbott JA: Use of atropine in patients with acute myocardial infarction and sinus bradycardia. Circulation 52:627–633, 1975.
60. Warren JV, Lewis RP: Beneficial effects of atropine in the prehospital phase of coronary care. Am J Cardiol 37:68–72, 1976.
61. Nathanson MH: Action of acetyl beta methylcholine on ventricular rhythms induced by adrenalin. Proc Soc Exp Biol Med 32:1297–1299, 1935.
62. Miller RR, Olson HG, Vera Z, et al: Clinical evaluation of the enhancement of vagal tone in acute myocardial infarction by edrophonium chloride: Effects on ventricular arrhythmias, His bundle electrocardiography and left ventricular function. Am Heart J 93:222–228, 1977.
63. Waxman MB, Downar E, Berman ND, et al: Phenylephrine (neosynephrine) terminated ventricular tachycardia. Circulation 50:656–664, 1974.
64. Waxman MB, Wald RW: Termination of ventricular tachycardia by an increase in cardiac vagal drive. Circulation 56:385–301, 1977.
65. Waxman MB, Cupps CL, Cameron DA: Modulation of an idioventricular rhythm by vagal tone. J Am Coll Cardiol 11:1052–1060, 1988.
66. Facchini M, De Ferrari GM, Bonazzi O, et al: Effect of reflex vagal activation on frequency of ventricular premature complexes. Am J Cardiol 68:349–354, 1991.
67. De Ferrari GM, Schwartz PJ: Autonomic nervous system and arrhythmias. Ann NY Acad Sci 601:247–262, 1990.
68. Schwartz PJ, La Rovere MT, Vanoli E: Autonomic nervous system and sudden cardiac death. Circulation 85(suppl. I):I77–I91, 1992.
69. Maroko PR, Kjekshus JK, Sobel BE, et al: Factors influencing infarct size following experimental coronary artery occlusions. Circulation 43:67–74, 1971.
70. El Sherif N: Reentrant ventricular arrhythmias in the late myocardial infarction period. 6. Effects of the autonomic nervous system. Circulation 58:103–110, 1978.

71. Wit AL, Rosen MR: Afterdepolarizations and triggered activity. In HA Fozzard, E Haber, RB Jennings, et al (eds): The Heart and Cardiovascular System. New York, NY, Raven Press, 1986, pp. 1343–1403.
72. Chadda KD, Banka VS, Helfant RH: Rate dependent ventricular ectopia following acute coronary occlusion. Circulation 49:654–659, 1974.
73. Pappano AJ, Inoue D: Development of different electrophysiological mechanisms for muscarinic inhibition of atria and ventricles. Fed Proc 43:2607–2612, 1984.
74. Prystowsky EN, Jackman WM, Rinkenberger RL, et al: Effect of autonomic blockade on ventricular refractoriness and atrioventricular nodal conduction in humans. Evidence supporting a direct cholinergic action on ventricular muscle refractoriness. Circ Res 49:511–518, 1981.
75. Litovsky SH, Antzelevitch C: Differences in the electrophysiological response of canine ventricular subendocardium and subepicardium to acetylcholine and isoproterenol. A direct effect of acetylcholine in ventricular myocardium. Circ Res 67:615–627, 1990.
76. De Ferrari GM, Zaza A: Drugs acting on cholinergic receptors. In BN Singh, VJ Dzau, P Van Houtten, et al (eds): Cardiovascular Pharmacology and Therapeutics. New York, NY, Churchill Livingstone, 1993, p. 125.
77. Satoh K, Yamashita S, Maruyiama M, et al: Comparison of the responses of the simian and canine coronary circulations to autonomic drugs. J Cardiovasc Pharmacol 4:820–828, 1982.
78. Van Winkle DM, Feigl EO: Acetylcholine causes coronary vasodilation in dogs and baboons. Circ Res 65:1580–1593, 1989.
79. Ludmer PL, Selwin AP, Shook TL, et al: Paradoxical vasoconstriction induced by acetylcholine in atherosclerotic coronary arteries. N Engl J Med 315:1046–1051, 1986.
80. Yasue H, Matsuyama K, Matsuyama K, et al: Responses of angiographically normal human coronary arteries to intracoronary injection of acetylcholine by age and segment. Possible role of early coronary atherosclerosis. Circulation 81:482–490, 1990.
81. De Ferrari GM, Mantica M, Vanoli E, et al: Scopolamine increases vagal tone and vagal reflexes in patients after myocardial infarction. J Am Coll Cardiol 22:1327, 1993.

Index